Update on Orthopedic Surgeries of the Lower Extremity Diseases and Injuries

Update on Orthopedic Surgeries of the Lower Extremity Diseases and Injuries

Editor

Woo Jong Kim

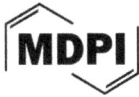

Basel • Beijing • Wuhan • Barcelona • Belgrade • Novi Sad • Cluj • Manchester

Editor
Woo Jong Kim
SoonChunHyang University
Cheonan Hospital
Cheonan
Republic of Korea

Editorial Office
MDPI
St. Alban-Anlage 66
4052 Basel, Switzerland

This is a reprint of articles from the Special Issue published online in the open access journal *Medicina* (ISSN 1648-9144) (available at: https://www.mdpi.com/journal/medicina/special_issues/Orthopedic_Surgeries_Diseases).

For citation purposes, cite each article independently as indicated on the article page online and as indicated below:

Lastname, A.A.; Lastname, B.B. Article Title. *Journal Name* **Year**, *Volume Number*, Page Range.

ISBN 978-3-7258-0745-1 (Hbk)
ISBN 978-3-7258-0746-8 (PDF)
doi.org/10.3390/books978-3-7258-0746-8

© 2024 by the authors. Articles in this book are Open Access and distributed under the Creative Commons Attribution (CC BY) license. The book as a whole is distributed by MDPI under the terms and conditions of the Creative Commons Attribution-NonCommercial-NoDerivs (CC BY-NC-ND) license.

Contents

About the Editor ix

Eui-Dong Yeo, Ki-Jin Jung, Yong-Cheol Hong, Chang-Hwa Hong, Hong-Seop Lee, Sung-Hun Won, et al.
A Tension-Band Wiring Technique for Direct Fixation of a Chaput Tubercle Fracture: Technical Note
Reprinted from: *Medicina* 2022, *58*, 1005, doi:10.3390/medicina58081005 1

Pei-Shao Liao, Ching-Chih Chiu, Yi-Hsiu Fu, Chia-Chun Hsia, Yu-Cih Yang, Kun-Feng Lee, et al.
Incidence of Hip Fractures among Patients with Chronic Otitis Media: The Real-World Data
Reprinted from: *Medicina* 2022, *58*, 1138, doi:10.3390/medicina58081138 7

Sung-Joon Yoon, Jun-Bum Kim, Ki-Jin Jung, Hee-Jun Chang, Yong-Cheol Hong, Chang-Hwa Hong, et al.
Evaluation of the Quality of Information Available on the Internet Regarding Chronic Ankle Instability
Reprinted from: *Medicina* 2022, *58*, 1315, doi:10.3390/medicina58101315 16

Dong Ryun Lee, Young Je Woo, Sung Gyu Moon, Woo Jong Kim and Dhong Won Lee
Comparison of Radiologic Results after Lateral Meniscal Allograft Transplantation with or without Capsulodesis Using an All-Soft Suture Anchor
Reprinted from: *Medicina* 2023, *59*, 1, doi:10.3390/medicina59010001 25

Dragos Apostu, Bianca Berechet, Daniel Oltean-Dan, Alexandru Mester, Bobe Petrushev, Catalin Popa, et al.
Low-Molecular-Weight Heparins (LMWH) and Synthetic Factor X Inhibitors Can Impair the Osseointegration Process of a Titanium Implant in an Interventional Animal Study
Reprinted from: *Medicina* 2022, *58*, 1590, doi:10.3390/medicina58111590 39

Sung Hwan Kim, Woo-Jong Kim, Eun Seok Park, Jun Yong Kim and Young Koo Lee
Iatrogenic Ankle Charcot Neuropathic Arthropathy after Spinal Surgery: A Case Report and Literature Review
Reprinted from: *Medicina* 2022, *58*, 1776, doi:10.3390/medicina58121776 53

Wen-Chin Su, Tzai-Chiu Yu, Cheng-Huan Peng, Kuan-Lin Liu, Wen-Tien Wu, Ing-Ho Chen, et al.
Use of an Intramedullary Allogenic Fibular Strut Bone and Lateral Locking Plate for Distal Femoral Fracture with Supracondylar Comminution in Patients over 50 Years of Age
Reprinted from: *Medicina* 2023, *59*, 9, doi:10.3390/medicina59010009 60

Zhimin Guo, Hui Liu, Deqing Luo, Taoyi Cai, Jinhui Zhang and Jin Wu
Application of Cortical Bone Plate Allografts Combined with Less Invasive Stabilization System (LISS) Plates in Fixation of Comminuted Distal Femur Fractures
Reprinted from: *Medicina* 2023, *59*, 207, doi:10.3390/medicina59020207 70

Annette Eidmann, Yama Kamawal, Martin Luedemann, Peter Raab, Maximilian Rudert and Ioannis Stratos
Demographics and Etiology for Lower Extremity Amputations—Experiences of an University Orthopaedic Center in Germany
Reprinted from: *Medicina* 2023, *59*, 200, doi:10.3390/medicina59020200 81

Seungha Woo, Youngho Lee and Doohoon Sun
A Pilot Experiment to Measure the Initial Mechanical Stability of the Femoral Head Implant in a Cadaveric Model of Osteonecrosis of Femoral Head Involving up to 50% of the Remaining Femoral Head
Reprinted from: *Medicina* 2023, *59*, 508, doi:10.3390/medicina59030508 89

Mustafa Yalın, Fatih Golgelioglu and Sefa Key
Intertrochanteric Femoral Fractures: A Comparison of Clinical and Radiographic Results with the Proximal Femoral Intramedullary Nail (PROFIN), the Anti-Rotation Proximal Femoral Nail (A-PFN), and the InterTAN Nail
Reprinted from: *Medicina* 2023, *59*, 559, doi:10.3390/medicina59030559 102

Håkan Alfredson, Markus Waldén, David Roberts and Christoph Spang
Combined Midportion Achilles and Plantaris Tendinopathy: A 1-Year Follow-Up Study after Ultrasound and Color-Doppler -Guided WALANT Surgery in a Private Setting in Southern Sweden
Reprinted from: *Medicina* 2023, *59*, 438, doi:10.3390/medicina59030438 115

Sung-Joon Yoon, Ki-Jin Jung, Yong-Cheol Hong, Eui-Dong Yeo, Hong-Seop Lee, Sung-Hun Won, et al.
Anatomical Augmentation Using Suture Tape for Acute Syndesmotic Injury in Maisonneuve Fracture: A Case Report
Reprinted from: *Medicina* 2023, *59*, 652, doi:10.3390/medicina59040652 123

Yong Bum Joo, Yoo Sun Jeon, Woo Yong Lee and Hyung Jin Chung
Risk Factors Associated with Intraoperative Iatrogenic Fracture in Patients Undergoing Intramedullary Nailing for Atypical Femoral Fractures with Marked Anterior and Lateral Bowing
Reprinted from: *Medicina* 2023, *59*, 735, doi:10.3390/medicina59040735 131

Lotan Raphael, Epstein Edna, Kaykov Irina and Hershkovich Oded
The Efficacy of Low-Dose Risperidone Treatment for Post-Surgical Delirium in Elderly Orthopedic Patients
Reprinted from: *Medicina* 2023, *59*, 1052, doi:10.3390/medicina59061052 144

Jun Young Lee, Sung Hwan Kim, Joo Young Cha and Young Koo Lee
Taekwondo Athlete's Bilateral Achilles Tendon Rupture: A Case Report
Reprinted from: *Medicina* 2023, *59*, 733, doi:10.3390/medicina59040733 153

Alberto Di Martino, Niccolò Stefanini, Matteo Brunello, Barbara Bordini, Federico Pilla, Giuseppe Geraci, et al.
Is the Direct Anterior Approach for Total Hip Arthroplasty Effective in Obese Patients? Early Clinical and Radiographic Results from a Retrospective Comparative Study
Reprinted from: *Medicina* 2023, *59*, 769, doi:10.3390/medicina59040769 160

Sung Hwan Kim, Young Hwan Kim, Joo Young Cha and Young Koo Lee
Correlations of Sesamoid Bone Subluxation with the Radiologic Measures of Hallux Valgus and Its Clinical Implications
Reprinted from: *Medicina* 2023, *59*, 876, doi:10.3390/medicina59050876 171

Young Yi and Sagar Chaudhari
Various Flexible Fixation Techniques Using Suture Button for Ligamentous Lisfranc Injuries: A Review of Surgical Options
Reprinted from: *Medicina* 2023, *59*, 1134, doi:10.3390/medicina59061134 183

Sung Hwan Kim, Jae Hyuck Choi, Sang Heon Lee and Young Koo Lee
The Superficial Peroneal Nerve Is at Risk during the "All Inside" Arthroscopic Broström Procedure: A Cadaveric Study
Reprinted from: *Medicina* **2023**, *59*, 1109, doi:10.3390/medicina59061109 195

Hiroki Okamura, Hiroki Ishikawa, Takuya Ohno, Shogo Fujita, Kei Nagasaki, Katsunori Inagaki and Yoshifumi Kudo
Type V Tibial Tubercle Avulsion Fracture with Suspected Complication of Anterior Cruciate Ligament Injury: A Case Report
Reprinted from: *Medicina* **2023**, *59*, 1061, doi:10.3390/medicina59061061 205

Matteo Filippini, Marta Bortoli, Andrea Montanari, Andrea Pace, Lorenzo Di Prinzio, Gianluca Lonardo, et al.
Does Surgical Approach Influence Complication Rate of Hip Hemiarthroplasty for Femoral Neck Fractures? A Literature Review and Meta-Analysis
Reprinted from: *Medicina* **2023**, *59*, 1220, doi:10.3390/medicina59071220 212

Danilo Jeremić, Nina Rajovic, Boris Gluscevic, Branislav Krivokapic, Stanislav Rajkovic, Nikola Bogosavljevic, et al.
Updated Meta-Analysis of Randomized Controlled Trials Comparing External Fixation to Intramedullary Nailing in the Treatment of Open Tibial Fractures
Reprinted from: *Medicina* **2023**, *59*, 1301, doi:10.3390/medicina59071301 230

Jeong-Kil Lee, Gi-Soo Lee, Sang-Bum Kim, Chan Kang, Kyong-Sik Kim and Jae-Hwang Song
A Comparative Analysis of Pain Control Methods after Ankle Fracture Surgery with a Peripheral Nerve Block: A Single-Center Randomized Controlled Prospective Study
Reprinted from: *Medicina* **2023**, *59*, 1302, doi:10.3390/medicina59071302 246

Dong Hwan Lee, Hwa Sung Lee, Chae-Gwan Kong and Se-Won Lee
Isolated Avulsion Fracture of the Tibial Tuberosity in an Adult Treated with Suture-Bridge Fixation: A Rare Case and Literature Review
Reprinted from: *Medicina* **2023**, *59*, 1565, doi:10.3390/medicina59091565 257

Hua-Yong Tay, Wen-Tien Wu, Cheng-Huan Peng, Kuan-Lin Liu, Tzai-Chiu Yu, Ing-Ho Chen, et al.
COVID-19 Infection Was Associated with the Functional Outcomes of Hip Fracture among Older Adults during the COVID-19 Pandemic Apex
Reprinted from: *Medicina* **2023**, *59*, 1640, doi:10.3390/medicina59091640 265

Jun Young Lee, Hyo Jun Lee, Sung Hoon Yang, Je Hong Ryu, Hyoung Tae Kim, Byung Ho Lee, et al.
Treatment of Soft Tissue Defects after Minimally Invasive Plate Osteosynthesis in Fractures of the Distal Tibia: Clinical Results after Reverse Sural Artery Flap
Reprinted from: *Medicina* **2023**, *59*, 1751, doi:10.3390/medicina59101751 276

Mustafa Yalın and Fatih Gölgelioğlu
A Comparative Analysis of Fasciotomy Results in Children and Adults Affected by Crush-Induced Acute Kidney Injury following the Kahramanmaraş Earthquakes
Reprinted from: *Medicina* **2023**, *59*, 1593, doi:10.3390/medicina59091593 287

Rodrigo Simões Castilho, João Murilo Brandão Magalhães, Bruno Peliz Machado Veríssimo, Carlo Perisano, Tommaso Greco and Roberto Zambelli
Minimally Invasive Peroneal Tenodesis Assisted by Peroneal Tendoscopy: Technique and Preliminary Results
Reprinted from: *Medicina* **2024**, *60*, 104, doi:10.3390/medicina60010104 300

Cesare Faldini, Leonardo Tassinari, Davide Pederiva, Valentino Rossomando, Matteo Brunello, Federico Pilla, et al.
Direct Anterior Approach in Total Hip Arthroplasty for Severe Crowe IV Dysplasia: Retrospective Clinical and Radiological Study
Reprinted from: *Medicina* **2024**, *60*, 114, doi:10.3390/medicina60010114 309

Isabella-Ionela Sanda, Samer Hosin, Dinu Vermesan, Bogdan Deleanu, Daniel Pop, Dan Crisan, et al.
Impact of Syndesmotic Screw Removal on Quality of Life, Mobility, and Daily Living Activities in Patients Post Distal Tibiofibular Diastasis Repair
Reprinted from: *Medicina* **2023**, *59*, 2048, doi:10.3390/medicina59122048 322

Rafał Wójcicki, Tomasz Pielak, Piotr Marcin Walus, Łukasz Jaworski, Bartłomiej Małkowski, Przemysław Jasiewicz, et al.
The Association of Acetabulum Fracture and Mechanism of Injury with BMI, Days Spent in Hospital, Blood Loss, and Surgery Time: A Retrospective Analysis of 67 Patients
Reprinted from: *Medicina* **2024**, *60*, 455, doi:10.3390/medicina60030455 335

About the Editor

Woo Jong Kim

Woo Jong Kim, who serves as a Professor and the Chief of the Foot and Ankle Service at the Department of Orthopedic Surgery at Soonchunhyang University Cheonan Hospital in South Korea, is a paragon of academic excellence, clinical expertise, and athletic prowess. With a Ph.D. in medicine, since 2021, Kim has played a transformative role in the medical community, not only by sharing knowledge as an Associate Professor but also by being a pioneer in orthopedic surgery, with a focus on foot and ankle disorders.

Beyond his significant contributions to medical science and education, Kim is celebrated for his exceptional career as a professional boxer. As the Vice Chairman of the Cheonan City Boxing Association, he has helped to raise the profile of boxing in South Korea. His commitment extends beyond the ring; he participates in sports medicine, serving as a team doctor for a professional soccer team and as an advisory doctor for the Hapkido Association. These roles highlight his dedication to improving athlete welfare and sports safety.

Kim's engagement with various prestigious medical societies underscores his commitment to his field. He is an active member of societies that focus on orthopedics, the foot and ankle, sports medicine, diabetic foot, fractures, osteoporosis, wound management, ultrasonography, and arthroscopy. His primary research interests are in treating sports injuries as well as fractures of the foot and ankle, significantly advancing knowledge and treatments in these areas through his extensive research and numerous publications.

Kim's diverse expertise not only showcases his multifaceted career but also demonstrates his substantial contributions to sports medicine, orthopedic surgery, and athlete health and safety. His work exemplifies a dedication to improving patient care, advancing medical knowledge, and promoting the well-being of athletes across disciplines.

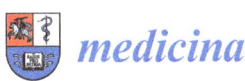

Technical Note

A Tension-Band Wiring Technique for Direct Fixation of a Chaput Tubercle Fracture: Technical Note

Eui-Dong Yeo [1,†], Ki-Jin Jung [2,†], Yong-Cheol Hong [2], Chang-Hwa Hong [2], Hong-Seop Lee [3], Sung-Hun Won [4], Sung-Joon Yoon [2], Sung-Hwan Kim [5], Jae-Young Ji [6], Dhong-Won Lee [7] and Woo-Jong Kim [2,*]

1. Veterans Health Service Medical Center, Department of Orthopaedic Surgery, Seoul 05368, Korea; angel_doctor@naver.com
2. Department of Orthopaedic Surgery, Soonchunhyang University Hospital Cheonan, 31, Suncheonhyang 6-gil, Dongam-gu, Cheonan 31151, Korea; c89546@schmc.ac.kr (K.-J.J.); ryanhong90@gmail.com (Y.-C.H.); chhong@schmc.ac.kr (C.-H.H.); yunsj0103@naver.com (S.-J.Y.)
3. Nowon Eulji Medical Center, Department of Foot and Ankle Surgery, Eulji University, 68, Hangeulbiseok-ro, Nowon-gu, Seoul 01830, Korea; sup4036@naver.com
4. Department of Orthopaedic Surgery, Soonchunhyang University Hospital Seoul, 59, Daesagwan-ro, Yongsan-gu, Seoul 04401, Korea; orthowon@schmc.ac.kr
5. Department of Orthopaedic Surgery, Soonchunhyang University Hospital Bucheon, 170, Jomaru-ro, Wonmi-gu, Gyeonggi-do, Bucheon-si 14584, Korea; sjk9528@naver.com
6. Department of Anesthesiology and Pain Medicine, Soonchunhyang University Hospital Cheonan, 31, Suncheonhyang 6-gil, Dongam-gu, Cheonan 31151, Korea; phmjjy@naver.com
7. Konkuk University Medical Center, Department of Orthopaedic Surgery, 120-1, Neungdong-ro, Gwangjin-gu, Seoul 05030, Korea; bestal@naver.com
* Correspondence: kwj9383@hanmail.net; Tel.: +82-41-570-2170
† These authors contributed equally to this work and are co-first authors.

Abstract: Few reports have described direct fixation of the Chaput tubercle; screw fixation is usually employed. Herein, we introduce a novel technique for Chaput tubercle fixation using tension-band wiring. This technique is applicable to fractured tubercles of various sizes and has the advantage that the fragment breakage that may occur during screw fixation is impossible. In addition, our technique increases fixation strength.

Keywords: ankle fracture; syndesmosis injury; Chaput tubercle; avulsion fracture; tension-band wiring

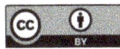

1. Introduction

Distal tibiofibular syndesmotic injury associated with ankle fracture accounts for 10% of all ankle fractures, and up to 20% are treated surgically as rotational ankle fractures [1–3]. Distal tibiofibular syndesmosis is critical for maintenance of ankle congruency and integrity during weight-bearing; unstable syndesmosis requires surgery [4,5]. Anatomical reduction of an ankle fracture with stabilization of any accompanying syndesmosis injury is essential to ensure good, long-term functional results and to prevent post-traumatic arthritis [1,6]. The anterior inferior tibiofibular ligament (AITFL) is the strongest of the four ligaments of the syndesmosis and plays a prime role in stability; it prevents displacement of the distal fibula outward from the mortis when an external rotation force is applied to the ankle joint [7,8]. The AITFL is attached to the anterior tibial tubercle on the distal tibial side (this tubercle is better known as the "Chaput tubercle"). Thus, a fracture of the tubercle is generally termed a "Chaput fracture", reflecting indirect injury of the syndesmosis [9]. Recent studies have suggested that direct fixation of fracture fragments is optimal for treating syndesmosis joint instability caused by a Chaput fracture [10,11]. Most direct fixation methods employ K-wires or screws [10–12], but this is impossible when the fracture fragments are small; in addition, the fixation strength is weaker than that of tension-band wiring (TBW) [13]. Here, we present a novel tension-band wiring technique that handles fracture fragments of various sizes and increases fixation strength. Such wiring is commonly performed in operating rooms.

2. Surgical Technique

This technical note was approved by the Institutional Review Board of Soonchunhyang University Cheonan Hospital (approval no. 2022–06–037, 2022-06-22). The patient provided written informed consent for the publication of this report and the accompanying images.

The procedure is performed under general or spinal anesthesia, or a lower extremity nerve block. The patient is placed supine, and the lower extremity is prepared and draped in the usual sterile manner. A tourniquet is inflated to ensure a bloodless surgical field. If a fibular fracture is also present, a curved anterolateral approach is chosen (Figure 1, dotted line). Through this line, first, reduction of the fibular fracture and, in most cases, plate fixation, and then approach to Chaput fragment are attempted. In the absence of a fibular fracture, a small anterolateral incision (2–3 cm) is created (solid line) directly over the palpable Chaput tubercle of the distal tibia. The anterolateral tibial fragment (the Chaput fracture) is identified and the fracture is cleared of debris. The fracture is reduced and temporarily fixed using small point-reduction forceps. The extent of reduction and the congruency of the articular surface are confirmed via intraoperative fluoroscopy. This also serves to ensure that the hardware is appropriately positioned and that the articular surface is not displaced. Then, two 1.2–1.6-mm (the diameter varies by the size of the fracture fragment) Kirschner (K)-wires are inserted proximally from the end edge of the Chaput fragment through the fracture site. These wires prevent fracture rotation and are later used to anchor a figure-of-eight wire distally. To ensure that the K-wires are fully seated on the end of the tubercle after the ends have been bent, they are pulled back slightly. Next, the medial incision site over the distal tibia is retracted to expose the anterolateral tibial border approximately 2 to 3 cm cephalad to the fracture site, and a ϕ 4.0-mm, cancellous, full-thread screw is inserted without tapping and without complete seating (Figure 2). Stainless-steel wires (ϕ 0.8 mm) are looped around the screw and the K-wires in a figure-of-eight manner (Figure 3). Then, the loops are tightened to ensure that they cling to the anteroinferior surface of the distal Chaput fragment and the steel wires are twisted at the points of insertion in the K-wires. Next, the two K-wires are cut obliquely, bent medially, and tapped into the medial malleolus; they are now fully seated. If the fracture fragment is small, thinner K-wires and steel wires are used. If a fracture fragment is impacted, it is possible to first attempt a bone graft. Figure 4 shows a postoperative plain X-ray of open reduction/internal fixation of a Chaput fracture using this technique (Figure 4). Axial computed tomography confirmed that both the reduction and the fixation were satisfactory (Figure 5). For this patient, a short leg splint was prescribed postoperatively for about 1–2 weeks. Then, the cast or range-of-motion (ROM) ankle walker brace was changed and the patient was instructed not to place weight on the limb for a further 4 weeks. ROM exercise commenced at 4 weeks after surgery, and then weight-bearing was gradually restored using the ROM ankle walker brace. After 6 weeks, full weight-bearing commenced, and the brace was removed at 8 weeks. A clinical union was confirmed 6 weeks after surgery and a radiologic union was confirmed on follow-up CT 3 months after surgery. The patient demographics and clinical analysis results are presented in Table 1.

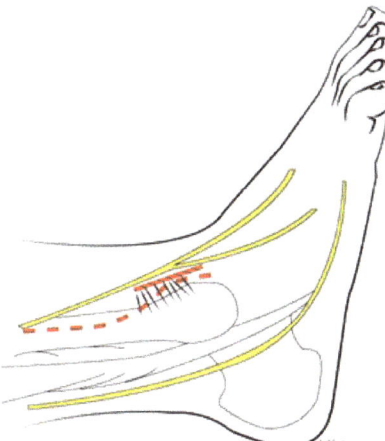

Figure 1. If a fibular fracture is also present, we take a curved anterolateral approach (dotted line). In the absence of such a fracture, a small anterolateral incision (about 2–3 cm) is created (solid line) directly over the palpable Chaput tubercle of the distal tibia.

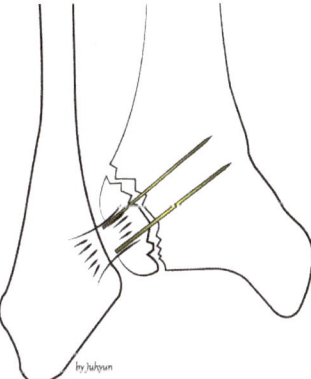

Figure 2. After the Chaput fracture has been reduced, two K-wires and screws are fixed.

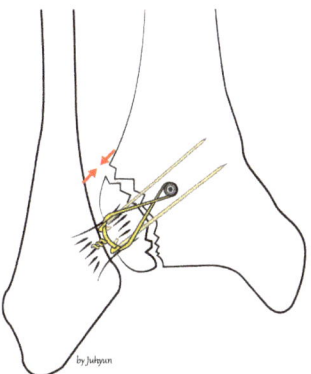

Figure 3. Stainless-steel wires are looped around the screw and the K-wires in a figure-of-eight manner.

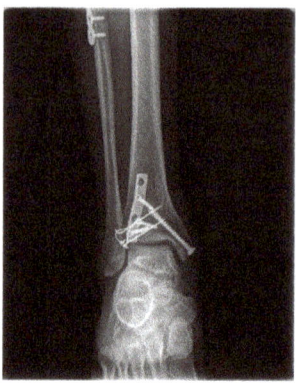

Figure 4. A postoperative, plain anteroposterior radiograph shows a Chaput fracture fixed using the new technique.

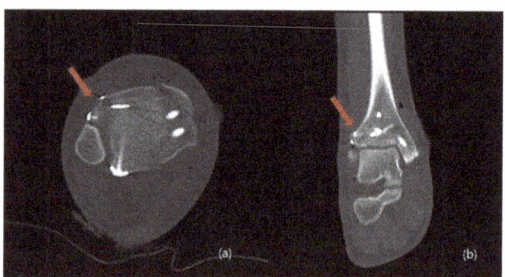

Figure 5. Postoperative axial (**a**) and coronal (**b**) computed tomography images show that the Chaput fracture exhibited good reduction, compression, and fixation (arrow).

Table 1. Patient demographics and results.

Pt. No.	Age	Sex	Cause	Lauge-Hansen Classification	Injury to Surgery Interval (hr)	* Procedure Time (min)	Injured Side	Follow-Up (mo)	OMAS		VAS Score		Interval to Union (wk)	Complications
									Pre	Post	Pre	Post		
1	57	F	S	SER IV	138	19	Left	9	30	80	8	1	14	None
2	76	F	S	SER IV	118	20	Left	14	25	85	7	0	15	None
3	56	F	S	SER II	98	18	Right	6	30	90	8	0	14	None
4	39	M	S	SER IV	87	18	Left	13	35	95	8	0	12	None
5	58	F	S	SER IV	282	19	Left	12	0	80	9	1	14	None
6	79	F	TA	PER IV	97	17	Left	6	0	70	8	0	16	None
7	16	M	TA	PER IV	68	18	Right	4	40	95	8	0	13	None
8	17	M	TA	PER II	39	18	Right	4	30	90	7	0	12	None
9	53	F	S	SER IV	258	16	Left	3	0	60	9	0	14	None
Mean	50.1	NA	NA	NA	131.7	18.1	NA	7.9	21.1	82.8	8	0.2	13.8	NA
SD	22.5	NA	NA	NA	83.5	1.2	NA	4.2	164	11.8	0.7	0.4	1.3	NA
p-value									0.007		0.006			

Abbreviations: Pt. No., patient number; OMAS, Olerud–Molander Ankle Score; VAS, visual analog scale; Pre, preoperative; Post, postoperative; F, female; M, male; S, slip down; TA, traffic accident; SER, supination external rotation; NA, not applicable; SD, standard deviation; * procedure time, tension-band wiring time. Statistical analysis was performed by a statistical expert. All calculations were made using SPSS, version 26.0, software (IBM Corp., Armonk, NY, USA). Quantitative variables are expressed as the mean ± standard deviation. The pre- and postoperative VAS and OMAS scores were compared using the Wilcoxon signed-rank test. A two-sided test with $p < 0.05$ was considered statistically significant.

3. Discussion

Several studies have reported the prognoses of Chaput fracture treatment. Haraguchi et al. [14] reported that the union rate of non-operated Chaput tubercle fractures was only 65%. Birnie et al. [15] reported that four patients (6.2%) of an AITL avulsion fracture group required additional surgery. Zhao et al. [16] performed open reduction/internal fixation on 15 adult patients with ankle fractures involving Tillaux–Chaput fractures. The mean AOFAS score was 87, with an excellent or good rate of 80%: excellent in nine cases, good in three, and fair in three. Bae et al. [11] performed direct avulsion fracture fixation on patients evidencing syndesmotic instability after malleolar fractures combined with AITL avulsion fractures. Syndesmotic stability was achieved by 45 (83.3%) of 54 patients; the remaining 9 (16.7%) required additional syndesmosis screw fixation.

Direct fixation of a fractured Chaput tubercle ensures not only bone-to-bone fixation of the anterior syndesmosis but also correct positioning of the fibula into the tibial incisura [17]. A few studies have found that inadequately treated bony avulsions of the tibiofibular syndesmosis can trigger translational or rotational malposition, which damages the structure of the ankle mortise [18,19]. After such a postoperative event, revision surgery should be urgently performed.

Several methods for direct fixation of Chaput fractures have been described. Chung et al. [10] reported good results after direct fixation of anteroinferior, tibiofibular, ligament avulsion fractures using K-wires, mini-screws, or absorbable suture materials. Six cases presented with Chaput fractures, including four of the modified Wagstaffe classification type III and two of type IV. However, the fixation materials were not described. Rammelt et al. [20] used plates, screws, and suture anchors. Gasparova et al. [12] found that screw fixation was optimal for monofragmented fractures, but plate fixation was best for multifragmentary fractures.

Historically, TBW has been recommended for AO patients when a fragment is too small for screw fixation into an avulsion fracture or when screw fixation is inadequate, such as in osteoporotic bone [21]. However, TBW has gradually become used to fix large fragments; it is increasingly recognized that TBW ensures good fusion rates and good functional results [22]. We reviewed the literature when applying TBW to treat Chaput fractures.

However, a limitation of this study is that the fixation strength of this technique was not compared with other devices in fixing the Chaput tubercle fragment. It is thought that cadaver studies for strength comparison are necessary.

Our technique is independent of the size of the fractured Chaput tubercle. Neither high-level surgical skill nor extensive experience are required.

4. Conclusions

This technique is applicable to fractured tubercles of various sizes. Additionally, it is advantageous when there is a possibility that fragment breakage may occur during other device fixation.

Author Contributions: Conceptualization, W.-J.K. and E.-D.Y.; methodology, Y.-C.H.; software, C.-H.H.; validation, W.-J.K. and Y.-C.H.; formal analysis, W.-J.K.; investigation, E.-D.Y. and H.-S.L.; resources, S.-J.Y.; data curation, Y.-C.H. and D.-W.L.; writing—original draft preparation, W.-J.K.; writing—review and editing, Y.-C.H.; visualization, S.-H.W.; supervision, J.-Y.J., K.-J.J. and S.-H.K.; project administration, S.-H.K. and J.-Y.J.; funding acquisition, K.-J.J. All authors have read and agreed to the published version of the manuscript.

Funding: The authors would like to thank the Soonchunhyang University Research Fund for support. (1022-0019). This research was supported by the Bio & Medical Technology Development Program of the Korea Medical Device Development Fund (KMDF) funded by the Ministry of Health and Welfare (202015X36-03).

Institutional Review Board Statement: The study was conducted according to the guidelines of the Declaration of Helsinki and approved by the Institutional Review Board and Human Research Ethics Committee of Soonchunhyang University Cheonan Hospital (IRB No. 2022-05-029).

Informed Consent Statement: Written informed consent has been obtained from the patient to publish this paper.

Data Availability Statement: Data sharing is not applicable to this article as no datasets were generated or analyzed during the current study.

Conflicts of Interest: The authors declare no conflict of interest.

Abbreviations

AITFL	anterior inferior tibiofibular ligament
TBW	tension-band wiring
K	Kirschner
ROM	range-of-motion

References

1. Egol, K.A.; Pahk, B.; Walsh, M.; Tejwani, N.C.; Davidovitch, R.I.; Koval, K.J. Outcome after unstable ankle fracture: Effect of syndesmotic stabilization. *J. Orthop. Trauma* **2010**, *24*, 7–11. [CrossRef] [PubMed]
2. Van den Bekerom, M.P.; Lamme, B.; Hogervorst, M.; Bolhuis, H.W. Which ankle fractures require syndesmotic stabilization? *J. Foot Ankle Surg.* **2007**, *46*, 456–463. [CrossRef] [PubMed]
3. Court-Brown, C.M.; McBirnie, J.; Wilson, G. Adult ankle fractures: An increasing problem? *Acta Orthop. Scand.* **1998**, *69*, 43–47. [CrossRef] [PubMed]
4. Bartoníček, J. Anatomy of the tibiofibular syndesmosis and its clinical relevance. *Surg. Radiol. Anat.* **2003**, *25*, 379–386. [CrossRef]
5. van Zuuren, W.J.; Schepers, T.; Beumer, A.; Sierevelt, I.; van Noort, A.; van den Bekerom, M.P.J. Acute syndesmotic instability in ankle fractures: A review. *Foot Ankle Surg.* **2017**, *23*, 135–141. [CrossRef] [PubMed]
6. Sagi, H.C.; Shah, A.R.; Sanders, R.W. The functional consequence of syndesmotic joint malreduction at a minimum 2-year follow-up. *J. Orthop. Trauma* **2012**, *26*, 439–443. [CrossRef]
7. Ogilvie-Harris, D.J.; Reed, S.C. Disruption of the ankle syndesmosis: Diagnosis and treatment by arthroscopic surgery. *Arthroscopy* **1994**, *10*, 561–568. [CrossRef]
8. Yuen, C.P.; Lui, T.H. Distal tibiofibular syndesmosis: Anatomy, biomechanics, injury and management. *Open Orthop. J.* **2017**, *11*, 670–677. [CrossRef]
9. Chaput, H. *Les Fractures Malléolaires du cou-de-pied et les Accidents du Travail*; Masson et Cie: Paris, France, 1907.
10. Chung, H.-J.; Bae, S.-Y.; Kim, M.-Y. Treatment of anteroinferior tibiofibular ligament avulsion fracture accompanied with ankle fracture. *J. Korean Foot Ankle Soc.* **2011**, *15*, 13–17.
11. Bae, K.J.; Kang, S.B.; Kim, J.; Lee, J.; Go, T.W. Reduction and fixation of anterior inferior tibiofibular ligament avulsion fracture without syndesmotic screw fixation in rotational ankle fracture. *J. Int. Med. Res.* **2020**, *48*, 300060519882550. [CrossRef]
12. Gasparova, M.; Falougy, H.E.; Kubikova, E.; Almasi, J. Isolated "Tillaux" fracture in adulthood: Rarity where the key of success is not to miss it. *Bratisl. Lek. Listy* **2020**, *121*, 533–536. [CrossRef] [PubMed]
13. Johnson, B.A.; Fallat, L.M. Comparison of tension-band wire and cancellous bone screw fixation for medial malleolar fractures. *J. Foot Ankle Surg.* **1997**, *36*, 284–289. [CrossRef]
14. Haraguchi, N.; Toga, H.; Shiba, N.; Kato, F. Avulsion fracture of the lateral ankle ligament complex in severe inversion injury: Incidence and clinical outcome. *Am. J. Sports Med.* **2007**, *35*, 1144–1152. [CrossRef] [PubMed]
15. Birnie, M.F.N.; van Schilt, K.L.J.; Sanders, F.R.K.; Kloen, P.; Schepers, T. Anterior inferior tibiofibular ligament avulsion fractures in operatively treated ankle fractures: A retrospective analysis. *Arch. Orthop. Trauma Surg.* **2019**, *139*, 787–793. [CrossRef] [PubMed]
16. Zhao, J.; Shu, H.; Li, W.; Liu, Y.; Shi, B.; Zheng, G. Clinical features and surgical effectiveness of ankle fractures involving Tillaux-Chaput in adults. *Chin. J. Reparative Reconstr. Surg.* **2015**, *29*, 288–291.
17. Rammelt, S.; Bartoníček, J.; Kroker, L.; Neumann, A.P. Surgical fixation of quadrimalleolar fractures of the ankle. *J. Orthop. Trauma* **2021**, *35*, e216–e222. [CrossRef]
18. Rammelt, S.; Boszczyk, A. Computed tomography in the diagnosis and treatment of ankle fractures: A critical analysis review. *JBJS Rev.* **2018**, *6*, e7. [CrossRef]
19. Marx, C.; Schaser, K.D.; Rammelt, S. Early corrections after failed ankle fracture fixation. *Z. Orthop. Unf.* **2021**, *159*, 323–331. [CrossRef]
20. Rammelt, S.; Bartoníček, J.; Schepers, T.; Kroker, L. Fixation of anterolateral distal tibial fractures: The anterior malleolus. *Oper. Orthop. Traumatol.* **2021**, *33*, 125–138. [CrossRef]
21. Muller, M.; Allgower, M.; Schneider, R.; Willenegger, H. Screws and plates and their application. *Man. Intern. Fixat.* **1991**, *3*, 179–290.
22. Kanakis, T.E.; Papadakis, E.; Orfanos, A.; Andreadakis, A.; Xylouris, E. Figure eight tension band in the treatment of fractures and pseudarthroses of the medial malleolus. *Injury* **1990**, *21*, 393–397. [CrossRef]

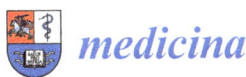

Article

Incidence of Hip Fractures among Patients with Chronic Otitis Media: The Real-World Data

Pei-Shao Liao [1,†], Ching-Chih Chiu [2,†], Yi-Hsiu Fu [3,†], Chia-Chun Hsia [2], Yu-Cih Yang [4], Kun-Feng Lee [2], Shang-Lin Hsieh [5,*] and Shu-Jui Kuo [5,6,*]

[1] Department of Otolaryngology Head and Neck Surgery, China Medical University Hospital, Taichung 404327, Taiwan
[2] Department of Education, China Medical University Hospital, Taichung 404327, Taiwan
[3] Department of Education, Taichung Veterans General Hospital, Taichung 407219, Taiwan
[4] Management Office for Health Data, China Medical University Hospital, Taichung 404327, Taiwan
[5] School of Medicine, China Medical University, Taichung 404328, Taiwan
[6] Department of Orthopedic Surgery, China Medical University Hospital, Taichung 404327, Taiwan
* Correspondence: neosolomon@msn.com (S.-L.H.); b90401073@gmail.com (S.-J.K.)
† These authors contributed equally to this work.

Abstract: Chronic otitis media (COM) has been considered as a localized disease, and its systemic impact is poorly understood. Whether COM-induced inflammation could be associated with systemic bone loss and hip fracture is unknown at present. Our study tried to determine the risk of hip fracture among COM patients. We selected the comparison individuals without the COM coding and paired the controls with COM patients by gender, age, and comorbidities (including osteoporosis) by about a one-to-two ratio. Our study showed that the incidence of hip fracture was 4.48 and 3.92 per 1000 person-years for comparison and COM cohorts respectively. The cumulative incidence of hip fracture is higher in the COM cohort ($p < 0.001$). After adjustment for gender, age, and comorbidities, the COM patients had a 1.11-fold (aHR = 1.11; 95% CI = 1.05–1.17) risk of hip fracture than the control subjects. Among COM patients, a history of hearing loss is associated with higher (aHR = 1.21; 95% CI = 1.20–1.42) fracture risk. Our study showed that COM patients, especially those with hearing loss, are susceptible to a higher risk for hip fracture.

Keywords: chronic otitis media; hearing loss; hip fracture; National Health Insurance Research Database; osteoporosis

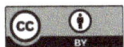

1. Introduction

Chronic otitis media (COM) is manifested by inflammation of the middle ear due to infectious or non-infectious processes, resulting in pathologic changes in the tympanic membrane [1]. The pathologic changes of the tympanic membrane secondary to COM include atelectasis, perforation, retraction, tympanosclerosis, and cholesteatoma [1,2]. COM is also an important etiology of acquired hearing loss and is the main disease in the field of otolaryngology [1]. COM can lead to potentially deadly complications such as mastoiditis, petrositis, labyrinthitis, meningitis, brain abscess, and thrombophlebitis [1]. Despite the potentially fatal nature of the complications mentioned above, these complications are local in nature and the systemic effects of COM are unknown currently.

Bone loss is a recognized consequence of systemic inflammatory processes, which could be explained by the perspective of evolution, disturbed energy expenditure and storage, and immunologic as well as neuroendocrine factors [3]. There is also a genetic linkage between auditory tract disease and bone loss. For example, FBXO11 is associated with the susceptibility to otitis media and affects osteoblastogenesis [4–6]. The correlations between inflammation, shared genetic factors, and the impact of COM on bone metabolism have not been rigorously determined.

The most devastating complication secondary to bone loss is hip fracture [7]. Hip fractures are accountable for 25% of geriatric fractures mandating hospitalization with high morbidity and mortality [8]. There is no available evidence demonstrating whether COM-induced inflammation could be associated with systemic bone loss and hip fracture. In our study, we want to investigate the incidence of hip fracture among subjects with COM. We thus conducted a nationwide population-based study, attempting to unravel the association between COM and hip fracture. We hypothesize that COM patients might be predisposed to a higher risk of hip fracture.

2. Materials and Methods

The Longitudinal Health Insurance Database (LHID) of the National Health Insurance Research Database (NHIRD) was employed for our study under the approval of the Institutional Review Board of China Medical University, Taichung, Taiwan (CMUH104-REC2–115). The LHID is composed of the registry data for the beneficiaries, inpatient and outpatient files, and the registry for drug prescriptions as well as medical services. The history of medical comorbidities of the insured individuals was retrieved from the inpatient and outpatient files. The International Classification of Diseases, 9th Revision, Clinical Modification (ICD-9-CM) system was applied as the disease-coding system in NHIRD. The original identification numbers were eliminated to safeguard the privacy of the insured citizens, and a scrambled number was offered to correlate the claim data to each individual before releasing the data for research purposes.

A population-based cohort study was established to determine the incidence of hip fracture (ICD-9-CM code 820.x) among the subjects with COM. All of the patients who were coded with COM (ICD-9-CM code 382.1–382.9) first in their lifetime from 1 January 2000 to 31 December 2013, were assessed. The date when the diagnosis of COM was initially coded was defined as the index date. The comparison individuals without the diagnostic coding of COM were chosen from the LHID and paired with COM patients by gender, age (exact year), and the coding of osteoporosis (ICD-9-CM 733.0 and 733.1) at the index date by about a one-to-two ratio. The comparison subjects were recruited on the same date as the paired COM patients. All of the enrolled individuals were followed until the withdrawal from the insurance, the advent of hip fracture, or until 31 December 2013. The comorbidities analyzed in our study included hypertension (ICD-9-CM code 401–405), diabetes (ICD-9-CM code 250), epilepsy (ICD-9-CM code 345, A225), ischemic heart disease (ICD-9-CM code 410–414), chronic obstructive pulmonary disease (COPD, ICD-9-CM code 491, 492, 493 and 496), stroke (ICD-9-CM code 430–438), liver cirrhosis (ICD-9-CM code 571 and 572), osteoporosis (ICD-9-CM code 733) and end-stage renal disease (ICD-9-CM code 585.6). The impact of hearing loss (ICD-9-CM code 389), vertigo (ICD-9-CM code 386), and tinnitus (ICD-9-CM code 388.3) on the occurrence of hip fractures among COM patients were also analyzed.

The incidence rate of hip fracture was expressed as events per 1,000 person-years. The chi-square test for categorical variables and the two-sample t-test for continuous variables were applied for between-group comparisons. The Kaplan–Meier method was utilized to plot the cumulative incidence of hip fractures, and the log-rank test was employed to determine the significance of between-group differences [9,10]. To demonstrate the risk of hip fracture for the COM and control cohorts, the crude and adjusted hazard ratios (cHRs and aHRs) and 95% confidence intervals (CIs) were calculated by employing the single- and multi-variable Cox proportional hazard models [11]. The SAS 9.4 software (SAS Institute, Cary, NC, USA) was applied for data analysis and the R software (R Foundation for Statistical Computing, Vienna, Austria) was employed to plot the incidence curves.

3. Results

There were 53,997 patients in the COM cohort and 107,865 individuals in the comparison cohort. The distribution of gender, age, and the percentage with the initial diagnosis of osteoporosis were comparable between the two cohorts. The mean age of COM and comparison cohorts were 27.8 ± 86.0 and 28.1 ± 84.4 years, respectively (Table 1). The prevalence of hypertension, diabetes, epilepsy, ischemic heart disease, chronic obstructive pulmonary disease, stroke, and liver cirrhosis were all higher in the COM cohort (all $p < 0.001$). The follow-up duration was 9.49 ±3.7 years for the COM cohort and 9.43 ± 3.7 years for the comparison cohort. The flow diagram for the subject recruitment process was shown in Figure 1.

Table 1. Demographic profiles for the COM and comparison cohorts.

	COM Cohort $n = 53,977$		Comparison Cohort $n = 107,865$		p-Value *
	n	%	n	%	
Gender					0.820
Female	27,443	50.8	54,885	50.9	
Male	26,554	49.2	52,980	49.1	
Age					0.999
<20	26,132	48.4	52,135	48.3	
20–44	12,896	23.8	25,792	23.9	
45–64	10,154	18.8	20,308	18.8	
≥65	4815	8.92	9630	8.93	
mean(SD) †	27.84 (86.0)		28.11 (84.4)		<0.001
Comorbidities					
Hypertension	11,988	22.2	21,349	19.7	<0.001
Diabetes	7024	13.0	12,033	11.1	<0.001
Epilepsy	453	0.84	638	0.59	<0.001
Ischemic heart disease	3854	7.14	6120	5.67	<0.001
COPD	10,639	20.3	14,314	13.2	<0.001
Stroke	2392	4.43	3899	3.61	<0.001
Liver cirrhosis	5576	10.3	8724	8.09	<0.001
Osteoporosis	1712	3.17	3422	3.17	0.983
End-stage renal disease	0	0	0	0	-

COM: chronic otitis media; COPD: Chronic obstructive pulmonary disease; SD: standard deviation. †: compared by two-sample t-test; *: compared by chi-square test unless marked by †.

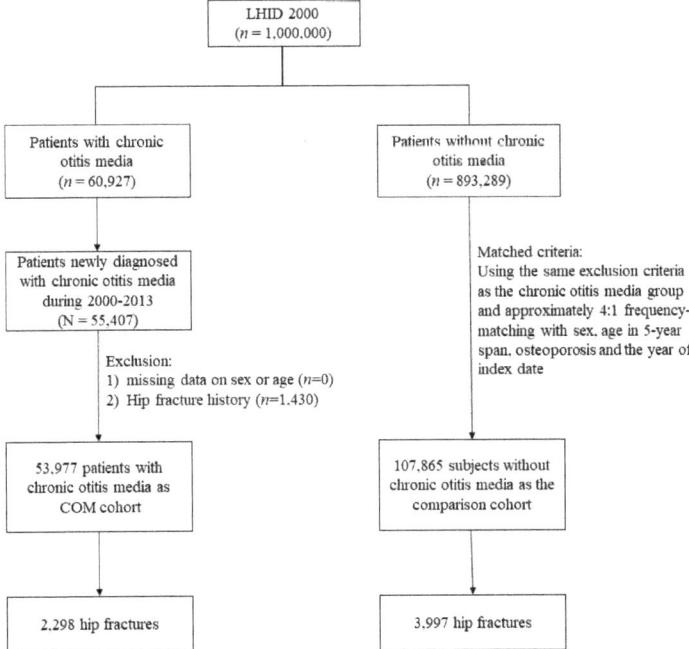

Figure 1. The flow diagram of the recruitment process.

There were 2298 hip fractures in the COM cohort with an incidence density of 4.48 per 1000 person-years. As for the comparison cohort, 3997 individuals suffered from hip fractures with an incidence density of 3.92 per 1000 person-years (Table 2). The cumulative incidence of hip fracture was higher in the COM cohort than in the comparison cohort (Figure 2, $p < 0.001$ for log-rank test). After adjustment for gender, age, and all of the enlisted comorbidities, the subjects in the COM cohort had a 1.11-fold risk of hip fracture than the individuals in the comparison cohort (aHR = 1.11; 95% CI = 1.05–1.17). Age, gender, hypertension, diabetes, epilepsy, chronic obstructive pulmonary disease, stroke, and osteoporosis were also associated with a higher incidence of hip fracture in our model.

Table 2. The incidence density of hip fracture stratified by the history of chronic otitis media, gender, age, and comorbidities.

Variable	Hip Fracture			Crude HR (95%CI)	# Adjusted HR (95%CI)
	Hip Fracture	PY	IR		
Chronic otitis media					
No	3997	1,018,072	3.92	1 (reference)	1 (reference)
Yes	2298	512,483	4.48	1.14 (1.08–1.20) ***	1.11 (1.05–1.17) ***
Gender					
Female	3175	777,192	4.08	1 (reference)	1 (reference)
Male	3120	753,363	4.14	1.01 (0.96–1.06)	1.07 (1.02–1.13) **
Age					
<20	2148	858,051	2.50	1 (reference)	1 (reference)
20–44	1113	332,276	3.34	1.37 (1.27–1.47) ***	1.32 (1.23–1.43) ***
45–64	1653	245,380	6.73	2.78 (2.61–2.96) ***	2.21 (2.04–2.39) ***
≥65	1381	94,848	14.5	6.14 (5.74–6.58) ***	4.10 (3.72–4.52) ***
Comorbidities					
Hypertension					
No	3826	1,259,598	3.03	1 (reference)	1 (reference)
Yes	2469	270,957	9.11	3.08 (2.88–3.19) ***	1.21 (1.12–1.30) ***
Diabetes					
No	4793	1,376,069	3.48	1 (reference)	1 (reference)
Yes	1502	154,486	9.72	2.82 (2.66–2.98) ***	1.22 (1.14–1.31) ***
Epilepsy					
No	6240	1,522,127	4.09	1 (reference)	1 (reference)
Yes	55	8428	6.52	1.60 (1.23–2.09) ***	1.44 (1.10–1.88) **
Ischemic heart disease					
No	5538	1,463,746	3.78	1 (reference)	1 (reference)
Yes	757	66,809	11.3	3.06 (2.84–3.31) ***	0.98 (0.89–1.07)
COPD					
No	4994	1,317,988	3.78	1 (reference)	1 (reference)
Yes	1301	212,567	6.12	1.62 (1.53–1.73) ***	1.19 (1.11–1.27) ***
Stroke					
No	5767	1,491,279	3.86	1 (reference)	1 (reference)
Yes	528	39,276	13.4	3.56 (3.25–3.89) ***	1.24 (1.12–1.37) ***
Liver cirrhosis					
No	5502	1,428,513	3.85	1 (reference)	1 (reference)
Yes	793	102,042	7.77	2.05 (1.90–2.21) ***	1.00 (0.92–1.09)
Osteoporosis					
No	5808	1,495,082	3.88	1 (reference)	1 (reference)
Yes	487	35,473	13.7	3.60 (3.28–3.95) ***	1.49 (1.34–1.65) ***
End-stage renal disease					
No	6295	1,530,555	4.11	1 (reference)	1 (reference)
Yes	–	–	–	–	–

COPD: chronic obstructive pulmonary disease; PY: person-years; IR: incidence rate per 1000 PYs; HR: hazard ratio; CI: confidence interval; ** $p < 0.01$, *** $p < 0.001$; # Adjusted for age, gender, and enlisted comorbidities.

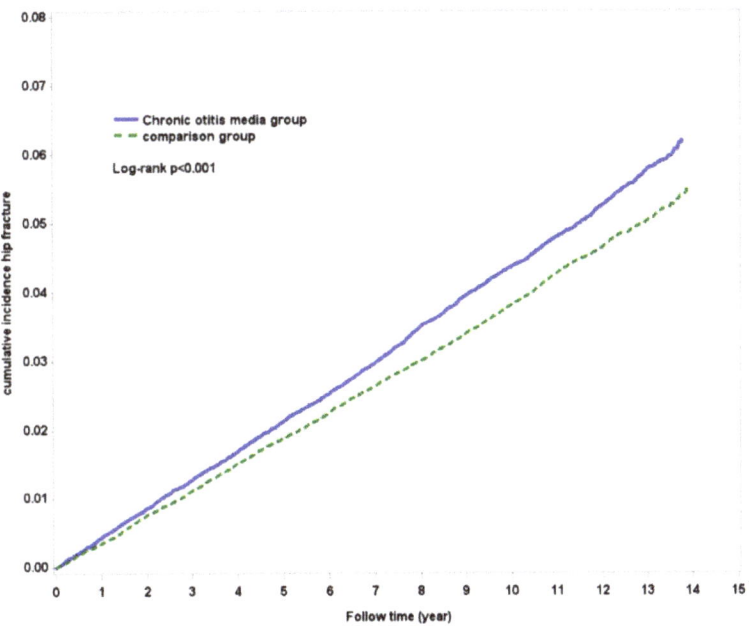

Figure 2. The incidence of hip fracture among COM and comparison cohorts. The dashed line indicates the comparison cohort, and the solid line indicates the COM cohort.

Table 3 showed that the impact of COM and on the risk of hip fracture was more pronounced among subjects with female gender (aHR = 1.17; 95% CI = 1.09–1.26), hypertension (aHR = 1.14; 95% CI = 1.05–1.24), diabetes (aHR = 1.19; 95% CI = 1.07–1.32), ischemic heart disease (aHR = 1.15; 95% CI = 1.00–1.33), and chronic obstructive pulmonary disease (aHR = 1.14; 95% CI = 1.02–1.27).

Table 3. Differential incidence rate and hazard ratio of hip fracture among the subjects with and without chronic otitis media stratified by gender, age, and comorbidities.

Variable	Chronic Otitis Media						Crude HR (95%CI)	# Adjusted HR (95%CI)
	No			Yes				
	Hip Fracture	PY	IR	Hip Fracture	PY	IR		
Gender								
Female	1980	517,377	3.82	1195	259,815	4.59	1.20 (1.11–1.29) ***	1.17 (1.09–1.26) ***
Male	2017	500,695	4.02	1103	252,668	4.36	1.08 (1.00–1.16) *	1.05 (0.97–1.13)
Age								
<20	1389	570,608	2.43	759	287,443	2.64	1.08 (0.99–1.18)	1.07 (0.98–1.17)
20–44	675	220,884	3.05	438	111,392	3.93	1.28 (1.14–1.45) ***	1.23 (1.09–1.39) ***
45–64	1045	163,603	6.38	608	81,777	7.43	1.16 (1.05–1.28) **	1.12 (1.01–1.24) *
≥65	888	62,977	14.10	493	31,871	15.46	1.09 (0.98–1.22)	1.06 (0.95–1.19)
Comorbidity								
Hypertension								
No	2492	844,254	2.95	1334	415,344	3.21	1.08 (1.01–1.16) *	1.08 (1.01–1.16) *
Yes	1505	173,818	8.65	964	97,139	9.92	1.14 (1.05–1.24) ***	1.14 (1.05–1.24) **
Diabetes								
No	3106	920,361	3.37	1687	455,708	3.70	1.09 (1.03–1.16) **	1.08 (1.02–1.15) **
Yes	891	97,711	9.11	611	56,775	10.7	1.18 (1.06–1.30) **	1.19 (1.07–1.32) ***

Table 3. Cont.

Variable	Chronic Otitis Media						Crude HR (95%CI)	# Adjusted HR (95%CI)
	No			Yes				
	Hip Fracture	PY	IR	Hip Fracture	PY	IR		
Epilepsy								
No	3964	1,013,163	3.91	2276	508,964	4.47	1.14 (1.08–1.20) ***	1.11 (1.05–1.17) ***
Yes	33	4909	6.72	22	3519	6.25	0.93 (0.54–1.60)	1.02 (0.59–1.77)
IHD								
No	3559	977,529	3.64	1979	486,216	4.07	1.11 (1.05–1.18) ***	1.10 (1.04–1.16) ***
Yes	438	40,543	10.8	319	26,267	12.1	1.12 (0.97–1.29)	1.15 (1.00–1.33) *
COPD								
No	3287	900,652	3.64	1707	417,335	4.09	1.12 (1.05–1.18) ***	1.10 (1.04–1.17) ***
Yes	710	117,420	6.04	591	95,148	6.21	1.02 (0.92–1.14)	1.14 (1.02–1.27) *
Stroke								
No	3675	994,043	3.69	2092	497,236	4.20	1.13 (1.07–1.20) ***	1.11 (1.05–1.17) ***
Yes	322	24,029	13.4	206	15,247	13.5	1.00 (0.84–1.20)	1.04 (0.87–1.24)
Liver cirrhosis								
No	3531	956,226	3.69	1971	472,287	4.17	1.12 (1.06–1.19) ***	1.11 (1.05–1.18) ***
Yes	466	61,846	7.53	327	40,196	8.13	1.08 (0.93–1.24)	1.08 (0.93–1.24)
Osteoporosis								
No	3688	994,420	3.70	2120	500,661	4.23	1.14 (1.08–1.20) ***	1.10 (1.05–1.16) ***
Yes	309	23,652	13.0	178	11,822	15.05	1.15 (0.95–1.38)	1.14 (0.94–1.37)
ESRD								
No	3997	1,018,072	3.92	2298	512,483	4.48	1.14 (1.08–1.20) ***	1.11 (1.05–1.17) ***
Yes	0	0	0	0	0	0	–	–

COPD: chronic obstructive pulmonary disease; ESRD: end-stage renal disease; IHD: ischemic heart disease; PYs: person-years; IR: incidence rate per 1000 PYs; HR: hazard ratio; CI: confidence interval; * $p < 0.05$, ** $p < 0.01$, *** $p < 0.001$; # Adjusted for age, gender, and the comorbidities enlisted in this table.

Among the COM patients, a history of hearing loss is associated with a higher (aHR = 1.21; 95% CI = 1.20–1.42) risk of hip fracture (Table 4).

Table 4. The subgroup analysis risk of hip fractures among the COM patients.

	Hip Fracture n = 2298	PY	IR	Crude HR (95%CI)	# Adjusted HR (95%CI)
Gender					
Female	1195	259,815	4.59	1 (reference)	1 (reference)
Male	1103	252,668	4.36	0.94 (0.87–1.03)	1.19 (1.05–1.34) **
Age					
<20	759	287,443	2.64	1 (reference)	1 (reference)
20–44	438	111,392	3.93	1.53 (1.36–1.72) ***	1.45 (1.22–1.71) ***
45–64	608	81,777	7.43	2.91 (2.61–3.24) ***	1.83 (1.44–2.33) ***
≥65	493	31,871	15.46	6.19 (5.52–6.94) ***	2.85 (2.13–3.80) ***
Outpatient frequencies					
≤3 (times)	1157	270,863	4.27	1 (reference)	1 (reference)
>3	1141	241,620	4.72	1.10 (1.01–1.19) *	0.93 (0.82–1.04)
Hospitalization frequencies					
<1 (times)	1953	449,444	4.34	1 (reference)	1 (reference)
≥1	345	63,039	5.47	1.25 (1.11–1.40) ***	1.12 (0.94–1.33)
Hearing loss					
No	1885	468,142	4.02	1 (reference)	1 (reference)
Yes	413	44,341	9.31	2.32 (2.08–2.58) ***	1.21 (1.20–1.42) *
Vertigo					
No	1832	456,977	4.00	1 (reference)	1 (reference)
Yes	466	55,506	8.39	2.10 (1.90–2.33) ***	1.00 (0.85–1.18)
Tinnitus					
No	1851	459,547	4.02	1 (reference)	1 (reference)
Yes	447	52,936	8.44	2.11 (1.90–2.34) ***	1.02 (0.86–1.20)

PY: person-years; IR: incidence rate per 1000 PYs; HR: hazard ratio; CI: confidence interval; * $p < 0.05$, ** $p < 0.01$, *** $p < 0.001$. # Adjusted for gender, age, outpatient and hospitalization frequencies, hearing loss, vertigo, and tinnitus.

4. Discussion

COM has been considered as a localized disease, and its systemic impact is poorly understood. In our study, we showed that the COM patients were subject to 1.11-fold the risk of suffering from hip fracture than the comparison individuals (95% CI = 1.05–1.17). The impact of COM was more prominent among the subjects of female gender, hypertension, diabetes, ischemic heart disease, and chronic obstructive pulmonary disease. Among the COM patients, the history of hearing loss furtherly increased the risk of hip fracture. These results indicate that COM is not merely a "localized" disease.

The pathophysiologic linkage between COM and osteoporotic hip fracture is not clear at present. However, the inflammation and genetic factor could potentially be the pathophysiologic linkage between COM and hip fracture.

As for inflammation, the "three-pillar theory" has been proposed to account for the bone loss under inflammation, including evolution, disturbed energy expenditure and storage, and immunologic as well as endocrine factors [3]. Inflammation has been shown to be involved in the pathogenesis of both auditory tract disease and systemic bone loss. Wang et al. have shown that the osteoporosis cohort displayed a 1.32-fold risk to suffer from acquired cholesteatoma compared with the control cohort (aHR = 1.32; 95% CI = 1.11–1.57), thus suggesting that otolaryngologists should examine the middle ear of osteoporotic patients [12]. Additionally, cholesteatoma is characterized by bone erosion in the middle ear, and increased expression of receptor activator for nuclear factor-κB ligand (RANKL) and osteoprotegerin (OPG) is found in tissues of cholesteatoma [13–15]. These results nicely demonstrated the correlation between bone loss and the inflammation of the auditory tract. In our study, we demonstrated that the COM patients had 1.11 times the risk of suffering from hip fracture when compared with the paired comparison individuals. Our study supplemented the previous publications in bridging the association between the inflammation of the auditory tract and bone disease.

A shared genetic factor could be the potential nexus between COM and systemic bone loss. Otitis media (recurrent acute otitis media, chronic otitis media with effusion) is largely associated with genetic susceptibility (40–70%) [16]. Mahmood et al. demonstrated the association between COM and the genetic loci of FBXO11 and TGIF1, both of which are involved in the transforming growth factor -beta (TGF-β) signaling via regulating the Smad proteins [17]. Smad proteins are involved in osteoclastogenesis via the RANKL–RANK interplay [18]. FBXO11 can inhibit the transcriptional activity of the p53 gene via promoting its neddylation as a function of Nedd8-ligase and affects its synergistic cooperation with phospho-Smad2 protein on TGF-β signaling [19]. Phospho-Smad2 could enhance the gene expression specific to osteoclast, resulting in inflammatory bone destruction [18]. Furthermore, p53 itself also suppresses osteoblastogenesis and thus results in reduced bone formation [6,20]. As for TGIF1, it has also been shown that TGIF1 knockout mice could develop COM with suppressed Smad expression in middle ear epithelial cells [21]. Vertigo and dizziness are the clinical manifestations of COM, and a previous study revealed that they could increase the risk of falling [22]. The associations between genetic factors, COM, precipitation to falling, and hip fracture warrant further investigations.

We also displayed that the history of hearing loss coincided with a higher risk of hip fracture among the COM patients. Previous studies have shown that osteoporosis was associated with decreased ossicle mass, decreased bone density of the cochlea, and disturbed sound transmission to the cochlea, which end up having a higher incidence of a sensorineural type of hearing loss [23,24]. Yoo et al. analyzed 2588 women and 2273 men aged over 50 years to determine the correlation between senile hearing loss and osteoporosis. The authors demonstrated that individuals with decreased femoral neck bone mineral density could sustain a 1.7-fold risk of suffering from hearing loss ($p < 0.01$) [20]. In our study, the history of hearing loss is associated with a higher (aHR = 1.21; 95% CI = 1.20–1.42) risk of suffering from hip fracture among COM patients. The shown impact of hearing loss on the onset of hip fracture among COM patients in our study supplemented the knowledge concerning the correlation between hearing loss and bone disease.

Our study is not free from limitations. First, the NHIRD did not include all the known risk factors for hip fracture. Some important risk factors, such as vitamin D deficiency and family history, could not be retrieved from the NHIRD. In fact, it is impossible and not necessary to include every known risk factor of hip fracture for analysis. The optimal way to determine the impact of COM on the occurrence of hip fracture was propensity score matching. The absence of propensity score matching would raise the concern that the association between COM and hip fracture might be secondary to the un-recognized medical comorbidities associated with COM. However, excessive matching could skew the generalizability of our findings, so we only paired the coding of osteoporosis in this study and rigorously adjusted all the retrieval comorbidity factors in our regression model instead. Our group has been dedicated to unraveling the association between diseases that can stimulate inflammatory responses and hip fracture. Our future work will continue to unravel more disease entities that could predispose patients to hip fracture. We hope that our work can help in optimizing the risk prediction of, or even prevent, hip fracture.

5. Conclusions

- ✓ The incidence of hip fracture was 4.48 and 3.92 per 1000 person-years for comparison and COM cohorts respectively. After adjustment for gender, age, and comorbidities, the COM patients had a 1.11-fold (aHR = 1.11; 95% CI = 1.05–1.17) risk of hip fracture than the control subjects.
- ✓ The cumulative incidence of hip fracture is higher in the COM cohort ($p < 0.001$) than in the comparison cohort.
- ✓ Among the COM patients, a history of hearing loss is associated with higher (aHR = 1.21; 95% CI = 1.20–1.42) fracture risk.

Author Contributions: Conceptualization, S.-J.K. and S.-L.H.; methodology, S.-J.K. and P.-S.L.; software, Y.-C.Y.; validation, P.-S.L., C.-C.C. and Y.-H.F.; formal analysis, Y.-H.F., C.-C.H. and K.-F.L.; investigation, S.-J.K., K.-F.L. and Y.-C.Y.; resources, S.-J.K., Y.-C.Y. and S.-L.H.; data curation, P.-S.L. and C.-C.C.; writing—original draft preparation, Y.-H.F., C.-C.H., and K.-F.L.; writing—review and editing, P.-S.L., C.-C.C. and S.-J.K.; visualization, S.-L.H.; supervision, S.-J.K. and S.-L.H.; project administration, P.-S.L. and C.-C.C.; funding acquisition, S.-J.K. All authors have read and agreed to the published version of the manuscript.

Funding: This research was funded by the Ministry of Health and Welfare Clinical Trial Center, Taiwan (MOHW109-TDU-B-212-114004), the Minister of Science and Technology, Taiwan (MOST 109-2314-B-039-018-MY3, MOST 108-2622-E-039-002-CC1, MOST 109-2321-B-039-002, and MOST 108-2221-E-039-006-MY3), China Medical University (CMU109-MF-82), and China Medical University Hospital (DMR-110-111, DMR-110-222, DMR-110-224, DMR-111-114, and DMR-111-230), and Tseng-Lien Lin Foundation, Taichung, Taiwan.

Institutional Review Board Statement: The study was conducted in accordance with the Declaration of Helsinki, and approved by the Institutional Review Board of China Medical University, Taichung, Taiwan (CMUH104-REC2-115 (CR4), date of approval: 5 July 2019).

Informed Consent Statement: Patient consent was waived under the agreement of the Institutional Review Board of China Medical University, Taichung, Taiwan because the identify of the subjects could not be identified.

Data Availability Statement: The data presented in this study are available on request from the corresponding author.

Conflicts of Interest: The authors declare no conflict of interest.

References

1. Park, M.; Lee, J.S.; Lee, J.H.; Oh, S.H.; Park, M.K. Prevalence and risk factors of chronic otitis media: The Korean National Health and Nutrition Examination Survey 2010–2012. *PLoS ONE* **2015**, *10*, e0125905. [CrossRef] [PubMed]
2. Nadol, J.B., Jr. Revision mastoidectomy. *Otolaryngol. Clin. N. Am.* **2006**, *39*, 723–740. [CrossRef] [PubMed]
3. Straub, R.H.; Cutolo, M.; Pacifici, R. Evolutionary medicine and bone loss in chronic inflammatory diseases—A theory of inflammation-related osteopenia. *Semin. Arthritis Rheum.* **2015**, *45*, 220–228. [CrossRef] [PubMed]

4. Segade, F.; Daly, K.A.; Allred, D.; Hicks, P.J.; Cox, M.; Brown, M.; Hardisty-Hughes, R.E.; Brown, S.D.; Rich, S.S.; Bowden, D.W. Association of the FBXO11 gene with chronic otitis media with effusion and recurrent otitis media: The Minnesota COME/ROM Family Study. *Arch. Otolaryngol. Head Neck Surg.* **2006**, *132*, 729–733. [CrossRef] [PubMed]
5. Rye, M.S.; Wiertsema, S.P.; Scaman, E.S.; Oommen, J.; Sun, W.; Francis, R.W.; Ang, W.; Pennell, C.E.; Burgner, D.; Richmond, P.; et al. FBXO11, a regulator of the TGFbeta pathway, is associated with severe otitis media in Western Australian children. *Genes Immun.* **2011**, *12*, 352–359. [CrossRef] [PubMed]
6. Wang, X.; Kua, H.Y.; Hu, Y.; Guo, K.; Zeng, Q.; Wu, Q.; Ng, H.H.; Karsenty, G.; de Crombrugghe, B.; Yeh, J.; et al. p53 functions as a negative regulator of osteoblastogenesis, osteoblast-dependent osteoclastogenesis, and bone remodeling. *J. Cell Biol.* **2006**, *172*, 115–125. [CrossRef] [PubMed]
7. Metcalfe, D. The pathophysiology of osteoporotic hip fracture. *McGill J. Med.* **2008**, *11*, 51–57. [CrossRef] [PubMed]
8. Carpintero, P.; Caeiro, J.R.; Carpintero, R.; Morales, A.; Silva, S.; Mesa, M. Complications of hip fractures: A review. *World J. Orthop.* **2014**, *5*, 402–411. [CrossRef] [PubMed]
9. Lai, S.W.; Liao, K.F.; Lin, C.L.; Lin, C.C.; Lin, C.H. Longitudinal data of multimorbidity and polypharmacy in older adults in Taiwan from 2000 to 2013. *Biomedicine* **2020**, *10*, 1–4. [CrossRef]
10. Lai, S.W.; Liao, K.F.; Lin, C.L.; Lin, C.H. Association between Parkinson's disease and proton pump inhibitors therapy in older people. *Biomedicine* **2020**, *10*, 1–4. [CrossRef]
11. Chiang, C.H.; Li, C.Y.; Hu, K.C.; Fu, Y.H.; Chiu, C.C.; Hsia, C.C.; Kuo, S.J.; Hung, C.H. The Association between Iron-Deficiency Anemia (IDA) and Septic Arthritis (SA): The Real-World Data. *Medicina* **2022**, *58*, 617. [CrossRef] [PubMed]
12. Wang, T.C.; Lin, C.C.; Lin, C.D.; Chung, H.K.; Wang, C.Y.; Tsai, M.H.; Kao, C.H. Increased Acquired Cholesteatoma Risk in Patients with Osteoporosis: A Retrospective Cohort Study. *PLoS ONE* **2015**, *10*, e0132447. [CrossRef] [PubMed]
13. Amar, M.S.; Wishahi, H.F.; Zakhary, M.M. Clinical and biochemical studies of bone destruction in cholesteatoma. *J. Laryngol. Otol.* **1996**, *110*, 534–539. [CrossRef] [PubMed]
14. Kuczkowski, J.; Sakowicz-Burkiewicz, M.; Izycka-Swieszewska, E. Expression of the receptor activator for nuclear factor-kappaB ligand and osteoprotegerin in chronic otitis media. *Am. J. Otolaryngol.* **2010**, *31*, 404–409. [CrossRef] [PubMed]
15. Jung, J.Y.; Chole, R.A. Bone resorption in chronic otitis media: The role of the osteoclast. *ORL J. Otorhinolaryngol. Relat. Spec.* **2002**, *64*, 95–107. [CrossRef]
16. Rye, M.S.; Blackwell, J.M.; Jamieson, S.E. Genetic susceptibility to otitis media in childhood. *Laryngoscope* **2012**, *122*, 665–675. [CrossRef]
17. Bhutta, M.F.; Lambie, J.; Hobson, L.; Goel, A.; Hafren, L.; Einarsdottir, E.; Mattila, P.S.; Farrall, M.; Brown, S.; Burton, M.J. A mouse-to-man candidate gene study identifies association of chronic otitis media with the loci TGIF1 and FBXO11. *Sci. Rep.* **2017**, *7*, 12496. [CrossRef]
18. Fennen, M.; Pap, T.; Dankbar, B. Smad-dependent mechanisms of inflammatory bone destruction. *Arthritis Res. Ther.* **2016**, *18*, 279. [CrossRef]
19. Tateossian, H.; Hardisty-Hughes, R.E.; Morse, S.; Romero, M.R.; Hilton, H.; Dean, C.; Brown, S.D. Regulation of TGF-beta signalling by Fbxo11, the gene mutated in the Jeff otitis media mouse mutant. *Pathogenetics* **2009**, *2*, 5. [CrossRef]
20. Abida, W.M.; Nikolaev, A.; Zhao, W.; Zhang, W.; Gu, W. FBXO11 promotes the Neddylation of p53 and inhibits its transcriptional activity. *J. Biol. Chem.* **2007**, *282*, 1797–1804. [CrossRef]
21. Tateossian, H.; Morse, S.; Parker, A.; Mburu, P.; Warr, N.; Acevedo-Arozena, A.; Cheeseman, M.; Wells, S.; Brown, S.D. Otitis media in the Tgif knockout mouse implicates TGFbeta signalling in chronic middle ear inflammatory disease. *Hum. Mol. Genet.* **2013**, *22*, 2553–2565. [CrossRef] [PubMed]
22. Schlick, C.; Schniepp, R.; Loidl, V.; Wuehr, M.; Hesselbarth, K.; Jahn, K. Falls and fear of falling in vertigo and balance disorders: A controlled cross-sectional study. *J. Vestib. Res.* **2016**, *25*, 241–251. [CrossRef] [PubMed]
23. Yoo, J.I.; Park, K.S.; Seo, S.H.; Park, H.W. Osteoporosis and hearing loss: Findings from the Korea National Health and Nutrition Examination Survey 2009–2011. *Braz. J. Otorhinolaryngol.* **2020**, *86*, 332–338. [CrossRef] [PubMed]
24. Kahveci, O.K.; Demirdal, U.S.; Yucedag, F.; Cerci, U. Patients with osteoporosis have higher incidence of sensorineural hearing loss. *Clin. Otolaryngol.* **2014**, *39*, 145–149. [CrossRef]

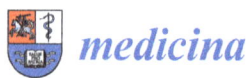

Article

Evaluation of the Quality of Information Available on the Internet Regarding Chronic Ankle Instability

Sung-Joon Yoon [1,†], Jun-Bum Kim [1,†], Ki-Jin Jung [1], Hee-Jun Chang [1], Yong-Cheol Hong [1], Chang-Hwa Hong [1], Byung-Ryul Lee [1], Eui-Dong Yeo [2], Hong-Seop Lee [3], Sung-Hun Won [4], Jae-Young Ji [5], Dhong-Won Lee [6] and Woo-Jong Kim [1,*]

[1] Department of Orthopaedic Surgery, Soonchunhyang University Hospital Cheonan, 31 Suncheonhyang 6-gil, Dongam-gu, Cheonan 31151, Korea
[2] Department of Orthopaedic Surgery, Veterans Health Service Medical Center, Seoul 05368, Korea
[3] Department of Foot and Ankle Surgery, Nowon Eulji Medical Center, Eulji University, 68 Hangeulbiseok-ro, Nowon-gu, Seoul 01830, Korea
[4] Department of Orthopaedic Surgery, Soonchunhyang University Hospital Seoul, 59 Daesagwan-ro, Yongsan-gu, Seoul 04401, Korea
[5] Department of Anesthesiology and Pain Medicine, Soonchunhyang University Hospital Cheonan, 31 Suncheonhyang 6-gil, Dongam-gu, Cheonan 31151, Korea
[6] Department of Orthopaedic Surgery, Konkuk University Medical Center, 120-1 Neungdong-ro, Gwangjin-gu, Seoul 05030, Korea
* Correspondence: kwj9383@hanmail.net; Tel.: +82-41-570-2170
† These authors contributed equally to this work.

Abstract: *Background and objectives*: Most Koreans obtain medical information from the Internet. Despite the vast amount of information available, there is a possibility that patients acquire false information or are dissatisfied. Chronic ankle instability (CAI) is one of the most common sports injuries that develops after an ankle sprain. Although the information available on the Internet related to CAI has been evaluated in other countries, such studies have not been conducted in Korea. *Materials and Methods*: The key term "chronic ankle instability" was searched on the three most commonly used search engines in Korea. The top 150 website results were classified into university hospital, private hospital, commercial, non-commercial, and unspecified websites by a single investigator. The websites were rated according to the quality of information using the DISCERN instrument, accuracy score, and exhaustivity score. *Results*: Of the 150 websites, 96 were included in the analysis. University and private hospital websites had significantly higher DISCERN, accuracy, and exhaustivity scores compared to the other websites. *Conclusions*: Accurate medical information is essential for improving patient satisfaction and treatment outcomes. The quality of websites should be improved to provide high-quality medical information to patients, which can be facilitated by doctors.

Keywords: chronic ankle instability; Internet medical information; website assessment

Citation: Yoon, S.-J.; Kim, J.-B.; Jung, K.-J.; Chang, H.-J.; Hong, Y.-C.; Hong, C.-H.; Lee, B.-R.; Yeo, E.-D.; Lee, H.-S.; Won, S.-H.; et al. Evaluation of the Quality of Information Available on the Internet Regarding Chronic Ankle Instability. *Medicina* **2022**, *58*, 1315. https://doi.org/10.3390/medicina58101315

Academic Editor: Vassilios S. Nikolaou

Received: 30 August 2022
Accepted: 19 September 2022
Published: 20 September 2022

Publisher's Note: MDPI stays neutral with regard to jurisdictional claims in published maps and institutional affiliations.

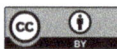

Copyright: © 2022 by the authors. Licensee MDPI, Basel, Switzerland. This article is an open access article distributed under the terms and conditions of the Creative Commons Attribution (CC BY) license (https://creativecommons.org/licenses/by/4.0/).

1. Introduction

According to the 2018 report by the International Telecommunication Union, the Internet usage rate in Korea is 95.1%, which is the highest in the world, and most people can use the Internet easily [1]. In addition, patients frequently use the Internet to access medical information. A study found that almost 90% and 65% of patients search the Internet to obtain information regarding their disease and its treatment [2]. Patients who obtain accurate medical information through the Internet tend to enter into good patient–physician relationships, which leads to better treatment outcomes [3,4]. Therefore, qualitative analyses of the quality of such websites are necessary to ensure that they provide accurate medical information to patients.

Chronic ankle instability (CAI) is one of the most common sports injuries that develops after an ankle sprain [5]. Ankle sprains are the most common musculoskeletal sports injuries, with a prevalence of about 25,000 to 30,000 people per day in the United States, accounting for about 15~25% of all sports injuries. There are no accurate statistics on ankle sprains in Korea, but it can be assumed that they are not much different from other countries. With acute lateral ankle sprains, good results can be obtained through conservative treatment in most cases, but it is known that some patients will develop CAI, i.e., re-injury or persistent symptoms resulting therefrom. Diminished range of motion (ROM), decreased strength, altered functional movement patterns, and impaired neuromuscular control are characteristics of CAI [6]. A decreased ankle dorsiflexion ROM increases instability, which directly cause the loss balance [7]. Additionally, in the presence of ankle instability, the proximal muscles of the lower limb may be affected [8]. A recent review found that 70% of individuals who experience an acute lateral ankle sprain may develop CAI over a short time period, and a prospective cohort study found that 40% of individuals develop CAI 1 year after a first-time lateral ankle sprain [9–11]. In CAI, unlike acute ankle sprain, if conservative treatment is ineffective, surgical treatment should be considered [6,12–15].

Since CAI is an important pathological condition that can cause discomfort and joint destruction in the long term, accurate information and understanding are essential for proper diagnosis and treatment [16]. Although the information available on the Internet related to CAI has been evaluated in other countries, such studies have not been conducted in Korea [17]. Therefore, we hypothesized that the quality of information would vary among websites and assessed the quality of Internet websites that provide information related to CAI.

2. Materials and Methods

2.1. Study Subjects and Criteria

This study was conducted at Soonchunhyang University Hospital, Cheonan, South Korea. According to Internet Trend (www.internettrend.co.kr (accessed on 29 August 2022)), a Korean log analysis website, the top three search engines (Naver, Google, and Daum) accounted for 56.10%, 34.73%, and 5.46% of the search traffic in 2021, respectively; the three search engines combined accounted for 96.29% of search traffic. Hence, these three search engines were searched for "chronic ankle instability" and the top 50 websites from each search engine were selected for analysis. In all, 150 websites were analyzed. Website contents that were not in text format, such as radio or TV broadcast materials and YouTube, were excluded from the study. Websites that could not be accessed, duplicate websites, and websites not related to CAI were also excluded. Figure 1 shows the method of selection and evaluation of websites.

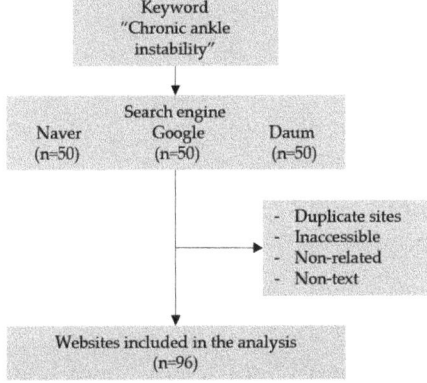

Figure 1. Method of selection and evaluation of websites.

2.2. Website Classification

Website authors were classified into university hospitals, private hospitals, commercial organizations (such as medical device company), non-commercial organizations (such as civic groups and government agencies), and others. In addition, they were classified by specialty: orthopedic surgeons, rehabilitation medicine specialists, other doctors, oriental doctors, and non-doctor authors.

2.3. Evaluation of Website Information

Although several studies have evaluated the medical information available on websites, there is no standard evaluation tool. In the present study, we used the DISCERN instrument, which is commonly used for the objective evaluation of websites (Table 1) [18]. DISCERN is a tool developed by Oxford University and British Library for qualitative evaluation of medical information and assigns a score of 1–5 for 16 items (total score: 16–80) [19–26]. We modified it to a score of 20. Because DISCERN does not evaluate the accuracy and exhaustivity of information, we used five additional items to evaluate these factors (Tables 2 and 3). Two orthopedic surgeons with training in podiatry and two sports rehabilitation medicine specialists independently evaluated the websites and assigned the scores.

Table 1. DISCERN questionnaire for the evaluation of consumer health information.

Question	Score
1. Are the aims clear?	1–5 points
2. Does it achieve its aims?	1–5 points
3. Is it relevant?	1–5 points
4. Is it clear what sources of information were used to compile the publication (other than the author or producer)?	1–5 points
5. Is it clear when the information used or reported in the publication was produced?	1–5 points
6. Is it balanced and unbiased?	1–5 points
7. Does it provide details of additional sources of support and information?	1–5 points
8. Does it refer to areas of uncertainty?	1–5 points
9. Does it describe how each treatment works?	1–5 points
10. Does it describe the benefits of each treatment?	1–5 points
11. Does it describe the risks of each treatment?	1–5 points
12. Does it describe what would happen if no treatment was used?	1–5 points
13. Does it describe how the treatment choices affect overall quality of life?	1–5 points
14. Is it clear that there may be more than one possible treatment choice?	1–5 points
15. Does it provide support for shared decision making?	1–5 points
16. Based on the answers to all of the above questions, rate the overall quality of the publication as a source of information about treatment choices	1–5 points
Total	16–80 points

Table 2. Accuracy score scale.

No inaccurate information	5 points
Rare inaccurate information without consequences	4 points
Frequent inaccurate information without consequences	3 points
One serious inaccuracy	2 points
Many serious inaccuracies	1 point

Table 3. Exhaustivity score scale.

Exhaustive subject coverage	5 points
Complete subject coverage but with few details	4 points
Partial coverage of subject with sufficient details	3 points
Partial coverage of subject with few details	2 points
Little coverage of the subject matter	1 point

2.4. Statistical Analysis

Statistical analysis was performed using SPSS (version 26.0; IBM Corp., Armonk, NY, USA). One-way analysis of variance and the Kruskal–Wallis test were performed, as appropriate. The significance level was set at $p < 0.05$.

3. Results

3.1. Website Classification

Of the 150 websites identified, 96 were included in the analysis. In total, 19.7%, 32.2%, 18.7%, 20.8%, and 8.3% were published by university hospitals, private hospitals, commercial organizations, non-commercial organizations, and other organizations, respectively (Figure 2). In addition, 28.1%, 21.8%, 20.8%, 16.6%, and 12.5% of the authors were orthopedic surgeons, rehabilitation medicine specialists, other doctors, oriental doctors, and non-doctors, respectively (Figure 3). University and private hospitals accounted over half of the authors (51.9%). Orthopedic surgeons and rehabilitation medicine specialists accounted for nearly half of the authors (49.9%). The combination these of these data is summarized in Table 4.

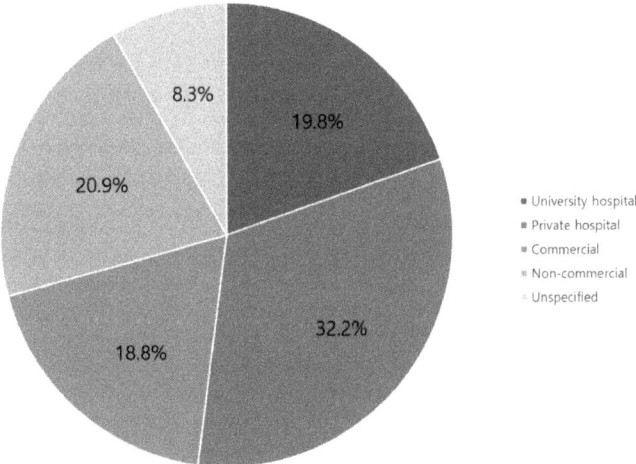

Figure 2. Summary of websites by website authors.

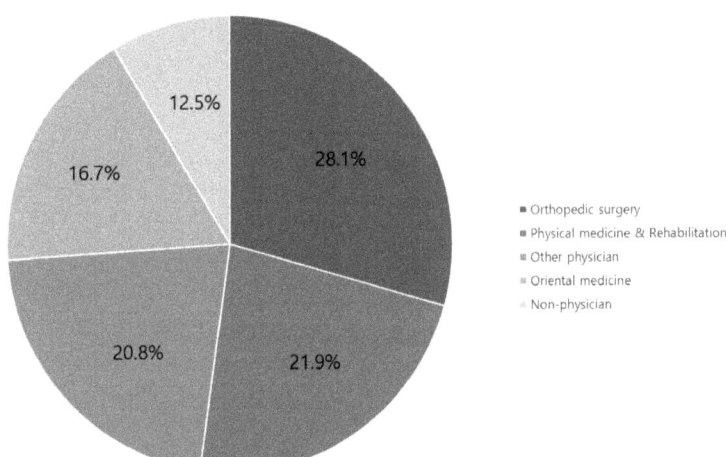

Figure 3. Summary of websites by specialty.

Table 4. Websites classified by authorship and specialty.

	Orthopedic Surgery	Physical Medicine and Rehabilitation	Other Physicians	Oriental Medicine	Non-Physician	Total
University hospital	16	3	-	-	-	19
Private hospital	8	12	4	7	-	31
Commercial	1	2	2	6	7	18
Non-commercial	2	3	9	1	5	20
Others	-	1	5	2	-	8
Total	27	21	20	16	12	-

3.2. Evaluation of Website Information

The mean DISCERN, accuracy, and exhaustivity scores assigned by the four evaluators were recorded. The website scores were compared to the mean score of the group to which the website was assigned. The converted DISCERN scores were 15.4, 14.6, 9.4, 8.7, and 6.3 for websites published by university hospitals, private hospitals, non-commercial organizations, commercial organizations, and others (Table 5). The accuracy scores were 4.6, 4.3, 3.8, 3.6, and 2.8 for websites published by university hospitals, private hospitals, non-commercial organizations, commercial organizations, and others (Table 6). The exhaustivity scores were 4.4, 4.1, 3.6, 3.4, and 2.1 for websites published by university hospitals, private hospitals, non-commercial organizations, commercial organizations, and others (Table 7). The DISCERN scores of the university and private hospital websites were significantly higher than those of the other three groups (non-commercial organization, commercial, and other sites) ($p = 0.04$); there were no statistically significant differences between the scores of university and private hospital websites ($p = 0.21$). In addition, the accuracy scores of university and private hospital sites were significantly higher than those of the other three groups ($p = 0.03$); there were no statistically significant differences between the accuracy scores of university and private hospital websites ($p = 0.33$). The exhaustivity scores of the university and private hospital websites were significantly higher than those of the other groups ($p = 0.04$); there were no statistically significant differences between the exhaustivity scores of university and private hospital websites ($p = 0.34$).

Table 5. DISCERN scores by website authors.

Website Authorship	DISCERN Score [1]
University hospital [2,3]	15.4 (0.77)
Private hospital [2,3]	14.6 (2.58)
Commercial [2]	9.4 (0.91)
Non-commercial [2]	8.7 (1.83)
Unspecified [2]	6.3 (0.86)

[1] Values are mean (SD). [2] University and private hospital websites scored significantly higher than those of the other three groups ($p = 0.04$). [3] There were no statistically significant differences between the scores of university and private hospital websites ($p = 0.21$).

Table 6. Accuracy scores by website authors.

Website Authorship	Accuracy Score [1]
University hospital [2,3]	4.6 (0.49)
Private hospital [2,3]	4.3 (0.62)
Commercial [2]	3.8 (0.87)
Non-commercial [2]	3.6 (0.72)
Unspecified [2]	2.8 (0.68)

[1] Values are mean (SD). [2] University and private hospital websites scored significantly higher than those of the other three groups ($p = 0.03$). [3] There were no statistically significant differences between the scores of university and private hospital websites ($p = 0.33$).

Table 7. Exhaustivity scores by website authors.

Website Authorship	Exhaustivity Score [1]
University hospital [2,3]	4.4 (0.63)
Private hospital [2,3]	4.1 (0.76)
Commercial [2]	3.6 (0.59)
Non-commercial [2]	3.4 (0.86)
Unspecified [2]	2.1 (0.92)

[1] Values are mean (SD). [2] University and private hospital websites scored significantly higher than those of the other three groups ($p = 0.04$). [3] There were no statistically significant differences between the scores of university and private hospital websites ($p = 0.34$).

4. Discussion

Several studies have reported that patient education and provision of accurate information improve treatment outcomes [27–29]. The Internet represents a cost-effective medium through which patients can be educated. Vast amounts of information are available on the Internet but it is essential to select accurate and reliable information [30–32]. In such an environment, the provision of correct medical information to patients by medical professionals is essential for a desirable patient–physician relationship, and plays a decisive role in improving patient satisfaction and treatment compliance [33]. However, unlike peer-reviewed academic journals, anyone can post information on websites, which can lead to patients obtaining low-quality medical information, poor decision making, and even treatment failure [25,34]. Because of the frequent use of Internet websites for patient education, several studies have evaluated the medical information available on the Internet; however, such studies have rarely been performed in Korea.

CAI is a major complication of acute ankle sprain that leads to discomfort during daily and sports activities [35]. Studies of online information related to lumbar disc herniation, lumbar stenosis, and cervical disc herniation have been published in the field of orthopedic surgery in Korea, but no previous study from Korea has evaluated the information related to CAI available on the Internet [16,18,36,37]. In addition, some of the aforementioned domestic studies conducted online information quality analyses using evaluation criteria arbitrarily created by the authors; thus, objectivity was not guaranteed and the criteria were applied only once. As a result, no follow-up studies were conducted and there is little possibility of revising or developing the evaluation criteria. By contrast, in this study, reliability and objectivity could be ensured by using the internationally standardized DISCERN instrument, which has also been used in other medical papers. Thus, this study should lead to follow-up research, rather than acting as a standalone study.

This study created accuracy and exhaustivity items; similar items have been constructed and analyzed in other studies to supplement DISCERN. It seems necessary to improve the DISCERN instrument [38,39]. As DISCERN is used as a standard to evaluate medical text, we excluded audiovisual materials, such as radio/TV broadcasts and YouTube videos; i.e., we used the DISCERN instrument as the sole evaluation standard [40]. In subsequent studies, standards that overcome the limitations of the DISCERN instrument, and the use of both audiovisual and written data will be needed [41]. University and private hospital websites had higher DISCERN, accuracy, and exhaustivity scores compared to other websites; these results are in line with previous studies [42,43]. However, some studies have suggested that academic institution websites, such as university hospital websites, may not necessarily provide high-quality information. Although it is extremely rare for an academic institution to provide inaccurate information, there is a tendency to omit information related to treatments that are not offered at the institution [44,45].

In this study, duplicate websites identified using the top three search engines were excluded. Comparing the order of presentation of websites within the search results for each search engine, and the total DISCERN, accuracy, and exhaustivity scores, would enable the evaluation of the ability of search engines to list websites that provide high-quality information first.

We analyzed the quality, accuracy, and exhaustivity of the information provided by websites to determine the quality of the information provided to patients. However, we did not evaluate the comprehensibility and readability of information, which are important for patient education. Information must not only be reliable; it must be understandable to patients [46]. We did not evaluate whether medical consumers with poor health literacy could easily understand the information, which is necessary for patient education. Future studies should evaluate comprehensibility and readability to allow a comprehensive evaluation of medical information for patient education. In the present study, the information provided by the websites was analyzed by two orthopedic surgeons trained in podiatry and two sports rehabilitation medicine specialists. A limitation of the present study is that the information was not evaluated by doctors from other departments; this should be addressed in future studies.

Many studies used qualitative evaluation methods and have developed certification systems for use in Korea to ensure the quality of medical information is of high quality [47]. As a method to provide high-quality Internet medical information to medical consumers, medical organizations could implement a "quality labeling system"; a representative example of this is the Health On the Net (HON) Foundation code [48]. However, due to the lack of awareness of such certification systems, many high-quality websites are not certified [25,34]. Some studies have also shown that certification systems do not guarantee the quality of online medical information [43]. As the amount of Internet medical information increases, medical consumers are experiencing difficulty obtaining reliable information. There is a research result that about 70% of patients hope to be recommended an appropriate medical sites to their doctors; medical organizations should play a central role in ensuring high-quality medical information [31].

Finally, detection bias in association with evaluations of individual websites should be reduced in future studies.

5. Conclusions

Accurate medical information should be obtained from the Internet to improve patient–physician relationships and treatment outcomes. However, regarding CAI, there is a lack of research on the quality of such information in Korea. Information provided by university and private hospital websites had the highest accuracy and quality scores. Efforts should be made to evaluate the quality of medical information provided by websites. It is expected to contribute to improving the quality of information regarding CAI on the Internet. Medical organizations and physicians should play a central role in improving the information available to patients.

Author Contributions: Conceptualization, W.-J.K. and, S.-J.Y.; methodology, J.-B.K.; software, K.-J.J.; validation, Y.-C.H.; formal analysis, H.-J.C.; investigation, C.-H.H.; resources, H.-S.L.; data curation, B.-R.L.; writing—original draft preparation, S.-J.Y.; writing—review and editing, W.-J.K.; visualization, J.-Y.J.; supervision, E.-D.Y.; project administration, S.-H.W.; funding acquisition, D.-W.L. All authors have read and agreed to the published version of the manuscript.

Funding: The authors would like to thank the Soonchunhyang University Research Fund for support (1022-0033).

Institutional Review Board Statement: Not applicable.

Informed Consent Statement: Not applicable.

Data Availability Statement: Data sharing is not applicable to this article as no datasets were generated or analyzed during the current study.

Conflicts of Interest: The authors declare no conflict of interest.

Abbreviation

CAI: chronic ankle instability.

References

1. International Telecommunication Union. Measuring the Information Society Report. 2018. Available online: https://www.itu.int/en/ITU-D/Statistics/Pages/publications/misr2018.aspx (accessed on 29 August 2022).
2. Kim, H.; Park, H.A. Selection Criteria and Utilization of Health Information on the Internet by Consumers. *J. Korean Soc. Med. Inform.* **2004**, *10*, 55–68. [CrossRef]
3. Tan, S.S.; Goonawardene, N. Internet Health Information Seeking and the Patient-Physician Relationship: A Systematic Review. *J. Med. Internet Res.* **2017**, *19*, e9. [CrossRef] [PubMed]
4. Shaw, J.M.; Mynors, G.; Kelham, C. Information for patients on medicines. *BMJ* **2005**, *331*, 1034–1035. [CrossRef] [PubMed]
5. Lin, C.I.; Houtenbos, S.; Lu, Y.H.; Mayer, F.; Wippert, P.M. The epidemiology of chronic ankle instability with perceived ankle instability- a systematic review. *J. Foot Ankle Res.* **2021**, *14*, 41. [CrossRef] [PubMed]
6. Donovan, L.; Hertel, J. A new paradigm for rehabilitation of patients with chronic ankle instability. *Phys. Sportsmed.* **2012**, *40*, 41–51. [CrossRef]
7. Romero Morales, C.; Calvo Lobo, C.; Rodríguez Sanz, D.; Sanz Corbalán, I.; Ruiz Ruiz, B.; López López, D. The concurrent validity and reliability of the Leg Motion system for measuring ankle dorsiflexion range of motion in older adults. *PeerJ* **2017**, *5*, e2820. [CrossRef]
8. Kazemi, K.; Arab, A.M.; Abdollahi, I.; López-López, D.; Calvo-Lobo, C. Electromyography comparison of distal and proximal lower limb muscle activity patterns during external perturbation in subjects with and without functional ankle instability. *Hum. Mov. Sci.* **2017**, *55*, 211–220. [CrossRef]
9. Herzog, M.M.; Kerr, Z.Y.; Marshall, S.W.; Wikstrom, E.A. Epidemiology of Ankle Sprains and Chronic Ankle Instability. *J. Athl. Train.* **2019**, *54*, 603–610. [CrossRef]
10. Hubbard, T.J. Ligament laxity following inversion injury with and without chronic ankle instability. *Foot Ankle Int.* **2008**, *29*, 305–311. [CrossRef]
11. Yeung, M.S.; Chan, K.M.; So, C.H.; Yuan, W.Y. An epidemiological survey on ankle sprain. *Br. J. Sports Med.* **1994**, *28*, 112–116. [CrossRef]
12. DiGiovanni, C.W.; Brodsky, A. Current concepts: Lateral ankle instability. *Foot Ankle Int.* **2006**, *27*, 854–866. [CrossRef] [PubMed]
13. Maffulli, N.; Ferran, N.A. Management of acute and chronic ankle instability. *J. Am. Acad. Orthop. Surg.* **2008**, *16*, 608–615. [CrossRef] [PubMed]
14. Ajis, A.; Maffulli, N. Conservative management of chronic ankle instability. *Foot Ankle Clin.* **2006**, *11*, 531–537. [CrossRef] [PubMed]
15. Karlsson, J.; Lansinger, O. Lateral instability of the ankle joint (1). Non-surgical treatment is the first choice–20 per cent may need ligament surgery. *Lakartidningen* **1991**, *88*, 1399–1402. [PubMed]
16. Kim, D.-W.; Sung, K.-S. Chronic Lateral Ankle Instability. *JKFAS* **2018**, *22*, 55–61. [CrossRef]
17. Schwarz, G.M.; Lisy, M.; Hajdu, S.; Windhager, R.; Willegger, M. Quality and readability of online resources on chronic ankle instability. *Foot Ankle Surg.* **2022**, *28*, 384–389. [CrossRef]
18. Hong, Y.C.; Kim, W.J.; Soh, J.W.; Chang, H.J.; Hong, C.H. Evaluation of the Source and Quality of Information Regarding Cervical Disc Herniation on Websites. *J. Korean Soc. Spine Surg.* **2020**, *27*, 77–83. [CrossRef]
19. Ademiluyi, G.; Rees, C.E.; Sheard, C.E. Evaluating the reliability and validity of three tools to assess the quality of health information on the Internet. *Patient Educ. Couns.* **2003**, *50*, 151–155. [CrossRef]
20. Bartels, U.; Hargrave, D.; Lau, L.; Esquembre, C.; Humpl, T.; Bouffet, E. Analysis of paediatric neuro-oncological information on the Internet in German language. *Klin. Padiatr.* **2003**, *215*, 352–357.
21. Commission of the European Communities. Brussels. eEurope 2002: Quality Criteria for Health Related Websites. *J. Med. Internet Res.* **2002**, *4*, e15.
22. Hargrave, D.; Bartels, U.; Lau, L.; Esquembre, C.; Bouffet, E. Quality of childhood brain tumour information on the Internet in French language. *Bull. Cancer* **2003**, *90*, 650–655.
23. Hargrave, D.R.; Hargrave, U.A.; Bouffet, E. Quality of health information on the Internet in pediatric neuro-oncology. *Neuro Oncol.* **2006**, *8*, 175–182. [CrossRef]
24. Lau, L.; Hargrave, D.R.; Bartels, U.; Esquembre, C.; Bouffet, E. Childhood brain tumour information on the Internet in the Chinese language. *Childs Nerv. Syst.* **2006**, *22*, 346–351. [CrossRef]
25. Lévêque, M.; Dimitriu, C.; Gustin, T.; Jamart, J.; Gilliard, C.; Bojanowski, M.W. Evaluation of neuro-oncology information for French speaking patients on the Internet. *Neurochirurgie* **2007**, *53*, 343–355. [CrossRef] [PubMed]
26. Meric, F.; Bernstam, E.V.; Mirza, N.Q.; Hunt, K.K.; Ames, F.C.; Ross, M.I.; Kuerer, H.M.; E Pollock, R.; Musen, M.; Singletary, S.E. Breast cancer on the world wide web: Cross sectional survey of quality of information and popularity of websites. *BMJ* **2002**, *324*, 577–581. [CrossRef] [PubMed]
27. Khoury, V.; Kourilovitch, M.; Massardo, L. Education for patients with rheumatoid arthritis in Latin America and the Caribbean. *Clin. Rheumatol.* **2015**, *34* (Suppl. 1), S45–S49. [CrossRef] [PubMed]
28. Schrieber, L.; Colley, M. Patient education. *Best Pract. Res. Clin. Rheumatol.* **2004**, *18*, 465–476. [CrossRef]
29. Traeger, A.C.; Lee, H.; Hübscher, M.; Skinner, I.W.; Moseley, G.L.; Nicholas, M.K.; Henschke, N.; Refshauge, K.M.; Blyth, F.M.; Main, C.J.; et al. Effect of Intensive Patient Education vs. Placebo Patient Education on Outcomes in Patients With Acute Low Back Pain: A Randomized Clinical Trial. *JAMA Neurol.* **2019**, *76*, 161–169. [CrossRef]

30. Dekkers, T.; Melles, M.; Groeneveld, B.S.; de Ridder, H. Web-Based Patient Education in Orthopedics: Systematic Review. *J. Med. Internet Res.* **2018**, *20*, e143. [CrossRef]
31. Pellisé, F.; Sell, P. Patient information and education with modern media: The Spine Society of Europe Patient Line. *Eur. Spine J.* **2009**, *18* (Suppl. 3), 395–401. [CrossRef]
32. Bartlett, E.E. Cost-benefit analysis of patient education. *Patient Educ. Couns.* **1995**, *26*, 87–91. [CrossRef]
33. Gross, D.P.; Ferrari, R.; Russell, A.S.; Battié, M.C.; Schopflocher, D.; Hu, R.W.; Waddell, G.; Buchbinder, R. A population-based survey of back pain beliefs in Canada. *Spine* **2006**, *31*, 2142–2145. [CrossRef] [PubMed]
34. Sproule, J.A.; Tansey, C.; Burns, B.; Fenelon, G. The Web: Friend or Foe of the Hand Surgeon? *Hand Surg.* **2003**, *8*, 181–185. [CrossRef]
35. Lopes, R.; Andrieu, M.; Cordier, G.; Molinier, F.; Benoist, J.; Colin, F.; Thès, A.; Elkaïm, M.; Boniface, O.; Guillo, S.; et al. Arthroscopic treatment of chronic ankle instability: Prospective study of outcomes in 286 patients. *Orthop. Traumatol. Surg. Res.* **2018**, *104*, S199–S205. [CrossRef]
36. Shim, D.M.; Jeung, U.O.; Kim, T.K.; Kim, J.W.; Park, J.Y.; Kweon, S.H.; Park, S.K.; Choi, B.S. Analysis of Homepages Relating to Lumbar Disc Surgery in Orthopaedic and Neurosurgical Hospitals. *J. Korean Orthop. Assoc.* **2008**, *43*, 166–170. [CrossRef]
37. Chang, H.-J.; Kim, J.-B.; Yoon, S.-J.; Kim, W.-J.; Jung, K.-J.; Kim, C.-H.; Park, J.-S.; Hong, C.-H. Analysis of the Quality of the Internet Web Sites Providing Informations and Treatment Options about Lumbar Stenosis. *J. Korean Soc. Spine Surg.* **2021**, *28*, 123–129. [CrossRef]
38. Cerminara, C.; Santarone, M.E.; Casarelli, L.; Curatolo, P.; El Malhany, N. Use of the DISCERN tool for evaluating web searches in childhood epilepsy. *Epilepsy Behav.* **2014**, *41*, 119–121. [CrossRef]
39. Weil, A.G.; Bojanowski, M.W.; Jamart, J.; Gustin, T.; Lévêque, M. Evaluation of the quality of information on the Internet available to patients undergoing cervical spine surgery. *World Neurosurg.* **2014**, *82*, e31–e39. [CrossRef]
40. Charnock, D.; Shepperd, S.; Needham, G.; Gann, R. DISCERN: An instrument for judging the quality of written consumer health information on treatment choices. *J. Epidemiol. Community Health* **1999**, *53*, 105–111. [CrossRef]
41. Kulasegarah, J.; McGregor, K.; Mahadevan, M. Quality of information on the Internet-has a decade made a difference? *Ir. J. Med. Sci.* **2018**, *187*, 873–876. [CrossRef]
42. Mathur, S.; Shanti, N.; Brkaric, M.; Sood, V.; Kubeck, J.; Paulino, C.; Merola, A.A. Surfing for scoliosis: The quality of information available on the Internet. *Spine* **2005**, *30*, 2695–2700. [CrossRef] [PubMed]
43. Morr, S.; Shanti, N.; Carrer, A.; Kubeck, J.; Gerling, M.C. Quality of information concerning cervical disc herniation on the Internet. *Spine J.* **2010**, *10*, 350–354. [CrossRef] [PubMed]
44. Eysenbach, G.; Powell, J.; Kuss, O.; Sa, E.R. Empirical studies assessing the quality of health information for consumers on the world wide web: A systematic review. *JAMA* **2002**, *287*, 2691–2700. [CrossRef] [PubMed]
45. John, A.K. A critical appraisal of internet resources on colorectal cancer. *Colorectal Dis.* **2006**, *8*, 217–223. [CrossRef]
46. Zraick, R.I.; Azios, M.; Handley, M.M.; Bellon-Harn, M.L.; Manchaiah, V. Quality and readability of internet information about stuttering. *J. Fluen. Disord.* **2021**, *67*, 105824. [CrossRef]
47. Fahy, E.; Hardikar, R.; Fox, A.; Mackay, S. Quality of patient health information on the Internet: Reviewing a complex and evolving landscape. *Australas. Med. J.* **2014**, *7*, 24–28. [CrossRef]
48. Boyer, C.; Selby, M.; Scherrer, J.R.; Appel, R.D. The Health On the Net Code of Conduct for medical and health Websites. *Comput. Biol. Med.* **1998**, *28*, 603–610. [CrossRef]

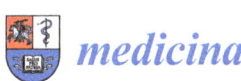

Article

Comparison of Radiologic Results after Lateral Meniscal Allograft Transplantation with or without Capsulodesis Using an All-Soft Suture Anchor

Dong Ryun Lee [1], Young Je Woo [1], Sung Gyu Moon [2], Woo Jong Kim [3] and Dhong Won Lee [1],*

[1] Department of Orthopaedic Surgery, KonKuk University Medical Center, Konkuk University School of Medicine, Seoul 05030, Republic of Korea
[2] Department of Radiology, KonKuk University Medical Center, Konkuk University School of Medicine, Seoul 05030, Republic of Korea
[3] Department of Orthopaedic Surgery, Soonchunhyang University Hospital Cheonan, Cheonan 31151, Republic of Korea
* Correspondence: osdoctorknee@kuh.ac.kr

Abstract: *Background and Objectives*: Studies analyzing magnetic resonance imaging (MRI) after simultaneously performing lateral meniscal allograft transplantation (MAT) and capsulodesis are currently rare. This study aimed to compare the MRI results between the group that performed lateral MAT alone and the group that performed both lateral MAT and capsulodesis simultaneously. *Materials and Methods*: A total of 55 patients who underwent lateral MAT with a 1-year follow-up MRI were included. The patients were divided into two groups according to the surgical procedure: group I (isolated lateral MAT, n = 26) and group C (combined lateral MAT and capsulodesis, n = 29). Differences between groups were compared regarding subjective knee scores, graft extrusion, graft signal, articular cartilage loss, and joint space width (JSW). *Results*: The subjective knee scores improved significantly in both groups (all, $p < 0.001$), and there were no significant differences in these scores between both groups at the 1-year follow-up. Group C showed less coronal graft extrusion at the 1-year follow-up (1.1 ± 1.7 mm vs. 2.4 ± 1.8 mm, $p < 0.001$). Pathologic coronal graft extrusion (≥ 3 mm) was found in seven (26.9%) patients in group I and three (10.3%) in group C. Concerning the graft signal, group C showed less grade 3 signal intensity in the posterior root of the graft. There were no significant differences in preoperative and postoperative cartilage status between groups. Regarding JSW, there were no significant differences in postoperative JSW between both groups. However, in group C, JSW significantly increased from 3.9 ± 0.4 mm to 4.5 ± 1.4 mm ($p = 0.031$). *Conclusions*: In lateral MAT, capsulodesis (open decortication and suture anchor fixation) could reduce graft extrusion without complications. In the future, large-volume and long-term prospective comparative studies are needed to confirm the clinical effects following capsulodesis.

Keywords: meniscal allograft transplantation; meniscal extrusion; capsulodesis; magnetic resonance imaging

1. Introduction

Meniscal allograft transplantation (MAT) reduces knee pain, improves knee function, and alleviates the degenerative progression of articular cartilage [1–5]. A recent systematic review by Novaretti et al. [6] stated that MAT showed good long-term survivorship rates, with a 10-year survival rate of 73.5% and a 15-year survival rate of 60.3%. However, it has been reported that graft extrusion frequently occurs after MAT, which leads to the abrasion of the articular cartilage and the aggravation of subchondral bone lesions in an inappropriate biomechanical environment [1,5,7–10].

The causes of graft extrusion after MAT include graft size mismatch before surgery, malposition of the graft during surgery, overtensioning of the meniscal suture, osteophytes, and overstuffing. Graft size reduction, anatomic placement of the graft, and peripheral

osteophyte excision have been performed to overcome graft extrusion [11–17]. Recently, surgeons have been performing capsulodesis, which reduces the space where the graft extrusion may occur by pulling the stretched lateral capsule to the lateral tibial plateau [18–20]. The capsulodesis includes a method using a suture anchor and another using transosseous sutures, and each surgeon has reported different results on whether it can reduce graft extrusion [18–20].

Studies analyzing magnetic resonance images (MRI) after simultaneously performing lateral MAT and capsulodesis are currently rare. It is believed that different results may be shown depending on the method of performing capsulodesis. Therefore, this study aimed to compare the MRI results between the group that performed lateral MAT alone and the group that performed both lateral MAT and capsulodesis (open decortication and suture anchor fixation) simultaneously. It was hypothesized that the group that simultaneously underwent lateral MAT and capsulodesis would show less graft extrusion and osteoarthritis progression on the MRI one year after MAT.

2. Materials and Methods

2.1. Patients

A total of 63 patients who underwent lateral MAT in our institute from March 2018 to July 2021 were retrospectively reviewed. The lateral MAT was indicated for patients with failed conservative treatment after subtotal or total meniscectomy for 6 months and with visual analog scale (VAS) scores ≥ 3 for pain. The patients who underwent MRI examination within 2 days postoperatively and were available for follow-up evaluation for ≥ 1 year were included. Exclusion criteria were axial limb malalignment $\geq 5°$, cruciate ligament deficiency, diffuse osteoarthritis categorized as more than grade 3 according to modified Outerbridge grade (MOG), joint obliteration on the Rosenberg view, and medial compartment osteoarthritis $\geq$ Kellgren-Lawrence grade 2. However, MAT was performed as a salvage operation in cases of localized MOG 3 or 4 lesions in which coverage by the meniscal graft could be expected. Finally, out of 63 patients, 55 were selected. The patients were divided into two groups according to the surgical procedure in a consecutive and non-random manner: group I (isolated lateral MAT, n = 26) with patients from March 2018 to June 2019, and group C (combined lateral MAT and capsulodesis, n = 29) with patients from July 2019 onward (Figure 1). Combined capsulodesis was started with a clinical suspicion that it could benefit graft stabilization. This retrospective comparative study was conducted following approval from the Ethics Committee of Konkuk University Medical Center (KUMC 2022-09-001).

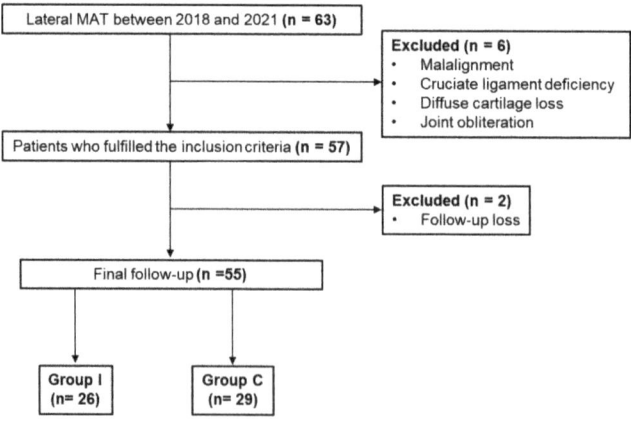

Figure 1. Flowchart of included patients in both groups.

2.2. Surgical Techniques

Lateral MAT was performed using the keyhole technique with modified instruments by a single experienced surgeon (D.W. Lee) [17]. The allografts were fresh-frozen and non-irradiated. After debridement of the peripheral rim of the remaining lateral meniscus, a mini arthrotomy was performed. A keyhole-shaped slot was made using our customized osteotome and dilator along the centers of the anterior and posterior root attachments under the lateral eminence of the tibial articular surface [17]. A posterolateral incision was made for meniscal sutures. To reach the posterolateral area, dissection was carefully performed between the inferior-to-iliotibial band and the superior-to-biceps femoris complex. Through an anteromedial portal, a suture passing wire with the loop positioned posteriorly for the leading suture for traction was passed through the posterolateral capsule in an in-to-outside fashion.

In patients undergoing capsulodesis, after palpating the lateral epicondyle, an oblique small stab wound was made anteriorly on the iliotibial band, and the articular capsule was exposed by bending the iliotibial band up and down. After exposing the rim of the lateral tibial plateau by longitudinally excising the articular capsule, a part of the cartilage and the cortical bone were removed gently in the 10 mm anterior and 10 mm posterior sections using a small rongeur to expose the cancellous bone. At the rim of the lateral tibial plateau, an all-soft suture anchor (Y-Knot, ConMed Linvatec, Largo, FL, USA) was inserted slightly anterior to the midbody level of the lateral meniscus (Figure 2). Two pairs of strands of suture anchor were pulled out of the joint to form an X shape at a point of 5–7 mm at the anterior and posterior margins of the incised articular capsule and then sutured (Figure 3A–D). The narrowing of the lateral space, in which the lateral joint capsule was attached to the lateral tibial plateau, was identified using arthroscopy, and stabilization of the lateral capsule was confirmed with probing (Figure 4). The bone bridge of the allograft was inserted into the keyhole-shaped slot to position the allograft into the joint. After confirming that the anterior and posterior allograft was in the appropriate position, the midbody was sutured using the inside-out method, the posterior horn using the Fast-Fix 360 system (Smith & Nephew Endoscopy, Andover, MA, USA), and the anterior horn using the outside-in method.

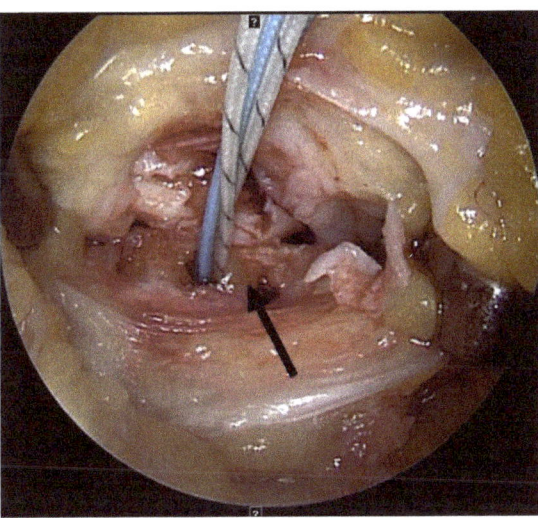

Figure 2. All-soft suture anchor is inserted slightly anterior to the midbody level of the lateral meniscus.

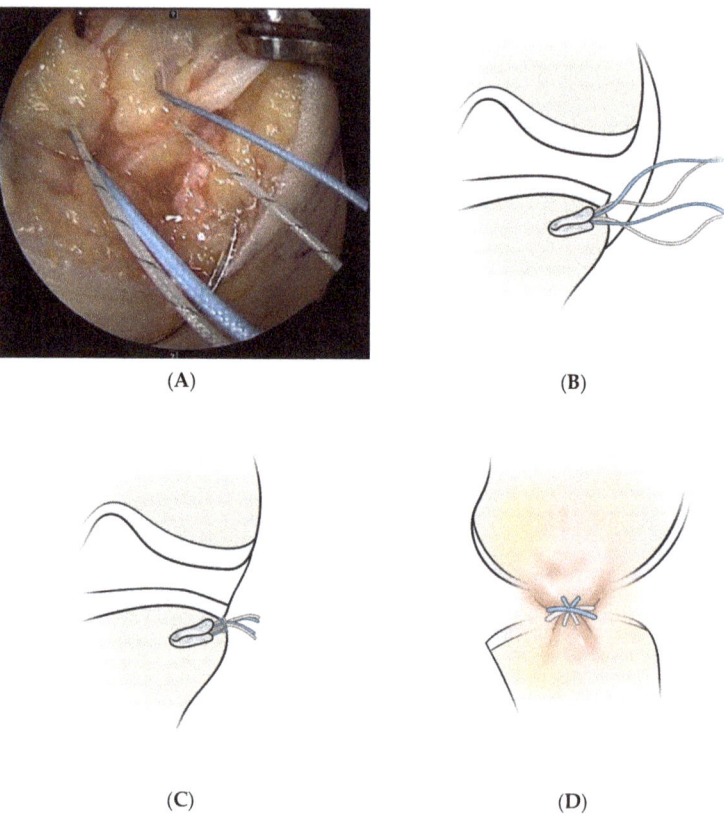

Figure 3. Capsulodesis using an all-soft suture anchor. (**A,B**) Two pairs of strands of suture anchor are pulled out of the lateral capsule. (**C,D**) They form an X shape and are tied. The lateral capsule is attached to the lateral tibial plateau after capsulodesis.

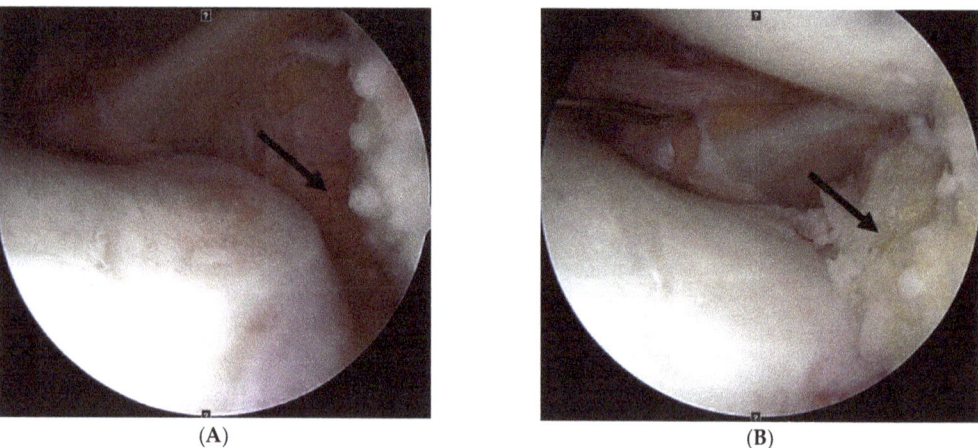

Figure 4. (**A**) The lateral capsule is displaced from the lateral tibial plateau previous to capsulodesis. (**B**) The lateral capsule is attached to the lateral tibial plateau after capsulodesis.

For postoperative rehabilitation, the same delayed rehabilitation protocol was applied to all patients [21]. The cast was fixed while applying a varus force for the first three weeks after the surgery, and the range of motion (ROM) exercise was started with the cast-off after three weeks. ROM was targeted at 90 degrees by six weeks and 120 degrees by 12 weeks. A lateral unloading brace (DonJoy OA Adjuster; DJO Global, Vista, CA, USA) was immediately put on while casting off and maintained until 12 weeks after surgery. Crutch walking was started immediately after surgery, and weight bearing was gradually performed until six weeks so that full weight bearing was possible. Isometric quadriceps muscle-strengthening and straight leg-raising exercises were begun immediately after surgery, and isokinetic exercise was performed in weeks 10–12. A gradual functional improvement exercise was performed so that the patients could return to light jogging at 4–5 months, noncontact sports at 7–9 months, and contact sports at 10–12 months. Only patients who met the criteria by performing muscle strength and functional tests were allowed to return to exercise.

2.3. Radiological Evaluation

The lateral joint space width (JSW) was measured from the Rosenberg. The measurements were performed on a picture archiving and communication system (PACS) workstation (Centricity RA 1000; GE Healthcare, Chicago, IL, USA). The absolute JSW was calculated from the lateral edge of the femoral condyle to the lateral edge of the tibial plateau [22–24] (Figure 5). Our previous study proved that only the lateral edge was observed to be significantly reduced without whole joint obliteration at the time of lateral meniscal allograft transplantation [24]. The relative JSW was calculated by dividing the absolute JSW of the involved knee by the absolute JSW of the uninvolved knee to better standardize the data. The progression of joint space narrowing (JSN) was assessed. Lower extremity alignment was assessed using the mechanical axis of the hip–knee–ankle angle on a standing anteroposterior scanogram.

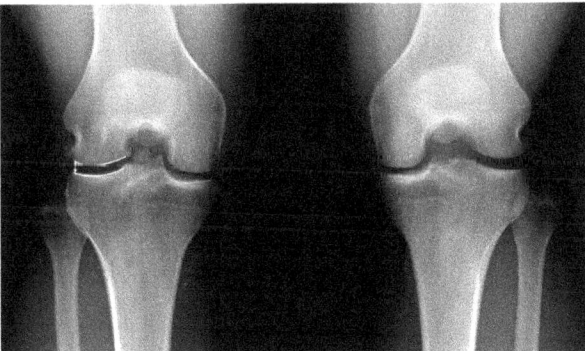

Figure 5. The absolute joint space width is measured from the lateral edge of the femoral condyle to the lateral edge of the tibial plateau (white arrow).

To evaluate graft position and the status of the cartilage of the lateral compartment, follow-up MRIs at 2 days and 12 months postoperatively were conducted. All patients signed an informed consent form prior to MRI examinations with a 3.0-T system apparatus (Signa HD; GE Healthcare, Milwaukee, WI, USA). Graft extrusion on the coronal plane at the level of the posterior border of the medial collateral ligament was measured from the lateral margin of the graft to the superolateral aspect of the tibial plateau (Figure 6). Pathologic extrusion was defined as graft extrusion ≥ 3 mm [14,25–29]. Graft extrusion on the sagittal plane was measured relative to the anterior horn and posterior horn. The absolute sagittal anterior horn extrusion was defined as the distance from the anterior margin of the proximal tibial articular surface to the anterior border of the anterior horn, and the relative sagittal anterior horn extrusion was calculated as the absolute anterior horn extrusion divided by the entire anterior horn [30] (Figure 7a). The posterior horn extrusion was similarly assessed (Figure 7b). Extrusion of the anterior horn outside the anterior border and of the posterior horn outside the posterior border of the tibial articular cartilage was defined as positive, whereas extrusion inside these borders was defined as negative. The axial trough angle on the axial plane was measured between the line drawn along the long axis of the keyhole-shaped slot and the line perpendicular to the trans posterior tibial condylar line [14,15,27].

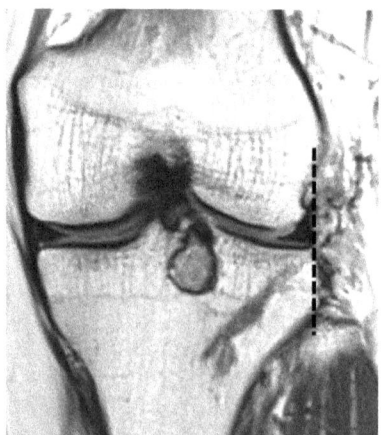

Figure 6. Graft extrusion on the coronal plane is defined as the distance between the lateral margin of the graft and the superolateral aspect of the tibial plateau. There is no graft extrusion.

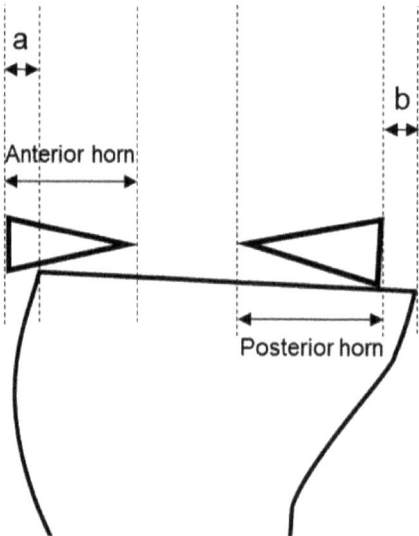

Figure 7. The absolute sagittal anterior horn extrusion (a) and posterior horn extrusion (b).

Graft signal was assessed using MRI at 12 months, postoperatively, and graded following Park et al. [31]: grade 0 (normal), grade 1 (globular increased signal intensity), grade 2 (linear signal intensity within the meniscal graft), and grade 3 (diffuse increased signal intensity or communicated to the articular surface) (Figure 8). This grading was applied for five sections: anterior root, anterior third of the meniscal graft, mid-body, posterior third of the meniscal graft, and posterior root.

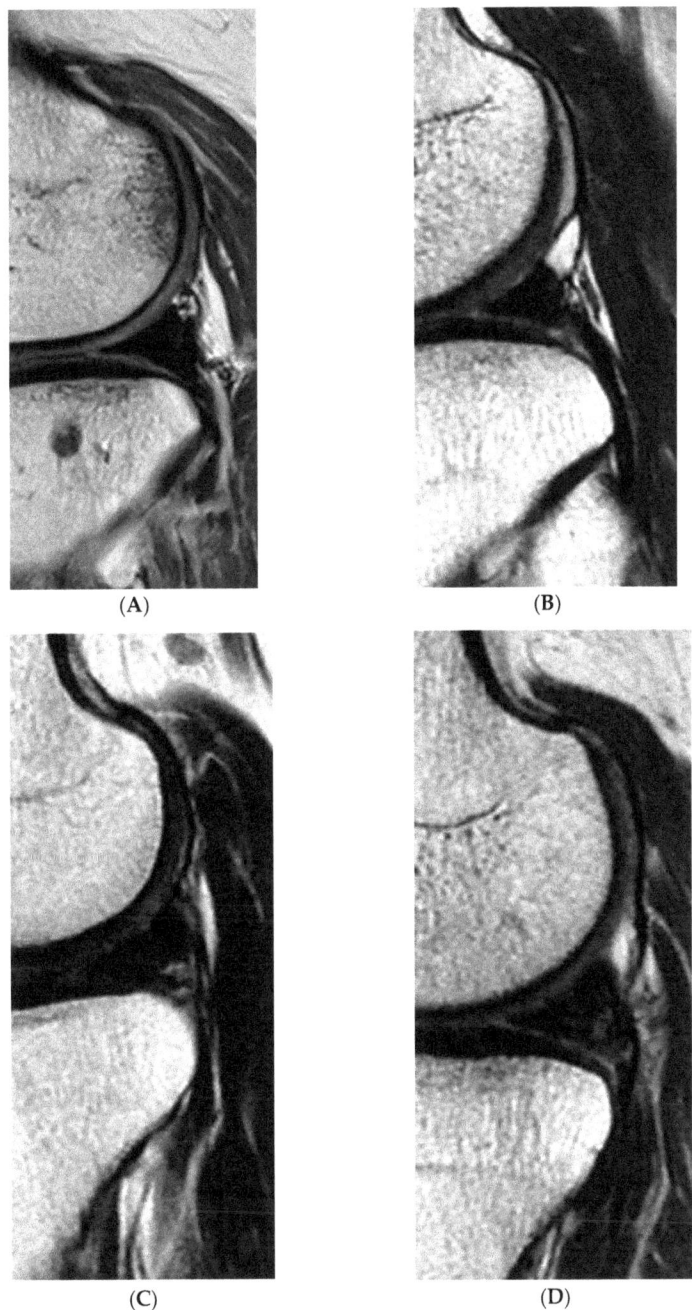

Figure 8. Graft signal. (**A**) Grade 0, (**B**) Grade 1, (**C**) Grade 2, and (**D**) Grade 3.

The cartilage status at the lateral compartment was assessed according to the MOG (grade 0, normal; grade 1, cartilage surface fibrillation; grade 2, <50% loss of cartilage thickness; grade 3, ≥50% loss of cartilage thickness; grade 4, exposed subchondral bone) [32–34]. The worst MOG of the lateral femoral condyle (LFC) and lateral tibial plateau (LTP) was used to present the overall status of the lateral compartment [35]. The cartilage status was categorized into three groups: low-grade (MOG ≤ 2) cartilage lesions on LFC or/and LTP; high-grade (MOG ≥ 3) cartilage lesions on either LFC or LTP; and high-grade cartilage lesions on both LFC and LTP [31].

Radiological measurements were independently performed by one experienced orthopedic surgeon and one experienced radiologist (D.W. Lee and S.G. Moon). Each examiner measured twice with a 6-week interval, and the mean value was used. In the grading system, if there were different results between the two examiners, the results were determined based on consensus.

2.4. Clinical Evaluation

The clinical outcomes were evaluated using the Lysholm score and International Knee Documentation Committee (IKDC) subjective knee score. Preoperative data and postoperative data at 12 months were compared.

2.5. Statistical Analysis

Statistical analysis was performed using the SPSS software (IBM SPSS Statistics 21; IBM Corp, Somers, NY, USA). In all analyses, statistical significance was set at $p < 0.05$. The independent t-test or Mann–Whitney U test was used to compare parametric variables between the two groups. Preoperative and postoperative parametric or non-parametric variables were compared using the paired t-test or Wilcoxon signed-rank test in each group. The intraobserver and interobserver reliabilities of measurements were presented with the intraclass correlation coefficient (ICC) [36]. To detect a difference of 2 mm in graft extrusion between group I and group C with a significance level of 5% and a power of 80%, the required sample size was 16 patients for each group. Therefore, the number of patients in the current study had sufficient statistical power [21,24].

3. Results

Preoperative demographic data showed no statistically significant differences between both groups and are summarized in Table 1. The Lysholm and IKDC subjective knee scores improved significantly in both groups (from 64.3 ± 10.1 and 55.5 ± 9.8 to 86.4 ± 7.2 and 82.2 ± 8.5 in group I, and from 65.7 ± 8.4 and 54.3 ± 10.7 to 87.3 ± 7.4 and 84.5 ± 8.1 in group C, all $p < 0.001$). There were no significant differences in these scores between both groups at the 1-year follow-up ($p = 0.650$ and 0.309, respectively).

All ICC values for intraobserver and interobserver reliabilities were >0.81 in radiologic measurements, which was considered to be excellent. Regarding the initial graft position verified by MRI 2 days after MAT, there were no significant differences at the axial trough angle, coronal position of the graft, and sagittal position of the anterior and posterior horns of the graft (Table 2). However, group C showed less coronal graft extrusion at the 1-year follow-up (1.1 ± 1.7 mm vs. 2.4 ± 1.8 mm, $p < 0.001$). Coronal graft extrusion increased significantly from 1.4 ± 1.6 mm to 2.7 ± 1.2 in group I ($p < 0.001$) and not in group C ($p = 0.223$) (Figure 9). Pathologic coronal graft extrusion (≥3 mm) was found in seven (26.9%) patients in group I and three (10.3%) in group C. In graft signal on MRI at 1-year follow-up, group C showed less grade 3 signal intensity in the posterior root of the graft (Table 3).

Table 1. Demographic data.

	Group I (n = 26)	Group C (n = 29)	p-Value
Age (yrs)	31.9 ± 8.3	32.6 ± 12.1	0.806
Sex (Male/Female)	14/12	16/13	0.772
Body Mass Index, kg/m^2	23.1 ± 4.2	22.8 ± 3.7	0.779
Period from meniscectomy to MAT, months	18.2 ± 7.3	17.3 ± 6.8	0.638
MRI follow-up duration, months	12.7 ± 1.8	13.2 ± 2.1	0.350
Preoperative Lysholm score	64.3 ± 10.1	65.7 ± 8.4	0.577
Preoperative IKDC subjective score	55.5 ± 9.8	54.3 ± 10.7	0.668
Preoperative mechanical axis (hip-knee-ankle), °	0.3 ± 1.7	0.1 ± 1.9	0.684
Preoperative JSW of lateral edge, mm	3.7 ± 0.5	3.9 ± 0.4	0.106
Preoperative MOG, n (%)			
Low grade	23 (88.5%)	25 (86.2%)	
High grade on either LFC or LTP	2 (7.7%)	3 (10.3%)	
High grade on both LFC and LTP	1 (3.8%)	1 (3.4%)	

MAT, meniscal allograft transplantation; JSW, joint space width; MOG, modified Outerbridge grade; MRI, magnetic resonance imaging.

Table 2. Graft extrusion.

	Group I (n = 26)	Group C (n = 29)	p-Value
Aixal trough angle (°) on MRI postoperative 2 days	4.3 ± 2.7	4.6 ± 2.2	0.652
Sagittal graft anterior horn extrusion on MRI postoperative 2 days			
Absolute value, mm	1.3 ± 1.6	1.4 ± 1.8	0.829
Relative value, %	14.5 ± 8.1	13.7 ± 8.4	0.721
Sagittal graft posterior horn extrusion on MRI postoperative 2 days			
Absolute value, mm	−1.3 ± 1.0	−1.1 ± 1.2	0.508
Relative value, %	9.9 ± 7.8	10.3 ± 7.1	0.843
Coronal graft extrusion on MRI postoperative 2 days, mm [a]	0.8 ± 1.6	0.4 ± 0.9	0.252
Coronal graft extrusion on MRI postoperative 1 year, mm [b]	2.4 ± 1.8	1.1 ± 1.7	<0.001
p-value *	<0.001	0.055	

MRI, magnetic resonance imaging. * Paired t-test (a and b).

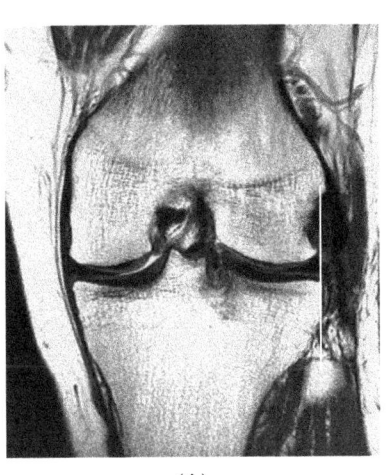
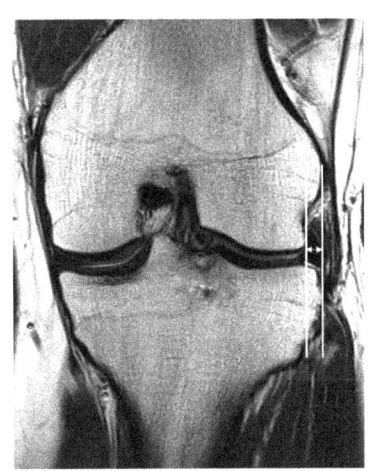

(A)   (B)

Figure 9. Cont.

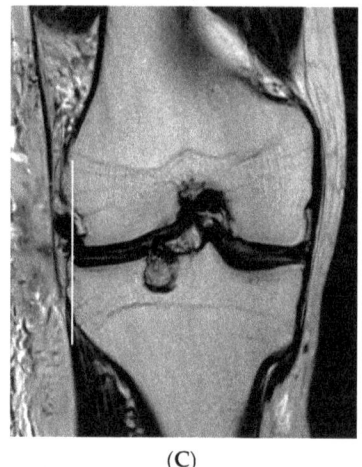
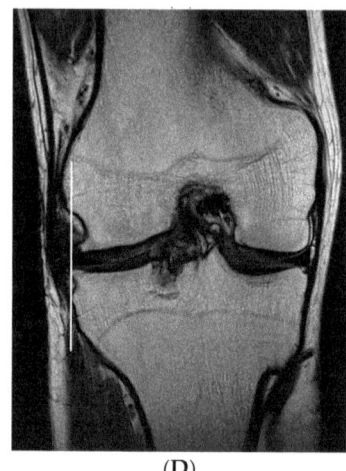

(C)   (D)

Figure 9. (**A**) Postoperative magnetic resonance image (MRI) at 2 days after lateral meniscal allograft transplantation (MAT) and (**B**) postoperative MRI at 1 year after the surgery in the patient who performed isolated lateral MAT. Graft extrusion increased from 0mm to 2.9mm. (**C**) Postoperative MRI at 2 days after lateral MAT and (**D**) postoperative MRI at 1 year after the surgery in the patient who performed lateral MAT + capsulodesis. Graft extrusion was not found until 1 year after the surgery.

Table 3. Graft Signal on MRI at 1-year follow-up.

Signal Intensity	Group I (n = 26)	Group C (n = 29)	p-Value
Anterior root, n (%)			
Grade 0–2	20 (76.9%)	27 (93.1%)	0.131
Grade 3	6 (23.1%)	2 (6.9%)	
Anterior one-third, n (%)			
Grade 0–2	22 (84.6%)	28 (96.6%)	0.178
Grade 3	4 (15.3%)	1 (3.4%)	
Mid-body, n (%)			
Grade 0–2	23 (88.5%)	29 (100%)	0.099
Grade 3	3 (11.5%)	0	
Posterior one-third, n (%)			
Grade 0–2	21 (80.8%)	28 (96.6%)	0.090
Grade 3	5 (19.2%)	1 (3.4%)	
Posterior root, n (%)			
Grade 0–2	19 (73.1%)	28 (96.6%)	0.020
Grade 3	7 (26.9%)	1 (3.4%)	

There were no significant differences in preoperative and postoperative cartilage status between both groups (Table 4). Regarding JSW, there were no significant differences in postoperative JSW between both groups (Table 5). However, in group C, JSW significantly increased from 3.9 ± 0.4 mm to 4.5 ± 1.4 mm ($p = 0.031$).

Table 4. Cartilage status.

	Group I (n = 26)	Group C (n = 29)	p-Value
Preoperative MOG, n (%)			0.941
Low grade	23 (88.5%)	25 (86.2%)	
High grade on either LFC or LTP	2 (7.7%)	3 (10.3%)	
High grade on both LFC and LTP	1 (3.8%)	1 (3.4%)	
At 1-year follow-up MOG, n (%)			0.404
Low grade	23 (88.5%)	28 (96.6%)	
High grade on either LFC or LTP	2 (7.7%)	1 (3.4%)	
High grade on both LFC and LTP	1 (3.8%)	0	

MOG, modified Outerbridge grade; low grade: MOG grade 0, 1, or 2; high grade: MOG 3 or 4; LFC, lateral femoral condyle; LTP, lateral tibial plateau.

Table 5. Changes in Joint Space Width of Lateral Edge on Rosenberg View.

	Group I (n =26)	Group C (n =29)	p-Value
Contralateral JSW, mm			
Preoperative	5.6 ± 2.3	5.7 ± 2.5	0.878
1 year postoperatively	5.5 ± 2.4	5.7 ± 2.8	0.779
p-value	0.879	0.892	
Absolute JSW, mm			
Preoperative	3.7 ± 0.5	3.9 ± 0.4	0.106
1 year postoperatively	4.0 ± 1.8	4.5 ± 1.4	0.253
p-value	0.417	0.031	
Relative JSW			
Preoperative	0.7 ± 0.5	0.7 ± 0.8	0.738
1 year postoperatively	0.7 ± 0.7	0.8 ± 0.9	0.602
p-value	0.889	0.656	

There were no complications related to the suture anchor. Group C showed no lateral capsular tear, meniscocapsular separation, or lateral tibial plateau bone edema.

4. Discussion

The main finding of the current study was that combined lateral MAT and capsulodesis (open decortication and suture anchor fixation) showed less coronal graft extrusion and a greater increase of lateral JSW at the 1-year follow-up compared with isolated lateral MAT. Additional capsulodesis also positively affected graft maturation in the posterior root.

Various efforts have been implemented to reduce graft extrusion after MAT, and recently, studies have reported positive results by applying a method of stabilizing the stretched lateral capsule during MAT. Masferrer-Pino et al. [19] found that major graft extrusion greater than 3 mm occurred in 73.3% of the group (n = 15) that performed the suture-only technique and 28.6% of the group (n = 14) that performed capsulodesis (trans-osseous suture). Masferrer-Pino et al. [20] also reported that major graft extrusion greater than 3 mm occurred in 41.4% of the group (n = 15) that performed the bony fixation technique and 53.3% of the group (n = 14) that performed capsulodesis (trans-osseous suture). Seo et al. [18] reported that when comparing the isolated lateral MAT group (n = 13) and the lateral MAT + capsulodesis using the suture anchor group (n = 10), the mean of graft extrusion in the MRI six months after surgery was 1.2 ± 2.1 mm and 2.6 ± 1.3 mm, respectively. The graft extrusion of the isolated MAT group increased by an average of 1.3 mm six months after surgery compared to before surgery, whereas that of the lateral MAT + capsulodesis group decreased by an average of 1.1 mm. In the present study, the coronal graft position was appropriately located in both groups without significant differences in MRI performed on the second day after surgery. The mean graft extrusion in group C was significantly smaller in MRI performed the first year after lateral MAT. In group I, the graft extrusion increased significantly from 0.8 ± 1.6 mm on the second day after surgery to 2.4 ± 1.8 mm in the first year after surgery, and in group C, it was found to be from 0.4 ± 0.9 mm to

1.1 ± 1.7 mm, which was non-significant. Pathologic graft extrusion occurred in 26.9% of the patients in group I and 10.3% in group C. It is thought that lateral capsular healing and graft incorporation could be promoted because the articular capsule was incised to diffusely decorate the rim of the tibial plateau before performing a procedure for attaching the lateral capsule to it, and capsulodesis was performed with a wide X-shaped attachment.

The cause of high signal intensity seen in MRI after MAT is believed to be extracellular matrix degeneration or fibrocartilaginous scar formation rather than tear [31,37]. The clinical significance of high signal intensity has not yet been elucidated. When the signal intensity was evaluated for the five sections of the graft on MRI one year after surgery in this study, there was a significant difference between the two groups in the posterior root section, and the grade 3 high signal intensity showed a high frequency in group I. As the cause of graft immaturity in the posterior root in group I, it can be considered that stress was more concentrated in the posterior root section, which played an essential role in load distribution due to greater graft extrusion compared to group C [28,38]. Park et al. [31] explained that when 138 MRIs were evaluated three years or more after MAT, grade 3 high signal intensity was observed in approximately one-third of them; in particular, the case of distorted contour with a grade 3 high signal intensity in the posterior third and posterior root was significantly associated with inferior outcomes.

We did not apply universal classification such as Kellgren-Lawrence grade to determine joint space narrowing of the lateral edge [39,40]. Lee et al. [24] revealed that joint cartilage is relatively well maintained when only the lateral edge, not the joint obliteration, is narrow in a considerable number of patients. They showed no significant differences in the ratio of lesions ≥ modified Outerbridge grade 3 between less and moderate joint space narrowing groups. Thus, we suggest that joint space narrowing of the lateral edge and cartilage destruction are not closely related. For this reason, there seems to be no difference in subjective clinical scores at short-term follow-up between the two groups in the current study. Moreover, we assume that the degree of graft extrusion in the first year after lateral MAT minimally affected the subjective clinical outcomes [5,21,41].

Capsulodesis may be an excellent attempt to reduce graft extrusion after MAT, but further biomechanical studies are needed to elucidate how this procedure will affect the physiological meniscal movement. Seo et al. [18] stated that one capsular tear and three meniscocapsular separations occurred among ten patients who underwent MAT + capsulodesis. They hypothesized that the occurrence of these complications might be a limitation of normal meniscal excrusion due to capsulodesis. In this study, no capsular tear or meniscocapsular separation occurred, which is thought to be the difference in the type of suture anchor and the suture method.

The current technique for lateral capsulodesis using an all-soft suture anchor seems to be a simple, reliable, and easy method to prevent graft extrusion. There is also less possibility of complications due to additional procedures. The all-soft suture anchor did not result in significant bone loss in the lateral tibial plateau and allowed for optimal postoperative MRI evaluation.

There are several limitations in this study. First, two different surgical methods were not randomly assigned because lateral capsulodesis was started with clinical suspicion that it could be beneficial for graft stabilization. A lateral MAT was not conducted frequently under strict criteria, and the current study had a relatively small sample size and could not perform a prospective randomized trial. However, the inclusion criteria for both groups were the same, and preoperative demography after retrospective analysis revealed that the two groups did not differ significantly. Second, since the result of MRI and clinical examinations in the first year are considered in this study, a longer follow-up is necessary to identify how graft extrusion affects long-term clinical outcomes. Third, it may be necessary to use two suture anchors, depending on the size of the tibia, but this study conducted capsulodesis using only one. Fourth, objective functional tests were not performed. It is necessary to analyze how graft extrusion affects motor function in closed kinetic chain situations as well as subjective function scores. Finally, there was no second-look arthroscopy; thus, the authors could not evaluate intra-articular biological conditions.

5. Conclusions

In lateral MAT, capsulodesis (open decortication and suture anchor fixation) could reduce graft extrusion without complications. In the future, large-volume and long-term prospective comparative studies are needed to confirm the clinical effect following capsulodesis.

Author Contributions: Conceptualization, D.W.L.; methodology, D.R.L. and W.J.K.; software, Y.J.W.; validation, D.R.L. and Y.J.W.; formal analysis, D.R.L. and S.G.M.; investigation, Y.J.W.; resources, W.J.K.; data curation, S.G.M.; writing—original draft preparation, D.R.L.; writing—review and editing, D.W.L.; visualization, W.J.K.; supervision, D.W.L.; project administration, D.W.L. All authors have read and agreed to the published version of the manuscript.

Funding: This research received no external funding.

Institutional Review Board Statement: The study was conducted in accordance with the Declaration of Helsinki and approved by the Institutional Review Board (or Ethics Committee) of Konkuk University Medical Center (KUMC 2022−09-001).

Informed Consent Statement: Informed consent was obtained from all subjects involved in the study.

Data Availability Statement: The data that support the findings of this study are available on request from the corresponding author.

Conflicts of Interest: The authors declare no conflict of interest.

References

1. Rosso, F.; Bisicchia, S.; Bonasia, D.E.; Amendola, A. Meniscal allograft transplantation: A systematic review. *Am. J. Sports Med.* **2015**, *43*, 998–1007. [CrossRef]
2. Samitier, G.; Alentorn-Geli, E.; Taylor, D.C.; Rill, B.; Lock, T.; Moutzouros, V.; Kolowich, P. Meniscal allograft transplantation. Part 2: Systematic review of transplant timing, outcomes, return to competition, associated procedures, and prevention of osteoarthritis. *Knee Surg. Sports Traumatol. Arthrosc.* **2015**, *23*, 323–333. [CrossRef]
3. Smith, N.A.; MacKay, N.; Costa, M.; Spalding, T. Meniscal allograft transplantation in a symptomatic meniscal deficient knee: A systematic review. *Knee Surg. Sports Traumatol. Arthrosc.* **2015**, *23*, 270–279. [CrossRef]
4. Samitier, G.; Alentorn-Geli, E.; Taylor, D.C.; Rill, B.; Lock, T.; Moutzouros, V.; Kolowich, P. Meniscal allograft transplantation. Part 1: Systematic review of graft biology, graft shrinkage, graft extrusion, graft sizing, and graft fixation. *Knee Surg. Sports Traumatol. Arthrosc.* **2015**, *23*, 310–322. [CrossRef]
5. Ha, J.K.; Shim, J.C.; Kim, D.W.; Lee, Y.S.; Ra, H.J.; Kim, J.G. Relationship between meniscal extrusion and various clinical findings after meniscus allograft transplantation. *Am. J. Sport. Med.* **2010**, *38*, 2448–2455. [CrossRef]
6. Novaretti, J.V.; Patel, N.K.; Lian, J.; Vaswani, R.; de Sa, D.; Getgood, A.; Musahl, V. Long-Term Survival Analysis and Outcomes of Meniscal Allograft Transplantation With Minimum 10-Year Follow-Up: A Systematic Review. *Arthroscopy* **2019**, *35*, 659–667. [CrossRef]
7. Kim, J.G.; Lee, Y.S.; Bae, T.S.; Ha, J.K.; Lee, D.H.; Kim, Y.J.; Ra, H.J. Tibiofemoral contact mechanics following posterior root of medial meniscus tear, repair, meniscectomy, and allograft transplantation. *Knee Surg. Sports Traumatol. Arthrosc.* **2013**, *21*, 2121–2125. [CrossRef]
8. Teichtahl, A.J.; Cicuttini, F.M.; Abram, F.; Wang, Y.; Pelletier, J.P.; Dodin, P.; Martel-Pelletier, J. Meniscal extrusion and bone marrow lesions are associated with incident and progressive knee osteoarthritis. *Osteoarthr. Cartil.* **2017**, *25*, 1076–1083. [CrossRef]
9. Bloecker, K.; Wirth, W.; Guermazi, A.; Hunter, D.J.; Resch, H.; Hochreiter, J.; Eckstein, F. Relationship Between Medial Meniscal Extrusion and Cartilage Loss in Specific Femorotibial Subregions: Data From the Osteoarthritis Initiative. *Arthritis Care Res.* **2015**, *67*, 1545–1552. [CrossRef]
10. Lee, B.S.; Bin, S.I.; Kim, J.M.; Kim, J.H.; Lim, E.J. Meniscal allograft subluxations are not associated with preoperative native meniscal subluxations. *Knee Surg. Sports Traumatol. Arthrosc.* **2017**, *25*, 200–206. [CrossRef]
11. Choi, N.H.; Yoo, S.Y.; Victoroff, B.N. Position of the bony bridge of lateral meniscal transplants can affect meniscal extrusion. *Am. J. Sport. Med.* **2011**, *39*, 1955–1959. [CrossRef] [PubMed]
12. Jeon, B.; Kim, J.M.; Kim, J.M.; Lee, C.R.; Kim, K.A.; Bin, S.I. An osteophyte in the tibial plateau is a risk factor for allograft extrusion after meniscus allograft transplantation. *Am. J. Sports Med.* **2015**, *43*, 1215–1221. [CrossRef] [PubMed]
13. Jang, S.H.; Kim, J.G.; Ha, J.G.; Shim, J.C. Reducing the size of the meniscal allograft decreases the percentage of extrusion after meniscal allograft transplantation. *Arthroscopy* **2011**, *27*, 914–922. [CrossRef]
14. Lee, S.R.; Kim, J.G.; Nam, S.W. The tips and pitfalls of meniscus allograft transplantation. *Knee Surg. Relat. Res.* **2012**, *24*, 137–145. [CrossRef]
15. Choi, N.H.; Choi, J.K.; Yang, B.S.; Lee, D.H.; Victoroff, B.N. Lateral Meniscal Allograft Transplant via a Medial Approach Leads to Less Extrusion. *Am. J. Sports Med.* **2017**, *45*, 2791–2796. [CrossRef]

16. Lee, D.W.; Park, J.H.; Chung, K.S.; Ha, J.K.; Kim, J.G. Arthroscopic Medial Meniscal Allograft Transplantation with Modified Bone Plug Technique. *Arthrosc. Tech.* **2017**, *6*, e1437–e1442. [CrossRef]
17. Lee, D.W.; Park, J.H.; Chung, K.S.; Ha, J.K.; Kim, J.G. Arthroscopic Lateral Meniscal Allograft Transplantation with the Key-Hole Technique. *Arthrosc. Tech.* **2017**, *6*, e1815–e1820. [CrossRef]
18. Seo, Y.J.; Choi, N.H.; Hwangbo, B.H.; Hwang, J.S.; Victoroff, B.N. Lateral Capsular Stabilization in Lateral Meniscal Allograft Transplantation. *Orthop. J. Sports Med.* **2021**, *9*, 23259671211028652. [CrossRef]
19. Masferrer-Pino, A.; Monllau, J.C.; Abat, F.; Gelber, P.E. Capsular fixation limits graft extrusion in lateral meniscal allograft transplantation. *Int. Orthop.* **2019**, *43*, 2549–2556. [CrossRef]
20. Masferrer-Pino, A.; Monllau, J.C.; Ibanez, M.; Erquicia, J.I.; Pelfort, X.; Gelber, P.E. Capsulodesis Versus Bone Trough Technique in Lateral Meniscal Allograft Transplantation: Graft Extrusion and Functional Results. *Arthroscopy* **2018**, *34*, 1879–1888. [CrossRef]
21. Lee, D.W.; Lee, J.H.; Kim, D.H.; Kim, J.G. Delayed Rehabilitation After Lateral Meniscal Allograft Transplantation Can Reduce Graft Extrusion Compared With Standard Rehabilitation. *Am. J. Sports Med.* **2018**, *46*, 2432–2440. [CrossRef]
22. Kellgren, J.H.; Lawrence, J.S. Radiological assessment of osteo-arthrosis. *Ann. Rheum. Dis.* **1957**, *16*, 494–502.
23. Lee, D.W.; Kim, M.K.; Jang, H.S.; Ha, J.K.; Kim, J.G. Clinical and radiologic evaluation of arthroscopic medial meniscus root tear refixation: Comparison of the modified Mason-Allen stitch and simple stitches. *Arthroscopy* **2014**, *30*, 1439–1446. [CrossRef]
24. Lee, D.W.; Lee, D.R.; Kim, M.A.; Lee, J.K.; Kim, J.G. Effect of Preoperative Joint Space Width on Lateral Meniscal Allograft Transplantation: Outcomes at Midterm Follow-up. *Orthop. J. Sports Med.* **2022**, *10*, 23259671221103845. [CrossRef]
25. Lerer, D.B.; Umans, H.R.; Hu, M.X.; Jones, M.H. The role of meniscal root pathology and radial meniscal tear in medial meniscal extrusion. *Skelet. Radiol.* **2004**, *33*, 569–574. [CrossRef]
26. Chung, J.Y.; Song, H.K.; Jung, M.K.; Oh, H.T.; Kim, J.H.; Yoon, J.S.; Min, B.H. Larger medial femoral to tibial condylar dimension may trigger posterior root tear of medial meniscus. *Knee Surg. Sports Traumatol. Arthrosc.* **2016**, *24*, 1448–1454. [CrossRef]
27. Ahn, J.H.; Kang, H.W.; Yang, T.Y.; Lee, J.Y. Multivariate Analysis of Risk Factors of Graft Extrusion After Lateral Meniscus Allograft Transplantation. *Arthroscopy* **2016**, *32*, 1337–1345. [CrossRef]
28. Kim, D.H.; Lee, G.C.; Kim, H.H.; Cha, D.H. Correlation between meniscal extrusion and symptom duration, alignment, and arthritic changes in medial meniscus posterior root tear: Research article. *Knee Surg. Relat. Res.* **2020**, *32*, 2. [CrossRef]
29. Makiev, K.G.; Vasios, I.S.; Georgoulas, P.; Tilkeridis, K.; Drosos, G.; Ververidis, A. Clinical significance and management of meniscal extrusion in different knee pathologies: A comprehensive review of the literature and treatment algorithm. *Knee Surg. Relat. Res.* **2022**, *34*, 35. [CrossRef]
30. Kim, N.K.; Bin, S.I.; Kim, J.M.; Lee, C.R.; Kim, J.H. Meniscal Extrusion Does Not Progress During the Midterm Follow-up Period After Lateral Meniscal Transplantation. *Am. J. Sport. Med.* **2017**, *45*, 900–908. [CrossRef]
31. Park, J.G.; Bin, S.I.; Kim, J.M.; Lee, B.S.; Lee, S.M.; Song, J.H. Increased MRI Signal Intensity of Allografts in the Midterm Period After Meniscal Allograft Transplant: An Evaluation of Clinical Significance According to Location and Morphology. *Orthop. J. Sports Med.* **2021**, *9*, 23259671211033598. [CrossRef]
32. Kijowski, R.; Blankenbaker, D.G.; Davis, K.W.; Shinki, K.; Kaplan, L.D.; De Smet, A.A. Comparison of 1.5- and 3.0-T MR imaging for evaluating the articular cartilage of the knee joint. *Radiology* **2009**, *250*, 839–848. [CrossRef]
33. Crema, M.D.; Roemer, F.W.; Marra, M.D.; Burstein, D.; Gold, G.E.; Eckstein, F.; Baum, T.; Mosher, T.J.; Carrino, J.A.; Guermazi, A. Articular cartilage in the knee: Current MR imaging techniques and applications in clinical practice and research. *Radiographics* **2011**, *31*, 37–61. [CrossRef]
34. Paunipagar, B.K.; Rasalkar, D. Imaging of articular cartilage. *Indian J. Radiol. Imaging* **2014**, *24*, 237–248. [CrossRef]
35. Lee, S.M.; Bin, S.I.; Kim, J.M.; Lee, B.S.; Suh, K.T.; Park, J.G. Meniscal Deficiency Period and High Body Mass Index Are Preoperative Risk Factors for Joint Space Narrowing After Meniscal Allograft Transplantation. *Am. J. Sports Med.* **2021**, *49*, 693–699. [CrossRef]
36. Landis, J.R.; Koch, G.G. The measurement of observer agreement for categorical data. *Biometrics* **1977**, *33*, 159–174. [CrossRef]
37. Lee, D.H.; Lee, B.S.; Chung, J.W.; Kim, J.M.; Yang, K.S.; Cha, E.J.; Bin, S.I. Changes in magnetic resonance imaging signal intensity of transplanted meniscus allografts are not associated with clinical outcomes. *Arthroscopy* **2011**, *27*, 1211–1218. [CrossRef]
38. Allaire, R.; Muriuki, M.; Gilbertson, L.; Harner, C.D. Biomechanical consequences of a tear of the posterior root of the medial meniscus. Similar to total meniscectomy. *J. Bone Jt. Surg. Am.* **2008**, *90*, 1922–1931. [CrossRef]
39. Cheung, J.C.; Tam, A.Y.; Chan, L.C.; Chan, P.K.; Wen, C. Superiority of Multiple-Joint Space Width over Minimum-Joint Space Width Approach in the Machine Learning for Radiographic Severity and Knee Osteoarthritis Progression. *Biology* **2021**, *10*, 1107. [CrossRef]
40. Tiulpin, A.; Saarakkala, S. Automatic Grading of Individual Knee Osteoarthritis Features in Plain Radiographs Using Deep Convolutional Neural Networks. *Diagnostics* **2020**, *10*, 932. [CrossRef]
41. Lee, S.M.; Bin, S.I.; Kim, J.M.; Lee, B.S.; Lee, C.R.; Son, D.W.; Park, J.G. Long-term Outcomes of Meniscal Allograft Transplantation With and Without Extrusion: Mean 12.3-Year Follow-up Study. *Am. J. Sport. Med.* **2019**, *47*, 815–821. [CrossRef] [PubMed]

Disclaimer/Publisher's Note: The statements, opinions and data contained in all publications are solely those of the individual author(s) and contributor(s) and not of MDPI and/or the editor(s). MDPI and/or the editor(s) disclaim responsibility for any injury to people or property resulting from any ideas, methods, instructions or products referred to in the content.

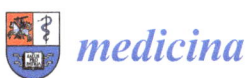

Article

Low-Molecular-Weight Heparins (LMWH) and Synthetic Factor X Inhibitors Can Impair the Osseointegration Process of a Titanium Implant in an Interventional Animal Study

Dragos Apostu [1], Bianca Berechet [2], Daniel Oltean-Dan [1], Alexandru Mester [3], Bobe Petrushev [2], Catalin Popa [4], Madalina Luciana Gherman [5], Adrian Bogdan Tigu [6], Ciprian Ionut Tomuleasa [7,8,9,*], Lucian Barbu-Tudoran [10], Horea Rares Ciprian Benea [1] and Doina Piciu [11]

[1] Department of Orthopedics, Traumatology and Pediatric Orthopaedics, University of Medicine and Pharmacy Cluj-Napoca, 400347 Cluj-Napoca, Romania
[2] Department of Gastroenterology, "Octavian Fodor" Institute of Gastroenterology and Hepatology, 400347 Cluj-Napoca, Romania
[3] Department of Oral Health, University of Medicine and Pharmacy Cluj-Napoca, 400012 Cluj-Napoca, Romania
[4] Department of Materials Science and Engineering, Technical University of Cluj-Napoca, 400114 Cluj-Napoca, Romania
[5] Experimental Center, University of Medicine and Pharmacy Cluj-Napoca, 400012 Cluj-Napoca, Romania
[6] Research Center for Advanced Medicine—MedFuture, Department of Translational Medicine, University of Medicine and Pharmacy Cluj-Napoca, 400347 Cluj-Napoca, Romania
[7] Department of Hematology, University of Medicine and Pharmacy Cluj-Napoca, 400012 Cluj-Napoca, Romania
[8] Department of Hematology, Ion Chiricuta Clinical Cancer Center, 400015 Cluj-Napoca, Romania
[9] Medfuture Research Center for Advanced Medicine, University of Medicine and Pharmacy Cluj-Napoca, 400012 Cluj-Napoca, Romania
[10] Electron Microscopy Center, Faculty of Biology and Geology, Babes-Bolyai University, 400006 Cluj-Napoca, Romania
[11] Nuclear Medicine Department, University of Medicine and Pharmacy Cluj-Napoca, 400012 Cluj-Napoca, Romania
* Correspondence: ciprian.tomuleasa@gmail.com

Abstract: *Background and objectives:* Cementless total hip arthroplasty is a common surgical procedure and perioperative thromboprophylaxis is used to prevent deep vein thrombosis or pulmonary embolism. Osseointegration is important for long-term implant survival, and there is no research on the effect of different thromboprophylaxis agents on the process of osseointegration. *Materials and Methods:* Seventy rats were allocated as follows: Group I (control group), Group II (enoxaparin), Group III (nadroparin), and Group IV (fondaparinux). Ovariectomy was performed on all subjects, followed by the introduction of an intramedullary titanium implant into the femur. Thromboprophylaxis was administered accordingly to each treatment group for 35 days postoperatively. *Results:* Group I had statistically significantly lower anti-Xa levels compared to treatment groups. Micro-CT analysis showed that nadroparin had lower values compared to control in bone volume (0.12 vs. 0.21, $p = 0.01$) and percent bone volume (1.46 vs. 1.93, $p = 0.047$). The pull-out test showed statistically significant differences between the control group (8.81 N) compared to enoxaparin, nadroparin, and fondaparinux groups (4.53 N, 4 N and 4.07 N, respectively). Nadroparin had a lower histological cortical bone tissue and a higher width of fibrous tissue (27.49 μm and 86.9 μm) at the peri-implant area, compared to control (43.2 μm and 39.2 μm), enoxaparin (39.6 μm and 24 μm), and fondaparinux (36.2 μm and 32.7 μm). *Conclusions:* Short-term administration of enoxaparin, nadroparin, and fondaparinux can reduce the osseointegration of titanium implants, with nadroparin having the most negative effect. These results show that enoxaparin and fondaparinux are preferred to be administered due to a lesser negative impact on the initial implant fixation.

Keywords: aseptic loosening; cementless hip arthroplasty; enoxaparin; fondaparinux; implant osseointegration; nadroparin

1. Introduction

Total hip replacement is a common procedure performed worldwide to treat hip osteoarthritis. This pathology affects 10 to 13% of people over 60 years old [1]. Total hip replacement implants are made from titanium alloys. The most frequently used titanium alloy in total hip replacements is $Ti_{90}Al_6V_4$, consisting of titanium, aluminium and vanadium. Although offering good results overall, complications of total hip replacement exist. The most frequent late complication of this type of this surgical procedure is a deficient implant fixation, called aseptic loosening, which leads to increased pain and disability [2]. Patients affected by this complication cannot weight-bear on the affected limb, thus leading to an important functional deficit. When aseptic loosening is present, revision surgery is required, which is expensive for the healthcare system [3]. Moreover, it is technically demanding, requires an experienced team, and is usually performed in tertiary-care hospitals. Additionally, the revision of the total hip replacement often results in a lower patient satisfaction rate than the primary hip replacement [4].

Aseptic loosening can be prevented with a more enhanced osseointegration process, represented by bone apposition at the titanium surface of the total hip arthroplasty implant [5,6]. This complex process is dependent on the processes of bone formation, performed by osteoblasts, and bone resorption, performed by osteoclasts. The process of osseointegration is regulated by many cellular pathways which modulate the activity of osteoblasts and osteoclasts [6]. Osteoblasts arise from mesenchymal stem cells (MSC) under the influence of cytokines, such as tumour necrosis factor (TNF) alpha, interleukin (IL) 1, IL-6 and IL-11. On the other hand, osteoclastogenesis is positively modulated by macrophage colony-stimulating factor (M-CSF) and transforming growth factor beta (TGF-β1). The more active the osteoblasts are compared to osteoclasts, the stronger the implant fixation will be and the lower the risk of aseptic loosening. The process of osseointegration is similar in the case of titanium intramedullary implants and titanium dental implants [7–9]. Our study group has proven that osseointegration can be influenced by many factors, including systemic drugs [10].

Low-molecular-weight heparins (LMWH) and synthetic factor X inhibitors are routinely administered postoperatively to prevent deep vein thrombosis (DVT) and pulmonary embolism. Among the most commonly used drugs to prevent DVT postoperatively following total hip replacement are enoxaparin, nadroparin, and fondaparinux.

Previous studies by Kock et al. and Osip et al. showed that LMWHs could inhibit osteoblastogenesis during in vitro experimental studies [11–14]. These studies were the first to prove that low-molecular-weight heparins have an impact on bone metabolism. One explanation is that LMWHs can alter the function of the cytokines involved in osteoblastogenesis and osteoclastogenesis [15]. As a result, the whole osseointegration process can be affected [15]. Numerous in vivo studies were performed to study the effects of LMWHs on bone biology. Enoxaparin, dalteparin, nadroparin and tinzaparin were shown to increase osteoclastogenesis and bone resorption by modulating M-CSF and TGF-β1, [16–22]. Additionally, researchers studied the effects of LMWHs on bone metabolism in the case of fracture healing. A study performed by Strett et al. showed that enoxaparin attenuated the bone repair process compared to the control group [23]. The result is confirmed by a more recent study by Li et al., which concluded that enoxaparin suppresses osteoblastogenesis [24]. On the other hand, other studies showed that LMWHs did not impair the fracture process [25,26].

Although previous studies showed that LMWHs have an impact on bone biology, the overall effect is still controversial. Moreover, we did not find any study to test the effects of LMWHs on the process of osseointegration of the titanium implant. We consider that in vivo studies are essential to test the osseointegration process of titanium implants because there is an implication of osteoclasts, osteoblasts and the titanium surface, which are impossible to replicate in the case of in vitro studies. We also consider it essential to know whether thromboprophylaxis agents can impair the titanium implant osseointegration. Clinical trials are challenging to be performed due to a lack of specific examinations for the osseointegration process in the clinical setting, which are available in an animal model. Moreover, the long follow-up to study the rate of aseptic loosening makes clinical trials more difficult to perform.

This study aims to test, for the first time in the literature, the impact of thromboprophylaxis agents on the process of osseointegration in vivo. For this study, we tested three of the most commonly used drugs in DVT prophylaxis: enoxaparin, nadroparin, and fondaparinux, in terms of early implant fixation in vivo.

2. Materials and Methods

2.1. Animal Model

The study received approval from the Ethical Commission of the local university (no. 210/02/04/2020). The experiments were performed at the Center of Experimental Medicine Cluj-Napoca and according to the European guidelines (directive 2010/63/EU). A total of 70 female albino Wistar rats of 8–10 weeks old and with a weight of 190 ± 30 mg were used. The animals were raised at the same animal facility without any genetic modification, while food and water were provided ad libitum. A veterinary doctor checked all of the subjects to be enrolled in the study to be clinically healthy. The subjects were randomized into four groups: Group I (OVX group, $n = 22$), Group II (OVX + enoxaparin, $n = 16$), Group III (OVX + nadroparin, $n = 16$), and Group IV (OVX + fondaparinux, $n = 16$).

2.2. Ovariectomy (OVX) Procedure

The procedures were performed on all subjects at the time of enrolment, and each subject's weight was determined preoperatively. General anaesthesia was induced with a mixture of 80–100 mg/kg of ketamine and 10–12.5 mg/kg of xylazine injected intraperitoneally. Skin preparation using betadine and sterile draping was performed. Following an abdominal midline incision, the ovaries were identified and excised with electrocautery (Figures 1a and 2). The abdominal wall was sutured, and a local antibiotic was applied. Postoperatively, analgesics were provided in the drinking water.

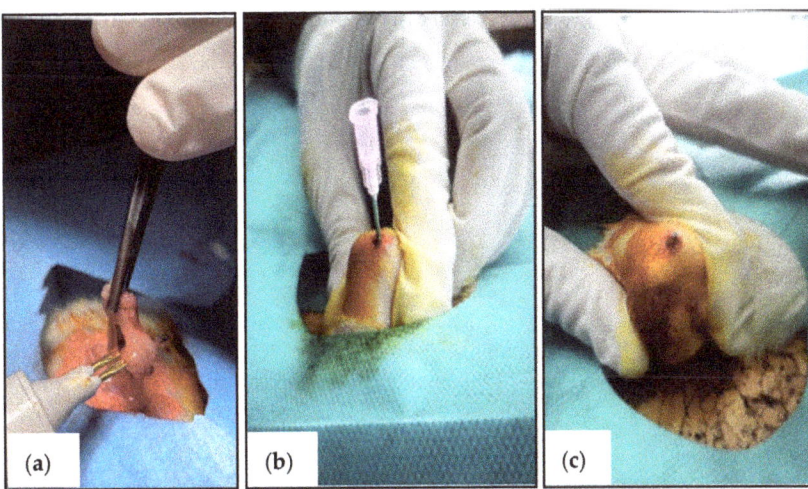

Figure 1. Intraoperative images: (**a**) Ovariectomy procedure; (**b**) Opening of the femoral canal; (**c**) Implantation of the titanium intramedullary nail.

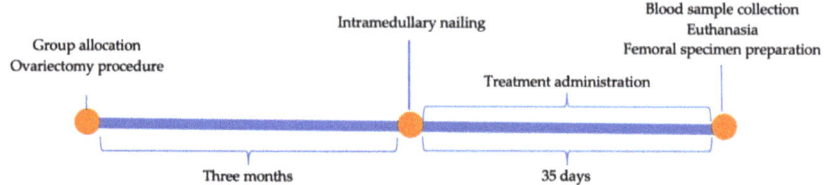

Figure 2. Project's timeline: group allocation, ovariectomy procedures, intramedullary nailing, treatment administration, blood sample collection, euthanasia, and femoral specimen preparation.

2.3. Intramedullary Nail

Three months after the ovariectomy procedure, bilateral femoral intramedullary nailing was performed in all subjects under general anaesthesia. Both legs were prepared, and sterile draping was performed. The femoral condyles were palpated, and using a sterile 18-gauge needle, and the femoral canal was opened percutaneously at the level of the femoral notch (Figures 1b and 2). Then, $Ti_{90}Al_6V_4$ alloy nails (Goodfellow Cambridge Ltd., Huntingdon, UK) with a diameter of 1 mm and 20 mm in length were introduced into the femur (Figure 1c). There was no need for a suture since the technique was entirely percutaneous. A local antibiotic was applied to the insertion site. Postoperatively, analgesics were provided in the drinking water.

2.4. Treatment

Starting on day one postoperatively, the subjects were weighted daily, and treatment was administered subcutaneously according to each group (Figure 2). Group I received saline subcutaneously daily for 35 days. Group II received enoxaparin 1 mg/kg subcutaneously daily for 35 days. Group III received receive nadroparin 10 mg/kg subcutaneously daily for 35 days and group IV received receive fondaparinux 0.1 mg/kg subcutaneously daily for 35 days.

2.5. Collection of Samples

Three months after the intramedullary nailing, blood samples were harvested. Under general anaesthesia, the subjects were euthanised. We looked for uterus atrophy and the absence of ovaries. Moreover, the bilateral femoral bones were collected and placed in 10% formaldehyde. The femurs underwent histological, micro-CT, and mechanical pull-out test examinations.

2.6. Serum Analysis

Using the ELISA method, we tested the rat coagulation factor Xa (NovusBiologicals®, Cambridge, UK). The calibration was performed using the following concentrations: 40 ng/mL, 20 ng/mL, 10 ng/mL, 5 ng/mL, 2.5 ng/mL, 1.25 ng/mL and 0.63 ng/mL. The samples were diluted five times. We used the TECAN Spark 10M (TECAN, Grödig, Austria) microplate reader.

2.7. Micro-CT Examination

Bruker Skyscan 1172® (Billerica, MA, USA) with a 50 mm image field width and 11 Mp X-ray camera was used at a resolution of 2000 × 2000 px for the micro-CT scanning. We analysed a region of interest of a round shape, and a diameter of 120 mm centred on the implant. The length of the area of interest was 600 slices (8.1 mm) starting from the distal metaphysis proximally. The Bruker CTAn® v.1.18. software was used to calculate bone volume (BV), percent bone volume (BV%), bone surface (BS), bone surface/volume ratio (BS/VR), tissue surface (TS), mean total cross-sectional bone area, trabecular number (TN), cross-sectional thickness, and trabecular diameter (TD). The measurements were performed while the examiner was unaware of group allocation.

2.8. Mechanical Pull-Out Test

An osteotomy of the femoral diaphysis in the proximal one third was sequentially performed until 5 mm of the intramedullary nail was exposed. The nail was tightened in a pneumatic grip, and the Zwick/Roell Z005® (Ulm, Germany) tensile testing device with a maximum test load of 5 kN was used to measure the force needed for nail extraction. The forces were measured in newtons at a low speed of 1 mm/min. The measurements were performed while the examiner was unaware of group allocation.

2.9. Histological Examination

Following the mechanical pull-out test, the femoral bones were decalcified and sectioned longitudinally along the implant site. Hematoxylin–eosin and Tricom Masson stainings were performed and analysed with a Leica DM750® (Wetzlar, Germany) microscope. We used ImageJ® software for the morphometric measurements. The thickness of the cortical bone at the peri-implant site was measured at five different points at about 20-0 μm apart. The same method was applied to measure the fibrous tissue at the peri-implant site. Two independent measurements were performed by different examiners who did not know the allocation within the groups, and the average was noted.

2.10. SEM/EDX Analysis

We tested a total of 12 samples equally divided into groups. The samples were fixed in glutaraldehyde (2.7% in PBS), dehydrated in alcohol, and infused with hexamethyldisilane. After sputter-coating with 7 nm of gold in an Agar Automatic Sputter-Coater B7341 (Essex, UK), samples were examined in a Hitachi SU8230 HRCFEG SEM (Tokyo, Japan).

2.11. Statistical Analysis

The sample size was calculated during the study design using the StatMate® software. For the sample size calculation, we used the results obtained from previous studies on titanium implant osseointegration following systemic administration [27,28]. The type I/II error rates we used during calculations were alpha values of 0.05 and power of the study of 80%. Moreover, we assumed a 20% mortality rate due to the two surgical interventions and general anaesthesia. The statistical analysis was performed using the GraphPad Prism 6.0® software, and we calculated means, standard deviations, frequencies, percentages, and correlation tests. The distribution was calculated using the Shapiro–Wilk test. The results were considered statistically significant if the p-value was less than 0.05.

3. Results

Of the seventy subjects included in the study, nine died throughout the process: seven died due to anaesthesia, and two died from infection. Five of the subjects belonged to Group I, one subject belonged to Group II, and three subjects belonged to Group IV.

3.1. Weight

All of the subjects were weighed during the study. The average weight before the ovariectomy procedure was 216 ± 22 g. The mean weight according to each group are as follows: 209.4 ± 17.5 g (Group I), 221.5 ± 23 g (Group II), 216 ± 25 g (Group III), and 222 ± 21 g (Group IV). Group I had a statistically significant lower weight compared to Groups II, III and IV ($p < 0.05$).

At the end of the study, the mean weight according to each group were as follows: 215 ± 16.5 g (Group I), 230 ± 20 g (Group II), 225 ± 27 g (Group III), and 229 ± 21 g (Group IV). Additionally, Group I had a statistically significantly lower weight than Groups II, III and IV ($p < 0.05$). Nevertheless, all of the subjects increased in weight during the study.

3.2. Serum Analysis

The rat coagulation factor Xa was calculated in all of the subjects at the end of the study (n = 61), as follows: 17 subjects in Group I, 15 subjects in Group II, 16 subjects in Group III and 13 subjects in Group IV. The results are available in Figure 3. Group I had statistically significantly lower levels than Groups II, III and IV ($p < 0.001$). There were no statistically significant differences between Groups II, III and IV.

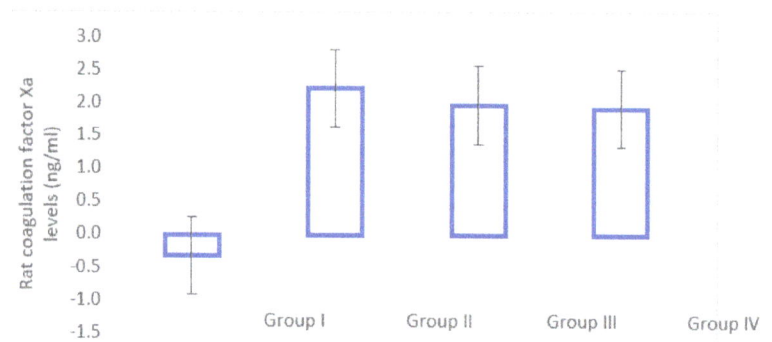

Figure 3. Rat coagulation factor Xa levels at the end of the study in Group I (control), Group II (enoxaparin), Group III (nadroparin) and Group IV (fondaparinux).

3.3. Micro-CT Examination

A total of 12 samples were analysed, equally divided within the groups. The results of the calculate bone volume (BV), percent bone volume (BV%), bone surface (BS), bone surface/volume ration (BS/VR), tissue surface (TS), mean total cross-sectional bone area, trabecular number (TN), cross-sectional thickness and trabecular diameter (TD) are available in Table 1. The only statistically significant differences observed were between Group I and Group III in terms of bone volume ($p = 0.001$) and percent bone volume ($p = 0.047$). Images obtained during micro-CT examinations are available in Figure 4.

Table 1. Results of micro-CT examination expressed in mean (± standard deviation).

Parameter	Group I (Control) n = 3	Group II (Enoxaparin) n = 3	Group III (Nadroparin) n = 3	Group IV (Fondaparinux) n = 3
Bone volume (BV)	0.21 (±0.02) [b]	0.20 (±0.04)	0.12 (±0.06) [a]	0.22 (±0.03)
Percent bone volume (BV%)	1.93 (±0.15) [b]	1.72 (±0.5)	1.46 (±0.2) [a]	1.75 (±0.4)
Bone surface (BS)	39.46 (±6.5)	38.54 (±7.5)	32.23 (±9.2)	40.21 (±4.8)
Tissue surface (TS)	43.21 (±2.4)	45.32 (±4.2)	56.56 (±7.1)	43.32 (±5.3)
Bone surface/volume ratio (BS/VR)	207.68	226.7	230.21	236.52
Mean total cross-sectional bone area	0.038 (±0.02)	0.034 (±0.025)	0.029 (±0.05)	0.036 (±0.045)
Cross-sectional thickness	0.013 (±0.002)	0.014 (±0.004)	0.010 (±0.004)	0.016 (±0.002)
Trabecular diameter	0.020 (±0.003)	0.023 (±0.0025)	0.016 (±0.005)	0.021 (±0.002)
Trabecular number	8.82 (±0.53)	9.2 (±0.63)	7.52 (±0.78)	8.26 (±0.32)

Note: [a] Statistically significant compared to Group I; [b] Statistically significant compared to Group IV.

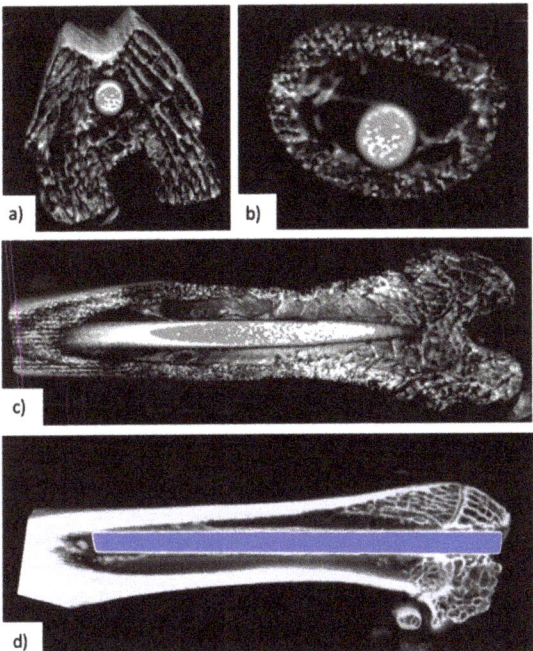

Figure 4. Images obtained following micro-CT examinations: (**a**) cross-sectional view of the intramedullary nail at the distal epiphysis; (**b**) cross-sectional view of the intramedullary nail at the middle of the femoral diaphysis; (**c**) longitudinal view of the intramedullary nail; (**d**) longitudinal view of the intramedullary nail with automatic detection of the metal implant by the software.

3.4. Mechanical Pull-Out Test

The mechanical pull-out test was performed in all of the subjects ($n = 61$). The average values of the maximum force needed to extract the intramedullary nail are available in Figure 5. The control group had the highest average force needed for intramedullary nail extraction, followed by enoxaparin. There were statistically significant differences between Group I and Group III ($p = 0.01$), Group I and Group IV ($p = 0.03$), as well as between Group I and Group II ($p = 0.04$). There were no statistically significant differences between the treatment groups.

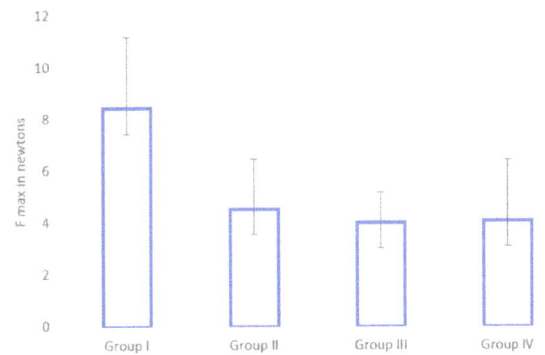

Figure 5. Mechanical pull-put test in Group I (control), Group II (enoxaparin), Group III (nadroparin) and Group IV (fondaparinux).

3.5. Histological Analysis

Histological analysis was performed on all of the subjects within the study ($n = 60$), except for one subject in Group IV whom we excluded after SEM/EDX analysis due to higher concentrations of calcium and phosphorus on the implant after its removal. Images from the measurements of the fibrous tissue and bone tissue are seen in Figures 6 and 7.

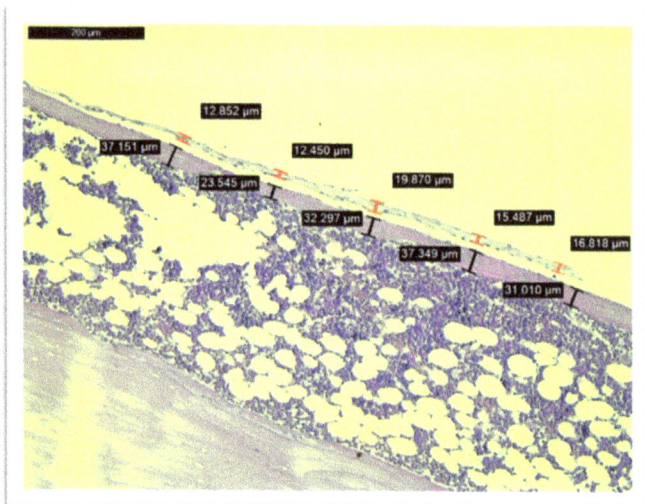

Figure 6. Histological measurements of cortical bone tissue and fibrous tissue in the peri-implant site within Group I (control).

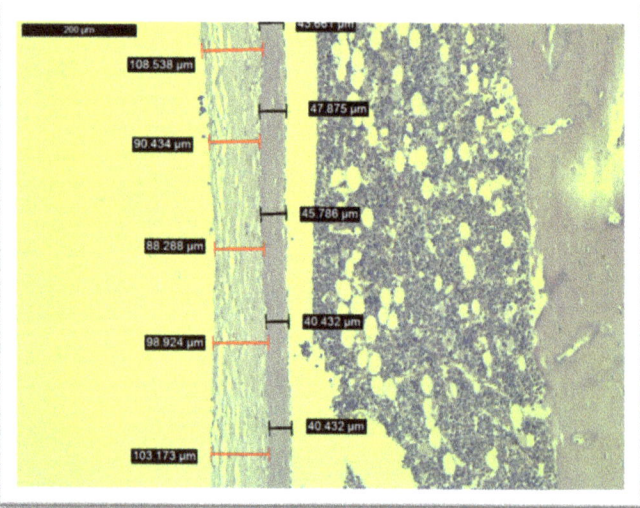

Figure 7. Histological measurements of cortical bone tissue and fibrous tissue in the peri-implant site within Group III (nadroparin).

In terms of cortical bone surrounding the implant site, the nadroparin group had the lowest width (see Figure 8). The only statistically significant result was obtained between Group I and Group III ($p = 0.0002$).

Regarding fibrous tissue surrounding the implant, the nadroparin group had the highest values (see Figure 9). The only statistically significant results were between Group II and Group III ($p = 0.02$) and between Group III and Group IV ($p = 0.04$).

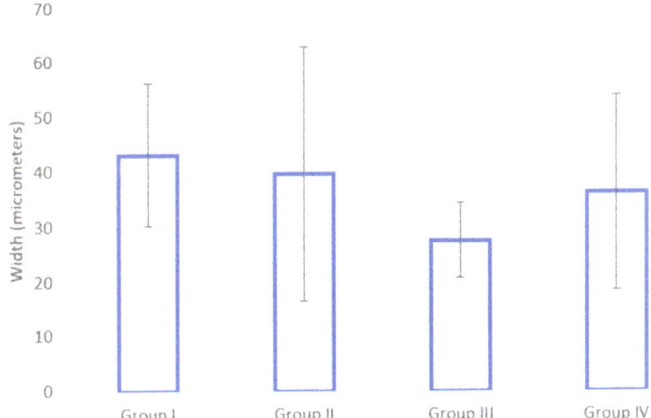

Figure 8. The average width of the cortical bone tissue at the peri-implant region.

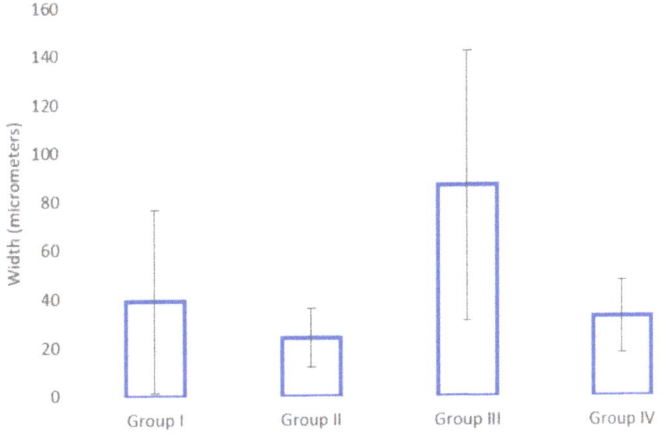

Figure 9. The average width of the fibrous tissue at the peri-implant region.

3.6. SEM/EDX Analysis

The SEM/EDX analysis was performed on a number of three titanium implants within each group, resulting in a total of twelve implants. Except for one case, the maximum Wt% of both calcium and phosphorus was 1.3%. There were no statistically significant differences between groups in terms of calcium and phosphorus concentrations.

Moreover, the EDX analysis of the titanium, aluminium, and vanadium showed an average concentration of 88.6%, 7.3%, and 3.8%, respectively. The images obtained from the SEM/EDX analysis are available in Figure 10.

There was one case belonging to Group IV (Figure 11), where the Wt% of calcium was 52.9% and 25.4% in the case of phosphorus.

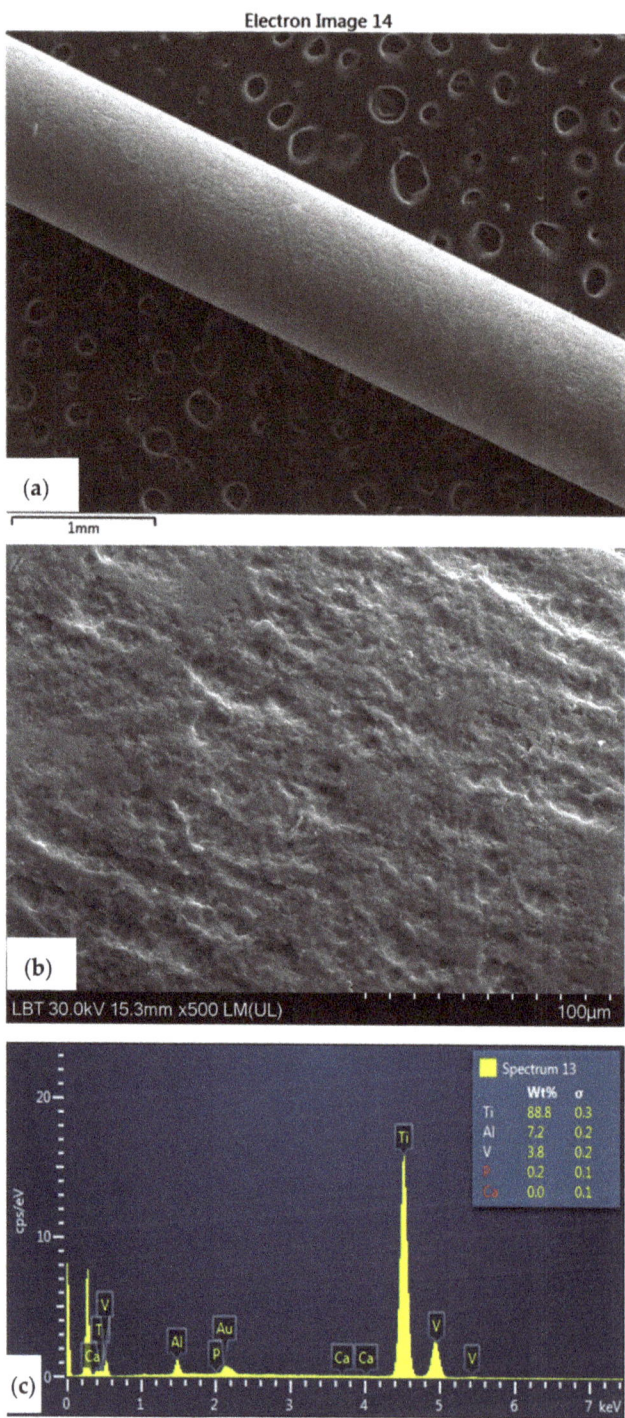

Figure 10. (a,b) Scanning electron microscopy image at different image magnification; (c) EDX analysis diagram.

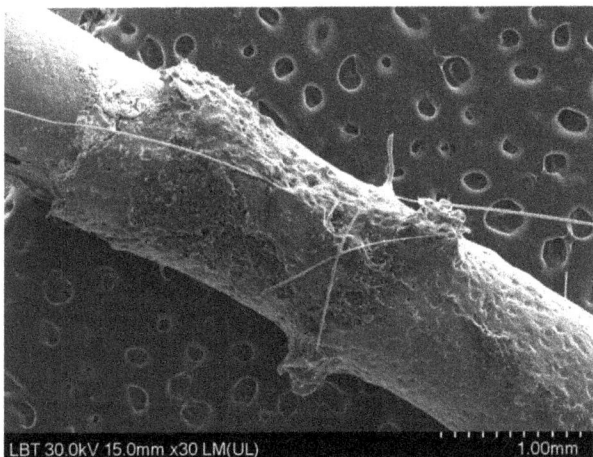

Figure 11. Scanning electron microscopy image of one case with an increased concentration on both calcium and phosphorus.

4. Discussion

To our knowledge, this is the first in vivo study to test and compare the effect of enoxaparin, nadroparin, and fondaparinux on the process of titanium implant osseointegration.

The rat animal model was used due to the high resemblance of bone metabolism compared to humans. They also represent the most commonly used animal model for the study of osseointegration. In clinical practice, patients requiring total hip arthroplasty are frequently osteoporotic and have a deficient bone metabolism [29]. Therefore, we decided to perform an ovariectomy to induce osteoporosis in our animal model. Additionally, when an osteoporotic animal model is used, there is a higher impact on the treatment involved, meaning a lower number of subjects is needed to obtain statistically significant results [30]. In the literature, osteoporosis is generally accepted to be obtained at three months; therefore, we performed the intramedullary implantation of the nails at 12 weeks. For this study, we used $Ti_{90}Al_6V_4$ alloy nails which resemble the alloy of cementless total hip arthroplasties. Moreover, throughout the study, we had no deaths due to pulmonary embolism because the surgical intervention was minimally invasive and the subjects could completely weight bear after the surgery.

The treatment was administered for 35 days after titanium nail implantation, which is the current protocol in our country. The doses were obtained from different studies in which deep vein thrombosis prophylaxis was performed in rat animal models using the three types of treatment [31–33]. In order to test the efficiency of the treatment administration, rat coagulation factor Xa was determined. Additionally, we performed the SEM/EDX analysis of the extracted implants to identify any bone tissue extracted along with the implant.

The anti-Xa levels were statistically significantly increased in the treatment groups compared to the control group, showing a good treatment administration. Nevertheless, we do not have an established therapeutic range in the animal model. As a result, the serum analysis does not provide information about the dosing.

The micro-CT analysis showed that nadroparin statistically significantly has a lower bone volume around the implant compared to the control group. Moreover, there were no statistically significant differences between the treatment groups. These results show the effect of these drugs in the osseointegration process of titanium implants. Moreover, despite other differences observed, the sample size in the case of micro-CT examinations was insufficient to provide other statistically significant results.

The pull-out test is an essential tool to assess the strength of the osseointegration process because it tests both the quantity and the quality of the implant fixation. During the pull-out test, all treatment groups showed a significantly lower force needed for implant extraction compared to the control group. This result shows a stronger implant fixation in the absence of treatment.

The histological analysis found a significantly lower cortical bone mass around the implant site in the case of nadroparin compared to the control group. Despite enoxaparin and fondaparinux also showing an overall lower cortical bone mass compared to the control, as well, the results were not statistically significant. Nevertheless, the biggest difference was when comparing the fibrous tissue around the implant site, which was significantly higher in the nadroparin group than in all other groups. The histological results show that nadroparin significantly reduces implant fixation than in all other groups.

We also performed the SEM/EDX analysis to determine whether bone tissue was still present on the implant surface after its extraction from the femoral bone during the pull-out test. The EDX analysis only showed small concentrations of calcium and phosphorus in all of the implants, except in one case, where there was a high concentration of calcium and phosphorus and was later excluded from the histological examination. These results show that most implants did not contain relevant concentrations of calcium or phosphorus following implant removal.

We have found no similar studies to compare our study's results. Nevertheless, other studies on bone metabolism showed that enoxaparin and nadroparin increase osteoclastogenesis, thus leading to an increased bone resorption process [16–22]. These results are according to our study, where the osseointegration process is impaired by enoxaparin and nadroparin. Other studies on fracture healing have shown that enoxaparin can impair bone growth compared to control, a result related to our study due to a deficient bone metabolism [23].

Bruker Skyscan 1172 micro-CT is a microfocus X-ray microtomography optimized for small samples offering good precision for osseointegration examination. The error and tolerance are insignificant since a standard method of determining the region of interest was used in all samples. The Zwick/Roell Z005® testing machine has a machine compliance correction, offering real-time modifications for the highest possible level of precision.

The study also has some limitations. The main limitation of our study is the inability to perform the histological analysis with the implant in situ. This could provide a better assessment of the histological bone–implant contact. During the implant removal, even though it is performed at low speeds, a quantity of bone and fibrous tissue could still be attached to the implant and therefore provide deficient information when the bone specimens are analysed. In order to test this hypothesis, we performed an SEM/EDX analysis which showed that only a small quantity of calcium and phosphorus had been removed along with the implants, with only one exception, which was later excluded. This result provides sufficient information to state that the implant removal during the pull-out test at low speed does not affect the histological analysis of the implant site.

Another limitation is the lack of a known therapeutic range for the anti-Xa coagulation factor level for us to know whether or not the dosing was correct. This limitation could influence the study's results due to potentially different concentrations of drugs. Additionally, a limitation of our study is the relatively low number of subjects for micro-CT analysis and SEM/EDX analysis.

Our study has shown, for the first time in the literature, that some low-molecular-weight heparins (LMWH) and synthetic factor X inhibitors can affect the process of osseointegration in vivo. An impaired osseointegration process can lead to aseptic loosening of cementless total hip arthroplasties. Our study's results are significant, especially due to the long-term follow-up needed to determine the association between aseptic loosening and the type of thromboprophylaxis drug in a clinical setting. We found no clinical studies to determine this association and we recommend further studies be performed in this direction, since our study has proven the implication of thromboprophylaxis agents on the process of osseointegration.

5. Conclusions

Short-term administration of enoxaparin, nadroparin, and fondaparinux can reduce the osseointegration of titanium implants, while nadroparin resulted in the highest quantity of fibrous tissue and the lowest quantity of cortical bone tissue surrounding the implant site. Further clinical research is needed to test the influence of thromboprophylaxis agents on the process of osseointegration.

Author Contributions: Conceptualization, D.A. and D.P.; methodology, D.A., B.B., D.O.-D., A.M. and M.L.G.; formal analysis, D.A., B.B., D.O.-D., A.M., M.L.G. and H.R.C.B.; investigation, A.B.T., B.P., C.P., L.B.-T. and H.R.C.B.; resources, D.A., D.P. and C.I.T.; data curation, D.A.; writing—original draft preparation, D.A.; writing—review and editing, D.P. and C.I.T.; supervision, D.P. and C.I.T.; project administration, D.A.; funding acquisition, D.A., D.P. and C.I.T. All authors have read and agreed to the published version of the manuscript.

Funding: This work was supported by a grant from the Romanian Ministry of Education and Research, CNCS-UEFISCDI, project number PN-III-P1-1.1-PD-2019-0124, within PNCDI III. The work was funded by an international grant awarded by the Novo Nordisk Haemophilia Foundation to the Romanian Hematology Society—Romania 4.

Institutional Review Board Statement: The study received approval from the Ethical Commission of the local university (no. 210/02/04/2020). The experiments were performed at the Center of Experimental Medicine Cluj-Napoca and according to the European guidelines (directive 2010/63/EU).

Conflicts of Interest: The authors declare no conflict of interest.

Abbreviations

BS	Bone surface
BS/VR	Bone surface/volume ratio
BV	Bone volume
BV%	Percent bone volume
DVT	Deep vein thrombosis
EDX	Energy-dispersive X-ray spectroscopy
IL	Interleukin
LMWH	Low-molecular-weight heparins
MSC	Mesenchymal stem cell
M-CSF	Macrophage colony-stimulating factor
OVX	Ovariectomy
SEM	Scanning electron microscope
TD	Trabecular diameter
TGF-β1	Transforming growth factor beta 1
TN	Trabecular number
TNF	Tumour necrosis factor
TS	Tissue surface

References

1. Zhang, Y.; Jordan, J.M. Epidemiology of Osteoarthritis. *Clin. Geriatr. Med.* **2010**, *26*, 355–369. [CrossRef]
2. Kochbati, R.; Rbai, H.; Jlailia, M.; Makhlouf, H.; Bouguira, A.; Daghfous, M.S. Predictive factors of aseptic loosening of cemented total hip prostheses. *Pan. Afr. Med. J.* **2016**, *24*, 260. [PubMed]
3. Vanhegan, I.S.; Malik, A.K.; Jayakumar, P.; Islam, S.; Haddad, F.S. A financial analysis of revision hip arthroplasty: The economic burden in relation to the national tariff. *J. Bone Jt. Surg. Br.* **2012**, *94*, 619–623. [CrossRef]
4. Adelani, M.A.; Crook, K.; Barrack, R.L.; Maloney, W.J.; Clohisy, J.C. What is the Prognosis of Revision Total Hip Arthroplasty in Patients 55 Years and Younger? *Clin. Orthop. Relat. Res.* **2014**, *472*, 1518–1525. [CrossRef] [PubMed]
5. Coelho, P.G.; Jimbo, R. Osseointegration of metallic devices: Current trends based on implant hardware design. *Arch. Biochem. Biophys.* **2014**, *561*, 99–108. [CrossRef] [PubMed]
6. Apostu, D.; Lucaciu, O.; Lucaciu, G.D.; Crisan, B.; Crisan, L.; Baciut, M.; Onisor, F.; Baciut, G.; Campian, R.S.; Bran, S. Systemic drugs that influence titanium implant osseointegration. *Drug Metab. Rev.* **2017**, *49*, 92–104. [CrossRef]
7. Minervini, G.; Del Mondo, D.; Russo, D.; Cervino, G.; D'Amico, C.; Fiorillo, L. Stem Cells in Temporomandibular Joint Engineering: State of Art and Future Perspectives. *J. Craniofacial Surg.* **2022**, *33*, 2181–2187. [CrossRef]

8. Minervini, G.; Romano, A.; Petruzzi, M.; Maio, C.; Serpico, R.; Lucchese, A.; Candotto, V.; Di Stasio, D. Telescopic overdenture on natural teeth: Prosthetic rehabilitation on (OFD) syndromic patient and a review on available literature. *J. Biol. Regul. Homeost. Agents* **2018**, *32* (Suppl. 1), 131–134.
9. Minervini, G.; Fiorillo, L.; Russo, D.; Lanza, A.; D'Amico, C.; Cervino, G.; Meto, A.; Di Francesco, F. Prosthodontic Treatment in Patients with Temporomandibular Disorders and Orofacial Pain and/or Bruxism: A Review of the Literature. *Prosthesis* **2022**, *4*, 253–262. [CrossRef]
10. Apostu, D.; Lucaciu, O.; Mester, A.; Oltean-Dan, D.; Gheban, D.; Benea, H.R.C. Tibolone, alendronate, and simvastatin enhance implant osseointegration in a preclinical in vivo model. *Clin. Oral Implant. Res.* **2020**, *31*, 655–668. [CrossRef]
11. Kock, H.J.; Handschin, A.E. Osteoblast Growth Inhibition by Unfractioned Heparin and by Low molecular Weight Heparins: An In-Vitro Investigation. *Clin. Appl. Thromb. Hemost.* **2002**, *8*, 251–255. [CrossRef] [PubMed]
12. Osip, S.L.; Butcher, M.; Young, E.; Yang, L.; Shaughnessy, S.G. Differential effects of heparin and low molecular weight heparin on osteoblastogenesis and adipogenesis in vitro. *Thromb. Haemost.* **2004**, *92*, 803–810. [CrossRef] [PubMed]
13. Bhandari, M.; Hirsh, J.; Weitz, J.I.; Young, E.; Venner, T.J.; Shaughnessy, S.G. The effects of standard and low molecular weight heparin on bone nodule formation in vitro. *Thromb. Haemost.* **1998**, *80*, 413–417. [CrossRef] [PubMed]
14. Mavrogenis, A.F.; Dimitriou, R.; Parvizi, J.; Babis, G.C. Biology of implant osseointegration. *J. Musculoskelet. Neuronal Interact.* **2009**, *9*, 61–71.
15. Kapetanakis, S.; Nastoulis, E.; Demesticha, T.; Demetriou, T. The Effect of Low Molecular Weight Heparins on Fracture Healing. *Open Orthop. J.* **2015**, *9*, 226–236. [CrossRef]
16. Sudrova, M.; Kvasnicka, J.; Kudrnova, Z.; Zenahlikova, Z.; Mazoch, J. Influence of long-term thromboprophylaxis with low molecular weight heparin (enoxaparin) on changes of bone metabolism markers in pregnant women. *Clin. Appl. Thromb.* **2011**, *17*, 508–513. [CrossRef]
17. Sarahrudi, K.; Kaizer, G.; Thomas, A. The influence of low molecular weight heparin on the expression of osteogenic growth factors in human fracture healing. *Int. Orthop.* **2011**, *36*, 1095–1098. [CrossRef]
18. Folwarczna, J.; Janiec, W.; Gavor, M. Effects of enoxaparin on bone histomorphometric parameters in rats. *Pol. J. Pharm.* **2004**, *56*, 451–457.
19. Wawrzynska, L.; Tomkowski, W.Z.; Przedlacki, J.; Hajduk, B.; Torbicki, A. Changes in bone density during long term administration of low molecular weights heparins or acenocoumarol for secondary prophylaxis of venous thromboembolism. *Pathophysiol. Haemost. Thromb.* **2003**, *33*, 64–67. [CrossRef]
20. Matziolis, G.; Perka, C.; Disch, A.; Zippel, H. Effects of fondaparinus compared with dalteparin, enoxaparin and unfractionated heparin on human osteoblasts. *Calcif. Tissue Int.* **2003**, *73*, 370–379. [CrossRef]
21. Folwarczna, J.; Sliwinski, L.; Janiec, W.; Pikul, M. Effects of standard heparin and low molecular weight heparins on the formation of murine osteoclasts in vitro. *Pharm. Rep* **2005**, *57*, 635–645.
22. Handschin, A.E.; Trenz, O.A.; Hoerstrup, S.; Kock, H.J.; Wanner, G.A.; Trentz, O. Effect of low molecular weight heparin (dalteparin) and fondaparinux (arixtra) on human osteoblasts in vitro. *Br. J. Surg.* **2005**, *92*, 177–183. [CrossRef] [PubMed]
23. Street, J.T.; Mc Grath, M.; Regan, K. Thromboprophylaxis using a low molecular weight heparin delays fracture repair. *Clin. Orthop.* **2000**, *381*, 278–289. [CrossRef] [PubMed]
24. Li, Y.; Liu, L.; Li, S.; Sun, H.; Zhang, Y.; Duan, Z.; Wang, D. Impaired bone healing by enoxaparin via inhibiting the differentiation of bone marrow mesenchymal stem cells towards osteoblasts. *J. Bone Miner. Metab.* **2022**, *40*, 9–19. [CrossRef] [PubMed]
25. Filho, M.S.; Vidigal, L.; Canova, A.R. The effects of low molecular weight heparin (enoxaparin) on bony callus formation in rats femurs—An experimental study. *Acta Orthop. Bras.* **2006**, *14*, 78–82.
26. Demirtas, A.; Azboy, I.; Bulut, M.; Ucar, B.Y.; Alabalik, U.; Necmioglou, N.M. Investigation of the effects of Enoxaparin, Fondaparinux, and Rivaroxaban used in thromboembolism prophylaxis on fracture healing in rats. *Eur. Rev. Med. Pharm. Sci.* **2013**, *17*, 1850–1856.
27. Duan, Y.; Ma, W.; Li, D.; Wang, T.; Liu, B. Enhanced osseointegration of titanium implants in a rat model of osteoporosis using multilayer bone mesenchymal stem cell sheets. *Exp. Ther. Med.* **2017**, *14*, 5717–5726. [CrossRef]
28. Ozaras, N.; Rezvani, A. Diffuse skeletal pain after administration of alendronate. *Indian J. Pharm.* **2010**, *42*, 245–246. [CrossRef]
29. Da Silva Mello, A.S.; dos Santos, P.L.; Marquesi, A.; Queiroz, T.P.; Margonar, R.; de Souza Faloni, A.P. Some aspects of bone remodeling around dental implants. *Rev. Clin. Periodoncia Implantol. Rehabil. Oral* **2016**, *11*, 49–53.
30. Oh, K.C.; Moon, H.S.; Lee, J.H.; Park, Y.B.; Kim, J.-H. Effects of alendronate on the peri-implant bone in rats. *Oral Dis.* **2015**, *21*, 248–256. [CrossRef]
31. Figuero-Filho, E.A.; Aydos, R.D.; Senefonte, F.R.; Ferreira, C.M.; Pereira, E.F.; de Oliveire, V.M.; de Menezes, G.P.; Bosio, M.A.C. Effects of enoxaparin and unfractioned heparin in prophylactic and therapeutic doses on the fertility of female Wistar rats. *Acta Cir. Bras.* **2014**, *29*, 410–416. [CrossRef] [PubMed]
32. Hiebert, L.M.; Ping, T.; Wice, S.M. Repeated doses of oral and subcutaneous heparins have similar antithrombotic effect in rat carotid arterial model of thrombosis. *J Cardiovasc. Pharm.* **2012**, *17*, 110–116. [CrossRef] [PubMed]
33. Miklosz, J.; Kalaska, B.; Kaminski, K.; Szczubialka, K.; Pawlak, D.; Nowakowska, M.; Mogielnicki, A. Heparin binding copolymer reverses the anticoagulant activity of low molecular weight heparins: Safety and efficacy data in rats. *Cardiovasc. Res.* **2018**, *114* (Suppl. 1), S95. [CrossRef]

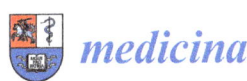

Case Report

Iatrogenic Ankle Charcot Neuropathic Arthropathy after Spinal Surgery: A Case Report and Literature Review

Sung Hwan Kim [1,†], Woo-Jong Kim [2,†], Eun Seok Park [1], Jun Yong Kim [1] and Young Koo Lee [1,*]

1. Department of Orthopaedic Surgery, Soonchunhyang University Hospital Bucheon, 170, Jomaru-ro, Wonmi-gu, Bucheon-si 14584, Republic of Korea
2. Department of Orthopaedic Surgery, Soonchunhyang University Hospital Cheonan, 31, Sooncheonhyang 6-gil, Dongnam-gu, Cheonan 31151, Republic of Korea
* Correspondence: brain0808@hanmail.net
† These authors contributed equally to this work and are co-first authors.

Abstract: Charcot neuropathic arthropathy is a relatively rare, chronic disease that leads to joint destruction and reduced quality of life of patients. Early diagnosis of Charcot arthropathy is essential for a good outcome. However, the diagnosis is often based on the clinical course and longitudinal follow-up of patients is required. Charcot arthropathy is suspected in patients with suggestive symptoms and an underlying etiology. Failed spinal surgery is not a known cause of Charcot arthropathy. Herein we report a patient with ankle Charcot neuropathic arthropathy that developed after failed spinal surgery. A 58-year-old man presented to the emergency room due to painful swelling of the left ankle for 2 weeks that developed spontaneously. He underwent spinal surgery 8 years ago that was associated with nerve damage, which led to weakness of great toe extension and ankle dorsiflexion, and sensory loss below the knee. CT and T2-weighted sagittal MRI showed a fine erosive lesion, subluxation, sclerosis, fragmentation, and large bone defects. Based on the patient's history and radiological findings, Charcot arthropathy was diagnosed. However, the abnormal blood parameters, positive blood cultures, and severe pain despite the decreased sensation suggested a diagnosis of septic arthritis. Therefore, diagnostic arthroscopy was performed. The ankle joint exhibited continued destruction after the initial surgery. Consequently, several repeat surgeries were performed over the next 2 years. Despite the early diagnosis and treatment of Charcot arthropathy, the destruction of the ankle joint continued. Given the chronic disease course and poor prognosis of Charcot arthropathy, it is essential to consider this diagnosis in patients with neuropathy.

Keywords: ankle; charcot neuropathic arthropathy; iatrogenic charcot; spinal surgery

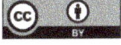

1. Introduction

Charcot neuropathic arthropathy was first reported by Jean-Martin Charcot in 1868 as a progressive joint disease characterized by gradual joint destruction [1]. It leads to painful or painless destruction of bones and joints in patients with neuropathy [2]. The pathophysiology of Charcot neuropathic arthropathy involves sensorineural, autonomic, and motor dysfunction, which lead to joint instability, osteopenia, microtrauma [3], acute localized inflammation, and bone destruction (e.g., subluxation, dislocation, and deformity) [4]. The joint deformity prevents the use of standard footwear and results in ulceration, deep infections, and even amputation [5]. The leading cause of Charcot arthropathy in previous decades was neurosyphilis; currently, the leading cause is diabetes mellitus [6]. Charcot arthropathy is often a chronic complication of diabetes mellitus with or without polyneuropathy [7]. Additionally, Charcot arthropathy may be caused by leprosy, spinal anesthesia, and spinal diseases [8]. A recent case report described a patient who developed knee Charcot arthropathy after spinal canal surgery [9]. However, there are no previous reports of ankle Charcot arthropathy caused by spinal surgery. Herein we describe a patient who developed ankle Charcot arthropathy after iatrogenic trauma during spinal surgery.

2. Case Presentation

2.1. Preoperative Evaluation

A 58-year-old man presented to the emergency room with painful swelling of the left ankle for 2 weeks that developed spontaneously. He had a history of spinal surgery and associated nerve damage 8 years ago, with residual weakness of great toe extension and ankle dorsiflexion and reduced sensation in the leg. He was able to ambulate for 50 m using a walker. The left ankle did not have a wound but was swollen, red, and warm (Figure 1). He complained of mild to moderate pain around the swollen left ankle. He had grade II great toe extension, ankle dorsiflexion and plantar flexion strength. Passive extension of the ankle was intact, with no limitation in the range of motion. There was partial sensory loss over the entire lower leg and foot. The patient had a sensory stimulus score of 2 below the ankle and 5 between the knee and ankle, compared to 10 at the normal. These deficits developed immediately after spinal surgery; the patient underwent rehabilitation therapy, which was unsuccessful. The blood glucose and HbA1c levels were 98 mg/dL (normal range: 60–99 mg/dL) and 5.5% (normal range: 4–6%), respectively. The erythrocyte sedimentation rate was 120 mm/hr (normal range: <5 mm/hr) and the C-reactive protein (CRP) level was 38.87 mg/dL (normal range: <0.5 mg/dL). A blood culture obtained in the emergency room showed the growth of methicillin-sensitive *Staphylococcus aureus* (MSSA). Radiographs showed erosion and subluxation of the distal tibiofibular joint and talus of both ankles (Figure 2). Computer tomography (CT) showed increased bone density around the ankle, indicating a chronic gliding mechanism. The tibial bone defect was similar in shape to the talar dome. In addition, multiple bony fragments were scattered in the distal tibia (Figure 3). T2-weighted coronal magnetic resonance imaging (MRI) revealed a cystic mass and joint destruction in the distal tibia with no erosion. There were no periarticular edema or bone marrow abnormalities (Figure 4). The patient was diagnosed with Charcot arthropathy based on the characteristic imaging findings of subluxation, sclerosis, fragmentation, and large bone defects. Although fine erosive lesions are less common in septic arthritis [2], the diagnosis of septic arthritis could not be excluded because of severe pain despite decreased sensations and abnormal blood parameters. Therefore, we performed arthroscopic surgery to exclude joint infection.

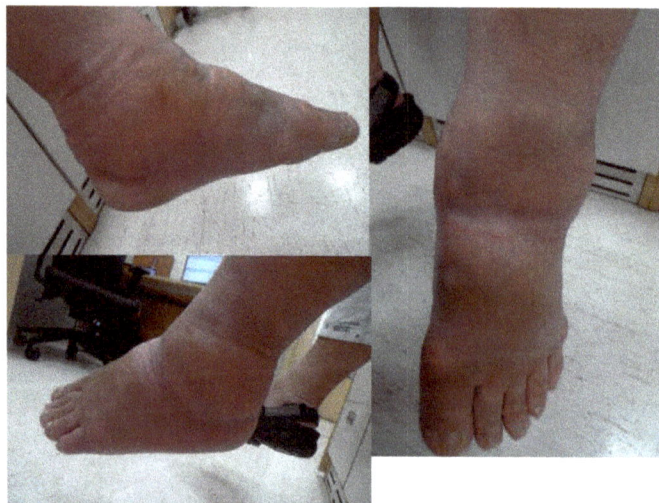

Figure 1. Left ankle at the time of presentation. There was no abrasion or laceration. The skin overlying the ankle joint was swollen and red.

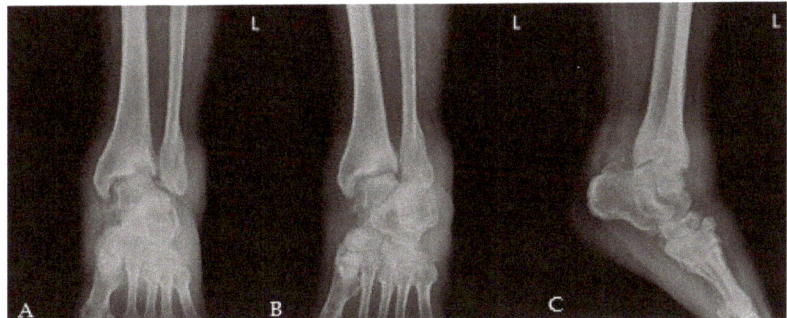

Figure 2. Initial left ankle X-ray. (**A**) Anteroposterior, (**B**) mortise, (**C**) lateral. Subluxations of the ankle joint and bony fragments were seen. An old healed fracture of the lateral malleolus was also visible.

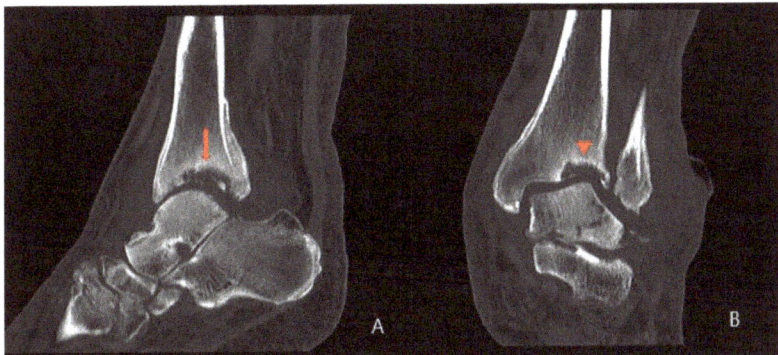

Figure 3. Initial left ankle: (**A**) sagittal and (**B**) coronal computer tomography scans. (**A**) Multiple bony fragments were scattered in the distal tibia (arrow). (**B**) The bone density was increased around the ankle and the tibial bone defect had a similar shape to the talar dome (arrowhead).

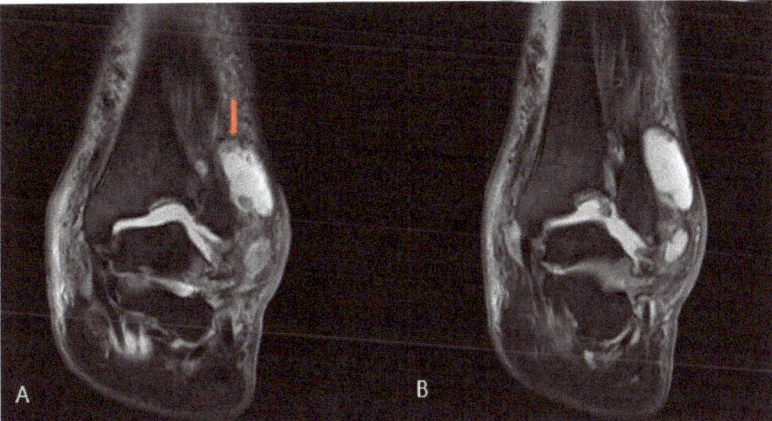

Figure 4. Initial left ankle T2-weighted coronal magnetic resonance imaging. (**A**) A cystic mass was seen near the distal fibula (arrow). (**B**) Joint destruction without bony erosion was seen in the distal tibia. There was no periarticular edema and the bone marrow was normal.

2.2. Surgical Procedure

Arthroscopic surgery was performed for examination and irrigation. Intraoperatively, bony fragments were scattered inside the ankle joint and the distal tibial articular surface was unevenly fragmented at the medial talar dome (Figure 5). The inflammatory tissue was debrided using a shaver and the free fragments were removed using forceps. The tissue culture obtained during surgery showed the growth of MSSA.

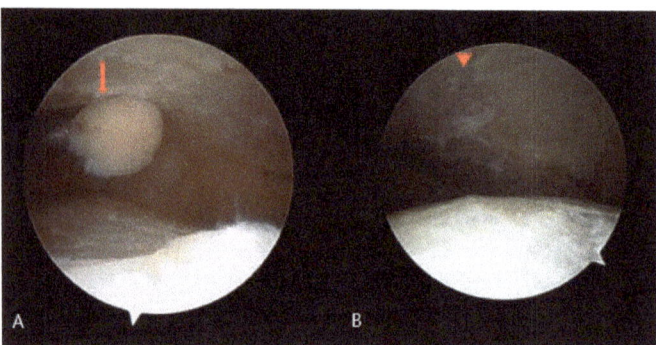

Figure 5. Findings during first arthroscopy. (**A**) Bony fragments were scattered inside the ankle. joint (arrow). (**B**) The distal tibial articular surface was unevenly fragmented at the level of the medial talar dome (arrowhead).

The CRP level remained high after the first surgery; therefore, the infectious diseases department was consulted and intravenous antibiotics were administered. Due to the persistently raised CRP level at 1 month after the first surgery, we performed a second surgery to insert an anti-bead and apply an external fixator. During the second surgery, soft tissue dissection revealed large quantities of fragile, chronic inflammatory tissue around the ankle (Figure 6). The tissue was removed by debridement and curettage. Then, an anti-bead was inserted and the Ilizarov apparatus was applied.

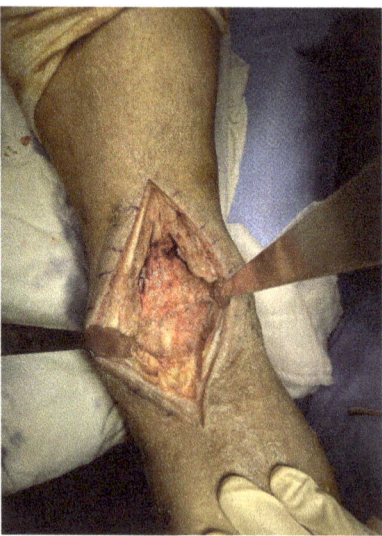

Figure 6. Intraoperative findings during the second surgery. A large quantity of fragile, chronic inflammatory tissue was observed around the ankle joint.

After the second operation, the patient was continued on intravenous antibiotics and the CRP level declined. Therefore, we performed anti-cement removal and tibiotalar fusion at 4 months after the second operation. After removal of the anti-bead inserted during the previous operation, rigid fixation using a locking screw and plate was performed, as well as a bone graft.

At the 1-year follow-up after the third operation, the patient exhibited talar subluxation at the site of ankle fusion. After discussion with the patient, subtalar fusion was performed. A bone graft was performed by harvesting auto bone in the left iliac area. The previously fused ankle joint showed talar subluxation. We performed decoration followed by grafting of the harvested auto-iliac bone. Staple and cannulated screws were used for rigid fixation. Finally, external fixation was applied using the Ilizarov fixator.

2.3. Postoperative Care

After the final surgery, the patient was regularly followed-up in the outpatient clinic; this is still ongoing. He has been advised to use a cam-walker and avoid weight bearing. The patient does not have significant pain but walking difficulty has persisted. The 1-year follow-up X-ray (Figure 7) showed no disruption of alignment but worsened bone collapse compared to the 2-month follow-up X-ray (Figure 8). The progressive bone collapse may require additional surgery. Although the patient has maintained alignment due to the avoidance of weight bearing, he may require amputation if subluxation or dislocation recurs.

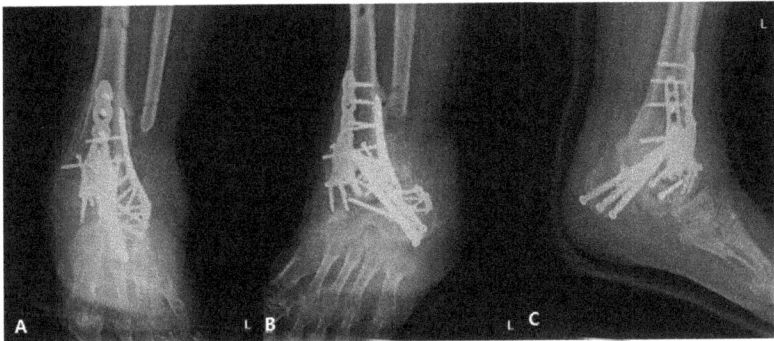

Figure 7. Left ankle X-ray. (**A**) Anteroposterior, (**B**) mortise, and (**C**) lateral images acquired 2 months after the final surgery. The images were obtained after removal of the external fixator.

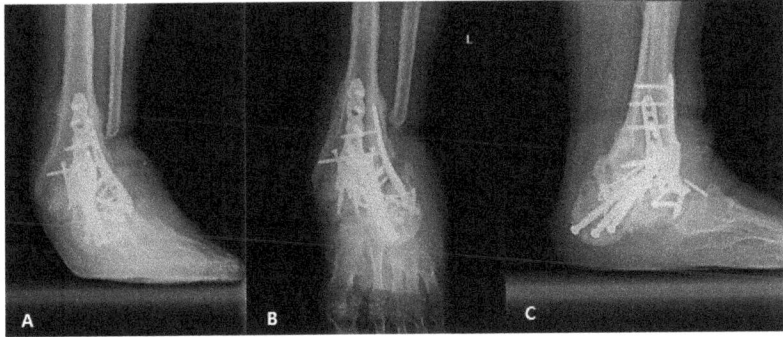

Figure 8. Left ankle X-ray. (**A**) Anteroposterior, (**B**) mortise, and (**C**) lateral images acquired 1 year after the final surgery. The X-ray showed progressive bone collapse but no worsening of alignment.

3. Discussion

Charcot neuropathic arthropathy has several causes, of which the most common is diabetes mellitus [10]. Other causes include several unrelated diseases that are complicated by nerve injury, including infection-related distal neuropathies (e.g., leprosy and syphilis), diseases of the spinal cord and nerve roots (e.g., tabes dorsalis, trauma, and syringomyelia), systemic diseases (e.g., Parkinson's disease, human immunodeficiency virus, sarcoidosis, rheumatoid disease, and psoriasis) [9], and toxins (e.g., ethanol and drug use) [11,12]. In our patient, the aforementioned causes were excluded based on the history, laboratory, and radiological findings. Our patient is similar to the previously reported case of knee Charcot neuropathic arthropathy that developed after nerve damage sustained during previous spinal surgery [7]. Our patient developed a superimposed infection that led to a high CRP level and growth of MSSA on the blood and tissue culture. The pathophysiology of Charcot neuropathic arthropathy involves increased blood flow to the bones due to damage to the sympathetic nerves, which results in bone resorption and weakening, ultimately leading to fractures and deformities [13]. Charcot neuropathic arthropathy is a chronic and progressive disease that is often difficult to diagnose [14]. The characteristic radiological findings of Charcot arthropathy include progressive bony destruction; however, there are no isolated laboratory or radiological findings that can confirm the diagnosis. Therefore, follow-up evaluation is often required [15]. Additionally, infection cannot be reliably excluded in cases with radiological findings of bony destruction. Therefore, laboratory and radiology examinations are often performed for patients with bony destruction [16]. In cases with infection, arthroscopy or incision and drainage and intravenous antibiotics, may be required. If the follow-up imaging reveals continued bone collapse despite no evidence of major trauma even after the infection has been treated, the possibility of Charcot neuropathic arthropathy should be considered [17]. The risk of Charcot arthropathy is particularly high in cases of neurological deficits, such as in our patient.

The limitation of this case report is that it describes a single case of Charcot arthropathy. Additionally, the pathophysiology of Charcot arthropathy was not explored. Despite early diagnosis and treatment of Charcot arthropathy, the disease continued to progress in our patient. The possibility of Charcot neuropathic arthropathy should be considered in patients with a history of neural trauma sustained during spinal surgery.

4. Conclusions

Spinal cord injury caused by neural trauma, such as failed spinal surgery, can cause Charcot neuropathic arthropathy. Therefore, such patients should be carefully evaluated for Charcot arthropathy, particularly in cases with severe bone collapse without a history of major trauma.

Author Contributions: Conceptualization, S.H.K. and Y.K.L.; methodology, S.H.K.; software, E.S.P.; validation, S.H.K. and E.S.P.; formal analysis, E.S.P.; investigation, Y.K.L.; resources, E.S.P.; data curation, J.Y.K.; writing—original draft preparation, S.H.K.; writing—review and editing, W.-J.K.; visualization, Y.K.L.; supervision, J.Y.K.; project administration, Y.K.L.; funding acquisition, S.H.K. All authors have read and agreed to the published version of the manuscript.

Funding: The authors would like to thank the Soonchunhyang University Research Fund for financial support (No. 2022-1004).

Institutional Review Board Statement: The study was conducted in accordance with the Declaration of Helsinki, and approved by the Institutional Review Board and Human Research Ethics Committee of Soonchunhyang University Bucheon Hospital (IRB No. 2022-09-018, 27 October 2022).

Informed Consent Statement: All of informed consent has been obtained from the patient to publish this paper.

Data Availability Statement: Data sharing is not applicable to this article because any datasets were made or analyzed during this study.

Conflicts of Interest: The authors declare that they have no conflict of interest.

Abbreviations

CRP	C-reactive protein
ESR	Erythrocyte sedimentation rate
CT	Computer tomography
MRI	Magnetic resonance imaging
MSSA	Methicillin-sensitive *Staphylococcus aureus*

References

1. Eichenholtz, S.N. Charcot joints. *J. Bone Jt. Surg.* **1962**, *44*, 1485.
2. Dardari, D. An overview of Charcot's neuroarthropathy. *J. Clin. Transl. Endocrinol.* **2020**, *22*, 100239. [CrossRef] [PubMed]
3. Rogers, L.C.; Frykberg, R.G.; Armstrong, D.G.; Boulton, A.J.; Edmonds, M.; Van, G.H.; Hartemann, A.; Game, F.; Jeffcoate, W.; Jirkovska, A.; et al. The Charcot foot in diabetes. *J. Am. Podiatr. Med. Assoc.* **2011**, *101*, 437–446. [CrossRef] [PubMed]
4. Sochocki, M.P.; Verity, S.; Atherton, P.J.; Huntington, J.L.; Sloan, J.A.; Embil, J.M.; Trepman, E. Health related quality of life in patients with Charcot arthropathy of the foot and ankle. *Foot Ankle Surg.* **2008**, *14*, 11–15. [CrossRef] [PubMed]
5. Wukich, D.K.; Sung, W.; Wipf, S.A.M.; Armstrong, D.G. The consequences of complacency: Managing the effects of unrecognized Charcot feet. *Diabet. Med.* **2011**, *28*, 195–198. [CrossRef] [PubMed]
6. Cianni, L.; Bocchi, M.B.; Vitiello, R.; Greco, T.; De Marco, D.; Masci, G.; Maccauro, G.; Pitocco, D.; Perisano, C. Arthrodesis in the Charcot foot: A systematic review. *Orthop. Rev.* **2020**, *12*, 8670. [CrossRef] [PubMed]
7. Cıvan, M.; Yazıcıoğlu, Ö.; Çakmak, M.; Akgül, T. Charcot arthropathy of the knee after unsuccessful spinal stenosis surgery: A case report. *Int. J. Surg. Case Rep.* **2017**, *36*, 22–25. [CrossRef] [PubMed]
8. Brown, C.W.; Jones, B.; Donaldson, D.H.; Akmakjian, J.; Brugman, J.L. Neuropathic (Charcot) Arthropathy of the Spine after Traumatic Spinal Paraplegia. *Spine* **1992**, *17*, S103–S108. [CrossRef] [PubMed]
9. Wukich, D.K.; Sung, W. Charcot arthropathy of the foot and ankle: Modern concepts and management review. *J. Diabetes Its Complicat.* **2009**, *23*, 409–426. [CrossRef] [PubMed]
10. Fabric, J.; Larsen, K.; Holstein, P.E. Long-term follow-up in diabetic Charcot feet with spontaneous onset. *Diabetes Care* **2000**, *23*, 796–800. [CrossRef] [PubMed]
11. McKay, D.J.; Sheehan, P.; DeLauro, T.M.; Iannuzzi, L.N. Vincristine-induced neuroarthropathy (Charcot's joint). *J. Am. Podiatr. Med. Assoc.* **2000**, *90*, 478–480. [CrossRef] [PubMed]
12. Arapostathi, C.; Tentolouris, N.; Jude, E.B. Charcot foot associated with chronic alcohol abuse. *BMJ Case Rep.* **2013**, *2013*, bcr2012008263. [CrossRef] [PubMed]
13. Jeffcoate, W.J.; Game, F.; Cavanagh, P.R. The role of proinflammatory cytokines in the cause of neuropathic osteoarthropathy (acute Charcot foot) in diabetes. *Lancet* **2005**, *366*, 2058–2061. [CrossRef] [PubMed]
14. Ramanujam, C.L.; Facaros, Z. An overview of conservative treatment options for diabetic Charcot foot neuroarthropathy. *Diabet. Foot Ankle* **2011**, *2*, 6418. [CrossRef] [PubMed]
15. Paliwal, V.K.; Singh, P.; Rahi, S.K.; Agarwal, V.; Gupta, R.K. Charcot knee secondary to lumbar spinal cord syringomyelia: Complication of spinal anesthesia. *J. Clin. Rheumatol.* **2012**, *18*, 207–208. [CrossRef] [PubMed]
16. Donegan, R.; Sumpio, B.; Blume, P.A. Charcot foot and ankle with osteomyelitis. *Diabet. Foot Ankle* **2013**, *4*, 21361. [CrossRef] [PubMed]
17. Illgner, U.; Wetz, H.H. Infections of Charcot Feet: Diagnostics and Treatment. *Clin. Res. Foot Ankle* **2014**, *S3*, 8. [CrossRef]

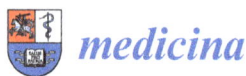

Article

Use of an Intramedullary Allogenic Fibular Strut Bone and Lateral Locking Plate for Distal Femoral Fracture with Supracondylar Comminution in Patients over 50 Years of Age

Wen-Chin Su [1], Tzai-Chiu Yu [1,2], Cheng-Huan Peng [1,2], Kuan-Lin Liu [1,2], Wen-Tien Wu [1,2,3], Ing-Ho Chen [1,2], Jen-Hung Wang [4] and Kuang-Ting Yeh [1,2,5,*]

[1] Department of Orthopedics, Hualien Tzu Chi Hospital, Buddhist Tzu Chi Medical Foundation, Hualien 970473, Taiwan
[2] School of Medicine, Tzu Chi University, Hualien 970374, Taiwan
[3] Institute of Medical Sciences, Tzu Chi University, Hualien 970374, Taiwan
[4] Department of Medical Research, Hualien Tzu Chi Hospital, Buddhist Tzu Chi Medical Foundation, Hualien 970473, Taiwan
[5] Graduate Institute of Clinical Pharmacy, Tzu Chi University, Hualien 970374, Taiwan
* Correspondence: micrograft@tzuchi.com.tw

Abstract: *Background and Objectives*: Distal femoral fracture is a severe injury that makes surgery challenging, particularly comminuted fractures in the supracondylar region. This study aimed to evaluate the outcomes of distal femoral fracture treated with the application of an intramedullary fibular allogenic bone strut in open reduction and internal fixation (ORIF) with precontoured locking plates in patients over 50 years of age. *Materials and Methods*: The study retrospectively enrolled 202 patients over 50 years of age with traumatic comminuted distal femoral fracture (AO/OTA 33-A3, 33-C2 and 33-C3) treated with ORIF with a locking plate from January 2016 to December 2019. The two groups were divided into patients who received an intramedullary allogenic bone strut and those who did not. Patients were followed for at least 1 year, with their function scores and radiographic data recorded. *Results*: A total of 124 patients were recruited, comprising 60 men and 64 women with an average age of 62.4 ± 8.5 years. The 36 patients who had received an intramedullary allogenic fibular bone strut reported lower postoperative pain scores at 1 month and lower postoperative Knee Society Scores (KSS) at 3 months than the control group. The application of an intramedullary allogenic fibular bone strut appeared to be significantly correlated with better 3-month postoperative KSS. *Conclusions*: The ORIF of distal femoral comminuted fracture with an intramedullary allogenic fibular bone strut can reduce pain and improve knee function in the early stages of postoperative rehabilitation and may reduce the time to union in patients over 50 years of age.

Keywords: distal femoral comminuted fracture; intramedullary allogenic fibular strut bone; knee society score; visual analogue scale for knee pain

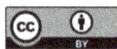

1. Introduction

Distal femoral fracture is a severe injury that is challenging to treat operatively. Less than 1% of all fracture patterns are accounted for in adult patients [1]. Incidents such as traffic accidents are the most common causes for such injuries in younger patients, whereas older adults or osteoporotic patients are likely to experience a higher rate of falls and knee contusions. This bimodal distribution introduces different treatment options along the distal femoral fracture [2]. Comminuted fracture, displaced fragments, and intra-articular involvement are often present. ORIF adequately realigns and reconstructs a smooth articular surface and provides immediate postoperative stability, fostering early rehabilitation [3]. Conservative treatment is indicated only for those unable to undergo surgery, such as patients with life-threatening conditions, medical comorbidities, or nondisplaced and stable fractures [4]. Precontoured locking compression plates are the most common implant type for distal femoral fracture; they provide better stability than dynamic condylar screws or angled blade plates and are thus ideal for osteoporotic or comminuted bone. Minimally invasive plate application can decrease damage to the fracture site's vascular supply [5]. Severe comminuted fracture patterns, poor bone quality, inadequate stabilization, insufficient blood supply, and infection can increase the nonunion rate. Nonunion rates ranged between 0% and 10% despite application of the locking plate [6]. Peschiera et al. noted that metaphyseal comminution, bone loss, and malalignment may contribute to a high nonunion rate and proposed that an allograft bone strut be considered when a medial cortical defect more than 2 cm in length is observed intraoperatively [7]. The use of allogenic bone graft has decreased due to challenges in allogenic bone graft procurement and the increased frequency of locking plate application; nevertheless, this method has been applied for decades. However, a biomechanical study has indicated that the use of intramedullary allogenic bone strut combined with locking plate provides superior mechanical stability in unstable osteoporotic proximal humeral fractures [8]. Suh et al. also documented that hybrid use of allogenic bone graft can provide global stability in total knee arthroplasty (TKA) supracondylar periprosthetic fracture [9].

Research has not explored the hybrid use of locking plates and allogenic bone strut in fresh distal femoral fracture. We conducted a single-center retrospective study to evaluate the perioperative trauma and surgical parameters, the functional outcomes as knee society score (KSS) and visual analogue scale (VAS) for knee pain, and the radiographic union status as radiographic union score of the femur (RUSF) of precontoured locking plates combined with allogenic bone strut use in comminuted distal femoral fracture.

2. Materials and Methods

The study was conducted in accordance with the Declaration of Helsinki and approved by the Research Ethics Committee of Hualien Tzu Chi Hospital, Buddhist Tzu Chi Medical Foundation. Our trauma center cares for 500,000 people in eastern Taiwan. This retrospective study enrolled 202 patients with new distal femoral fracture between January 2016 and December 2019 and followed the participants for at least 1 year. Eligibility criteria were as follows: patients over 50 years of age with a new traumatic comminuted distal femoral fracture (AO/OTA 33-A3, 33-C2 and 33-C3) treated with ORIF with a locking plate. An intramedullary allogenic bone strut application was determined mainly by two factors: (1) the preference and experience of the surgeon individually and (2) the existence or absence of allogenic bone strut in the bone bank at the time point of surgery. The exclusion criteria were as follows: patients with pathologic or concomitant fractures, active malignancy, or infection. The traumatic mechanism of injury and preoperative and postoperative VAS scores were recorded. Outcome measurements included postoperative radiological union and knee function with KSS. Adequate radiologic bone union was defined as the detection of callus bridging in three out of four cortices at the fracture site as observed through anterolateral and lateral radiography. We also used RUSF for evaluation of callus formation of the four cortices of the follow-up radiographs of the patients. RUSF was based on the assessment of healing at each cortex (i.e., medial and lateral cortices on the anteroposterior plain film as well as anterior and posterior cortices on the lateral film) [10].

2.1. Surgical Technique

The objectives of distal femoral fracture management are to achieve anatomic reduction of the joint surface and restore the limb's length, rotation, and mechanical axis. The patient was positioned in the supine position with a cushion placed under the ipsilateral buttock. The original lateral approach was administered, and an incision was made in the iliotibial band parallel to the fiber. Vastus lateralis muscle fascia was incised and retracted anteromedially. Care was taken to avoid excess periosteal stripping. The Swashbuckler approach was used in the case of intra-articular comminuted fracture [11]. The surgical incision was extended in the lateral parapatellar approach, and the capsulotomy technique was performed upon approaching the articular surface. Fracture fragments should first be identified through radiography or computed tomography. Adequate reduction of large bone fragments should be completed with the fixation of interfragmentary screws, wire, or Kirschner wire (K-wire). In the presence of severe comminution, an intramedullary allogenic bone strut can be inserted through the gap between comminuted fragments. Indirect reduction of the medial comminuted fragment or oblique medial cortex is then achieved. Further medialization of the bone strut by the K-wire "joystick" manipulation technique can reduce the medial comminuted cortex to its original position and augment the medial column in the case of massive medial cortical bone defect (Figure 1). A bone strut can sometimes be inserted through the intercondylar notch [12]. If the comminuted condyle is too fragile to be reduced in size, the bone strut can be advanced distally for the indirect reduction of the distal femoral articular block and facilitation of distal screw purchase. Temporary fixation with K-wire and a reduction clamp can be used to align the mechanical axis and lateral distal femoral angle. If the limb length, rotation, and mechanical axis are restored, the precontoured locking plate can be applied to neutralize the fracture (Figure 2). We presented short- and long-term radiographic follow-up of a 49-year-old female patient (Figure 3) and a 19 -year-old male patient (Figure 4), and they both had good postoperative function recovery and bone union.

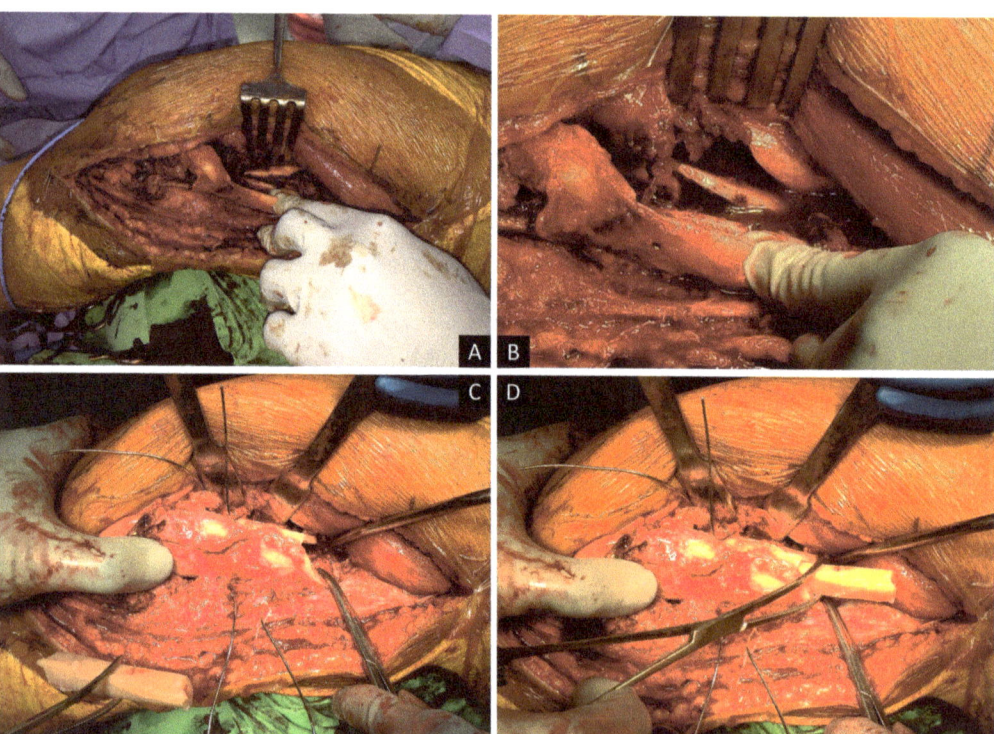

Figure 1. This is a 49-year-old female patient without any systemic disease admitted to our emergency department due to a traffic accident. Distal femoral fracture with AO33-C2 was diagnosed (Figure 3). Severe comminution of metaphysis with large bone defect was noted (**A**,**B**). We repositioned all the bone fragments (**C**) and an allogenic fibular strut was chosen for restoration of the fractured bone. Wire was applied as an outer restriction for fragment reposition (**D**). Allogenic bone strut supplied an inner supportive structure and wire was tied. Last, a precontoured locking plate was applied and proximal screws were inserted with minimal invasive technique.

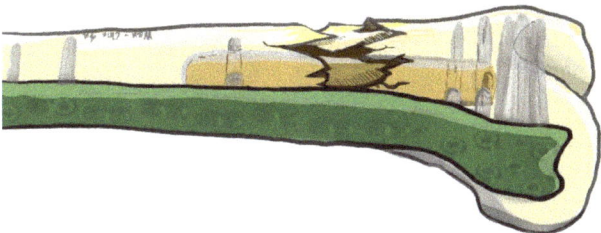

Figure 2. This figure shows the intramedullary application of the strut bone for distal femoral fracture. The strut bone provides fixation stability and medial cortex support.

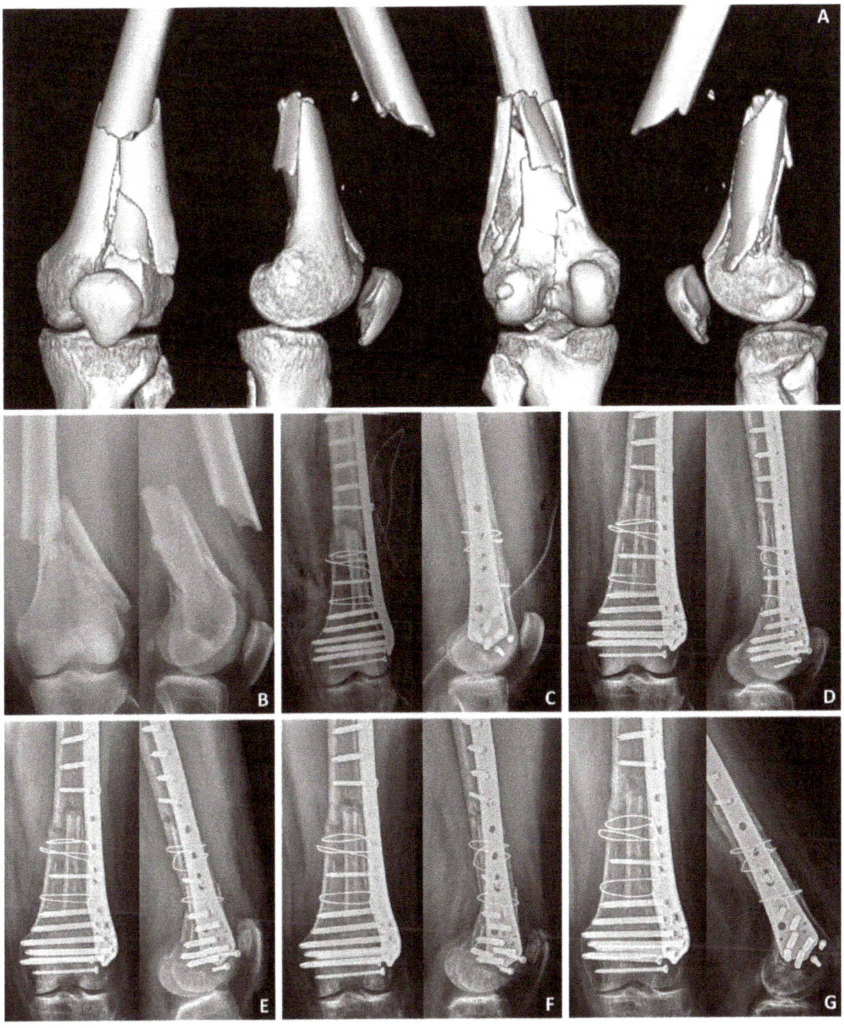

Figure 3. Radiography and computed tomography of the 49-year-old female patient with comminuted distal femoral fracture and good surgical result. (**A**) CT; (**B**) Pre-OP; (**C**) Post-OP; (**D**) Post-OP 1 month; (**E**) Post-OP 3 months; (**F**) Post-OP 6 months; (**G**) Post-OP 1 year.

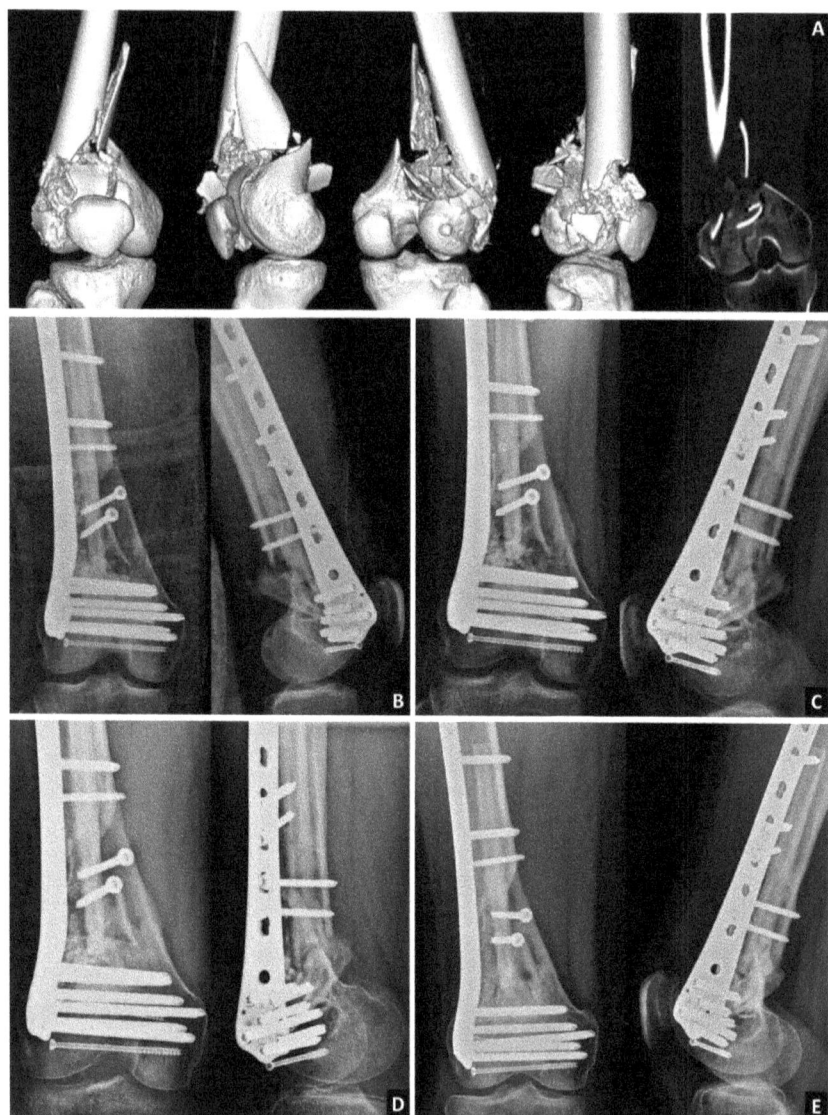

Figure 4. A 19-year-old male patient was involved in a traffic accident. Distal femoral open fracture with a 4 cm open wound at the anterolateral side of the distal femur. Computed tomography showed a severe comminuted metaphysis, AO 33-C2. After adequate debridement and irrigation, an allogenic fibular strut was applied. Medial cortex was fixed on the fibular strut. Allogenic TKA bone chip was stuff in the bone defect. (**A**) CT; (**B**) Post-OP; (**C**) Post-OP 3 months; (**D**) Post-OP 6 months; (**E**) Post-OP 1 year.

2.2. Source, Preparation and Storage of the Allogenic Bone Strut

The allogenic fibular strut bone was harvested from a brain-dead donor diagnosed by two different doctors. The donor was screened for syphilis (STS-RPR), HIV antibody (EIA), hepatitis B (HBs antigen), hepatitis C (anti-HCV antibody) and blood culture preoperatively. If all the laboratory screening tests were normal, allograft harvest could be administered. After the allogenic bone strut was retrieved and cleaned by normal saline solution, bacteria culture was swabbed immediately on each bone graft. The bone graft was packed in three layers of sterile plastic bags and stored in the bone bank at −70 °C. The bone graft could be applied to the orthopedic surgery after all the intraoperative bacteria culture data were negative for bacterial growth.

2.3. Statistical Analysis

Statistical analysis was performed using SPSS for Windows, version 23.0 (IBM, Armonk, NY, USA). Descriptive statistics (means, standard deviations, ranges, coefficients of variation, and proportions) were calculated, and an independent t-test was used for comparisons. A generalized linear model (GLM) was used to evaluate risk factors associated with KSS at 3 months and 1 year postoperative.

3. Results

A total of 202 patients were enrolled in the study between January 2016 and December 2019. Four patients expired during hospitalization due to comorbidities. An additional 74 patients did not engage in regular follow-up care, and their data were thus incomplete. The remaining 124 patients comprised 60 men and 64 women with an average age of 62.4 ± 8.5 years (Table 1).

Table 1. Demographic data of the included patients ($n = 124$).

Variable	Without Fibular Strut	With Fibular Strut	Total	p-Value
N	84	40	124	
Age	61.3 ± 9.7	64.9 ± 9.9	62.4 ± 8.5	0.065
Gender	-	-	-	0.082
Male	38 (45.2%)	14 (35.0%)	52 (41.9%)	
Female	46 (54.8%)	26 (65.0%)	72 (58.1%)	
Mechanism	-	-	-	0.073
Fall from height	26 (31.0%)	18 (45.0%)	44 (35.5%)	
Traffic accident	58 (69.0%)	22 (55.0%)	80 (64.5%)	
AO Type	-	-	-	0.086
A3	21 (25.0%)	16 (40.0%)	37 (29.8%)	
C	63 (75.0%)	24 (60.0%)	87 (70.2%)	
Blood loss	666.4 ± 152.5	475.6 ± 92.8	580.3 ± 135.1	0.102
Length of Stay	15.9 ± 5.8	10.0 ± 2.2	12.1 ± 10.0	0.144

Data are presented as n or mean ± standard deviation.

Traffic accidents were the cause of fracture for 80 patients. In total, 37 patients had AO/OTA type A3 fracture and the other 87 had AO/OTA type C1-3 fracture. The mean intraoperative blood loss was 580.3 ± 135.1 mL, and the mean length of hospital stay was 12.1 ± 10.0 days. We divided the patients into two groups based on their use or nonuse of an intramedullary allogenic fibular bone strut. Eighty-four patients received ORIF without intramedullary allogenic fibular bone strut and 40 patients received ORIF with intramedullary allogenic fibular bone strut (Table 1). In the postoperative evaluation of the distal femoral fracture, postoperative 1-month VAS ($p = 0.043$) score and postoperative 3-month KSS were significantly lower in the group that received the intramedullary allogenic fibular bone strut ($p < 0.001$; Table 2).

Postoperative 3-month RUSFs were significantly better in the group that received the intramedullary allogenic fibular bone strut ($p = 0.021$; Table 2), while postoperative 1-year RUSFs were slightly better in the group that received the intramedullary allogenic fibular bone strut with marginal significance ($p = 0.064$; Table 2). The mean bone union period was 7.4 ± 2.2 months with no significant difference between groups (Table 2). We performed a risk analysis between postoperative 3-month KSS and postoperative 1-year KSS. According to the GLM results, the use of intramedullary allogenic fibular bone strut is significantly correlated with better postoperative 3-month KSS ($p < 0.001$); old age and male sex are significantly correlated with poorer postoperative 1-year KSS ($p = 0.007$ and 0.009; Table 3).

Table 2. Postoperative functional evaluation of both groups (n = 124).

Variable	Without Fibular Strut	With Fibular Strut	Total	p-Value
VAS for knee pain (2W)	4.9 ± 1.1	5.1 ± 0.7	4.9 ± 0.9	0.328
VAS for knee pain (1M)	2.5 ± 1.0	2.0 ± 0.9	2.3 ± 0.9	0.043 *
Knee society score (3M)	66.4 ± 3.6	77.7 ± 1.5	69.7 ± 6.1	<0.001 *
Knee society score (1Y)	84.4 ± 5.0	85.8 ± 3.2	84.8 ± 4.6	0.209
Radiographic union score of the femur (3M)	6.4 ± 2.3	8.3 ± 2.2	7.0 ± 2.1	0.021 *
Radiographic union score of the femur (1Y)	9.5 ± 1.8	10.3 ± 1.3	9.8 ± 1.5	0.064
Union period (M)	7.7 ± 2.5	6.9 ± 0.9	7.4 ± 2.2	0.105

Data are presented as n or mean ± standard deviation. * p-value < 0.05 was considered statistically significant after test. VAS: visual analogue scale; M: month; Y: year.

Table 3. Factors associated with knee society score at 3 months and 1year after operation among patients (n = 124).

Variable	Knee Society Score (3M)		Knee society Score (1Y)	
	β (95% CI)	p-Value	β (95% CI)	p-Value
Intercept	65.76 (62.32, 69.21)	<0.001 *	88.69 (83.99, 93.39)	<0.001 *
Age	−0.02 (−0.06, 0.02)	0.365	−0.08 (−0.14, −0.02)	0.007 *
Gender	-	-	-	-
Male	1.15 (−0.32, 2.62)	0.123	−2.69 (−4.70, −0.68)	0.009 *
Female	References	NA	References	NA
Mechanism	-	-	-	-
Fall down	0.38 (−1.19, 1.95)	0.630	2.00 (−0.13, 4.14)	0.066
Traffic accident	References	NA	References	NA
LOS	0.05 (−0.02, 0.13)	0.129	−0.02 (−0.12, 0.08)	0.665
AO Type	-	-	-	-
A3	References	NA	References	NA
C	−0.25 (−1.92, 1.43)	0.770	0.13 (−2.16, 2.42)	0.912
Locking Plate	-	-	-	-
No	References	NA	References	NA
Yes	0.36 (−1.54, 2.25)	0.709	1.02 (−1.57, 3.60)	0.436
Application of fibular strut graft	-	-	-	-
No	References	NA	References	NA
Yes	12.04 (10.46, 13.63)	<0.001 *	1.04 (−1.12, 3.20)	0.341

Data are presented as odds ratio (95% CI). * p-value < 0.05 was considered statistically significant after test. M: month; Y: year.

4. Discussion

Minimally invasive osteosynthesis is the current preferred distal femoral fracture treatment strategy. The previous technique, which entailed substantial stripping of the periosteum and destruction of surrounding soft tissue, can disrupt the vascular supply, contributing to delayed union or nonunion [13,14]. Despite the frequent application of minimally invasive plate osteosynthesis, nonunion rates of distal femoral fracture remain at 0–10% [15]. Researchers have demonstrated that the predisposal of fresh distal femoral fracture to nonunion is due to metaphyseal bone defects, an inability to obtain adequate bony fixation, and a failure to augment bone grafts to address metaphyseal comminution [16]. Kubiak et al. revealed that rigid fixation by locking plates may restrict fracture healing under the principle of secondary healing [17]. As reported by Peschiera et al., malreduction caused by axial defects and medial cortical bone defects are the major risk factors of nonunion [7]. Patients in whom these two problems were unaddressed were reported to have a nonunion rate of approximately 12%. Peschiera et al. also proposed the application of medial support, such as a bone strut allograft or medial buttress plate, for medial cortical defects over 2 cm in length.

The use of an intramedullary allogenic bone strut can resolve the aforementioned causes of nonunion. First, an intramedullary allogenic bone strut can reduce the rate of malreduction. It is difficult to align the comminuted distal femoral fracture using a minimally invasive technique. If a long allogenic bone strut is inserted into the diaphysis and metaphysis, the strut can realign and reduce the displaced and comminuted fragments. Second, bone defects caused by metaphyseal comminution can be corrected with additional bone graft struts. Poor screw purchase may be encountered when the locking screw is applied at a comminuted metaphysis and condyle. Better screw purchase can be obtained between the locking plate and bone strut of this loose area and can provide augmented fixation and early stability. Third, intramedullary allogenic bone struts can function as a substitute for medial cortical bone defects and provide additional screw purchase stability. The use of a medial buttress plate for this defect can help prevent periosteal stripping at the medial distal femur.

According to a biomechanical study on TKA periprosthetic distal femoral fracture by Chen et al., locking plate fixation with intramedullary allograft provided better construct stiffness and less fracture micromotion and implant stress than the use of a locking plate alone. An allogenic bone strut can aid in partial knee load transmission and decrease the moment arm between the allograft and condyles, which can reduce the mechanical demands of the lateral less invasive stabilization system and help stabilize osteosynthesis [18].

Concerns may arise over the substantial stripping of the periosteum and destruction to surrounding soft tissue during insertion of the intramedullary allogenic bone strut. Because we addressed the problems of metaphyseal bone defects, an inability to obtain adequate bony fixation, and a failure to augment bone grafts in cases of metaphyseal comminution, cases of nonunion were absent in our data set. Although the application of an intramedullary allogenic bone strut had no significant associations, the data indicated that application may decrease union time. In addition, both short-term VAS and KSS were found to have statistically significant relationships in the intramedullary allogenic bone strut group. According to the results, excellent biochemical stability is produced by better construct stiffness and less fracture micromotion and implant stress, and greater relief of postoperative pain and early rehabilitation and range of motion can be achieved. Older adults can anticipate a better prognosis and less postoperative comorbidity due to timely rehabilitation. In addition, a lower ORIF revision rate and reduction in social and financial burden can be expected.

This retrospective study has several limitations. First, the sample was small and nonrandomized. Second, data on comprehensive comorbidities with the potential to influence fusion time, such as diabetes mellitus and smoking history, were not recorded. We also did not evaluate the local bone density status of the knee of the patients. In addition, the small sample size did not allow us to evaluate the AO classification subtype. The distal femur bone stock could not be classified precisely because some patients did not undergo preoperative computed tomography.

Nonetheless, the study demonstrated the efficacy of the intramedullary allogenic fibular bone strut among patients over 50 years of age with distal femoral fracture with comminution of the supracondylar region, especially in the early recovery stage. Future studies will focus on the comparison of this structure with other kinds of ORIF structures.

5. Conclusions

ORIF of comminuted distal femoral fracture with intramedullary allogenic bone fibular strut can reduce pain and improve knee function in the early stages of postoperative rehabilitation and may reduce union time. We particularly recommend intramedullary allogenic bone strut application for older patients.

Author Contributions: Conceptualization, T.-C.Y. and I.-H.C.; methodology, K.-T.Y.; software, J.-H.W.; validation, C.-H.P., K.-L.L. and W.-T.W.; formal analysis, J.-H.W.; investigation, C.-H.P.; resources, K.-L.L.; data curation, W.-C.S.; writing—original draft preparation, W.-C.S.; writing—review and editing, K.-T.Y.; visualization, I.-H.C.; supervision, W.-T.W. All authors have read and agreed to the published version of the manuscript.

Funding: This research received no external funding.

Institutional Review Board Statement: The study was conducted in accordance with the Declaration of Helsinki and approved by the Research Ethics Committee of Hualien Tzu Chi Hospital, Buddhist Tzu Chi Medical Foundation (IRB110-231A, 10 November 2021).

Informed Consent Statement: Informed consent was obtained from all subjects involved in the study.

Data Availability Statement: Data are contained within the article.

Conflicts of Interest: The authors declare no conflict of interest.

References

1. Gwathmey, F.W., Jr.; Jones-Quaidoo, S.M.; Kahler, D.; Hurwitz, S.; Cui, Q. Distal femoral fractures: Current concepts. *J. Am. Acad. Orthop. Surg.* **2010**, *18*, 597–607. [CrossRef] [PubMed]
2. Martinet, O.; Cordey, J.; Harder, Y.; Maier, A.; Bühler, M.; Barraud, G.E. The epidemiology of fractures of the distal femur. *Injury* **2000**, *31*, C62–C63. [CrossRef] [PubMed]
3. Stoffel, K.; Sommer, C.; Lee, M.; Zhu, T.Y.; Schwieger, K.; Finkemeier, C. Double fixation for complex distal femoral fractures. *EFORT Open Rev.* **2022**, *7*, 274–286. [CrossRef] [PubMed]
4. von Keudell, A.; Shoji, K.; Nasr, M.; Lucas, R.; Dolan, R.; Weaver, M.J. Treatment options for distal femur fractures. *J. Orthop. Trauma.* **2016**, *2*, S25–S27. [CrossRef] [PubMed]
5. Kayali, C.; Agus, H.; Turgut, A. Successful results of minimally invasive surgery for comminuted supracondylar femoral fractures with LISS: Comparative study of multiply injured and isolated femoral fractures. *J. Orthop. Sci.* **2007**, *12*, 458–465. [CrossRef] [PubMed]
6. Henderson, C.E.; Kuhl, L.L.; Fitzpatrick, D.C.; Marsh, J.L. Locking plates for distal femur fractures: Is there a problem with fracture healing? *J. Orthop. Trauma* **2011**, *25*, S8–S14. [CrossRef] [PubMed]
7. Peschiera, V.; Staletti, L.; Cavanna, M.; Saporito, M.; Berlusconi, M. Predicting the failure in distal femur fractures. *Injury* **2018**, *49*, S2–S7. [CrossRef] [PubMed]
8. Hsiao, C.K.; Tsai, Y.J.; Yen, C.Y.; Lee, C.H.; Yang, T.Y.; Tu, Y.K. Intramedullary cortical bone strut improves the cyclic stability of osteoporotic proximal humeral fractures. *BMC Musculoskele Disord.* **2017**, *18*, 64. [CrossRef] [PubMed]
9. Suh, D.; Ji, J.H.; Heu, J.Y.; Kim, J.Y.; Chi, H.; Lee, S.W. Use of an intramedullary fibular strut allograft and dual locking plate in periprosthetic fractures above total knee arthroplasty: New application of a well-known treatment method in trauma. *Eur. J. Trauma Emerg. Surg.* **2022**, *48*, 4105–4111. [CrossRef] [PubMed]
10. Chen, Y.H.; Liao, H.J.; Lin, S.M.; Chang, C.H.; Rwei, S.P.; Lan, T.Y. Radiographic outcomes of the treatment of complex femoral shaft fractures (AO/OTA 32-C) with intramedullary nailing: A retrospective analysis of different techniques. *J. Int. Med. Res.* **2022**, *50*, 3000605221103974. [CrossRef]
11. Raja, B.S.; Gowda, A.K.S.; Baby, B.K.; Chaudhary, S.; Meena, P.K. Swashbuckler approach for distal femur fractures: A systematic review. *J. Clin. Orthop. Trauma* **2021**, *24*, 101705. [CrossRef] [PubMed]
12. Levack, A.E.; Gadinsky, N.; Gausden, E.B.; Klinger, C.; Helfet, D.L.; Lorich, D.G. The Use of Fibular Allograft in Complex Periarticular Fractures Around the Knee. *Oper. Tech. Orthop.* **2018**, *28*, 141–151. [CrossRef] [PubMed]
13. Schütz, M.; Müller, M.; Krettek, C.; Höntzsch, D.; Regazzoni, P.; Ganz, R.; Haas, N. Minimally invasive fracture stabilization of distal femoral fractures with the LISS: A prospective multicenter study. Results of a clinical study with special emphasis on difficult cases. *Injury* **2001**, *32*, SC48–SC54. [CrossRef] [PubMed]
14. Ricci, W.M.; Loftus, T.; Cox, C.; Borrelli, J. Locked plates combined with minimally invasive insertion technique for the treatment of periprosthetic supracondylar femur fractures above a total knee arthroplasty. *J. Orthop. Trauma* **2006**, *20*, 190–196. [CrossRef] [PubMed]
15. Ricci, W.M.; Streubel, P.N.; Morshed, S.; Collinge, C.A.; Nork, S.E.; Gardner, M.J. Risk factors for failure of locked plate fixation of distal femur fractures: An analysis of 335 cases. *J. Orthop. Trauma* **2014**, *28*, 83–89. [CrossRef] [PubMed]

16. Ebraheim, N.A.; Martin, A.; Sochacki, K.R.; Liu, J. Nonunion of distal femoral fractures: A systematic review. *Orthop. Surg.* **2013**, *5*, 46–50. [CrossRef] [PubMed]
17. Kubiak, E.N.; Fulkerson, E.; Strauss, E.; Egol, K.A. The evolution of locked plates. *J. Bone Joint Surg. Am.* **2006**, *88*, S189–S200.
18. Chen, S.H.; Chiang, M.C.; Hung, C.H.; Lin, S.C.; Chang, H.W. Finite element comparison of retrograde intramedullary nailing and locking plate fixation with/without an intramedullary allograft for distal femur fracture following total knee arthroplasty. *Knee* **2014**, *21*, 224–231. [CrossRef] [PubMed]

Disclaimer/Publisher's Note: The statements, opinions and data contained in all publications are solely those of the individual author(s) and contributor(s) and not of MDPI and/or the editor(s). MDPI and/or the editor(s) disclaim responsibility for any injury to people or property resulting from any ideas, methods, instructions or products referred to in the content.

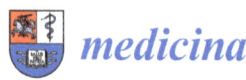

Article

Application of Cortical Bone Plate Allografts Combined with Less Invasive Stabilization System (LISS) Plates in Fixation of Comminuted Distal Femur Fractures

Zhimin Guo, Hui Liu, Deqing Luo, Taoyi Cai, Jinhui Zhang and Jin Wu *

Department of Orthopaedics, The 909th Hospital, School of Medicine, Xiamen University, Zhangzhou 363000, China
* Correspondence: wujin1983@xmu.edu.cn; Tel.: +86-0596-2931538

Abstract: *Background and Objectives:* At present, the management of comminuted distal femur fractures remains challenging for orthopedic surgeons. The aim of this study is to report a surgical treatment for comminuted distal femur fractures using supplementary medial cortical bone plate allografts in conjunction with the lateral less invasive stabilization system (LISS) plates. *Materials and Methods:* From January 2009 to January 2014, the records of thirty-three patients who underwent supplementary medial cortical bone plate allografts combined with lateral LISS plates fixation were reviewed. Clinical and radiographic data were collected during regular postoperative follow-up visits. Functional outcomes were determined according to the special surgery knee rating scale (HSS) used at the hospital. *Results:* Thirty patients were followed for 13 to 73 months after surgery, with an average follow-up time of 31.3 months. The mean time to bone union was 5.4 months (range of 3–12 months) and the mean range of knee flexion was 105.6° (range of 80–130°). Of the remaining patients, 10 had a score of "Excellent", while 10 had a score of "Good". Three patients had superficial or deep infections, one patient had nonunion that required bone grafting, and one patient had post-traumatic knee arthritis. *Conclusions:* Based on these promising results, we propose that supplementary medial cortical bone plate allografts combined with lateral LISS plate fixation may be a good treatment option for comminuted distal femur fractures. This treatment choice not only resulted in markedly improved stability on the medial side of the femur, but also satisfactory outcomes for distal femoral fractures.

Keywords: distal femur fracture; cortical bone plate allografts; LISS plates

Citation: Guo, Z.; Liu, H.; Luo, D.; Cai, T.; Zhang, J.; Wu, J. Application of Cortical Bone Plate Allografts Combined with Less Invasive Stabilization System (LISS) Plates in Fixation of Comminuted Distal Femur Fractures. *Medicina* **2023**, *59*, 207. https://doi.org/10.3390/medicina59020207

Academic Editor: Woo Jong Kim

Received: 6 December 2022
Revised: 11 January 2023
Accepted: 12 January 2023
Published: 20 January 2023

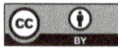

Copyright: © 2023 by the authors. Licensee MDPI, Basel, Switzerland. This article is an open access article distributed under the terms and conditions of the Creative Commons Attribution (CC BY) license (https://creativecommons.org/licenses/by/4.0/).

1. Introduction

Distal femoral fractures comprise approximately 3–6% of all femoral fractures [1]. Up to now, effective treatment of comminuted distal femur fractures remains difficult for orthopedic surgeons. These fractures are often unstable and comminuted, typically resulting either from falls in female patients older than 75 years or as a result of the high-energy activities common amongst adolescent boys and men aged 15 to 24 years [2]. Classification of distal femur fractures was first described by Müller et al. and expanded in the AO/OTA classification [3,4]. These classifications are based on fracture location and pattern and are useful in determining treatment and prognosis. With the development of improved internal fixation devices, operative treatment can now produce better results than nonoperative treatment. This is especially true for comminuted supracondylar and intercondylar femur fractures [5].

A complete set of instruments and familiarity with their use are required for surgical treatment of comminuted distal femur fractures. Condylar buttress plates, dynamic condylar screws (DCS), intramedullary nailing, LISS plates, and external fixation were introduced to facilitate the treatment of these types of fractures [6–9]. However, the spectrum of injuries is so great that no single implant has been found to be suitable for every case.

Moreover, patient outcomes with these types of fractures are generally unsatisfactory due to the proximity of the fracture to the knee joint [10], meaning that regaining full knee motion and function may be difficult, and significant complications such as malunion, nonunion, infection, malrotation, and implant failure occur at relatively high rates in many reports [11–15].

Given these challenges, this study investigated a surgical treatment strategy for comminuted distal femur fractures. The fractures included in this study were in accordance with AO/OTA classification, consisting of patients with either type A3 fractures involving distal shaft comminution, type C2 fractures involving metaphyseal comminution, or type C3 fractures characterized by metaphyseal and intra-articular comminution. The approach described here features the use of a supplementary medial cortical bone plate allograft in conjunction with a lateral LISS plate. Therapeutic effects were assessed in patients, with an average follow-up time of 31.3 months.

2. Patient and Method

2.1. Clinical Data

This study was a retrospective analysis of existing clinical cases and was approved by the institutional review board. Written informed consent was obtained preoperatively for all patients. Thirty-three patients (twenty males and thirteen females) were enrolled in the study between January 2009 and January 2014. All patients were diagnosed according to clinical presentation, X-ray, and computer tomography (CT) scans. Study participants were evaluated postoperatively every 1–2 months in the outpatient clinic.

2.2. Preoperative Preparation

Proximal tibial skeletal traction was performed immediately after all patients with closed fractures were admitted to the hospital. Patients with Gustilo I and Gustilo II open fractures first underwent debridement and suturing, after which they received proximal tibial skeletal traction. In two patients with a Gustilo III fracture, limited internal fixation combined with external fixation was implemented following debridement. All patients with open fractures received postoperative intravenous antibiotics for 24 to 48 h. X-ray and CT examinations were used to visualize fracture displacement and the presence of fragments when determining the surgical strategy for each patient. All patients underwent surgical treatment as soon as their condition had stabilized.

2.3. Surgical Procedure

Prophylactic antibiotics were given 30 min prior to surgery. No tourniquet was used. The patient was placed under either general or spinal anesthesia and then positioned in a supine position with a bolster under the knee to acquire 20–30° of flexion. This was performed in order to relax the deforming force of the gastrocnemius. For type A3 fractures, a 4–5 cm lateral incision was made just proximal to the joint line. A distal femoral LISS plate (AO, Synthes Inc., West Chester, PA, USA) was slipped under the vastus lateralis proximally and provisionally fixed distally using K wires. Close reduction was accomplished using traction and external manipulation and confirmed under fluoroscopy. During the procedure, specific attention was paid to limb alignment and length. When the position of the LISS plate was deemed satisfactory, three to six locking screws were inserted in the distal and proximal part of the bone, respectively.

For type C2 and C3 fractures, an incision was made on the lateral condyle of the femur and elongated to the tibial tubercle to fully expose the anterior and lateral aspects of the femoral condyle. Intercondylar fractures were then reduced and fixed with cannulated screws (AO) to form the supracondylar fracture. These fractures were then treated as type A3 fractures. For patients with implant failure after surgery, the lateral parapatellar approach was used to remove the implant. After the fracture was fully exposed, any scar tissue and sclerotic bone was excised, and the medullary cavity was reamed. An appropriate length LISS plate was then used to fix the fracture, and autologous iliac bone was implanted.

A suitable width cortical bone plate allograft (Xin Kang Chen Medical Technology Development Co., Ltd., Beijing, China) was selected and trimmed with a wire saw. The sharp edge of the cortical bone plate allograft was filed with a bone file, and the tip was rounded and obtuse. A 4–5 cm anteromedial incision was made along the anterior margin of the pes anserinus, following the adductor canal. The fascial envelope surrounding the vastus medialis along the posterior margin of the muscle was then incised. Blunt dissection was used to elevate the muscle off the periosteum and the intermuscular septum from the adductor tubercle to the intact proximal femoral shaft. Next, a periosteal elevator was used to strip the region between the periosteum and adductor muscles of the thigh. The prepared cortical bone plate allograft was implanted via the anteromedial incision and placed on the opposite side of the LISS plate. The LISS plate and cortical bone plate allograft were fixed in place with cortical bone screws. At least two screws were used at the distal and proximal ends of the bone plate. Finally, the open wound was rinsed and the incisions were closed, with a suction drain at the surgical site.

2.4. Postoperative Management

All patients received postoperative intravenous antibiotics for 24 h. Suction drains were removed on day 2–3. Active and passive range-of-motion exercises were then started. Full weight-bearing activity was allowed after a bridging callus was observed on radiographs.

2.5. Outcome Assessment

Outcomes after surgery were evaluated according to HSS scores, which rely on a 100-point scoring system that assesses pain (30 points), function (22 points), range of motion (18 points), muscle strength (10 points), flexion deformity (10 points), and joint stability (10 points). Overall, "Excellent" was classified as a cumulative score of 85 or more, "Good" as 70 to 84, "Fair" as 60 to 69, and "Poor" as 60 or less. Postoperative functional results were obtained regularly. Postoperative radiological parameters, including X-rays and CT scans, were taken every four weeks to evaluate bony fusion.

3. Results

Detailed clinical patient parameters are shown in Table 1. The average age at enrollment was 44.5 years (range was 18–78 years). Follow-up visits were conducted with thirty patients between 13 and 73 months post-operation, with an average follow-up time of 31.3 months. One patient stopped responding after a 3-month follow-up visit, and two patients lost connection at the 6-month follow-up visit. Twenty-nine patients suffered from closed fractures and four had open fractures (1 Gustilo I, 1 Gustilo II, 1 Gustilo IIIA, and 1 Gustilo IIIB). According to the AO/ASIF system, 33 fractures were classified as the following: A3 (n = 10), C2 (n = 13), and C3 (n = 10). The causes of injury included traffic accidents (20 patients, 60.6%), heavy object crush injuries (5 patients, 15.1%), falls from a significant height (6 patients, 18.2%), and implant failure (2 patients, 6.1%). Eight patients presented with complicated injury. Two patients had fractures associated with an ipsilateral tibial fracture (including one popliteal artery injury patient), two with a hemopneumothorax, two with a traumatic brain injury, two with contralateral tibial and fibula fractures, and one with an ipsilateral patella fracture. Due to the severity of associated hemopneumothorax and traumatic brain injury, neurosurgical or thoracic treatments were performed on patients before attending the lower limb fractures [16].

The mean time to bone union (formation of a circumferential bridging callus across the fracture) was 5.4 months (range was 3–12 months). Three patients stopped visits and ceased communication during the follow-up period (Patients 21, 28, and 33). Outcomes for the remaining patients were "Excellent" for 10 and "Good" for 10, making the percentage of combined "Excellent" and "Good" scores 67.7%. The mean range of knee flexion was

105.6° (range of 80–130°). More specifically, 2 patients had an 80° range, 4 patients had a 90° range, 7 had a 100° range, 12 had a 110° range, and 5 had a ≥120° range of knee flexion. All patients achieved full knee extension. Three patients had weakness in their quadriceps, but all others attained full quadricep strength. Six patients had the implant removed (Table 2).

Table 1. Clinical parameters of the patients.

Patients No	Gender	Age (Years)	Causes of Injury	Injury Type	Fracture Type	Other Injury
1	Male	40	Heavy object crushes	Closed fracture	C2	-
2	Male	61	Implant failure	Closed fracture	A3	-
3	Male	18	Fall from height	Closed fracture	A3	-
4	Male	35	Traffic accident	Closed fracture	C2	-
5	Male	29	Heavy object crushes	Closed fracture	C3	-
6	Female	69	Fall from height	Closed fracture	C2	-
7	Female	40	Traffic accident	Closed fracture	C3	-
8	Male	41	Fall from height	Closed fracture	C2	Traumatic brain injury
9	Female	22	Traffic accident	Closed fracture	C2	-
10	Male	21	Traffic accident	Open fracture	C3, Gustilo III b	Ipsilateral tibial fracture
11	Male	30	Traffic accident	Closed fracture	C2	Contralateral tibial and fibula fracture
12	Female	34	Traffic accident	Open fracture	A3, Gustilo I	-
13	Male	23	Heavy object crushes	Closed fracture	A3	-
14	Female	69	Implant failure	Closed fracture	C3	-
15	Female	31	Traffic accident	Closed fracture	C2	-
16	Male	40	Traffic accident	Closed fracture	C2	Ipsilateral tibial fracture
17	Male	23	Traffic accident	Closed fracture	A3	-
18	Female	59	Traffic accident	Closed fracture	C3	Hemopneumothorax
19	Male	55	Traffic accident	Closed fracture	C3	-
20	Female	71	Fall from height	Closed fracture	A3	-
21	Female	47	Heavy object crushes	Closed fracture	C2	Ipsilateral patella fracture
22	Male	33	Traffic accident	Open fracture	A3, Gustilo III a	-
23	Male	42	Traffic accident	Closed fracture	C2	Traumatic brain injury
24	Male	51	Traffic accident	Closed fracture	C3	-
25	Female	56	Traffic accident	Closed fracture	C2	Contralateral tibial and fibula fracture
26	Male	59	Traffic accident	Closed fracture	A3	-
27	Female	67	Fall from height	Closed fracture	C3	-
28	Female	42	Heavy object crushes	Closed fracture	C2	Hemopneumothorax
29	Male	53	Traffic accident	Open fracture	A3, Gustilo II	-
30	Male	46	Traffic accident	Closed fracture	C3	Contralateral tibial and fibula fracture
31	Male	33	Traffic accident	Closed fracture	C2	-
32	Male	78	Traffic accident	Closed fracture	A3	-
33	Female	51	Fall from height	Closed fracture	C3	-

One patient had a deep infection five days after the operation and underwent a secondary surgery (implant removal and external fixation). There were two patients who had minor surgical complications, including one superficial wound infection and one partial wound dehiscence. After debridement and suturing, both patients' complications were resolved. One patient with nonunion required bone grafting without hardware exchange. Post-traumatic arthritis was seen in one patient at the final follow-up, which was based on the radiologic assessment (Table 2). Typical cases are shown in Figure 1 (Patient 2), Figure 2 (Patient 5), and Figure 3 (Patient 10).

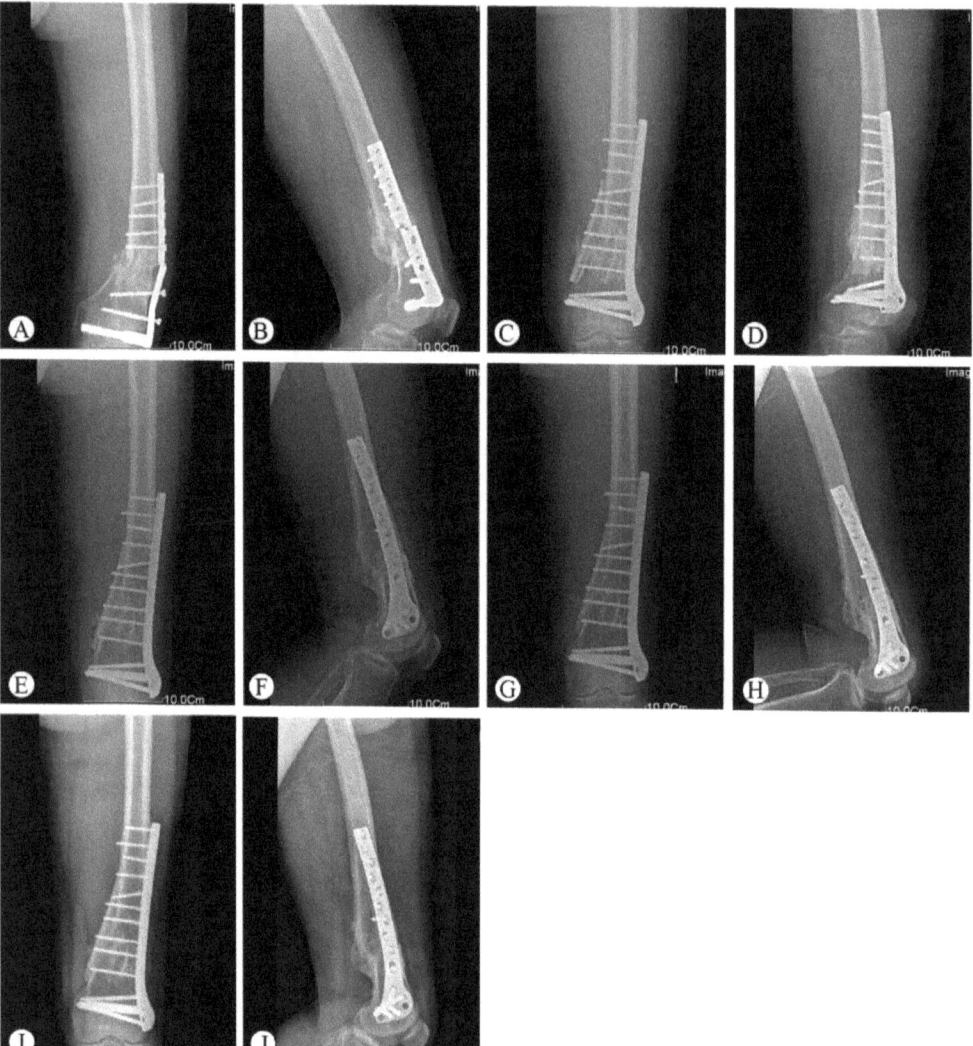

Figure 1. Representative images of Patient 2 (61-year-old male patient with a type A3 fracture that had been initially treated with dynamic condylar screws). (**A,B**) Implant breakage was observed seven months after surgery. (**C,D**) X-ray at 5 months after operation. Bone union was observed. (**E,F**) Follow-up X-ray at 36 months. (**G,H**) Follow-up X-ray at 60 months. (**I,J**) Follow-up X-ray at 73 months.

Table 2. Outcomes of the patients.

Patients No	Follow-Up (Months)	Bone Union (Months)	Knee Range of Motion	Outcomes *	Complications
1	14	4	110°	Good	-
2	73	5	100°	Fair	Quadricep strength grade 3
3	14	8	80°	Poor	Deep infection, secondary surgery
4	26	5	100°	Excellent	-
5	33	5	90°	Fair	Quadricep strength grade 4
6	29	6	110°	Excellent	-
7	28	7	100°	Good	-
8	35	6	110°	Excellent	-
9	22	3	110°	Good	-
10	69	9	80°	Poor	Quadricep strength grade 4
11	19	3	130°	Excellent	-
12	28	5	110°	Good	-
13	15	4	100°	Good	-
14	17	6	90°	Fair	-
15	26	7	110°	Fair	Superficial infection
16	31	5	120°	Excellent	-
17	43	4	130°	Excellent	-
18	19	5	100°	Fair	-
19	54	12	90°	Fair	Nonunion, secondary surgery
20	27	3	110°	Excellent	-
21	Lost to follow-up	-	-	-	-
22	50	8	110°	Good	-
23	25	5	120°	Excellent	-
24	60	4	110°	Good	Post-traumatic arthritis
25	24	5	110°	Good	-
26	17	4	110°	Excellent	-
27	42	6	110°	Good	-
28	Lost to follow-up	-	-	-	-
29	45	4	90°	Good	Superficial infection
30	26	4	100°	Fair	-
31	13	4	100°	Fair	-
32	33	5	120°	Excellent	-
33	Lost to follow-up	-	-	-	-

* Based on knee rating scale of the Hospital for Special Surgery.

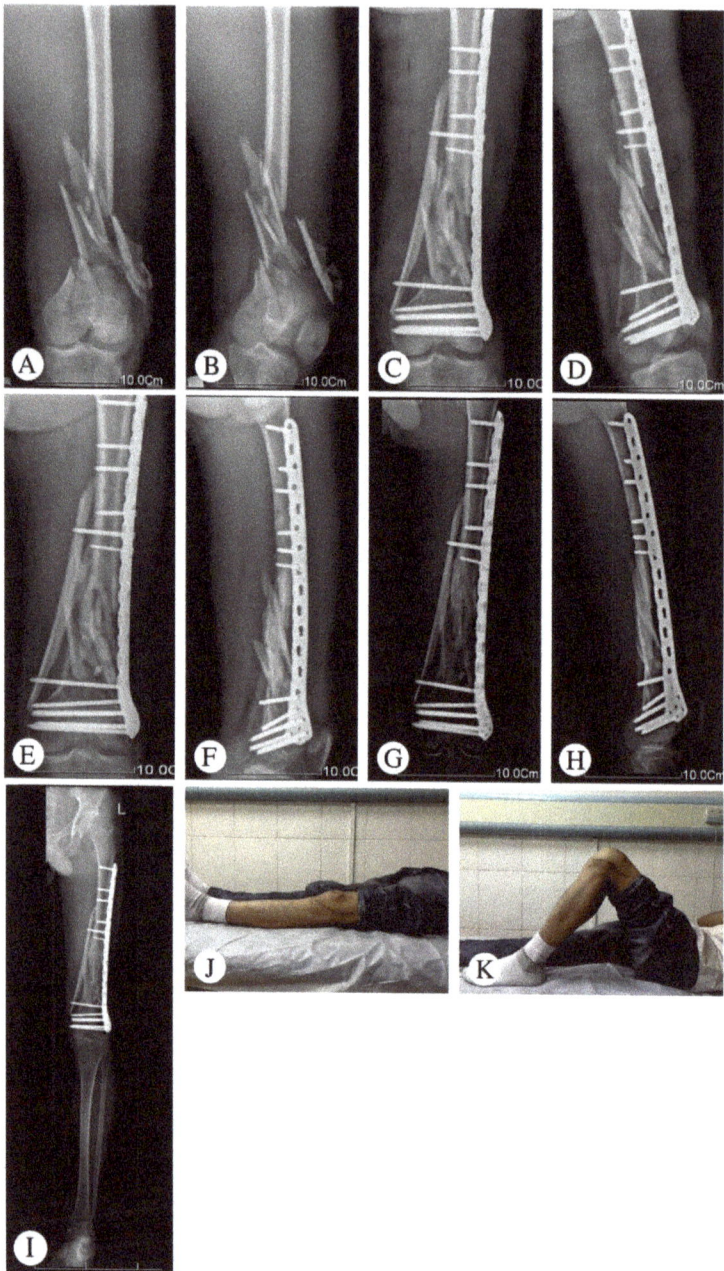

Figure 2. Representative images of Patient 5 (29-year-old male who suffered a heavy object crush to his left thigh). (**A,B**) X-ray at admission. (**C,D**) X-ray 5 days after the operation. (**E,F**) Follow-up X-ray at 3 months. (**G,H**) Follow-up X-ray at 30 months. (**I**) Full-length radiography showing the lower limb at a 33-month follow-up visit. Limb alignment and length was good. (**J,K**) Range of knee joint motion at a 33-month follow-up visit. The patient achieved full knee extension. However, the range of knee flexion was only 90°.

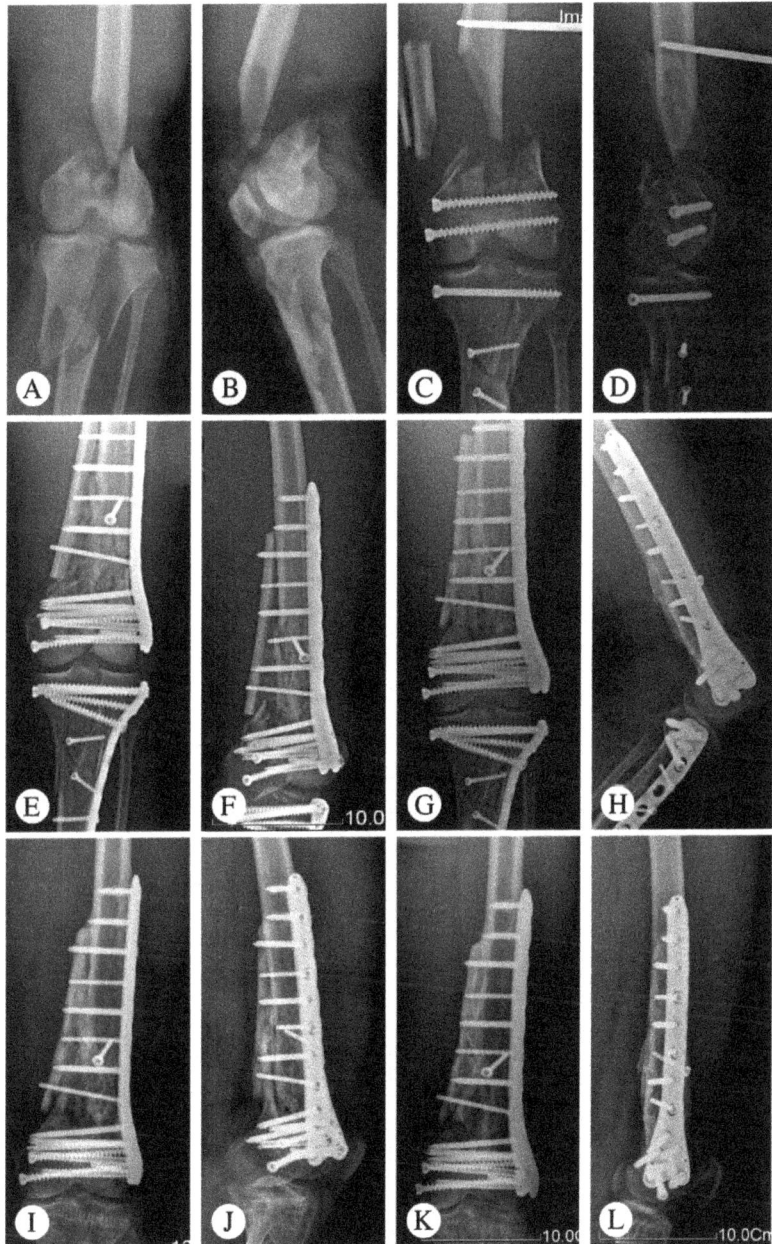

Figure 3. Representative images of Patient 10 (21-year-old male patient with a Gustilo IIIB fracture resulting from a traffic accident). (**A,B**) X-ray at admission. (**C,D**) X-ray after emergency operation. Limited internal fixation combined with external fixation was utilized. (**E,F**) X-ray 3 months after an interfixation operation. (**G,H**) Follow-up X-ray at 9 months. (**I,J**) Follow-up X-ray at 12 months. Removal of the tibial implant. (**K,L**) Follow-up X-ray at 69 months.

4. Discussion

Comminuted distal femur fractures are frequently associated with severe comminution, substantial soft tissue injury, and bone defects. Prior to the 1970s, nonoperative management was the treatment of choice [2]. With the steady improvement of surgical techniques and implants, operative fixation has gained widespread acceptance. Historically, these fractures were treated with condylar buttress plates [6]. Gradually, retrograde nails and DCS took the place of condylar buttress plates. This shift was due to their superior biomechanical design that resulted in decreased varus collapse events when compared with the results using standard condylar buttress plates [17]. The indication of DCS is non-comminuted periarticular fractures without coronal splits and with good bone quality [18]. Recently, locking plates have become the main treatment for comminuted distal femur fractures, particularly for supracondylar and intercondylar comminuted femur fractures. With the increased number of fixation screws used in the distal femur metaphysis, locking plates provide increased biomechanical resistance and stability [19]. However, perioperative and postoperative complications such as malunion, nonunion, implant failure, malrotation, and infection are still common with this approach [14,15].

The main reasons for implant failure are primarily due to the following problems: (1) high bending stress exerted on the laterally placed plates in the presence of marked cortical defects and (2) locking plates are usually implanted using the minimally invasive percutaneous plate osteosynthesis (MIPPO) technique. Since the MIPPO technique is relatively short range and intraoperative fluoroscopy has a limited range, there is a high incidence (approximately 30%) of axial malalignment after surgery. Axial malalignment results in increased load on the plate, which can cause implant failure. Here, implant failure was found in two patients over the age of 60 who had been initially treated with a single-side plate and screws, followed by additional operations as needed. The current treatment approach for implant failure features scar tissue removal and large amounts of autologous iliac bone grafts, as well as implant replacement. Bilateral autologous iliac bone grafts have often been applied to repair cortical defects, which can increase surgical trauma and the chance of infection. Furthermore, the stability immediately following the structural allograft cannot support early postoperative functional exercise, which is important for recovery. Therefore, we performed a medial implant of the cortical bone plate allograft integrated with a lateral LISS plate for the two patients with implant failures. Patient 2 was a 61-year-old male patient with a type A3 fracture that had been initially treated using dynamic condylar screws. The implant failure was observed seven months following surgery and required reoperation. After treatment with a cortical bone plate allograft combined with LISS plate fixation, bone union was observed five months later (Figure 1).

Types C2, C3, and partial A3 fractures of the distal femoral are prone to induce nonunion and implant failure, particularly in the cases of severe cortical defects in the medial femur. On the basis of lateral LISS plate implantation using MIPPO technology, a suitable length and width allogeneic cortical bone plate was implanted from the medial epicondyle of the femur, which achieved an integrated fixation of the triangular support and avoided excessive elevation of the periosteum at the fracture site. For severe comminuted fractures and/or periprosthetic fractures of the distal femur, double plating with autogenous bone grafting executed via a modified Olerud extensile approach was also used. Although acceptable clinical outcomes were achieved, there are some limitations to this approach, including excessive elevation of the periosteum, large trauma (tibial tuberosity osteotomy), and lack of integrated fixation [20]. Recently, a double-plating technique was used for the treatment of supracondylar femur fractures. Based on promising follow-up results, they recommended this technique specifically for patients with poor bone quality, comminuted fractures, and very low periprosthetic fractures [21]. However, no detailed functional outcomes were described in their results, and some important points needed to be clarified [22].

The application of allogeneic cortical bone plates in repairing bone defects has been frequently reported, and satisfactory clinical results have been achieved with this approach [23,24]. Moreover, allogeneic cortical bone plates were used in the treatment of periprosthetic fractures of the femur [25] and distal femoral nonunion [26]. However, there are not many relevant reports about the use of allogeneic cortical bone plates in the treatment of comminuted fractures of the distal femur. In our study, an allogeneic cortical bone plate was used in the treatment of comminuted distal femur fractures, which has the following advantages: (1) wide scope of application; (2) the union of the allogeneic cortical bone plate and host bone can reconstruct cortical defects of the medial femur, and when combined with an autologous iliac bone graft, this treatment has a strong osteoinductive effect and can promote bone healing; (3) LISS plates and allogeneic cortical bone plates were implanted using MIPPO technology, which minimized periosteal elevation and disruption of blood supply at the fracture site, which not only increased fixation rigidity, but also contributed to fracture healing; (4) allogeneic cortical bone plates are a biomechanically sound alternative to metal plates fixed with screws, and could markedly improve stability and rigidity after lateral LISS plate fixation; (5) utilization of an LISS plate and allogeneic cortical bone plate presented firm integrated fixation of the triangular support. Furthermore, knee function exercises were conducted soon after the operation, resulting in overall better therapeutic outcomes.

Taken together, we believed that a cortical bone plate allograft combined with the LISS plate fixation technique may be an option for the treatment of comminuted distal femur fractures and is beneficial for early weight-bearing following surgery. However, there are some limitations to this study, including its retrospective nature with old data, the relatively small group of patients studied, and a combining of young and old populations. A long-term RCT study with a larger number of patients and control groups that include other fixation methods should be performed to further validate our findings here.

5. Conclusions

Biomechanical and clinical studies suggested early weight-bearing may be performed immediately following surgical treatment of comminuted distal femur fractures, that fixation failure was associated with medial comminution, and that medial comminution should be managed with additional fixation [27]. Thus, we recommend that a cortical bone plate allograft combined with the LISS plate fixation technique be used for treatment of comminuted distal femur fractures, especially indicated in cases of severe medial femur cortical defects and implant failure after surgery.

Author Contributions: J.W. and Z.G., operation. H.L. and T.C., paper preparation. D.L. and J.Z., follow-up. All authors have read and agreed to the published version of the manuscript.

Funding: This research was funded by the General Program of PLA Nanjing Military Area Command, grant number 20XLS21.

Institutional Review Board Statement: The study was conducted in accordance with the Declaration of Helsinki and approved by the Institutional Review Board of the 909th Hospital, School of Medicine, Xiamen University (protocol code 6725 and 8 May 2008).

Informed Consent Statement: Informed consent was obtained from all subjects involved in the study. Written informed consent was obtained from the patient(s) to publish this paper.

Data Availability Statement: The analyzed datasets of this study are available from the corresponding author on reasonable request.

Conflicts of Interest: The corresponding author declares, on behalf of all the authors, that there is no conflict of interest.

References

1. Court-Brown, C.M.; Caesar, B. Epidemiology of adult fractures: A review. *Injury* **2006**, *37*, 691–697. [CrossRef] [PubMed]
2. Martinet, O.; Cordey, J.; Harder, Y.; Maier, A.; Bühler, M.; Barraud, G.E. The epidemiology of fractures of the distal femur. *Injury* **2000**, *31*, 62–63. [CrossRef]

3. Müller, M.E.; Nazarian, S.; Koch, P.; Schatzker, J. *The Comprehensive Classification of Fractures of Long Bones*; Springer: Berlin/Heidelberg, Germany; New York, NY, USA, 1990.
4. Marsh, J.L.; Slongo, T.F.; Agel, J.; Broderick, J.S.; Creevey, W.; DeCoster, T.A.; Prokuski, L.; Sirkin, M.S.; Ziran, B.; Henley, B.; et al. Fracture and dislocation classification compendium—2007: Orthopaedic Trauma Association classification, database and outcomes committee. *J. Orthop. Trauma.* **2007**, *21*, S1–S133. [CrossRef]
5. Johnson, K.D. Internal fixation of distal femoral fractures. *Instr. Course. Lect.* **1987**, *36*, 437–448. [PubMed]
6. Davison, B.L. Varus collapse of comminuted distal femur fractures after: Open reduction and internal fixation with a lateral condylar buttress plate. *Am. J. Orthop.* **2003**, *32*, 27–30. [PubMed]
7. Narsaria, N.; Singh, A.K.; Rastogi, A.; Singh, V. Biomechanical analysis of distal femoral fracture fixation: Dynamic condylar screw versus locked compression plate. *J. Orthop. Sci.* **2014**, *19*, 770–775. [CrossRef]
8. Kulkarni, S.G.; Varshneya, A.; Kulkarni, G.S.; Kulkarni, M.G.; Kulkarni, V.S.; Kulkarni, R.M. Antegrade interlocking nailing for distal femoral fractures. *J. Orthop. Surg.* **2012**, *20*, 48–54. [CrossRef]
9. Smith, T.O.; Hedges, C.; MacNair, R.; Wimhurst, J.A. The clinical and radiological outcomes of the LISS plate for distal femoral fractures: A systematic review. *Injury* **2009**, *40*, 1049–1063. [CrossRef]
10. Ali, F.; Saleh, M. Treatment of isolated complex distal femoral fractures by external fixation. *Injury* **2000**, *31*, 139–146. [CrossRef]
11. Wang, M.T.; An, V.V.G.; Sivakumar, B.S. Non-union in lateral locked plating for distal femoral fractures: A systematic review. *Injury* **2019**, *50*, 1790–1794. [CrossRef]
12. Rollo, G.; Pichierri, P.; Grubor, P.; Marsilio, A.; Bisaccia, M.; Grubor, M.; Pace, V.; Lanzetti, R.M.; Giaracuni, M.; Filipponi, M.; et al. The challenge of nonunion and malunion in distal femur surgical revision. *Med. Glas.* **2019**, *16*. ahead of print. [CrossRef]
13. Von Keudell, A.; Shoji, K.; Nasr, M.; Lucas, R.; Dolan, R.; Weaver, M.J. Treatment Options for Distal Femur Fractures. *J. Orthop. Trauma.* **2016**, *30*, S25–S27. [CrossRef] [PubMed]
14. Henderson, C.E.; Kuhl, L.L.; Fitzpatrick, D.C.; Marsh, J.L. Locking plates for distal femur fractures: Is there a problem with fracture healing? *J. Orthop. Trauma.* **2011**, *25*, S8–S14. [CrossRef]
15. Buckley, R.; Mohanty, K.; Malish, D. Lower limb malrotation following MIPO technique of distal femoral and proximal tibial fractures. *Injury* **2011**, *42*, 194–199. [CrossRef]
16. Dumitru, M.; Vrinceanu, D.; Banica, B.; Cergan, R.; Taciuc, I.A.; Manole, F.; Popa-Cherecheanu, M. Management of Aesthetic and Functional Deficits in Frontal Bone Trauma. *Medicina* **2022**, *58*, 1756. [CrossRef] [PubMed]
17. Hartin, N.L.; Harris, I.; Hazratwala, K. Retrograde nailing versus fixed-angle blade plating for supracondylar femoral fractures: A randomized controlled trial. *ANZ J. Surg.* **2006**, *76*, 290–294. [CrossRef]
18. Canadian Orthopaedic Trauma Society. Are Locking Constructs in Distal Femoral Fractures Always Best? A Prospective Multicenter Randomized Controlled Trial Comparing the Less Invasive Stabilization System with the Minimally Invasive Dynamic Condylar Screw System. *J. Orthop. Trauma.* **2016**, *30*, 1–6. [CrossRef] [PubMed]
19. Frigg, R.; Appenzeller, A.; Christense, R.; Frenk, A.; Gilbert, S.; Schavan, R. The development of the distal femur less invasive stabilization system (LISS). *Injury* **2001**, *32*, SC24-31. [CrossRef]
20. Khalil, A.-S.; Ayoub, M.A. Highly unstable complex C3-type distal femur fracture: Can double plating via a modified Olerud extensile approach be a standby solution? *J. Orthopaed. Traumatol.* **2012**, *13*, 179–188. [CrossRef]
21. Steinberg, E.L.; Elis, J.; Steinberg, Y.; Salai, M.; Ben-Tov, T. A double-plating approach to distal femur fracture: A clinical study. *Injury* **2017**, *48*, 2260–2265. [CrossRef]
22. Kumar, P.; Patel, S.; Kumar, V.; Rajnish, R.K.; Hooda, A. A double-plating approach to distal femur fracture: A clinical study; how apt is the technique? How strong is the evidence? *Injury* **2018**, *49*, 737–738. [CrossRef]
23. Shih, H.N.; Shih, L.Y.; Cheng, C.Y.; Hsu, K.Y.; Chang, C.H. Reconstructing humerus defects after tumor resection using an intramedullary cortical allograft strut. *Chang. Gung. Med. J.* **2002**, *25*, 656–662. [PubMed]
24. Van Houwelingen, A.P.; McKee, M.D. Treatment of osteopenic humeral shaft nonunion with compression plating, humeral cortical allograft struts, and bone grafting. *J. Orthop. Trauma.* **2005**, *19*, 36–42. [CrossRef] [PubMed]
25. Wang, J.W.; Wang, C.J. Supracondylar fractures of the femur above total knee arthroplasties with cortical allograft struts. *J. Arthroplast.* **2002**, *17*, 365–372. [CrossRef] [PubMed]
26. Wang, J.W.; Weng, L.H. Treatment of distal femoral nonunion with internal fixation, cortical allograft struts, and autogenous bone-grafting. *J. Bone. Joint. Surg. Am.* **2003**, *85*, 436–440. [CrossRef]
27. Keenan, O.J.F.; Ross, L.A.; Magill, M.; Moran, M.; Scott, C.E.H. Immediate weight-bearing is safe following lateral locked plate fixation of periprosthetic distal femoral fractures. *Knee. Surg. Relat. Res.* **2021**, *33*, 19. [CrossRef] [PubMed]

Disclaimer/Publisher's Note: The statements, opinions and data contained in all publications are solely those of the individual author(s) and contributor(s) and not of MDPI and/or the editor(s). MDPI and/or the editor(s) disclaim responsibility for any injury to people or property resulting from any ideas, methods, instructions or products referred to in the content.

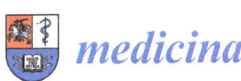

Article

Demographics and Etiology for Lower Extremity Amputations—Experiences of an University Orthopaedic Center in Germany

Annette Eidmann, Yama Kamawal, Martin Luedemann, Peter Raab, Maximilian Rudert and Ioannis Stratos *

Department of Orthopaedic Surgery, Julius-Maximilians University Wuerzburg, Koenig-Ludwig-Haus, Brettreichstrasse 11, 97074 Wuerzburg, Germany
* Correspondence: i-stratos.klh@uni-wuerzburg.de

Abstract: *Background and Objectives*: Currently, the worldwide incidence of major amputations in the general population is decreasing whereas the incidence of minor amputations is increasing. The purpose of our study was to analyze whether this trend is reflected among orthopaedic patients treated with lower extremity amputation in our orthopaedic university institution. *Materials and Methods*: We conducted a single-center retrospective study and included patients referred to our orthopaedic department for lower extremity amputation (LEA) between January 2007 and December 2019. Acquired data were the year of amputation, age, sex, level of amputation and cause of amputation. T test and Chi^2 test were performed to compare age and amputation rates between males and females; significance was defined as $p < 0.05$. Linear regression and multivariate logistic regression models were used to test time trends and to calculate probabilities for LEA. *Results*: A total of 114 amputations of the lower extremity were performed, of which 60.5% were major amputations. The number of major amputations increased over time with a rate of 0.6 amputation/year. Men were significantly more often affected by LEA than women. Age of LEA for men was significantly below the age of LEA for women (men: 54.8 ± 2.8 years, women: 64.9 ± 3.2 years, $p = 0.021$). Main causes leading to LEA were tumors (28.9%) and implant-associated complications (25.4%). Implant-associated complications and age raised the probability for major amputation, whereas malformation, angiopathies and infections were more likely to cause a minor amputation. *Conclusions*: Among patients in our orthopaedic institution, etiology of amputations of the lower extremity is multifactorial and differs from other surgical specialties. The number of major amputations has increased continuously over the past years. Age and sex, as well as diagnosis, influence the type and level of amputation.

Keywords: lower extremity amputation; major amputation; minor amputation; orthopaedic surgery

1. Introduction

Even though lower extremity amputation (LEA) is one of the oldest surgical techniques, dating back to the time of Hippocrates and beyond, it is still part of daily routine for many surgical specialties [1].

Causes leading to LEA differ between countries and geographic regions. In the western world, up to 75% of all LEAs are associated with diabetes mellitus (DM) and peripheral arterial disease (PAD) [2–4]. In less developed countries, amputations are more often due to trauma, infection and tumors [5–7]. Because of LEA's high socioeconomic impact as well as the relevant effect on the amputees themselves, efforts have been made to analyze and reduce amputation rates. Population-based data show a trend towards declining rates for major amputations in Europe and worldwide in the last decades, but increasing rates for minor amputations at the same time [2–4,8–14]. Generally, major amputations are defined as amputations proximal to, or through the ankle joint, whereas minor amputations are amputations distal to the ankle joint. Most of the aforementioned studies focus on

DM- and PAD-associated lower limb amputations. These diseases represent the largest group and thus have the greatest impact, especially in times of a worldwide increasing prevalence of DM [15]. Other causes for LEA are either excluded in these studies or are not further differentiated.

In orthopaedic surgery, LEA is also an important part of the surgical practice. In our daily routine, despite the trend to minimal and less-invasive operation techniques, there is an impression that the importance of lower limb amputations, especially of major amputations, had been increasing. As the population is getting older and patients are often multimorbid with a complex surgical history, the options for surgical treatment sometimes are limited to the most radical one, i.e., an amputation. Nevertheless, the main causes leading to LEA in orthopaedic patients tend to be a result of main diagnoses other than DM and PAD. As those diagnoses represent only a small number, regarding the overall population, they are excluded in the existing population-based studies. In the existing literature, no data exist about demographics, etiology and especially time trends of amputations in orthopaedic patients, which are not mainly due to DM and PAD. Therefore, it is unclear if the general trend of decreasing major amputation rates can also be assumed for orthopaedic patients.

The purpose of this study was to analyze the demographics and etiology for LEA in a collective of orthopaedic patients. Our hypothesis was that, contrary to the general trend, the number of amputations, especially major amputations, had been increasing over time. The results of this single-institution study may be used as a possible indicator for trends in this surgical discipline.

2. Materials and Methods

2.1. Study Design

The present study is a single-center retrospective study. A total of 106 patients treated between 2007 and 2019 were included.

2.2. Study Population

We retrospectively analyzed all digital patient-records of our orthopaedic hospital from amputated patients. To identify these patients, we searched for amputation-specific surgical codes (operating procedure keys (OPS): 5-864.0-9, 5-864.a/x/y, 5-865.0-9 and 5-865.x/y according to the classification of the "German Billing System for Inpatients" (DRG)). All patients who underwent any LEA between January 2007 and December 2019 were included in the study. Year of amputation, age, sex, level of amputation (exarticulation of the hip/transfemoral/exarticulation knee/transtibial/exarticulation ankle/midfoot/metatarsals/toe) and main diagnosis leading to amputation were collected and analyzed. Revisions on the same limb and on the same level of amputation were excluded from the analysis. Any additional amputation on the same patient was counted as separate amputation. As major amputations we defined amputations proximal to, or through the ankle joint, whereas minor amputation was defined as any amputation distal to the ankle joint. Causes for amputations were determined by the main diagnosis directly leading to the amputation according to the DRG system. Secondary diagnoses were not included. Following causes for amputation were classified: tumor, implant-associated complications (e.g., failed total joint replacements and osteosynthesis due to infection or fracture), angiopathies (DM- and PAD-related), malformation, infection (without implant- and DM/PAD-associated infections) and others (e.g., due to trauma).

2.3. Ethics Approval

All data used for analysis were part of the routine medical documentation. Ethical approval was waived by the local Ethics Committee of University of Würzburg in view of the retrospective nature of the study (Protocol number 20210125 02).

2.4. Statistics

Results are shown as means and standard error of the mean (S.E.M.). T test and Chi^2 test were performed to compare age and amputation rates between males and females; significance was defined as $p < 0.05$. To test time trends for major and minor amputations, linear regression was used, followed by likelihood ratio test to test for statistical significance. To calculate probabilities for LEA, multivariate logistic regression models were performed using age, level of amputation and indication as variables. A commercially available and a free statistical software program (Prism 8, GraphPad, CA, USA; jamovi version 1.6.9, the jamovi project (2020)) were used for statistical analysis and data visualization.

3. Results

Between 2007 and 2019, 114 amputations of the lower extremity were performed on 106 patients. A total of 60.5% (n = 69) were major and 39.5% (n = 45) were minor amputations. Of these, 61.4% (n = 70) of the patients were male, 38.6% (n = 44) were female. Men were significantly more often affected by LEA than women ($p = 0.015$) and the age at amputation was significantly younger for men than for women (men: 54.8 ± 2.8 years, women: 64.9 ± 3.2 years, $p = 0.021$) (Table 1).

Table 1. Gender and age distribution of lower extremity amputations. Distribution of gender and age of all LEA, major and minor amputations. Data are given as Means ± S.E.M.; * p = level of significance for the comparison female versus male for all LEA (χ^2 test); ** p = level of significance for the comparison female versus male for the factor age (t test).

	Female	Male	Total	
Amputations [n]	44	70	114	* $p = 0.015$
Major [n]	28	41	69	
Minor [n]	16	29	45	
Age [years]	64.9 ± 3.2	54.8 ± 2.8	58.7 ± 2.1	** $p = 0.021$

Main causes leading to LEA were tumors (28.9%) and implant-associated complications (25.4%), followed by angiopathies (21.1%), malformations (9.6%), infections (9.6%) and others (5.3%) (Table 2). All implant-associated complications and most tumors led to major amputation. Implant-associated complications increased the probability of a transfemoral amputation and of an exarticulation of the hip. Tumors are associated with a high chance of an amputation around the knee. Malformations, angiopathies and infections are more likely to cause a minor amputation (Figure 1 and Table 3).

Table 2. Causes for lower extremity amputation.

Indication	Major [n]	Minor [n]	Total [n;(%)]
Tumor	29	4	33 (28.9)
Implant-associated complications	29	0	29 (25.4)
Angiopathies	7	17	24 (21.1)
Malformation	0	11	11 (9.6)
Infection	2	9	11 (9.6)
Others	2	4	6 (5.3)

Increasing age significantly raises the probability of a major amputation, especially of a transfemoral amputation or an exarticulation of the hip (Figures 2 and 3 and Table 3).

Time trend from 2007 to 2019 shows a significantly increasing number of major amputations (on average 0.6 new major amputations per year) and an almost constant number of minor amputations at the same time (on average 0.04 new minor amputations per year) (Figure 4).

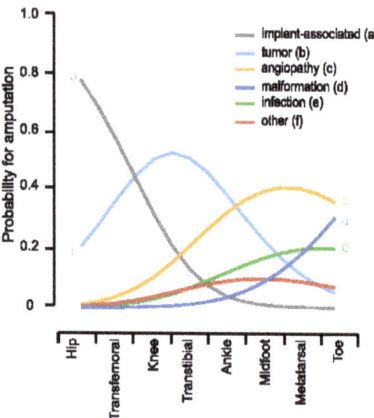

Figure 1. Multivariate logistic regression analysis for the level of amputation: The diagram illustrates the probability for amputation by cause in relation to the level of amputation.

Table 3. Model fit measures for logistic regression analysis. Akaike information criterion (AIC), Bayesian information criterion (BIC), McFadden's pseudo-R2 (R^2McF), degrees of freedom (df), probability (p). * p = level of significance for each comparison (left column) for all LEA (χ^2 test).

Model	Deviance	AIC	BIC	R^2_{McF}	Overall Model Test		
					χ^2	df	p
Age vs. Level of Amputation	392	420	458	0.046	18.9	7	* p = 0.009
Cause for amputation vs. Level of amputation	277	297	324	0.261	97.6	5	* p < 0.001
Major amputations vs. Age	148	152	157	0.035	5.41	1	* p = 0.020

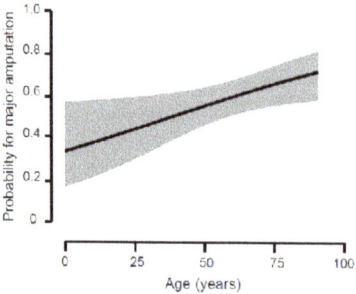

Figure 2. Logistic regression analysis for the probability of major amputation: The diagram shows the probability for a major amputation in relation to age. Conditional estimates plot with 95% confidence interval.

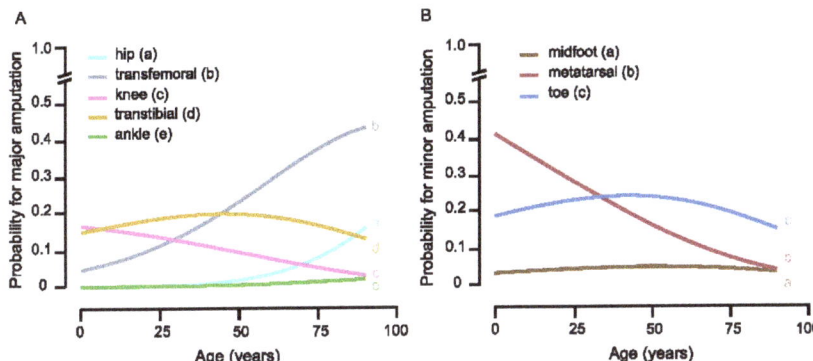

Figure 3. Multivariate logistic regression analysis for the level of amputation: The diagrams illustrate the probability for different levels of amputation in relation to age of amputation. (**A**) probability for major amputation. (**B**) probability for minor amputation.

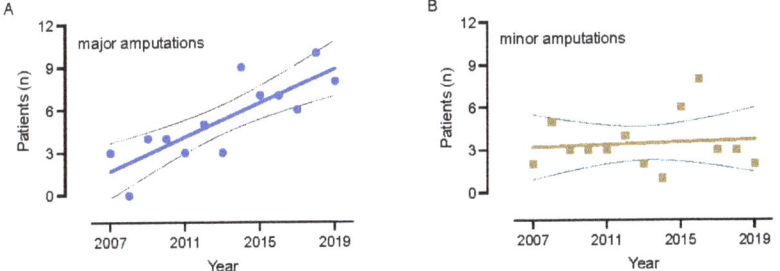

Figure 4. Linear regression analysis for major (**A**) and minor (**B**) amputations over time. During the study period from 20017 to 2019, major amputations are increasing significantly, while minor amputations stay at a constant level. Linear regression equation for major: y = 0.5989x − 1200; R^2(major) = 0.675, linear regression equation for minor: y = 0.0440x − 85.02; R^2(minor) = 0.008; likelihood ratio test: p = 0.0006 for major.

4. Discussion

In this retrospective single-center analysis, we showed that in a cohort of orthopaedic patients, etiology of amputations of the lower extremity is multifactorial and differs from other surgical specialties. Most common diagnoses leading to LEA in our collective of patients are tumors and implant-related complications, in contrast to the worldwide leading position of PAD/DM-related amputations [2,3]. Age and sex, as well as diagnosis, influence the type and level of amputation. Our time trends show an increasing number of major amputations with stable minor amputation rates during the observed period.

Most patients needing LEA in our population were males. Various studies have demonstrated that male sex is a risk factor for amputation, in the diabetic as well as in the non-diabetic population [4,9,11,14,16–19]. Additionally, males are significantly younger at the time of amputation compared to females as shown in the current study and other population-based studies [4,8,19,20]. This might be explained due to general demographic factors like a higher average age for women as well as lifestyle factors with a higher predisposition for certain comorbidities like DM and PAD [20,21].

Average age for amputation in our study is at 58.7 years. Other studies show 10 to 15 years' higher mean values [3,11,20]. This difference can be explained due to the fact that these studies analyze patients with overrepresented comorbidities like DM and PAD. These comorbidities are typically found in older patients. Our orthopaedic patients are diagnosed more frequently with musculoskeletal tumors, which can affect children and adolescents, or malformations, which are usually treated by amputation during early infancy. Thus, amputations among orthopaedic patients are not automatically an issue concerning only aged patients.

Nevertheless, increasing age has been shown to be a risk factor for major amputation, especially transfemoral amputation and exarticulation of the hip. This finding in our collective is also in line with other studies [4,11]. Currently, amputation is in most cases not the first line therapy for tumors; most tumor-associated amputations in our collective were due to relapses or complications like failed extremity-preserving techniques. Thus, the probability of amputation rises with age. The same can be assumed for implant-associated amputations. Most of them are salvage procedures after failed total joint replacements, mostly after a multi-annual patient history with multiple previous revision procedures [22].

Most studies from Europe and other "western countries" have shown declining rates for major amputations [2–4,8–13], which is contrary to the increasing major amputations found in our collective. Most amputations in the western world are associated with PAD and DM. Thus, implementing efficient therapies for DM and PAD can lead not only to a decrease of amputation rates in DM/PAD-related amputation rates, but to a decrease in the overall amputation rates. Interventional novelties in the field of angiology, improved recanalization techniques for PAD, better DM disease prevention programs as well as specialized diabetic foot care have led to this success [23–25]. Despite this process, there is still need for limb-preserving efforts: the goal of reducing DM-associated amputations by half within five years, which was set in the St. Vincent's Declaration of 1989, is still not reached [26].

According to a recent publication from Kröger et al., a decrease of major amputation rates has been observed in Germany between 2005 and 2014, whereas the overall number of amputations has increased by 3.5%. After exclusion of tumors and other musculoskeletal diseases, the increase of LEA is only 1.1% [8], which implies that musculoskeletal disorders relevantly contribute to LEA. The authors also state particularly that the number of major-amputations have not decreased for patients with tumors and other musculoskeletal disorders. Similar conclusions can be made according to the study from Walter et. al. [4]. In 2019 in Germany, 80% of minor amputations were due to PAD and DM, but only 69.2% of major amputations. This implies that the impact of "other" diagnosis like tumors, musculoskeletal disorders and complications due to implants is higher in the group of major amputations.

In the USA, Kalbaugh et al. have shown a change of indications leading to amputation between 2006 and 2016 [19]. The number of tumors, which are responsible for about 1% of all amputations, has been stable over time, but in the group of "infections", an increase from 8% to 24% has been detected.

In our population, the increase of major amputations referred to an increase of implant-related complications. The number of primary total joint replacements in Germany has been at a constant high level in previous years [27], thus leading to an increasing number of revision surgeries, which might rise even more in the future. This is not only due to the high prevalence of protheses, but also to the ageing population [28]. A consequence of increasing revision rates is an increasing number of failed total joint replacements, usually after numerous previous operations and mostly due to chronic infection with loss of function, defects of bone and soft tissue. Thus, it is not surprising that amputations due to periprosthetic complications are increasing, although this remains a salvage procedure. Nevertheless, even small increases should be taken seriously, as major amputation after total joint replacement is a catastrophic procedure for both patient and surgeon.

Our study has several limitations. We analyzed only a small group of patients which were treated in our institution. Therefore, this sample might not be representative for orthopaedic patients in general due to selection bias. In Germany, LEA are performed by several surgical disciplines. Thus, possible confounders could be regional structural conditions like the specialization of our hospital, the availability of specialized vascular surgeons within reach, as well as changes in procedures or surgical staff. Thus, data represent only a cohort of orthopaedic patients and cannot easily be generalized to the German population. A population-based analysis would be necessary, but using diagnoses and procedure codes from hospital or insurance data makes it difficult if not impossible to differentiate certain groups in the way we did. Nevertheless, musculoskeletal tumors remain rare diseases and consequently, amputations due to tumors are even more sparse. Consequently, in that context, the number of patients reported in this study is not small for a single institution. A good way to enlarge the study population would be a multi-center analysis.

Because the study population was small, we did not perform age and sex adjustment. Thus, changes in the absolute number of amputations might be due to changes in the affected age groups. Nevertheless, the impact on hospitals and health care systems remains the same.

5. Conclusions

Among patients in our orthopaedic institution, etiology of amputations of the lower extremity is multifactorial and differs from other surgical specialties. The number of major amputations has increased continuously over the past years. Age and sex, as well as diagnosis, influence the type and level of amputation.

Author Contributions: Conceptualization, M.R. and I.S.; Data curation, A.E. and I.S.; Formal analysis, A.E.; Investigation, A.E. and I.S.; Methodology, A.E.; Project administration, I.S.; Resources, A.E.; Software, I.S.; Supervision, I.S.; Validation, A.E., Y.K., M.L. and P.R.; Writing—original draft, A.E.; Writing—review & editing, Y.K., M.L., P.R., M.R. and I.S. All authors have read and agreed to the published version of the manuscript.

Funding: This publication was supported by the Open Access Publication Fund of the University of Wuerzburg.

Institutional Review Board Statement: Ethical approval was waived by the local Ethics Committee of University of Würzburg (protocol number 20210125 02).

Informed Consent Statement: According to the local Ethics Committee of University of Würzburg there is no need for "Consent to Participate" or "Consent to Publish" in view of the retrospective nature of the study. All performed medical procedures were part of the regular medical care.

Data Availability Statement: The datasets generated during the current study are available from the corresponding author on reasonable request.

Conflicts of Interest: The authors declare no conflict of interest.

References

1. Markatos, K.; Karamanou, M.; Saranteas, T.; Mavrogenis, A.F. Hallmarks of amputation surgery. *Int. Orthop. (SICOT)* **2019**, *43*, 493–499. [CrossRef] [PubMed]
2. Behrendt, C.; Sigvant, B.; Szeberin, Z.; Beiles, B.; Eldrup, N.; Thomson, I.A.; Venermo, M.; Altreuther, M.; Menyhei, G.; Nordanstig, J.; et al. International Variations in Amputation Practice: A VASCUNET Report. *Eur. J. Vasc. Endovasc. Surg.* **2018**, *56*, 391–399. [CrossRef] [PubMed]
3. Spoden, M.; Nimptsch, U.; Mansky, T. Amputation rates of the lower limb by amputation level–observational study using German national hospital discharge data from 2005 to 2015. *BMC Health Serv. Res.* **2019**, *19*, 8.
4. Walter, N.; Alt, V. Rupp, Lower Limb Amputation Rates in Germany. *Medicina* **2022**, *58*, 101. [CrossRef]
5. Gebreslassie, B.; Gebreselassie, K.; Esayas, R. Patterns and causes of amputation in Ayder Referral Hospital, Mekelle, Ethiopia: A three-year experience. *Ethiop J. Health Sci.* **2018**, *28*, 31–36. [CrossRef]
6. Thanni, L.O.A.; Tade, A.O. Extremity amputation in Nigeria—A review of indications and mortality. *Surgeon* **2007**, *5*, 213–217. [CrossRef]
7. Chalya, P.L.; Mabula, J.B.; Dass, R.M.; Ngayomela, I.H.; Chandika, A.B.; Mbelenge, N.; Gilyoma, J.M. Major limb amputations: A tertiary hospital experience in northwestern Tanzania. *J. Orthop. Surg. Res.* **2012**, *7*, 16. [CrossRef]
8. Kröger, K.; Berg, C.; Santosa, F.; Malyar, N.; Reinecke, H. Lower limb amputation in Germany: An analysis of data from the German Federal Statistical Office between 2005 and 2014. *Dtsch. Ärzteblatt Int.* **2017**, *114*, 130. [CrossRef]
9. Lopez-de-Andres, A.; Jiménez-García, R.; Aragón-Sánchez, J.; Jiménez-Trujillo, I.; Hernández-Barrera, V.; Méndez-Bailón, M.; de Miguel-Yanes Jose Mª Perez-Farinos, N.; Carrasco-Garrido, P. National trends in incidence and outcomes in lower extremity amputations in people with and without diabetes in Spain, 2001–2012. *Diabetes Res. Clin. Practice* **2015**, *108*, 499–507. [CrossRef]

10. Santosa, F.; Moysidis, T.; Kanya, S.; Babadagi-Hardt, Z.; Luther, B.; Kröger, K. Decrease in Major Amputations in Germany. *Int. Wound J.* **2015**, *12*, 276–279. [CrossRef]
11. Lombardo, F.L.; Maggini, M.; Bellis, A.D.; Seghieri, G.; Anichini, R.; Herder, C. Lower Extremity Amputations in Persons with and without Diabetes in Italy: 2001–2010. *PLoS ONE.* **2014**, *9*, e86405. [CrossRef] [PubMed]
12. Jørgensen, M.E.; Almdal, T.P.; Faerch, K. Reduced incidence of lower-extremity amputations in a Danish diabetes population from 2000 to 2011. *Diabet. Med.* **2014**, *31*, 443–447. [CrossRef] [PubMed]
13. Kurowski, J.R.; Nedkoff, L.; Schoen, D.E.; Knuiman, M.; Norman, P.E.; Briffa, T.G. Temporal trends in initial and recurrent lower extremity amputations in people with and without diabetes in Western Australia from 2000 to 2010. *Diabetes Res. Clin. Practice* **2015**, *108*, 280–287. [CrossRef] [PubMed]
14. Lopez-de-Andres, A.; Jimenez-Garcia, R.; Hernandez-Barrera, V.; de Miguel-Diez, J.; de Miguel-Yanes, J.; Omaña-Palanco, R.; Carabantes-Alarcon, D. Trends of Non-Traumatic Lower-Extremity Amputation and Type 2 Diabetes: Spain, 2001–2019. *JCM* **2022**, *11*, 1246. [CrossRef]
15. Saeedi, P.; Petersohn, I.; Salpea, P.; Malanda, B.; Karuranga, S.; Unwin, N.; Colagiuri, S.; Guariguata, L.; Motala, A.A.; Ogurtsova, K.; et al. Global and regional diabetes prevalence estimates for 2019 and projections for 2030 and 2045: Results from the International Diabetes Federation Diabetes Atlas, 9th edition. *Diabetes Res. Clin. Practice* **2019**, *157*, 107843. [CrossRef]
16. Armstrong, D.G.; Lavery, L.A.; van Houtum William, H.; Harkless, L.B. The impact of gender on amputation. *J. Foot Ankle Surg.* **1997**, *36*, 66–69. [CrossRef]
17. Tang, Z.; Chen, H.; Zhao, F. Gender Differences of Lower Extremity Amputation Risk in Patients With Diabetic Foot. *Int. J. Low. Extrem. Wounds* **2014**, *13*, 197–204. [CrossRef]
18. Vamos, E.P.; Bottle, A.; Edmonds, M.E.; Valabhji, J.; Majeed, A.; Millett, C. Changes in the Incidence of Lower Extremity Amputations in Individuals With and Without Diabetes in England Between 2004 and 2008. *Diabetes Care* **2010**, *33*, 2592–2597. [CrossRef]
19. Kalbaugh, C.A.; Strassle, P.D.; Paul, N.J.; McGinigle, K.L.; Kibbe, M.R.; Marston, W.A. Trends in Surgical Indications for Major Lower Limb Amputation in the USA from 2000 to 2016. *Eur. J. Vasc. Endovasc. Surg.* **2020**, *60*, 88–96. [CrossRef]
20. Narres, M.; Kvitkina, T.; Claessen, H.; Droste, S.; Schuster, B.; Morbach, S.; Rümenapf, G.; van Acker, K.; Icks, A.; Grabowski, A. Incidence of lower extremity amputations in the diabetic compared with the non-diabetic population: A systematic review. *PLoS ONE* **2017**, *12*, e0182081. [CrossRef]
21. Peek, M.E. Gender Differences in Diabetes-related Lower Extremity Amputations. *Clin. Orthop. Relat. Res.* **2011**, *469*, 1951–1955. [CrossRef]
22. Jones, R.E.; Russell, R.D.; Huo, M.H. Alternatives to revision total knee arthroplasty. *J. Bone Jt. Surg.* **2012**, *94*, 137–140. [CrossRef]
23. Goodney, P.P.; Beck, A.W.; Nagle, J.; Welch, H.G.; Zwolak, R.M. National trends in lower extremity bypass surgery, endovascular interventions, and major amputations. *J. Vasc. Surg.* **2009**, *50*, 54–60. [CrossRef] [PubMed]
24. Goodney, P.P.; Tarulli, M.; Faerber, A.E.; Schanzer, A.; Zwolak, R.M. Fifteen-Year Trends in Lower Limb Amputation, Revascularization, and Preventive Measures Among Medicare Patients. *JAMA Surg.* **2015**, *150*, 84–86. [CrossRef]
25. Faglia, E.; Mantero, M.; Caminiti, M.; Caravaggl, C.; Giglio, R.D.; Pritelli, C.; Clerici, G.; Fratino, P.; Cata, P.D.; Paola, L.D.; et al. Extensive use of peripheral angioplasty, particularly infrapopliteal, in the treatment of ischaemic diabetic foot ulcers: Clinical results of a multicentric study of 221 consecutive diabetic subjects. *J. Int. Med.* **2002**, *252*, 225–232. [CrossRef]
26. Diabetes Care and Research in Europe: The Saint Vincent Declaration. *Diabet. Med.* **1990**, *7*, 360. [CrossRef]
27. Bleß, H.-H.; Kip, M. *Weißbuch Gelenkersatz*; Springer: Berlin/Heidelberg, Germany. [CrossRef]
28. Wengler, A.; Nimptsch, U.; Mansky, T. Hip and Knee Replacement in Germany and the USA. *Dtsch. Aerzteblatt Online* **2014**, *111*, 407–416. [CrossRef]

Disclaimer/Publisher's Note: The statements, opinions and data contained in all publications are solely those of the individual author(s) and contributor(s) and not of MDPI and/or the editor(s). MDPI and/or the editor(s) disclaim responsibility for any injury to people or property resulting from any ideas, methods, instructions or products referred to in the content.

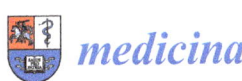

Article

A Pilot Experiment to Measure the Initial Mechanical Stability of the Femoral Head Implant in a Cadaveric Model of Osteonecrosis of Femoral Head Involving up to 50% of the Remaining Femoral Head

Seungha Woo, Youngho Lee and Doohoon Sun *

Department of Orthopedic Surgery, Daejeon Sun Hospital, 29 Mokjung-ro, Jung-gu, Daejeon 34811, Republic of Korea
* Correspondence: sunosdoctor@gmail.com; Tel.: +82-422-208-460; Fax: +82-422-208-464

Abstract: *Background and Objectives:* Currently, only patients with osteonecrosis of the femoral head (ONFH), who had bone defects involving 30–33.3% of the remaining femoral head, are indicated in hip resurfacing arthroplasty (HRA). In an experimental cadaver model of ONFH involving up to 50% of the remaining femoral head, the initial stability of the femoral head implant (FHI) at the interface between the implant and the remaining femoral head was measured. *Materials and Methods:* The ten specimens and the remaining ten served as the experimental group and the control group, respectively. We examined the degree of the displacement of the FHI, the bonding strength between the FHI and the retained bone and that at the interface between the FHI and bone cement. *Results:* Changes in the degree of displacement at the final phase from the initial phase were calculated as 0.089 ± 0.036 mm in the experimental group and 0.083 ± 0.056 mm in the control group. However, this difference reached no statistical significance (p = 0.7789). Overall, there was an increase in the degree of displacement due to the loading stress, with increased loading cycles in both groups. In cycles of up to 6000 times, there was a steep increase. After cycles of 8000 times, however, there was a gradual increase. Moreover, in cycles of up to 8000 times, there was an increase in the difference in the degree of displacement due to the loading stress between the two groups. After cycles of 8000 times, however, such difference remained almost unchanged. *Conclusions:* In conclusion, orthopedic surgeons could consider performing the HRA in patients with ONFH where the bone defects involved up to 50% of the remaining femoral head, without involving the femoral head–neck junction in the anterior and superior area of the femoral head. However, more evidence-based studies are warranted to justify our results.

Keywords: bone defect; femoral head; osteonecrosis of femoral head; resurfacing arthroplasty; stability

1. Introduction

Osteonecrosis of the femoral head (ONFH), also referred to as avascular necrosis, is defined as a pathologic condition arising from an ischemic injury that is characterized by both a crucial disruption of blood supply to the bone and an increase in the intraosseous pressure. Subsequently, this results in the degradation of the organic elements of the bone and the marrow, thus commonly leading to a collapse of subchondral bone in the femoral head [1–4]. As such, ONFH is a debilitating, progressive joint disease of idiopathic origin; it is an interesting topic from both clinical and economic perspectives [5–7]. Over the past few years, there has been an increase in the prevalence of ONFH [8]. Moreover, it has been diagnosed with increasing frequency in young adults and has a significant socioeconomic impact [9]. The annual number of patients who are hospitalized for the treatment of ONFH is estimated at 10,000–20,000 in the US [5]. It is a serious disease entity that may affect the quality of life in patients with ONFH [10]. Still, however, little is known about the risk factors associated with its pathogenesis and pathophysiology, although they include the long-term use of chronic steroids, smoking, alcoholism, hip trauma and prior hip surgery [11,12]. This makes it difficult to define surgical methods and curative effects [1,13]. It is, therefore, crucial to obtain a better understanding of the pathogenesis of and make therapeutic approaches to ONFH [8]. Despite recent advancements in diagnostic modalities, effective treatments have been elusive and a majority of cases of ONFH eventually result in a collapse of the femoral head. Most of the surgical modalities for patients with ONFH aim to prevent the collapse of the subchondral bone, although their clinical outcomes have been reported to be inconsistent [1,13]. Core decompression may be effective for the treatment of early-stage ONFH, although femoral osteotomy, vascularized or non-vascularized bone grafting and total hip arthroplasty (THA) may also be attempted for that of advanced ONFH [14].

Patients with ONFH account for 5–12% of those undergoing THA in the US [1]. If treated conservatively, >80% of affected hips would progress to femoral collapse and the destruction of the hip joint within four years of initial diagnosis; this often requires THA [15]. In the early stage of ONFH, joint-preserving surgical techniques are often considered. However, this causes problems, such as a significant failure rate and morbidity [16–19]. THA is often a mainstay of treatment in patients with osteonecrosis of the hip [18]. However, it may be not an attractive treatment option for younger patients; it would be desirable to avoid or delay THA. This is not only because most of the younger patients would outlive the current state-of-the art implants, but also because it has been suggested that such patients are less satisfied with its clinical outcomes [17,20]. It is therefore imperative that effective treatment modalities be developed, which would be essential for preventing the collapse of affected femoral heads or prolonging the interval between initial diagnosis and THA [7]. To date, diverse small animal models using rats or rabbits have been used to develop new treatment modalities for ONFH. Thus, these animal models induce ONFH by systematic insult, including steroid administration or steroid combined with another adjunct agent [21–27]. It would also be mandatory, however, to improve the relevance of animal models of ONFH in a clinical setting.

Both hemi-resurfacing arthroplasty and metal-on-metal hip resurfacing arthroplasty (HRA) are alternatives to conventional THA for patients with ONFH [28–30]. Hemi-resurfacing and total resurfacing arthroplasty are referred to as the prosthetic replacement of the femoral side only and that of both the femoral head and the acetabular surface, respectively [31]. According to a US nationwide study, the frequency of THA was the highest (90%), followed by HRA (0.2%) and osteotomy (1%) [32]. Both hemi-resurfacing arthroplasty and HRA are potentially advantageous in preserving bone and the loading of the proximal femur, lowering a risk of dislocation and eliminating the polyethylene debris that may cause osteolysis as compared with conventional THA [30,33,34]. Consequently, HRA is considered an appropriate option for young and active patients with ONFH [35].

However, there are things to consider regarding the indications of HRA in the context of regulatory requirements enforced by the US Food and Drug Administration (FDA). In 2006, the US FDA approved the clinical use of a metal-on-metal (MoM) resurfacing implant for primary HRA. This is based on the pre-market approval (PMA) process in 2385 patients with non-inflammatory or inflammatory arthritis receiving the Birmingham Hip Resurfacing (BHR) System (Smith & Nephew Orthopaedics, Memphis, TN) [36,37]. Later, in 2007 and 2009, the US FDA approved the clinical use of two additional MoM resurfacing implants, such as the Cormet™ Hip Resurfacing System (Corin, Tampa, FL, USA) and the Conserve® Plus Total Hip Resurfacing System (MicroPort Orthopedics, Boston, MA, USA), respectively, in patients with non-inflammatory degenerative or inflammatory arthritis [38,39]. Since then, the US FDA has cleared a variety of implants for marketing through the 510(k) process [40]. According to the US FDA, however, patients with ONFH who had a necrotic area involving >50% of the femoral head are contraindicated in the use of MoM implants [41].

Given the above background, we created an experimental cadaver model of ONFH involving 50% of the remaining femoral head. We conducted this study to measure the initial stability of the FHI at the interface between the implant and the remaining femoral head.

2. Materials and Methods

2.1. Experimental Materials and Setting

We conducted the current biomechanical study using ten pairs of specimens from ten cadavers ($n = 10$). The specimens were preserved in a frozen state ($-20\ °C$), and were gradually defrosted at room temperature for 24 h. A total of 20 specimens were equally divided into the experimental group ($n = 10$) and the control group ($n = 10$).

Inclusion criteria for the current experiment were a lack of pathologic bone lesions and the Singh index > 5. The Singh index is a typical classification system for the bone density of the femoral neck based on the qualitative visibility of the trabecular patterns [42].

The experimental procedures are schematically shown in Figure 1.

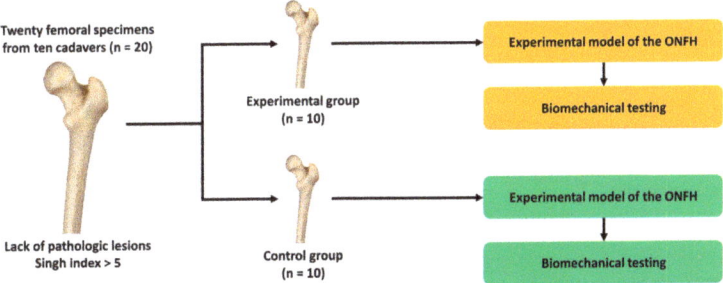

Figure 1. Experimental schema. Abbreviation: ONFH, osteonecrosis of femoral head.

2.2. Creation of an Experimental Model of ONFH

With a free-hand technique at an angle of 135° to the axis of the femoral shaft on the anterior–posterior plane and in parallel with the central axis of the femoral neck, we placed the femoral guide pin on the lateral plane. This was followed by the femoral reaming using a cannulated sleeve and a chamfering reamer with an appropriate size. After saline irrigation, we confirmed a lack of notching and inappropriate exposure of the cancellous bone at the femoral head–neck junction. Then, we dissected 50% of the antero-superior area of the remaining femoral head, and thereby caused bone defects in the experimental group. To consistently make bone defects, we mapped the area in dissecting the area of the femoral head (Figure 2).

Then, we placed an MoM implant (Durom®; Zimmer Inc., Warsaw, IN, USA) in the bone defect area and then fixed it using low-viscosity bone cement (Surgical Simplex® P; Stryker Howmedica Osteonics Corp., Rutherford, NJ, USA) for both groups. In the experimental group, however, we performed the same maneuver after restoring the bone defect area using a sufficient amount of low-viscosity bone cement.

2.3. Assessment of the Biomechanical Stability of the Specimen

We transected the specimen at the isthmus and then fixed it using a resin fixative (Vertex Self-Curing; Vertex-Dental B.V., Soesterberg, The Netherlands) (Figure 3A). We placed it on the machine at a valgus angle of 30°, thus attempting to preventing the fracture of the femoral neck while repeatedly applying a mechanical load to it.

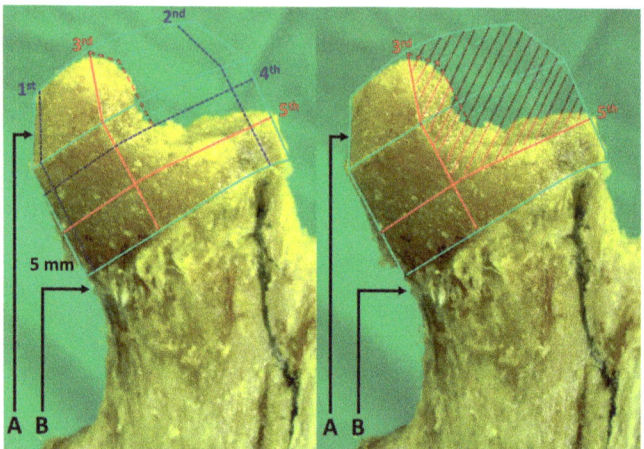

Figure 2. Anatomic specimens of the femur obtained from ten cadavers. Note: A: Femoral head, B: Femoral neck. We drew the 1st and 2nd lines along the midline of the femoral neck on the anterior–posterior and lateral plane, respectively. Then, we drew the 3rd line that crosses the 1st and 2nd lines from postero-superior to infero-anterior directions. We also drew the 4th line, that was vertical to the 3rd line and then crossed the center of the femoral head. In parallel with the 4th line, we drew the 5th line at 5 mm proximal to the head–neck junction. Finally, we dissected 50% of the antero-superior part of the remaining femoral head based on the 3rd and 5th lines.

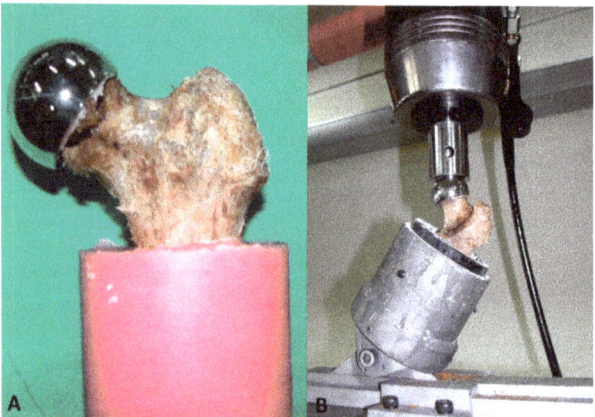

Figure 3. The preparation of the femoral specimens. (**A**) The femoral specimen was inserted in the resin block along the anatomical axis. (**B**) The femoral specimen with the femoral head implant was placed in a custom-made jig for the loading–unloading test.

We measured the biomechanical stability of the specimen using the dynamic testing machine based on the biaxial fluid pressure (Instron 8500®; Instron Corp., Norwood, MA, USA), for which we repeatedly applied a loading stress at a constant rate of 2 Hz [43,44]. The magnitude of loading stress ranged between 60 and 300 kg; it was five times higher as compared with the non-loading condition. The loading and displacement were measured at a sampling rate of 20 Hz using MAX^{TM} software (Instron Corp.) in a total of 15,000 cycles (Figure 3B) [45]. Then, we measured the strength against the displacement of the FHI due to the loading stress [46,47]. In each cycle of loading, we measured the degree of the displacement of the FHI through a scatter plotting analysis using a load versus displacement graph [48,49]. In measuring the bond strength, we defined the initial and final phase of loading as that applied to the specimen in cycles ranging from 1 to 5000 times and 10,000 to 15,000 times, respectively. Thus, we compared differences in changes in the bond strength at the final phase from the initial phase between the two groups, for which we maintained the degree of loading stress consistently throughout the experiment. Therefore, the magnitude of bond strength was solely dependent on the degree of the displacement of the FHI.

2.4. Scanning Electron Microscopy (SEM)

After selecting four pairs of the specimen obtained from the same cadavers in both groups, we prepared cross-sectional samples by pulling the diamond saw across the center of the bone defects on the coronal plane. Thus, we attempted to measure the bond strength at the largest bone defects (Figure 4).

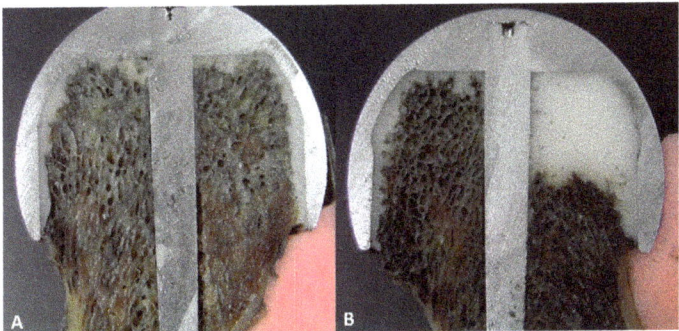

Figure 4. Cross sections of the femoral specimens. (**A**) In the control group, bone cements were used to fill the gap between bone and the implant. There were no other bone defects filled with bone cement. (**B**) In the experimental group, bone defects were used to sufficiently fill 50% of the bone defects. There were no other bone defects.

The samples were completely frozen in a refrigerator ($-80\ ^\circ$C) for 24 h and then underwent a freeze-drying process at a temperature of $-77\ ^\circ$C for two days. We therefore prepared dry femoral samples. This was followed by SEM to examine the bond strength both at the bone–cement interface and at the implant–cement interface.

2.5. Statistical Analysis

Statistical analysis was carried out using the SPSS version 25.0 (IBM Corp., Armonk, NY, USA). All data were presented as mean ± SD (SD: standard deviation). We compared differences in the size of the FHI and changes in the bond strength at the final phase from the initial phase between the two groups using the Student's t-test. A p-value of <0.05 was considered statistically significant.

3. Results

3.1. Size of the FHI

The mean size of the FHI was 49.4 ± 2.1 (range, 44–53) mm in the experimental group and 49.1 ± 1.8 (range, 43–52) mm in the control group. However, this difference reached no statistical significance ($p = 0.7356$).

3.2. Results of the Biomechanical Study

Overall, there was an increase in the degree of displacement due to the loading stress with increased loading cycles in both groups. In cycles of up to 6000 times, there was a steep increase. After cycles of 8000 times, however, there was a gradual increase. Moreover, in cycles of up to 8000 times, there was an increase in the difference in the degree of displacement due to the loading stress between the two groups. After cycles of 8000 times, however, such difference remained almost unchanged (Figure 5).

The degree of displacement at each phase is represented in Table 1. Changes in the degree of displacement at the final phase from the initial phase were calculated as 0.089 ± 0.036 mm in the experimental group and 0.083 ± 0.056 mm in the control group. However, this difference reached no statistical significance ($p = 0.7789$) (Figure 6).

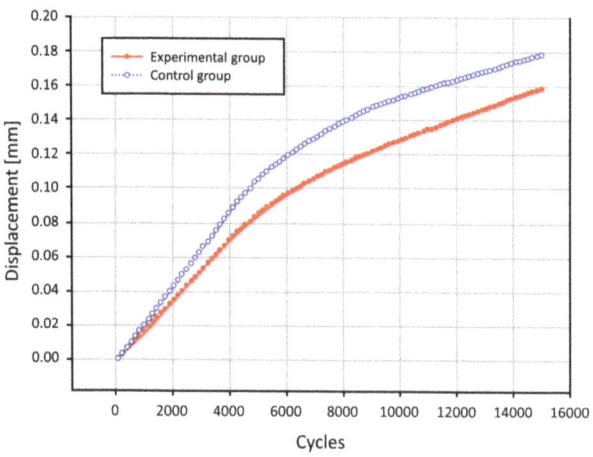

Figure 5. The degree of the displacement of the femoral head implant.

Table 1. The degree of displacement at each phase.

	Values					
#	Experimental Group (n = 10)			Control Group (n = 10)		
	Initial Phase	Final Phase	Δ	Initial Phase	Final Phase	Δ
1	0.237	0.450	0.213	0.051	0.121	0.07
2	0.032	0.066	0.034	0.078	0.190	0.112
3	0.069	0.151	0.082	0.055	0.140	0.085
4	0.031	0.061	0.03	0.109	0.240	0.131
5	0.123	0.251	0.128	0.025	0.073	0.048
6	0.098	0.199	0.01	0.140	0.308	0.168
7	0.042	0.090	0.048	0.075	0.146	0.071
8	0.077	0.172	0.095	0.045	0.104	0.059
9	0.088	0.201	0.113	0.068	0.162	0.094
10	0.062	0.143	0.081	0.052	0.103	0.051

Note: #, specimen identification number; Δ, changes in the degree of displacement at the final phase from the initial phase. All the values are presented at a unit of mm.

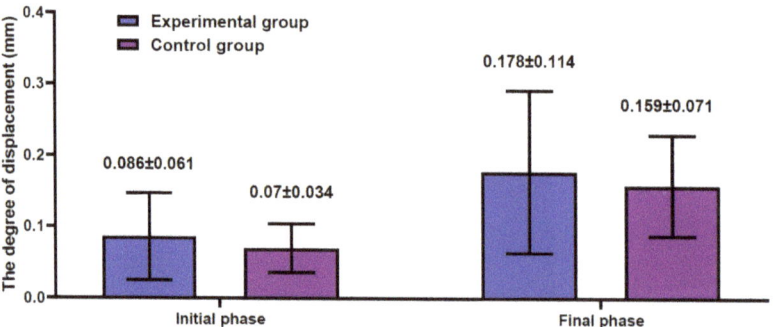

Figure 6. Changes in the degree of displacement at the final phase from the initial phase.

3.3. The Bond Strength at the Bone–Cement Interface

With SEM, all the four pairs of the femoral specimens, obtained from both groups, showed no gap at the bone–cement interface (Figure 7). However, there was a gap of approximately 0.2 mm in size at the interface between the FHI and the bone cement (Figure 8).

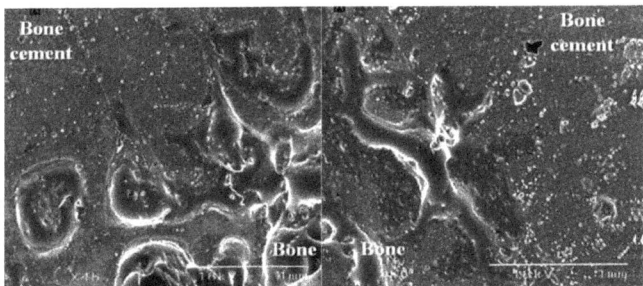

Figure 7. Scanning electron microscopy of the interface between the bone and bone cement. There was no gap between the bone and bone cement in all four pairs of the femoral specimens.

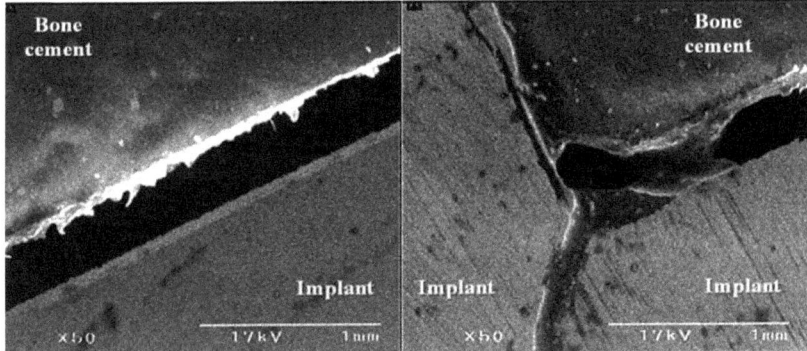

Figure 8. Scanning electron microscopy of the interface between the femoral head implant and bone cement.

4. Discussion

An appropriate experimental model of the human disease is a prerequisite for a clinical trial to assess the efficacy and safety of a novel treatment model in the setting of ONFH [1]. From this context, an animal model of ONFH played a key role in performing a pre-clinical trial to identify more effective treatments, whereas a cellular model was used to clarify the pathogenesis and pathophysiology of ONFH [50]. Nevertheless, many experimental models do not share the same physiological and metabolic characteristics with humans [51,52].

It is mandatory for orthopedic surgeons to obtain a complete understanding of human anatomy; anatomy is a basic medical discipline by which they can achieve improvements in their training. Moreover, cadaveric studies may allow orthopedic surgeons to study the characteristics of many diseases and anatomical structures that are vulnerable to damages, such as bone, muscle and ligament [53].

Cadaveric studies are also useful in performing an assessment of the biomechanics of anatomical structures, thus allowing orthopedic surgeons to develop new surgical techniques [53].

Biomechanical cadaveric studies can be performed when it is not easy to handle the movement or force of interest in the joint or soft tissue in vivo. This enables orthopedic surgeons to assess biomechanical characteristics and properties. Indeed, biomechanical cadaveric studies play a role in performing a pre-clinical assessment of new surgical techniques and implant designs [54–56]. This justifies the current biomechanical cadaveric study.

Mont MA et al. performed a systematic review of the previous published literature on untreated asymptomatic ONFH, thus showing that >25% involvement of the femoral head served as a risk factor of femoral head collapse [57]. Indeed, the HRA can be performed for patients aged < 50 years old who had necrotic lesions involving <30–33.3% of the femoral head [58,59].

To summarize, our results are as follows: First, changes in the degree of displacement at the final phase from the initial phase were calculated as 0.089 ± 0.036 mm in the experimental group and 0.083 ± 0.056 mm in the control group. However, this difference reached no statistical significance ($p = 0.7789$). Second, overall there was an increase in the degree of displacement due to the loading stress, with increased loading cycles in both groups. In cycles of up to 6000 times, there was a steep increase. After cycles of 8000 times, however, there was a gradual increase in it. Moreover, in cycles of up to 8000 times there was an increase in the difference in the degree of displacement due to the loading stress between the two groups. After cycles of 8000 times, however, such difference remained almost unchanged. Third, with SEM, all the four pairs of the femoral specimens, obtained from both groups, showed no gap at the bone–cement interface. However, there was a gap of approximately 0.2 mm in size at the interface between the FHI and bone cement.

However, our results cannot be generalized; further studies based on computational modeling are warranted to corroborate them. The necessity of computational modeling of musculoskeletal structures cannot be overlooked; it may be useful in not only providing the data about musculoskeletal structures, but also in simulating injuries and outcomes of surgical operations [60]. Thus, computational modeling and personalized simulations may provide fundamental insights into a better understanding of the pathophysiologic mechanisms underlying injuries. This can contribute to not only reducing the necessity of human or animal experiments, but also enabling orthopedic surgeons to implement novel treatment strategies or to make a plan for surgery [61]. To date, sophisticated approaches to the computational modeling of musculoskeletal structures have emerged. Indeed, such a model has been employed in studies about a specific type of implant or surgical procedure [62]. This is because a meticulous preoperative strategy based on computational modeling is of paramount importance when orthopedic surgeons choose the optimal type of implant [63].

The usefulness of computational modeling in the context of ONFH deserves special attention. It is more advantageous in predicting the whole process without actually performing the surgery as compared with a traditional static analysis [64].

Computational modeling with finite element analysis (FEA) plays a key role in the association with the design and development of a medical device [65]. More specifically, it can be used to assess the deformation field, strain field and stress field of the femoral head and support device [64]. It would, therefore, be worthwhile to explore the value of the FEA in the context of an MoM implant. Of note, the previous literature has simulated a loading by adopting a gait cycle reflecting the actual condition of an implant user [66–70].

An MoM implant is equipped with a higher stability and a lower risk of dislocations. It is harder as compared with ceramic materials; its advantages include a lower rate of fracture failure under high loads and a 20- to 100-fold lower rate of wear as compared with conventional metal-on-polyethylene implants [71]. Due to these benefits, an MoM implant may be used for younger and more active patients [72].

Efforts have been made to decrease the surface contact area (SCA) and to lower the rate of adhesion wear and the coefficient of friction [73]. A dimple is surface texturing that belongs to one such effort made for diverse types of mechanical components; it plays a role in trapping wear debris, preventing the abrasive wear of SCA and generating hydrodynamic pressure to provide additional lift [74,75]. Both theoretical and experimental studies have shown that surface texturing has a positive effect in improving the tribological performance of a device [76–79].

Jamari J. et al. assessed the effect of dimples on the rate of wear in the context of THA. These authors performed the FEA based on the prediction model with or without dimples. After simulations using 3D physiological loading of the joint under normal walking conditions, Jamari J. et al. showed that the dimples were effective in lowering the contact pressure and wear [80].

To date, orthopedic research has been driven by both biomechanical studies and clinical trials [81–84]. A cadaveric biomechanical study remains a useful method in that it allows surgeons, engineers and researchers to achieve results similar to in vivo clinical studies without endangering patients [53,85]. From this context, the current results are of significance in that this is a pilot experiment using a cadaveric model of the ONFH involving up to 50% of the remaining femoral head in Korea for future clinical studies. However, more efforts should be made to translate the current results into clinical practice.

5. Conclusions

In conclusion, our results indicate that orthopedic surgeons could consider performing the HRA in patients with ONFH where the bone defects involve up to 50% of the remaining femoral head without involving the femoral head–neck junction in the anterior and superior area of the femoral head. However, more evidence-based studies are warranted to justify our results.

Author Contributions: Conceptualization, S.W., Y.L. and D.S.; data curation, S.W. and Y.L.; formal analysis, S.W. and Y.L.; investigation, S.W. and Y.L.; methodology, S.W. and Y.L.; project administration, D.S.; resources, S.W. and Y.L.; supervision, D.S.; visualization, S.W. and Y.L.; writing—original draft, S.W. and Y.L.; writing—review and editing, S.W., Y.L. and D.S. All authors will be informed about each step of manuscript processing, including submission, revision, revision reminder, etc., via emails from the assigned Assistant Editor. All authors have read and agreed to the published version of the manuscript.

Funding: This research received no external funding.

Institutional Review Board Statement: We obtained the ethical approval of the current study from the Internal Institutional Review Board (IRB) of the Korea National Institute of Bioethics Pol-504 icy (IRB approval #: P01-202101-15-019; date of approval: 23 March 2021) and conducted it in compliance with the relevant guidelines and applicable laws. But a written informed consent was waived because this is a cadaveric study.

Informed Consent Statement: Not applicable.

Data Availability Statement: All data generated or analysed during this study are included in this published article.

Conflicts of Interest: The authors declare no conflict of interest.

References

1. Cardín-Pereda, A.; García-Sánchez, D.; Terán-Villagrá, N.; Alfonso-Fernández, A.; Fakkas, M.; Garcés-Zarzalejo, C.; Pérez-Campo, F.M. Osteonecrosis of the Femoral Head: A Multidisciplinary Approach in Diagnostic Accuracy. *Diagnostics* **2022**, *12*, 1731. [CrossRef]
2. Murab, S.; Hawk, T.; Snyder, A.; Herold, S.; Totapally, M.; Whitlock, P.W. Tissue Engineering Strategies for Treating Avascular Necrosis of the Femoral Head. *Bioengineering* **2021**, *8*, 200. [CrossRef]
3. Konarski, W.; Poboży, T.; Śliwczyński, A.; Kotela, I.; Krakowiak, J.; Hordowicz, M.; Kotela, A. Avascular Necrosis of Femoral Head—Overview and Current State of the Art. *Int. J. Environ. Res. Public Health* **2022**, *19*, 7348. [CrossRef] [PubMed]
4. Petek, D.; Hannouche, D.; Suva, D. Osteonecrosis of the femoral head: Pathophysiology and current concepts of treatment. *EFORT Open Rev.* **2019**, *4*, 85–97. [CrossRef]
5. Bejar, J.; Peled, E.; Boss, J.H. Vasculature deprivation-induced osteonecrosis of the rat femoral head as a model for therapeutic trials. *Theor. Biol. Med. Model* **2005**, *2*, 24. [CrossRef]
6. Choi, H.R.; Steinberg, M.E.; Y Cheng, E. Osteonecrosis of the femoral head: Diagnosis and classification systems. *Curr. Rev. Musculoskelet. Med.* **2015**, *8*, 210–220. [CrossRef]

7. Rezus, E.; Tamba, B.I.; Badescu, M.C.; Popescu, D.; Bratoiu, I.; Rezus, C. Osteonecrosis of the Femoral Head in Patients with Hypercoagulability—From Pathophysiology to Therapeutic Implications. *Int. J. Mol. Sci.* **2021**, *22*, 6801. [CrossRef] [PubMed]
8. Fu, D.; Qin, K.; Yang, S.; Lu, J.; Lian, H.; Zhao, D. Proper mechanical stress promotes femoral head recovery from steroid-induced osteonecrosis in rats through the OPG/RANK/RANKL system. *BMC Musculoskelet. Disord.* **2020**, *21*, 281. [CrossRef]
9. Paderno, E.; Zanon, V.; Vezzani, G.; Giacon, T.A.; Bernasek, T.L.; Camporesi, E.M.; Bosco, G. Evidence-Supported HBO Therapy in Femoral Head Necrosis: A Systematic Review and Meta-Analysis. *Int. J. Environ. Res. Public Health* **2021**, *18*, 2888. [CrossRef] [PubMed]
10. Wang, A.; Ren, M.; Wang, J. The pathogenesis of steroid-induced osteonecrosis of the femoral head: A systematic review of the literature. *Gene* **2018**, *671*, 103–109. [CrossRef]
11. Tsai, S.W.; Wu, P.K.; Chen, C.F.; Chiang, C.C.; Huang, C.K.; Chen, T.H.; Liu, C.L.; Chen, W.M. Etiologies and outcome of osteonecrosis of the femoral head: Etiology and outcome study in a Taiwan population. *J. Chin. Med. Assoc.* **2016**, *79*, 39–45. [CrossRef] [PubMed]
12. Kunze, K.N.; Sullivan, S.W.; Nwachukwu, B.U. Updates on Management of Avascular Necrosis Using Hip Arthroscopy for Core Decompression. *Front Surg.* **2022**, *9*, 662722. [CrossRef] [PubMed]
13. Karasuyama, K.; Motomura, G.; Ikemura, S.; Fukushi, J.I.; Hamai, S.; Sonoda, K.; Kubo, Y.; Yamamoto, T.; Nakashima, Y. Risk factor analysis for postoperative complications requiring revision surgery after transtrochanteric rotational osteotomy for osteonecrosis of the femoral head. *J. Orthop. Surg. Res.* **2018**, *13*, 6. [CrossRef] [PubMed]
14. Maruyama, M.; Nabeshima, A.; Pan, C.C.; Behn, A.W.; Thio, T.; Lin, T.; Pajarinen, J.; Kawai, T.; Takagi, M.; Goodman, S.B.; et al. The effects of a functionally-graded scaffold and bone marrow-derived mononuclear cells on steroid-induced femoral head osteonecrosis. *Biomaterials* **2018**, *187*, 39–46. [CrossRef]
15. Bakircioglu, S.; Atilla, B. Hip preserving procedures for osteonecrosis of the femoral head after collapse. *J. Clin. Orthop. Trauma* **2021**, *23*, 101636. [CrossRef]
16. Tripathy, S.K.; Goyal, T.; Sen, R.K. Management of femoral head osteonecrosis: Current concepts. *Indian J. Orthop.* **2015**, *49*, 28–45. [CrossRef]
17. Zhang, Q.Y.; Li, Z.R.; Gao, F.Q.; Sun, W. Pericollapse Stage of Osteonecrosis of the Femoral Head: A Last Chance for Joint Preservation. *Chin. Med. J.* **2018**, *131*, 2589–2598. [CrossRef]
18. Kuroda, Y.; Nankaku, M.; Okuzu, Y.; Kawai, T.; Goto, K.; Matsuda, S. Percutaneous autologous impaction bone graft for advanced femoral head osteonecrosis: A retrospective observational study of unsatisfactory short-term outcomes. *J. Orthop. Surg. Res.* **2021**, *16*, 141. [CrossRef]
19. Jie, K.; Feng, W.; Li, F.; Wu, K.; Chen, J.; Zhou, G.; Zeng, H.; Zeng, Y. Long-term survival and clinical outcomes of non-vascularized autologous and allogeneic fibular grafts are comparable for treating osteonecrosis of the femoral head. *J. Orthop. Surg. Res.* **2021**, *16*, 109. [CrossRef]
20. Ma, J.; Sun, W.; Gao, F.; Guo, W.; Wang, Y.; Li, Z. Porous Tantalum Implant in Treating Osteonecrosis of the Femoral Head: Still a Viable Option? *Sci. Rep.* **2016**, *6*, 28227. [CrossRef]
21. Yang, L.; Boyd, K.; Kaste, S.C.; Kamdem Kamdem, L.; Rahija, R.J.; Relling, M.V. A mouse model for glucocorticoid-induced osteonecrosis: Effect of a steroid holiday. *J. Orthop. Res.* **2009**, *27*, 169–175. [CrossRef]
22. Sugano, N.; Kubo, T.; Takaoka, K.; Ohzono, K.; Hotokebuchi, T.; Matsumoto, T.; Igarashi, H.; Ninomiya, S. Diagnostic criteria for non-traumatic osteonecrosis of the femoral head. A multicentre study. *J. Bone Joint Surg. Br.* **1999**, *81*, 590–595. [CrossRef] [PubMed]
23. Iwakiri, K.; Oda, Y.; Kaneshiro, Y.; Iwaki, H.; Masada, T.; Kobayashi, A.; Asada, A.; Takaoka, K. Effect of simvastatin on steroid-induced osteonecrosis evidenced by the serum lipid level and hepatic cytochrome P4503A in a rabbit model. *J. Orthop. Sci.* **2008**, *13*, 463–468. [CrossRef] [PubMed]
24. Ichiseki, T.; Matsumoto, T.; Nishino, M.; Kaneuji, A.; Katsuda, S. Oxidative stress and vascular permeability in steroid-induced osteonecrosis model. *J. Orthop. Sci.* **2004**, *9*, 509–515. [CrossRef]
25. Yamamoto, T.; Hirano, K.; Tsutsui, H.; Sugioka, Y.; Sueishi, K. Corticosteroid enhances the experimental induction of osteonecrosis in rabbits with Shwartzman reaction. *Clin. Orthop. Relat. Res.* **1995**, *316*, 235–243. [CrossRef]
26. Wu, X.; Yang, S.; Duan, D.; Zhang, Y.; Wang, J. Experimental osteonecrosis induced by a combination of low-dose lipopolysaccharide and high-dose methylprednisolone in rabbits. *Jt. Bone Spine* **2008**, *75*, 573–578. [CrossRef]
27. Qin, L.; Zhang, G.; Sheng, H.; Yeung, K.W.; Yeung, H.Y.; Chan, C.W.; Cheung, W.H.; Griffith, J.; Chiu, K.H.; Leung, K.S. Multiple bioimaging modalities in evaluation of an experimental osteonecrosis induced by a combination of lipopolysaccharide and methylprednisolone. *Bone* **2006**, *39*, 863–871. [CrossRef]
28. Calkins, T.E.; Suleiman, L.I.; Culvern, C.; Alazzawi, S.; Kazarian, G.S.; Barrack, R.L.; Haddad, F.S.; Della Valle, C.J. Hip resurfacing arthroplasty and total hip arthroplasty in the same patient: Which do they prefer? *Hip Int.* **2021**, *31*, 328–334. [CrossRef]
29. Clough, E.J.; Clough, T.M. Metal on metal hip resurfacing arthroplasty: Where are we now? *J. Orthop.* **2020**, *23*, 123–127. [CrossRef]
30. Park, C.W.; Lim, S.J.; Kim, J.H.; Park, Y.S. Hip resurfacing arthroplasty for osteonecrosis of the femoral head: Implant-specific outcomes and risk factors for failure. *J. Orthop. Translat.* **2020**, *21*, 41–48. [CrossRef]
31. Kabata, T.; Maeda, T.; Tanaka, K.; Yoshida, H.; Kajino, Y.; Horii, T.; Yagishita, S.; Tsuchiya, H. Hemi-resurfacing versus total resurfacing for osteonecrosis of the femoral head. *J. Orthop. Surg.* **2011**, *19*, 177–180. [CrossRef]

32. Sodhi, N.; Acuna, A.; Etcheson, J.; Mohamed, N.; Davila, I.; Ehiorobo, J.O.; Jones, L.C.; Delanois, R.E.; Mont, M.A. Management of osteonecrosis of the femoral head. *Bone Jt. J.* **2020**, *102-B*, 122–128. [CrossRef]
33. Ball, S.T.; Le Duff, M.J.; Amstutz, H.C. Early results of conversion of a failed femoral component in hip resurfacing arthroplasty. *J. Bone Joint Surg. Am.* **2007**, *89*, 735–741. [CrossRef] [PubMed]
34. Murray, D.W.; Grammatopoulos, G.; Gundle, R.; Gibbons, C.L.; Whitwell, D.; Taylor, A.; Glyn-Jones, S.; Pandit, H.G.; Ostlere, S.; Gill, H.S.; et al. Hip resurfacing and pseudotumour. *Hip Int.* **2011**, *21*, 279–283. [CrossRef]
35. Tai, C.L.; Chen, Y.C.; Hsieh, P.H. The effects of necrotic lesion size and orientation of the femoral component on stress alterations in the proximal femur in hip resurfacing—A finite element simulation. *BMC Musculoskelet. Disord.* **2014**, *15*, 262. [CrossRef]
36. Su, E.P.; Ho, H.; Bhal, V.; Housman, L.R.; Masonis, J.L.; Noble, J.W., Jr.; Hopper, R.H., Jr.; Engh, C.A., Jr. Results of the First U.S. FDA-Approved Hip Resurfacing Device at 10-Year Follow-up. *J. Bone Joint Surg. Am.* **2021**, *103*, 1303–1311. [CrossRef] [PubMed]
37. Food and Drug Administration. P040033: Birmingham Hip Resurfacing (BHR) System. 2006. Available online: http://www.accessdata.fda.gov/cdrh_docs/pdf4/p040033a.pdf (accessed on 9 February 2023).
38. Gross, T.P.; Liu, F.; Webb, L.A. Clinical outcome of the metal-on-metal hybrid Corin Cormet 2000 hip resurfacing system: An up to 11-year follow-up study. *J. Arthroplast.* **2012**, *27*, 533–538.e1. [CrossRef]
39. Mogensen, S.L.; Jakobsen, T.; Christoffersen, H.; Krarup, N. High Re-Operation Rates Using Conserve Metal-On-Metal Total Hip Articulations. *Open Orthop. J.* **2016**, *10*, 41–48. [CrossRef] [PubMed]
40. Samuel, A.M.; Rathi, V.K.; Grauer, J.N.; Ross, J.S. How do Orthopaedic Devices Change After Their Initial FDA Premarket Approval? *Clin. Orthop. Relat. Res.* **2016**, *474*, 1053–1068. [CrossRef] [PubMed]
41. Waewsawangwong, W.; Ruchiwit, P.; Huddleston, J.I.; Goodman, S.B. Hip arthroplasty for treatment of advanced osteonecrosis: Comprehensive review of implant options, outcomes and complications. *Orthop. Res. Rev.* **2016**, *8*, 13–29.
42. Yamamoto, N.; Sukegawa, S.; Kitamura, A.; Goto, R.; Noda, T.; Nakano, K.; Takabatake, K.; Kawai, H.; Nagatsuka, H.; Kawasaki, K.; et al. Deep Learning for Osteoporosis Classification Using Hip Radiographs and Patient Clinical Covariates. *Biomolecules* **2020**, *10*, 1534. [CrossRef] [PubMed]
43. Gao, S.; Hu, G. Experimental Study on Biaxial Dynamic Compressive Properties of ECC. *Materials* **2021**, *14*, 1257. [CrossRef] [PubMed]
44. Juvonen, T.; Nuutinen, J.P.; Koistinen, A.P.; Kröger, H.; Lappalainen, R. Biomechanical evaluation of bone screw fixation with a novel bone cement. *Biomed. Eng. Online* **2015**, *14*, 74. [CrossRef] [PubMed]
45. Faris, M.A.; Abdullah, M.M.A.B.; Muniandy, R.; Abu Hashim, M.F.; Błoch, K.; Jeż, B.; Garus, S.; Palutkiewicz, P.; Mohd Mortar, N.A.; Ghazali, M.F. Comparison of Hook and Straight Steel Fibers Addition on Malaysian Fly Ash-Based Geopolymer Concrete on the Slump, Density, Water Absorption and Mechanical Properties. *Materials* **2021**, *14*, 1310. [CrossRef]
46. Xu, H.Z.; Wang, X.Y.; Chi, Y.L.; Zhu, Q.A.; Lin, Y.; Huang, Q.S.; Dai, L.Y. Biomechanical evaluation of a dynamic pedicle screw fixation device. *Clin. Biomech.* **2006**, *21*, 330–336. [CrossRef] [PubMed]
47. Nourisa, J.; Rouhi, G. Biomechanical evaluation of intramedullary nail and bone plate for the fixation of distal metaphyseal fractures. *J. Mech. Behav. Biomed. Mater.* **2016**, *56*, 34–44. [CrossRef]
48. Motavalli, M.; Whitney, G.A.; Dennis, J.E.; Mansour, J.M. Investigating a continuous shear strain function for depth-dependent properties of native and tissue engineering cartilage using pixel-size data. *J. Mech. Behav. Biomed. Mater.* **2013**, *28*, 62–70. [CrossRef] [PubMed]
49. Gomez, A.D.; Zou, H.; Shiu, Y.T.; Hsu, E.W. Characterization of regional deformation and material properties of the intact explanted vein by microCT and computational analysis. *Cardiovasc. Eng. Technol.* **2014**, *5*, 359–370. [CrossRef]
50. Li, Z.; Shao, W.; Lv, X.; Wang, B.; Han, L.; Gong, S.; Wang, P.; Feng, Y. Advances in experimental models of osteonecrosis of the femoral head. *J. Orthop. Translat.* **2023**, *39*, 88–99. [CrossRef]
51. Xu, J.; Gong, H.; Lu, S.; Deasey, M.J.; Cui, Q. Animal models of steroid-induced osteonecrosis of the femoral head-a comprehensive research review up to 2018. *Int. Orthop.* **2018**, *42*, 1729–1737. [CrossRef] [PubMed]
52. Zheng, L.Z.; Liu, Z.; Lei, M.; Peng, J.; He, Y.X.; Xie, X.H.; Man, C.W.; Huang, L.; Wang, X.L.; Fong, D.T.; et al. Steroid-associated hip joint collapse in bipedal emus. *PLoS ONE* **2013**, *8*, e76797. [CrossRef] [PubMed]
53. Dal Fabbro, G.; Agostinone, P.; Lucidi, G.A.; Pizza, N.; Maitan, N.; Grassi, A.; Zaffagnini, S. The Cadaveric Studies and the Definition of the Antero-Lateral Ligament of the Knee: From the Anatomical Features to the Patient-Specific Reconstruction Surgical Techniques. *Int. J. Environ. Res. Public Health* **2021**, *18*, 12852. [CrossRef] [PubMed]
54. Kwak, D.-S.; Kim, Y.D.; Cho, N.; In, Y.; Kim, M.S.; Lim, D.; Koh, I.J. Restoration of the Joint Line Configuration Reproduces Native Mid-Flexion Biomechanics after Total Knee Arthroplasty: A Matched-Pair Cadaveric Study. *Bioengineering* **2022**, *9*, 564. [CrossRef] [PubMed]
55. Liu, A.; Sanderson, W.J.; Ingham, E.; Fisher, J.; Jennings, L.M. Development of a specimen-specific in vitro pre-clinical simulation model of the human cadaveric knee with appropriate soft tissue constraints. *PLoS ONE* **2020**, *15*, e0238785. [CrossRef]
56. Vanaclocha, A.; Vanaclocha, V.; Atienza, C.M.; Clavel, P.; Jordá-Gómez, P.; Barrios, C.; Saiz-Sapena, N.; Vanaclocha, L. Bionate Lumbar Disc Nucleus Prosthesis: Biomechanical Studies in Cadaveric Human Spines. *ACS Omega* **2022**, *7*, 46501–46514. [CrossRef] [PubMed]

57. Mont, M.A.; Zywiel, M.G.; Marker, D.R.; McGrath, M.S.; Delanois, R.E. The natural history of untreated asymptomatic osteonecrosis of the femoral head: A systematic literature review. *J. Bone Joint Surg. Am.* **2010**, *92*, 2165–2170. [CrossRef]
58. Kaushik, A.P.; Das, A.; Cui, Q. Osteonecrosis of the femoral head: An update in year 2012. *World J. Orthop.* **2012**, *3*, 49–57. [CrossRef] [PubMed]
59. Della Valle, C.J.; Nunley, R.M.; Raterman, S.J.; Barrack, R.L. Initial American experience with hip resurfacing following FDA approval. *Clin. Orthop. Relat. Res.* **2009**, *467*, 72–78. [CrossRef]
60. Liacouras, P.C.; Wayne, J.S. Computational modeling to predict mechanical function of joints: Application to the lower leg with simulation of two cadaver studies. *J. Biomech. Eng.* **2007**, *129*, 811–817. [CrossRef]
61. Weickenmeier, J.; Butler, C.A.M.; Young, P.G.; Goriely, A.; Kuhl, E. The mechanics of decompressive craniectomy: Personalized simulations. *Comput. Methods Appl. Mech. Eng.* **2017**, *314*, 180–195. [CrossRef]
62. Scifert, C.F.; Noble, P.C.; Brown, T.D.; Bartz, R.L.; Kadakia, N.; Sugano, N.; Johnston, R.C.; Pedersen, D.R.; Callaghan, J.J. Experimental and computational simulation of total hip arthroplasty dislocation. *Orthop. Clin. North Am.* **2001**, *32*, 553–567. [CrossRef] [PubMed]
63. Peng, M.J.; Chen, H.Y.; Hu, Y.; Ju, X.; Bai, B. Finite Element Analysis of porously punched prosthetic short stem virtually designed for simulative uncemented Hip Arthroplasty. *BMC Musculoskelet. Disord.* **2017**, *18*, 295. [CrossRef]
64. Yi, W.; Tian, Q.; Dai, Z.; Liu, X. Mechanical behaviour of umbrella-shaped, Ni-Ti memory alloy femoral head support device during implant operation: A finite element analysis study. *PLoS ONE* **2014**, *9*, e100765. [CrossRef]
65. Goel, V.K.; Nyman, E. Computational Modeling and Finite Element Analysis. *Spine* **2016**, *41* (Suppl. 7), S6–S7. [CrossRef]
66. Ammarullah, M.I.; Santoso, G.; Sugiharto, S.; Supriyono, T.; Wibowo, D.B.; Kurdi, O.; Tauviqirrahman, M.; Jamari, J. Minimizing Risk of Failure from Ceramic-on-Ceramic Total Hip Prosthesis by Selecting Ceramic Materials Based on Tresca Stress. *Sustainability* **2022**, *14*, 13413. [CrossRef]
67. Jamari, J.; Ammarullah, M.I.; Santoso, G.; Sugiharto, S.; Supriyono, T.; van der Heide, E. In Silico Contact Pressure of Metal-on-Metal Total Hip Implant with Different Materials Subjected to Gait Loading. *Metals* **2022**, *12*, 1241. [CrossRef]
68. Ammarullah, M.I.; Afif, I.Y.; Maula, M.I.; Winarni, T.I.; Tauviqirrahman, M.; Akbar, I.; Basri, H.; van der Heide, E.; Jamari, J. Tresca Stress Simulation of Metal-on-Metal Total Hip Arthroplasty during Normal Walking Activity. *Materials* **2021**, *14*, 7554. [CrossRef] [PubMed]
69. Jamari, J.; Ammarullah, M.I.; Santoso, G.; Sugiharto, S.; Supriyono, T.; Prakoso, A.T.; Basri, H.; van der Heide, E. Computational Contact Pressure Prediction of CoCrMo, SS 316L and Ti6Al4V Femoral Head against UHMWPE Acetabular Cup under Gait Cycle. *J. Funct. Biomater.* **2022**, *13*, 64. [CrossRef]
70. Jamari, J.; Ammarullah, M.I.; Santoso, G.; Sugiharto, S.; Supriyono, T.; Permana, M.S.; Winarni, T.I.; van der Heide, E. Adopted walking condition for computational simulation approach on bearing of hip joint prosthesis: Review over the past 30 years. *Heliyon* **2022**, *8*, e12050. [CrossRef]
71. Hu, C.Y.; Yoon, T.R. Recent Updates for Biomaterials Used in Total Hip Arthroplasty. *Biomater. Res.* **2018**, *22*, 33. [CrossRef]
72. Harun, M.N.; Wang, F.C.; Jin, Z.M.; Fisher, J. Long-Term Contact-Coupled Wear Prediction for Metal-on-Metal Total Hip Joint Replacement. *Proc. Inst. Mech. Eng. Part J J. Eng. Tribol.* **2009**, *223*, 993–1001. [CrossRef]
73. Choudhury, D.; Lackner, J.; Fleming, R.A.; Goss, J.; Chen, J.; Zou, M. Diamond-like Carbon Coatings with Zirconium-Containing Interlayers for Orthopedic Implants. *J. Mech. Behav. Biomed. Mater.* **2017**, *68*, 51–61. [CrossRef] [PubMed]
74. Basri, H.; Syahrom, A.; Ramadhoni, T.S.; Prakoso, A.T.; Ammarullah, M.I. The Analysis of the Dimple Arrangement of the Artificial Hip Joint to the Performance of Lubrication. *IOP Conf. Ser. Mater. Sci. Eng.* **2019**, *620*, 1–10. [CrossRef]
75. Basri, H.; Syahrom, A.; Prakoso, A.T.; Wicaksono, D.; Amarullah, M.I.; Ramadhoni, T.S.; Nugraha, R.D. The Analysis of Dimple Geometry on Artificial Hip Joint to the Performance of Lubrication. *J. Phys. Conf. Ser.* **2019**, *1198*, 1–10. [CrossRef]
76. Ammarullah, M.I.; Saad, A.P.; Syahrom, A. Contact Pressure Analysis of Acetabular Cup Surface with Dimple Addition on Total Hip Arthroplasty Using Finite Element Method. *IOP Conf. Ser. Mater. Sci. Eng.* **2021**, *1034*, 1–11. [CrossRef]
77. Wang, W.; He, Y.; Li, Y.; Wei, B.; Hu, Y.; Luo, J. Investigation on Inner Flow Field Characteristics of Groove Textures in Fully Lubricated Thrust Bearings. *Ind. Lubr. Tribol.* **2018**, *70*, 754–763. [CrossRef]
78. Pratap, T.; Patra, K. Mechanical Micro-Texturing of Ti-6Al-4V Surfaces for Improved Wettability and Bio-Tribological Performances. *Surf. Coat. Technol.* **2018**, *349*, 71–81. [CrossRef]
79. Choudhury, D.; Vrbka, M.; Bin Mamat, A.; Stavness, I.; Roy, C.K.; Mootanah, R.; Krupka, I. The impact of surface and geometry on coefficient of friction of artificial hip joints. *J. Mech. Behav. Biomed. Mater.* **2017**, *72*, 192–199. [CrossRef]
80. Jamari, J.; Ammarullah, M.I.; Saad, A.P.M.; Syahrom, A.; Uddin, M.; van der Heide, E.; Basri, H. The Effect of Bottom Profile Dimples on the Femoral Head on Wear in Metal-on-Metal Total Hip Arthroplasty. *J. Funct. Biomater.* **2021**, *12*, 38. [CrossRef] [PubMed]
81. Jain, A.K. Research in orthopedics: A necessity. *Indian J. Orthop.* **2009**, *43*, 315–317. [CrossRef] [PubMed]
82. Lu, C.; Buckley, J.M.; Colnot, C.; Marcucio, R.; Miclau, T. Basic research in orthopedic surgery: Current trends and future directions. *Indian J. Orthop.* **2009**, *43*, 318–323. [PubMed]
83. Nayar, S.K.; Dein, E.J.; Bernard, J.A.; Zikria, B.A.; Spiker, A.M. Basic Science Research Trends in Orthopedic Surgery: An Analysis of the Top 100 Cited Articles. *HSS J.* **2018**, *14*, 333–337. [CrossRef] [PubMed]

84. Madry, H.; Grässel, S.; Nöth, U.; Relja, B.; Bernstein, A.; Docheva, D.; Kauther, M.D.; Katthagen, J.C.; Bader, R.; van Griensven, M.; et al. The future of basic science in orthopaedics and traumatology: Cassandra or Prometheus? *Eur. J. Med. Res.* **2021**, *26*, 56. [CrossRef]
85. Maletsky, L.; Shalhoub, S.; Fitzwater, F.; Eboch, W.; Dickinson, M.; Akhbari, B.; Louie, E. In Vitro Experimental Testing of the Human Knee: A Concise Review. *J. Knee Surg.* **2016**, *29*, 138–148. [PubMed]

Disclaimer/Publisher's Note: The statements, opinions and data contained in all publications are solely those of the individual author(s) and contributor(s) and not of MDPI and/or the editor(s). MDPI and/or the editor(s) disclaim responsibility for any injury to people or property resulting from any ideas, methods, instructions or products referred to in the content.

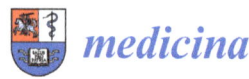

Article

Intertrochanteric Femoral Fractures: A Comparison of Clinical and Radiographic Results with the Proximal Femoral Intramedullary Nail (PROFIN), the Anti-Rotation Proximal Femoral Nail (A-PFN), and the InterTAN Nail

Mustafa Yalın [1,*], Fatih Golgelioglu [1] and Sefa Key [2]

[1] Department of Orthopedics and Traumatology, Fethi Sekin City Hospital, Elazığ 23280, Turkey; fatihgolgelioglu@gmail.com

[2] Department of Orthopedics and Traumatology, Faculty of Medicine, Firat University, Elazığ 23190, Turkey; sefa_key@hotmail.com

* Correspondence: mustiyalin1988@gmail.com

Abstract: *Background and Objectives:* The aim of this study was to evaluate retrospectively the radiological and functional outcomes of closed reduction and internal fixation for intertrochanteric femoral fractures (IFF) using three different proximal femoral nails (PFN). *Materials and Methods:* In total, 309 individuals (143 males and 166 females) who underwent surgery for IFF using a PFN between January 2018 and January 2021 were included in the study. Our surgical team conducted osteosynthesis using the A-PFN® (TST, Istanbul, Turkey) nail, the PROFIN® (TST, Istanbul, Turkey), and the Trigen InterTAN (Smith & Nephew, Memphis, TN, USA) nail. The PFNs were compared based on age, gender, body mass index (BMI), length of stay (LOS) in intensive care, whether to be admitted to intensive care, mortality in the first year, amount of transfusion, preoperative time to surgery, hospitalisation time, duration of surgery and fluoroscopy, fracture type and reduction quality, complication ratio, and clinical and radiological outcomes. The patients' function was measured with the Harris Hip Score (HHS) and the Katz Index of Independence in Activities of Daily Living (ADL). *Results:* Pain in the hip and thigh is the most common complication, followed by the V-effect. The Z-effect was seen in 5.7% of PROFIN patients. A-PFN was shown to have longer surgical and fluoroscopy durations, lower HHS values, and much lower Katz ADL Index values compared to the other two PFNs. The V-effect occurrence was significantly higher in the A-PFN group (36.7%) than in the InterTAN group. The V-effect was seen in 33.1% of 31A2-type fractures but in none of the 31A3-type fractures. *Conclusions:* InterTAN nails are the best choice for IFFs because they have high clinical scores after surgery, there is no chance of Z-effect, and the rate of V-effect is low.

Keywords: intertrochanteric femoral fractures; proximal femoral nail; Z-effect; V-effect

1. Introduction

Over a million individuals suffer from hip fractures every year, making it one of the most prevalent orthopaedic injuries [1,2]. Nearly half of all hip fractures are intertrochanteric femur fractures (IFFs), which are more common in the elderly and are often the consequence of low-energy traumas [3]. In order to achieve a satisfactory reduction and to facilitate the patients' early recovery, surgical treatment is required for such kinds of fractures [4]. The dynamic hip screw (DHS) implant, which was previously regarded as the gold standard therapy for stable intertrochanteric fractures, was shown to be inadequate for the stabilisation of fractures of the unstable kind [5]. As opposed to extramedullary devices such as DHS, proximal femoral nails (PFN) have a biomechanical advantage because of their closer location to the vector of force line and shorter moment arm [6]. Moreover, based on the results of several reports, intramedullary fixation may be preferable to extramedullary fixation for patients since there is a lower risk of implant failure and reoperation, and functional scores are higher [7–9]. It is possible to implant a PFN with a minimally invasive procedure. By performing a closed reduction of the fracture, the haematoma is maintained, and the surgeon can do a minimally invasive procedure with minimum soft-tissue dissection, thereby minimizing surgical trauma, blood loss, infection, and wound complications [10,11].

Bone healing is significantly aided by the interfragmentary linear compression provided by the lag screw in the majority of PFNs. One or two lag screws, integrated or locked lag screws, and a wedge block that offers rotational stability are some of the PFN designs on the industry [12]. Clinical and radiological evaluations of two distinct PFNs have been the subject of several published papers [12–15]. Even though PFNs such as A-PFN, PROFIN, and InterTAN are widely used in our country, very few studies have compared the radiological and clinical results of these three PFNs. Hence, the aim of the current study was to compare three distinct PFNs in terms of radiological and functional results in patients treated with closed reduction and internal fixation for IFFs.

2. Materials and Methods

A retrospective observational study was conducted, which included the evaluation of clinical data. After receiving approval from the local ethics committee (22 May 2021), patients who underwent surgery for IFFs between January 2018 and January 2021 were reviewed. All patients provided a written informed consent form in compliance with the hospital's ethical committee's norms. Individuals with unilateral isolated IFF who were mobile enough to undertake everyday tasks prior to the injury, were at least 18 years old, and whose follow-up period was at least 1 year participated in the study. Non-trochanteric fractures, pathologic fractures, polytrauma patients, bilateral simultaneous fractures, previous intertrochanteric fractures in the contralateral leg, impaired muscle strength, mental disorders including dementia and follow-up less than a year were the exclusion criteria. A total of 309 individuals (143 males and 166 females) who met the inclusion criteria were included in the study. Preoperative pelvic or hip images were employed to categorise fractures using the AO (Arbeitsgemeinschaft für Osteosynthesefragen) classification system. Surgeons have implanted three distinct PFNs, comprising InterTAN, PROFIN, and A-PFN (Figure 1). The PFNs were contrasted on several variables, including age, gender, body mass index (BMI), energy of trauma, length of staying (LOS) in intensive care, whether to be admitted to intensive care, mortality in the first year, amount of transfusion, preoperative time to surgery, hospitalisation time, duration of surgery and fluoroscopy, fracture type and reduction quality, complication ratio, and clinical and radiological outcomes. The functionality of patients was determined with the Harris Hip Score (HHS) and the Katz Index of Independence in Activities of Daily Living (ADL). For evaluating a person's ADL, a modified version of Katz's questionnaire [16] was used, which included six questions regarding self-care and four questions related to mobility. Respondents who were not capable of performing an activity without assistance or without significant trouble were labelled as limited regarding that activity. The number of limits was then written down, and a score between 0 and 10 was given. The reliability and validity of self-reported limitations on the Katz ADL were also investigated by Reijneveld et al. [17], who found that, in terms of clinical care, their findings support the idea that assessing self-reported ADL provides an acceptable, reliable, and valid measure of functional status. An experienced orthopaedic surgeon (SK) who was not participating in the patient's care reviewed the patient's radiological outcomes, including reduction quality, fracture union, and radiological complications including V-effect, Z-effect, and varus collapse. Postoperative reduction quality was evaluated by utilising Baumgartner reduction metrics, as revised by Fogagnolo et al. [18].

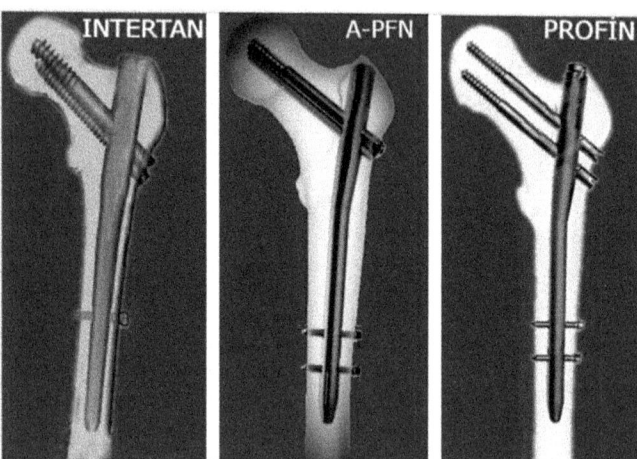

Figure 1. The medical images demonstrate the structural system of the three proximal femoral nails.

The kind of implant we employed for a patient was governed by the hospital's budget and the Ministry of Health's purchasing rules, both of which have changed over time. Hospital administration was charged for the type of nail. Neither doctors nor patients were responsible for this decision and were aware of the type of nail used just before the operation.

2.1. Characteristics of PFNs

2.1.1. InterTAN (Intertrochanteric Antegrade Nail)

The titanium alloy used in the production of InterTAN PFN allows for a proximal 4° valgus offset. The nail features a trapezoidal cross-section with a 17 mm proximal diameter and a 10 to 11.5 mm grooved distal tip diameter. InterTAN PFNs are available with either a 125° or 130° collodiaphyseal angle (CDA). A lag screw of 11 mm and a compression screw of 7 mm were used. The tip of the nail was secured by a single screw that was locked in either a dynamic or static configuration. With the combined proximal screw system, it was possible to achieve interfragmentary compression of up to 15 mm. The InterTAN nail is designed with an interlocking lag nail system that helps minimise femoral head movement and prevents the femoral head from collapsing [7].

2.1.2. A-PFN (Antirotational Proximal Femoral Nail)

A-PFN (TST Medical Devices, Istanbul, Turkey®) is available in two different lengths: 160 and 220 mm. The top portion of the proximal nail features a 6° valgus angle (mediolateral curvature) with a diameter of 15 mm. This nail is available in four different diameters: 9, 10, 11, and 12; it has a lag screw that compresses the fractures and a wedge block that provides rotational stability for femoral fractures. The 10 mm wide thread and 125° angle of the lag screw are consistent with the CDA. The wedge block is in the groove on the lower portion of the lag screw. The distal end of the nail has two locking holes appropriate for either dynamic or static fixations, as well as a slot [19].

2.1.3. PROFIN (Proximal Femoral Intramedullary Nail)

PROFIN PFN is a titanium alloy tube with a cannulated and flat design. It features a proximal valgus offset of 6° and a distal grooved shape, and it is attached with two 8.5 mm lag screws with 135° CDA. The surgical compression of interfragmentary fractures was also possible with this system. The nail has a 16 mm diameter at its proximal end and three separate distal diameters measuring 10, 11, and 12 mm. Both dynamic and static fixation with 4.5 mm locking screws are possible via the two distal holes [20].

2.2. Surgical Procedure

Every patient received 1 g of parenteral cefuroxime sodium 60 min prior to surgical incision. All procedures were carried out under general or regional anaesthesia. All procedures were performed by the same surgical team consisting of five surgeons with five years of expertise in orthopaedic trauma, with the patient laying supine on a traction table after a closed reduction under fluoroscopic guidance. Nailing was performed by utilizing a minimally invasive technique after a closed reduction was achieved under fluoroscopic control. Each of the three PFN kinds was inserted through the trochanter major. By installing the lag screw in InterTAN and employing the integrated compression screw, interfragmentary compression was achieved. Interfragmentary compression was accomplished in PROFIN by inserting two different lag screws into the nail. A lag screw and wedge block placed through the nail were used to generate interfragmentary compression in the A-PFN. Our surgical team performed osteosynthesis with the A-PFN® (TST, Istanbul, Turkey) nail, the PROFIN® (TST, Istanbul, Turkey), and the Trigen InterTAN (Smith & Nephew, Memphis, TN, USA) nail. All three PFNs likewise had the distal hole statically locked. In order to prevent venous thromboembolism (VTE), low molecular weight heparin was administered to all patients when they were admitted to the hospital. VTE prophylaxis administration was stopped twelve hours before the procedure, and then it was restarted six hours following the operation. All individuals were provided with precisely the same postoperative care. At 24 h postoperatively, all patients were given 4 × 1 gramme of cefazolin sodium intravenously as prophylaxis. Each patient was given enoxaparin for 14 days postoperatively to prevent thromboembolism, with the dosage based on their body mass index. Patients were encouraged to walk with a walker and start weight bearing as tolerated on the first postoperative day, when they also began quadricep exercises. Individuals were recommended to begin partial weight bearing two weeks following the procedure. A physiotherapist who also worked in the intensive care unit (ICU) helped give passive range-of-motion exercises to ICU patients while they were lying in bed. Walking and range-of-motion exercises were maintained after patients were admitted to the clinic. Upon radiological confirmation of fracture healing, patients were given clearance to begin full weight bearing. The duration of the surgery was determined to be the time from the first incision made on the patient following closed reduction of the fracture and the complete closure of the wound. Fluoroscopy time was calculated based on the total number of exposures taken at the conclusion of the procedure. Healing of a bone fracture was described as the development of cortical integrity, including at least three cortices or a bridging callus.

Clinical and radiographic assessments were performed on all patients by the same surgical team two weeks, three months, and six months following surgery, and once yearly afterwards. Hip and thigh pain was defined as a mild pain that responded to paracetamol treatment. It was considered a complication if it persisted at the third-month follow-up and was questioned by the same surgical team at each follow-up. Severe pain that did not respond to painkillers was investigated in terms of implant failure. Using the CDA of the patient's contralateral hip, the degree of varus collapse was determined. When the same surgical team that conducted the operation encountered complications during the postoperative follow-up, they advised further surgery to the patients if considered reasonable.

2.3. Statistics

For statistical purposes, IBM SPSS Statistics 22 (IBM SPSS, Turkey) was used to evaluate the study's findings. Using the Shapiro–Wilk test, the conformance of the study's parameters to the normal distribution was determined while the data were analysed. The results of the Shapiro–Wilk test as well as the histogram graphics and boxplot findings were considered while it was decided which test to apply. Because of their length, histogram and boxplot findings are not included in the final draft. In addition to descriptive statistical methods (mean, standard deviation, and frequency), the Kruskal–Wallis test was used to compare parameters that did not exhibit normal distribution in the comparison of quantitative data, and the Dunn's test was used to identify the group responsible for the difference. Using the chi-square test, the Fisher–Freeman–Halton test, and the continuity (Yates) correction, qualitative data were compared. Significance was evaluated at the $p < 0.05$ level.

3. Results

The study was conducted on a total of 309 cases—143 (46.3%) men and 166 (53.7%) women—aged between 23 and 95 between January 2018 and January 2021. The Shapiro–Wilk test, which was used to determine whether the parameters of the study matched a normal distribution, provided the findings shown in Table 1. The mean age of the patients was 77.34 ± 7.99 years. Tables 2 and 3 present the descriptive features of the patients. Simple falls are the most prevalent cause of injury across all categories. The average time between admission and surgery was 2.26 days. The average length of time between surgery and discharge was 4.95 days. The mean duration of surgery was 65.45 min, and the 1-year mortality rate was 27.5%. In 66.3% of the patients, anatomical reduction was achievable, whereas 7.8% of the reductions were of poor quality. Approximately 39.5% of patients had at least one complication, with 31-A2 fractures being the most prevalent kind of fracture.

Table 1. Normality test results according to type of nail groups and in total.

	Type of PFN	Shapiro–Wilk-Tests of Normality-p
Age	A-PFN	0.392
	InterTAN	0.066
	PROFIN	0.633
	Total	0.026 *
BMI	A-PFN	0.023 *
	InterTAN	0.006 *
	PROFIN	0.032 *
	Total	0.001 *
ASA score	A-PFN	0.000 *
	InterTAN	0.000 *
	PROFIN	0.000 *
	Total	0.000 *
Time from admission to surgery (days)	A-PFN	0.000 *
	InterTAN	0.000 *
	PROFIN	0.000 *
	Total	0.000 *
İntensive care stay (days)	A-PFN	0.000 *
	InterTAN	0.000 *
	PROFIN	0.001 *
	Total	0.000 *
Red blood cell transfusion (units)	A-PFN	0.000 *
	InterTAN	0.000 *
	PROFIN	0.000 *
	Total	0.000 *
Time from surgery to discharge (days)	A-PFN	0.003 *
	InterTAN	0.000 *
	PROFIN	0.000 *
	Total	0.000 *
Duration of surgery (min)	A-PFN	0.020 *
	InterTAN	0.019 *
	PROFIN	0.042 *
	Total	0.000 *
Fluoroscopy time (min)	A-PFN	0.170
	InterTAN	0.028 *
	PROFIN	0.489
	Total	0.000 *

* $p < 0.05$.

Table 2. The descriptive features of the patients.

		Min–Max	Mean ± SD (Median)
Age		23–95	77.34 ± 7.99 (76)
Body mass index		23–32	26.35 ± 1.91 (26)
Intensive care stay (days)		1–12	2.95 ± 1.51 (3)
		n	%
Gender	Male	143	46.3
	Female	166	53.7
Intensive care	Absence	211	68.3
	Presence	98	31.7
Mortality (in 1 year)	Absence	224	72.5
	Presence	85	27.5
ASA score		1–4	2.74 ± 0.86 (3)
Time from admission to surgery (days)		1–5	2.26 ± 1.56 (2)
Red blood cell transfusion (units)		0–3	0.29 ± 0.48 (0)
Time from surgery to discharge (days)		1–15	4.95 ± 1.87 (5)
Duration of surgery (min)		50–90	65.45 ± 7.83 (64)
Fluoroscopy time (min)		27–65	40.76 ± 8.3 (38)
Harris Hip Score		33–97	72.15 ± 13.89 (75)
Katz ADL Index		1–6	4.2 ± 1.12 (4)

Table 3. The descriptive features of the patients.

		n	%
Type of PFN	A-PFN	107	34.6
	InterTAN	98	31.7
	PROFIN	104	33.7
Energy of trauma	Simple fall	256	82.8
	Traffic accident	25	8.1
	Falling from high	28	9.1
Fracture side	Right	116	37.5
	Left	193	62.5
Reduction quality	Acceptable	80	25.9
	Anatomic	205	66.3
	Poor	24	7.8
Fracture classification (AO)	31A1	104	33.7
	31A2	179	57.9
	31A3	26	8.4
Anaesthesia type	General	62	20.1
	Spinal	247	79.9
Presence of complications	Absent	187	60.5
	Present	122	39.5
Complications (n = 122)	Cut-Out	10	8.2
	Hip and Thigh Pain	79	64.8
	Deep tissue infection	4	3.3
	Double screw back	1	0.8
	Hardware breakage	1	0.8
	Superficial infection	9	7.4
	Varus Collapse	14	11.5
	Urinary System infection	6	4.9
	V-effect	30	24.6
	Z-effect	6	4.9
	Non-union	1	0.8

A-PFN was shown to have longer surgical and fluoroscopy durations compared to the other two PFNs (Table 4). Based on the post hoc evaluations, A-PFN had considerably lower HHS values compared to the other two PFNs (Table 5). Comparing the Katz ADL Index values revealed a substantial difference between A-PFN and InterTAN, with A-PFN having much lower Katz ADL Index values compared to InterTAN (Table 5).

Table 4. Evaluation of general characteristics among proximal femoral nail subgroups.

		Type of PFN			p
		A-PFN	InterTAN	PROFIN	
		(Min–Max)–(Mean ± SD (Median))	(Min–Max)–(Mean ± SD (Median))	(Min–Max)–(Mean ± SD (Median))	
Age		(65–92)–(77.81 ± 6.64 (76))	(23–95)–(76.6 ± 9.64 (76))	(56–95)–(77.55 ± 7.57 (77.5))	[1] 0.799
Body mass index		(24–30)–(26.45 ± 1.68 (26))	(23–32)–(26.29 ± 1.93 (26))	(23–32)–(26.32 ± 2.12 (26))	[1] 0.521
Intensive care stay (days)		(1–5)–(2.66 ± 1 (2))	(1–12)–(3.52 ± 2.06 (3))	(1–6)–(2.81 ± 1.35 (2))	[1] 0.101
ASA score		(1–4)–(2.83 ± 0.69 (3))	(1–4)–(2.65 ± 0.93 (3))	(1–4)–(2.73 ± 0.95 (3))	[1] 0.405
Time from admission to surgery(days)		(1–5)–(2.25 ± 1.61 (1))	(1–5)–(2.32 ± 1.55 (2))	(1–5)–(2.21 ± 1.52 (2))	[1] 0.777
Red blood cell transfusion (units)		(0–1)–(0.32 ± 0.47 (0))	(0–3)–(0.31 ± 0.55 (0))	(0–1)–(0.26 ± 0.44 (0))	[1] 0.645
Time from surgery to discharge (days)		(2–7)–(4.76 ± 1.12 (5))	(2–15)–(5.1 ± 2.34 (5))	(1–13)–(5 ± 1.98 (5))	[1] 0.970
Duration of surgery (mins)		(64–90)–(74.11 ± 4.19 (74))	(50–71)–(60.46 ± 4.67 (60))	(50–85)–(61.24 ± 5.02 (60.5))	[1] 0.000 *
Fluoroscopy time (mins)		(40–65)–(50.55 ± 4.33 (50))	(27–49)–(35.15 ± 4.08 (36))	(27–47)–(35.97 ± 4.3 (36))	[1] 0.000 *
Harris Hip Score		(35–94)–(70.84 ± 13.59 (71))	(33–95)–(75.5 ± 13.42 (78))	(37–97)–(70.33 ± 14.19 (75))	[1] 0.010 *
Katz ADL Index		(2–6)–(4.02 ± 1.08 (4))	(1–6)–(4.45 ± 1.15 (4))	(2–6)–(4.16 ± 1.1 (4))	[1] 0.020 *
		n (%)	n (%)	n (%)	
Gender	Male	49 (%45.8)	47 (%48)	47 (%45.2)	[2] 0.918
	Female	58 (%54.2)	51 (%52)	57 (%54.8)	
İntensive care	Absent	72 (%67.3)	71 (%72.4)	68 (%65.4)	[2] 0.539
	Present	35 (%32.7)	27 (%27.6)	36 (%34.6)	
Mortality (in 1 year)	Absent	73 (%68.2)	75 (%76.5)	76 (%73.1)	[2] 0.407
	Present	34 (%31.8)	23 (%23.5)	28 (%26.9)	
Energy of trauma	Simple fall	89 (%83.2)	80 (%81.6)	87 (%83.7)	[2] 0.912
	Traffic accident	8 (%7.5)	10 (%10.2)	7 (%6.7)	
	Falling from high	10 (%9.3)	8 (%8.2)	10 (%9.6)	
Fracture side	Right	42 (%39.3)	35 (%35.7)	39 (%37.5)	[2] 0.872
	Left	65 (%60.7)	63 (%64.3)	65 (%62.5)	
Reduction quality	Acceptable	27 (%25.2)	21 (%21.4)	32 (%30.8)	[2] 0.088
	Anatomic	70 (%65.4)	74 (%75.5)	61 (%58.7)	
	Poor	10 (%9.3)	3 (%3.1)	11 (%10.6)	
Anaesthesia type	General	18 (%16.8)	21 (%21.4)	23 (%22.1)	[2] 0.581
	Spinal	89 (%83.2)	77 (%78.6)	81 (%77.9)	

[1] Kruskal–Wallis test. [2] Chi-square test. * $p < 0.05$.

Table 5. Post hoc evaluations of proximal femoral nail subtypes.

	A-PFN-InterTAN	A-PFN-PROFIN	InterTAN-PROFIN
Duration of surgery (min)	0.000 *	0.000 *	0.492
Fluoroscopy time (min)	0.000 *	0.000 *	0.483
Harris Hip Score	0.031 *	0.019 *	0.846
Katz ADL Index	0.006 *	0.308	0.080
ASA Score	0.008 *	0.014 *	0.589
Fracture classification (AO)	0.014 *	0.000 *	0.023 *

* $p < 0.05$.

Hip and thigh pain, in particular, stands out as the most common complication. Hip and thigh pain was reported by 29 individuals in PROFIN, 22 in InterTan, and 28 in A-PFN. The V-effect ranked as the second most frequent complication. The V-effect was detected by 9 individuals in PROFIN, 3 in InterTAN, and 18 in A-PFN. We detected the Z-effect in 6 of 104 patients treated with PROFIN. In one patient each, hardware breakage, double screw-back, and non-union were detected (Table 6).

Table 6. Evaluation of complication occurrence among proximal femoral nail subgroups.

		Type of Proximal Femoral Nail			p
		A-PFN	InterTAN	PROFIN	
		n (%)	n (%)	n (%)	
Presence of complications	Absent	58 (%54.2)	68 (%69.4)	61 (%58.7)	[1] 0.076
	Present	49 (%45.8)	30 (%30.6)	43 (%41.3)	
Complications	Cut-Out	3 (%6.1)	3 (%10)	4 (%9.3)	[2] 0.766
	Hip and thigh pain	28 (%57.1)	22 (%73.3)	29 (%67.4)	[1] 0.309
	Deep tissue infection	2 (%4.1)	1 (%3.3)	1 (%2.3)	-
	Double screw back	0 (%0)	0 (%0)	1 (%2.3)	-
	Hardware breakage	0 (%0)	0 (%0)	1 (%2.3)	-
	Superficial infection	3 (%6.1)	5 (%16.7)	1 (%2.3)	-
	Varus collapse	7 (%14.3)	2 (%6.7)	5 (%11.6)	[2] 0.673
	Urinary system infection	1 (%2)	2 (%6.7)	3 (%7)	-
	V-effect	18 (%36.7)	3 (%10)	9 (%20.9)	[1] 0.022 *
	Z-effect	0 (%0)	0 (%0)	6 (%14)	-
	Non-union	0 (%0)	1 (%3.3)	0 (%0)	-

[1] Chi-square test. [2] Fisher–Freeman–Halton test. * $p < 0.05$.

The incidence of the V-effect differed significantly ($p:0.022$; $p < 0.05$) depending on the PFN subtype (Table 6). Pairwise comparisons revealed that the incidence of the V-effect in the A-PFN group (36.7%) was significantly higher than in the InterTAN group (10%) ($p < 0.05$) (Table 7). The Z-effect could not be statistically evaluated among the PFN subgroups since it is just a potential complication in the PROFIN group.

Table 7. Post hoc evaluations of the V-effect among nail subtypes.

	A-PFN-InterTAN	A-PFN-PROFIN	InterTAN-PROFIN
V-effect	0.019 *	0.152	0.180

* $p < 0.05$.

4. Discussion

A noteworthy aspect of the current study is the comparison of the three most prevalent PFN models that have been used in our country in recent times. Other notable aspects of the current study also include the complication rates and the association of complications with implant type and fracture type.

The literature reports failure rates of up to 56%, depending on fracture severity and implant design, despite the improvements in operational treatment [21]. Pain, immobility, and the need for further surgery may all result from a failed fixation [22]. Unstable fractures (AO OTA 31-A2 and A3 type) which are multi-fragmentary or have a displaced femoral neck may be especially difficult to fix [23]. Even after the fracture has been reduced and stabilised, there is still a greater risk of failure, especially varus collapse, which may cause pain, functional impairments, and implant failure [24,25].

Yaozeng et al. [26] demonstrated that 90.1% of individuals experienced hip and thigh pain due to the gluteus medius muscle being scraped following nail insertion. However,

Kumbaracı et al. [13] discovered in their study that, even though 72% of patients had thigh or hip pain, it had no impact on functional results. Quartley et al. conducted a meta-analysis in 2022 comparing the InterTAN implant to different existing nails for unstable fractures and concluded that the InterTAN nail reduced implant-related failure, re-intervention rates, and hip and thigh pain without impacting recovery results [27]. The current study did not reveal any significant difference in hip and thigh pain between implant types. In their 2019 study, Duramaz et al. [28] reported a hip and thigh pain prevalence of 21.8%, which was similar to the current study's prevalence of 25.5%, and this prevalence seemed to have no influence on functional or radiological outcomes either.

Employing PFN with two independent lag screws to treat IFFs sometimes leads to issues such as Z-effect or reverse Z-effect [29]. There was a total of six individuals who suffered the Z-effect following PROFIN; however, no patients experienced the reverse Z-effect. The InterTAN nail is designed to improve rotational stability for hip fracture patients by using two interlocking lag screws (not independent) near the proximal end to construct a locking mechanism [27]. It is possible that this might help prevent problems such as femoral neck erosion, varus collapse, and unnatural shortening [30,31]. The current study's findings showing that InterTAN-treated individuals did not experience the Z-effect are in line with the existing literature. Ertürer et al. [29] claimed in 2012 that the Z-effect may be avoided by using two screws of equal size to distribute the strains on the hip. All patients in the current study who had PROFIN had a longer superior lag screw than an inferior lag screw, and the Z-effect occurred in 6% of individuals in the current study. Investigation into the biomechanics of this theory is clearly required.

The average surgery duration with the A-PFN nail was 55.19 ± 15.51 min, according to the 2018 study by Karakuş et al. [19]. Lin et al. [32] reported a mean operative time of 78.5 min in their study of 231 patients. In the current study, the mean duration of surgery following the application of an A-PFN nail was 74.11 ± 4.19 min, which was longer than that recorded in the literature. We believe that this is due to the fact that our surgeons had challenges during the insertion of the compression screws owing to technical issues with the implant set, resulting in an increase in the frequency and duration of fluoroscopy. Based on data from 2019, Duramaz et al. [28] found that InterTAN surgeries took an average of 61.6 min, while PROFIN surgeries took an average of 64.6 min. The present analysis confirmed the literature-reported values of 60.4 min for InterTAN and 61.2 min for PROFIN.

HHS was the most reported functional outcome for patients with intertrochanteric fractures, as reported in multiple studies [33–39], and in these reports, no statistically significant differences in HHS were found among PFN groups. Similar to the current study, a 2015 study by Uzer et al. [12] compared HHS values between patients who had InterTAN and PROFIN nails and found no significant difference. The mean HHS levels were also quite similar to those seen in the current study. Compared to InterTAN and PROFIN, A-PFN patients had significantly lower HHS and Katz ADL values in the current study. In their 2018 study, Karakuş et al. [19] evaluated their patients in groups based on age; the mobility scores of patients who received A-PFN were found to be in line with the Katz ADL values of patients in the current study. Evaluating the complication rates of PFNs reveals a statistically significant difference only in terms of the V-effect. Some of the reasons for the poor clinical results in A-PFN patients may be due to the prolonged duration of the surgery, in our perspective.

When the fracture line extends all the way to the greater trochanteric tip, an iatrogenic complication known as the "V-effect" might occur following fixation with PFN in IFFs (Figure 2). Hu et al. [40] were the first to provide a detailed description of the V-effect in the academic literature. The V-effect might be regarded as the result of two mechanisms. The first component is the placement of the guide wire to the fracture line, which continues towards the trochanteric point, instead of the guide wire's point of entry in accordance with the PFN model. Second, since the guide wire penetrates the intramedullary area in the incorrect way, the drilling performed on it produces a hinge impact rather than an intramedullary hole for PFN [41]. The varus of the femoral neck with respect to the femoral shaft seems to be a direct result of the V-effect. This is related to a large extent to the fact that PFN generates separation in the fracture zone, which eventually reaches the apex of the great trochanter. Based on the results of the current study, 9.7% of participants experienced the V-effect. This was consistent with the 9.4% incidence of the V-effect reported by Eceviz et al. [41] in their 2021 study. They also discovered that InterTAN nails had the lowest occurrence of the V-effect compared to PROFIN nails. Consistent with the previous research, the present study found that the V-effect was most prevalent in the A-PFN group and least prevalent in the InterTAN group. As the second most common complication in the current study, the V-effect was found in 32.9% of 31A2-type fractures but in none of the 31A3-type fractures, leading us to conclude that surgeons should be careful when operating on 31A2-type fractures. Hu et al. [40] advised having an assistant hold the greater trochanter while the surgeon performs reaming at a high rotational speed. Consequently, the proximal femur may have to be widened so that the PFN may be implanted at a more advantageous angle. It was concluded that the V-effect, which contributes to hip varus deformity and non-union, was avoidable. There is a lack of data about the clinical outcomes of patients diagnosed with the V-effect. Several individuals having perfect images did not recover to their former well-being level, while other individuals with the V-effect on images had no noticeable symptoms. Not all of our patients with the V-effect had varus collapse. Clinical results may be affected by the V-effect; hence, further long-term follow-up clinical studies evaluating varus progression in patients with the V-effect and examining this phenomenon are needed.

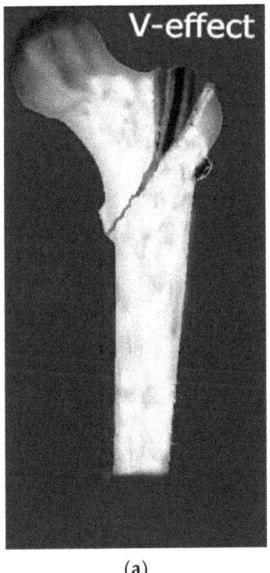 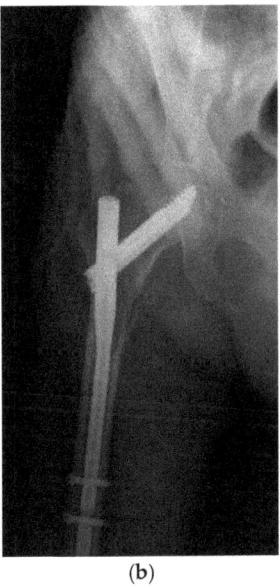

(a) (b)

Figure 2. The "V-effect", an iatrogenic complication of proximal femoral nail fixation in intertrochanteric femoral fractures, may develop when the fracture line extends all the way to the greater trochanteric tip. (a) An illustration of the "V-effect". (b) Observation of the V-effect in a patient who underwent surgery with A-PFN nail.

Several limitations exist in the current study. First, it is a retrospective study restricted to a single tertiary institution in our country; therefore, it has intrinsic drawbacks. Second, the most significant drawback of the research is the wide age range of individuals with hip fractures evaluated. Third, bone mineral density examinations, which could be beneficial in determining the durability of PFNs versus bone density scores, were also not regularly conducted for individuals with hip fractures. Fourth, the study did not identify postoperative complication treatment or surgical techniques. The strength of the study lies in its assessment of the clinical and radiological outcomes of three commonly applied PFN types in our country. The study's other strengths are its large sample size, its analysis of variations in complication occurrence among implant types, and its contribution to the literature on the V-effect, a rarely mentioned complication that surgeons may encounter frequently.

5. Conclusions

Consequently, when the three implant types are compared based on their complication rates and clinical outcomes, the InterTAN nail comes out on top. We consider that InterTAN nails will be an ideal choice for femur fractures due to their relatively short surgery and fluoroscopy times, high postoperative clinical scores, lack of Z-effect probability, and low V-effect rates, which were mentioned rarely in the literature. Multi-centred prospective studies comparing the three kinds of nails with larger patient populations are needed.

Author Contributions: Conceptualisation, M.Y. and S.K.; methodology, M.Y.; software, F.G.; validation, M.Y., F.G. and S.K.; formal analysis, M.Y.; investigation, M.Y.; resources, F.G.; data curation, M.Y.; writing—original draft preparation, M.Y.; writing—review and editing, M.Y.; visualisation, F.G.; supervision, S.K.; project administration, M.Y. All authors have read and agreed to the published version of the manuscript.

Funding: This research received no external funding.

Institutional Review Board Statement: The study was conducted in accordance with the Declaration of Helsinki and approved by the Institutional Review Board (or Ethics Committee) of Fırat University Faculty of Medicine (22 May 2021).

Informed Consent Statement: Informed consent was obtained from all subjects involved in the study.

Data Availability Statement: Not applicable.

Conflicts of Interest: The authors declare no conflict of interest.

Abbreviations

AO = Arbeitsgemeinschaft für Osteosynthesefragen; IFF = intertrochanteric femoral fracture; PFN = proximal femoral nail; A-PFN = antirotational proximal femoral nail; PROFIN = proximal femoral intramedullary nail; BMI = body mass index; LOS = length of stay; HHS = Harris Hip Score; ADL = activities of daily living; CDA = collo-diaphyseal angle; ICU = intensive care unit; VTE = venous thromboembolism.

References

1. Huette, P.; Abou-Arab, O.; Djebara, A.E.; Terrasi, B.; Beyls, C.; Guinot, P.G.; Havet, E.; Dupont, H.; Lorne, E.; Ntouba, A.; et al. Risk factors and mortality of patients undergoing hip fracture surgery: A one-year follow-up study. *Sci. Rep.* **2020**, *10*, 9607. [CrossRef] [PubMed]
2. Svedbom, A.; Hernlund, E.; Ivergård, M.; Compston, J.; Cooper, C.; Stenmark, J.; McCloskey, E.V.; Jönsson, B.; Kanis, J.A. Osteoporosis in the European Union: A compendium of country-specific reports. *Arch. Osteoporos.* **2013**, *8*, 137. [CrossRef] [PubMed]
3. Fischer, H.; Maleitzke, T.; Eder, C.; Ahmad, S.; Stöckle, U.; Braun, K.F. Management of proximal femur fractures in the elderly: Current concepts and treatment options. *Eur. J. Med. Res.* **2021**, *26*, 86. [CrossRef] [PubMed]
4. Sharma, V.; Babhulkar, S.; Babhulkar, S. Role of gamma nail in management of pertrochanteric fractures of femur. *Indian J. Orthop.* **2008**, *42*, 212–216. [CrossRef]
5. Zhang, K.; Zhang, S.; Yang, J.; Dong, W.; Wang, S.; Cheng, Y.; Al-Qwbani, M.; Wang, Q.; Yu, B. Proximal femoral nail vs. dynamic hip screw in treatment of intertrochanteric fractures: A meta-analysis. *Med. Sci. Monit.* **2014**, *20*, 1628–1633. [CrossRef] [PubMed]
6. Lu, Y.; Uppal, H.S. Hip Fractures: Relevant Anatomy, Classification, and Biomechanics of Fracture and Fixation. *Geriatr. Orthop. Surg. Rehabil.* **2019**, *10*, 2151459319859139. [CrossRef]
7. Zheng, X.L.; Park, Y.C.; Kim, S.; An, H.; Yang, K.H. Removal of a broken trigen intertan intertrochanteric antegrade nail. *Injury* **2017**, *48*, 557–559. [CrossRef]
8. Yu, X.; Wang, H.; Duan, X.; Liu, M.; Xiang, Z. Intramedullary versus extramedullary internal fixation for unstable intertrochanteric fracture, a meta-analysis. *Acta Orthop. Traumatol. Turc.* **2018**, *52*, 299–307. [CrossRef]

9. Li, A.B.; Zhang, W.J.; Wang, J.; Guo, W.J.; Wang, X.H.; Zhao, Y.M. Intramedullary and extramedullary fixations for the treatment of unstable femoral intertrochanteric fractures: A meta-analysis of prospective randomized controlled trials. *Int. Orthop.* **2017**, *41*, 403–413. [CrossRef]
10. Mereddy, P.; Kamath, S.; Ramakrishnan, M.; Malik, H.; Donnachie, N. The AO/ASIF proximal femoral nail antirotation (PFNA): A new design for the treatment of unstable proximal femoral fractures. *Injury* **2009**, *40*, 428–432. [CrossRef]
11. Nherera, L.; Trueman, P.; Horner, A.; Watson, T.; Johnstone, A.J. Comparison of a twin interlocking derotation and compression screw cephalomedullary nail (InterTAN) with a single screw derotation cephalomedullary nail (proximal femoral nail antirotation): A systematic review and meta-analysis for intertrochanteric fractures. *J. Orthop. Surg. Res.* **2018**, *13*, 46. [CrossRef] [PubMed]
12. Uzer, G.; Elmadağ, N.M.; Yıldız, F.; Bilsel, K.; Erden, T.; Toprak, H. Comparison of two types of proximal femoral hails in the treatment of intertrochanteric femur fractures. *Ulus. Travma Acil Cerrahi Derg.* **2015**, *21*, 385–391. [CrossRef] [PubMed]
13. Kumbaraci, M.; Karapinar, L.; Turgut, A. Comparison of Second and Third-Generation Nails in the Treatment of Intertrochanteric Fracture: Screws versus Helical Blades. *Eurasian J. Med.* **2017**, *49*, 7–11. [CrossRef] [PubMed]
14. Stern, R.; Lübbeke, A.; Suva, D.; Miozzari, H.; Hoffmeyer, P. Prospective randomised study comparing screw versus helical blade in the treatment of low-energy trochanteric fractures. *Int. Orthop.* **2011**, *35*, 1855–1861. [CrossRef] [PubMed]
15. D'Arrigo, C.; Carcangiu, A.; Perugia, D.; Scapellato, S.; Alonzo, R.; Frontini, S.; Ferretti, A. Intertrochanteric fractures: Comparison between two different locking nails. *Int. Orthop.* **2012**, *36*, 2545–2551. [CrossRef]
16. Katz, S.; Ford, A.B.; Moskowitz, R.W.; Jackson, B.A.; Jaffe, M.W. Studies of Illness in the Aged. The Index of ADL: A Standardized Measure of Biological and Psychosocial Function. *JAMA* **1963**, *185*, 914–919. [CrossRef]
17. Reijnveld, S.A.; Spijker, J.; Dijkshoorn, H. Katz' ADL index assessed functional performance of Turkish, Moroccan, and Dutch elderly. *J. Clin. Epidemiol.* **2007**, *60*, 382–388. [CrossRef] [PubMed]
18. Fogagnolo, F.; Kfuri, M., Jr.; Paccola, C.A. Intramedullary fixation of pertrochanteric hip fractures with the short AO-ASIF proximal femoral nail. *Arch. Orthop. Trauma Surg.* **2004**, *124*, 31–37. [CrossRef]
19. Karakus, O.; Ozdemir, G.; Karaca, S.; Cetin, M.; Saygi, B. The relationship between the type of unstable intertrochanteric femur fracture and mobility in the elderly. *J. Orthop. Surg. Res.* **2018**, *13*, 207. [CrossRef]
20. Soylemez, M.S.; Uygur, E.; Poyanli, O. Effectiveness of distally slotted proximal femoral nails on prevention of femur fractures during and after intertrochanteric femur fracture surgery. *Injury* **2019**, *50*, 2022–2029. [CrossRef]
21. Haidukewych, G.J.; Israel, T.A.; Berry, D.J. Reverse obliquity fractures of the intertrochanteric region of the femur. *J. Bone Joint Surg. Am.* **2001**, *83*, 643–650. [CrossRef]
22. Liu, P.; Jin, D.; Zhang, C.; Gao, Y. Revision surgery due to failed internal fixation of intertrochanteric femoral fracture: Current state-of-the-art. *BMC Musculoskelet. Disord.* **2020**, *21*, 573. [CrossRef] [PubMed]
23. Roberts, K.C.; Brox, W.T.; Jevsevar, D.S.; Sevarino, K. Management of hip fractures in the elderly. *J. Am. Acad. Orthop. Surg.* **2015**, *23*, 131–137. [CrossRef] [PubMed]
24. Tawari, A.A.; Kempegowda, H.; Suk, M.; Horwitz, D.S. What makes an intertrochanteric fracture unstable in 2015? Does the lateral wall play a role in the decision matrix? *J. Orthop. Trauma* **2015**, *29* (Suppl. S4), S4–S9. [CrossRef]
25. Lichtblau, S. The unstable intertrochanteric hip fracture. *Orthopedics* **2008**, *31*, 792–797. [CrossRef] [PubMed]
26. Yaozeng, X.; Dechun, G.; Huilin, Y.; Guangming, Z.; Xianbin, W. Comparative study of trochanteric fracture treated with the proximal femoral nail anti-rotation and the third generation of gamma nail. *Injury* **2010**, *41*, 1234–1238. [CrossRef]
27. Quartley, M.; Chloros, G.; Papakostidis, K.; Saunders, C.; Giannoudis, P.V. Stabilisation of AO OTA 31-A unstable proximal femoral fractures: Does the choice of intramedullary nail affect the incidence of post-operative complications? A systematic literature review and meta-analysis. *Injury* **2022**, *53*, 827–840. [CrossRef]
28. Duramaz, A.; İlter, M.H. The impact of proximal femoral nail type on clinical and radiological outcomes in the treatment of intertrochanteric femur fractures: A comparative study. *Eur. J. Orthop. Surg. Traumatol.* **2019**, *29*, 1441–1449. [CrossRef]
29. Ertürer, R.E.; Sönmez, M.M.; Sarı, S.; Seçkin, M.F.; Kara, A.; Öztürk, I. Intramedullary osteosynthesis of instable intertrochanteric femur fractures with Profin® nail in elderly patients. *Acta Orthop. Traumatol. Turc.* **2012**, *46*, 107–112. [CrossRef]
30. Ruecker, A.H.; Rupprecht, M.; Gruber, M.; Gebauer, M.; Barvencik, F.; Briem, D.; Rueger, J.M. The treatment of intertrochanteric fractures: Results using an intramedullary nail with integrated cephalocervical screws and linear compression. *J. Orthop. Trauma* **2009**, *23*, 22–30. [CrossRef]
31. Huang, Y.; Zhang, C.; Luo, Y. A comparative biomechanical study of proximal femoral nail (InterTAN) and proximal femoral nail antirotation for intertrochanteric fractures. *Int. Orthop.* **2013**, *37*, 2465–2473. [CrossRef] [PubMed]
32. Lin, P.H.; Chien, J.T.; Hung, J.P.; Hong, C.K.; Tsai, T.Y.; Yang, C.C. Unstable intertrochanteric fractures are associated with a greater hemoglobin drop during the perioperative period: A retrospective case control study. *BMC Musculoskelet. Disord.* **2020**, *21*, 244. [CrossRef]
33. Gavaskar, A.S.; Tummala, N.C.; Srinivasan, P.; Gopalan, H.; Karthik, B.; Santosh, S. Helical Blade or the Integrated Lag Screws: A Matched Pair Analysis of 100 Patients With Unstable Trochanteric Fractures. *J. Orthop. Trauma* **2018**, *32*, 274–277. [CrossRef] [PubMed]
34. Yu, W.; Zhang, X.; Zhu, X.; Hu, J.; Liu, Y. A retrospective analysis of the InterTan nail and proximal femoral nail anti-rotation-Asia in the treatment of unstable intertrochanteric femur fractures in the elderly. *J. Orthop. Surg. Res.* **2016**, *11*, 10. [CrossRef]
35. Zehir, S.; Şahin, E.; Zehir, R. Comparison of clinical outcomes with three different intramedullary nailing devices in the treatment of unstable trochanteric fractures. *Ulus. Travma Acil Cerrahi Derg.* **2015**, *21*, 469–476. [CrossRef] [PubMed]

36. Tekin, K.Ü.; Okan, T.; Seyhan, M.; Gereli, A.; Alper, K. Comparison of Third Generation Proximal Femoral Nails in Treatment of Reverse Oblique Intertrochanteric Fractures. *Bezmialem Sci.* **2019**, *7*, 271.
37. İmerci, A.; Aydogan, N.H.; Tosun, K. A comparison of the InterTan nail and proximal femoral fail antirotation in the treatment of reverse intertrochanteric femoral fractures. *Acta Orthop. Belg.* **2018**, *84*, 123–131.
38. Zhang, C.; Xu, B.; Liang, G.; Zeng, X.; Zeng, D.; Chen, D.; Ge, Z.; Yu, W.; Zhang, X. Optimizing stability in AO/OTA 31-A2 intertrochanteric fracture fixation in older patients with osteoporosis. *J. Int. Med. Res.* **2018**, *46*, 1767–1778. [CrossRef]
39. Zhao, F.; Guo, L.; Wang, X.; Zhang, Y. Benefit of lag screw placement by a single- or two-screw nailing system in elderly patients with AO/OTA 31-A2 trochanteric fractures. *J. Int. Med. Res.* **2021**, *49*, 3000605211003766. [CrossRef]
40. Hu, S.J.; Yu, G.R.; Zhang, S.M. Surgical treatment of basicervical intertrochanteric fractures of the proximal femur with cephalomeduallary hip nails. *Orthop. Surg.* **2013**, *5*, 124–129. [CrossRef]
41. Eceviz, E.; Cevik, H.B. The V-effect in fixation of intertrochanteric fractures with proximal femoral nails. *Orthop. Traumatol. Surg. Res.* **2021**, *107*, 102863. [CrossRef] [PubMed]

Disclaimer/Publisher's Note: The statements, opinions and data contained in all publications are solely those of the individual author(s) and contributor(s) and not of MDPI and/or the editor(s). MDPI and/or the editor(s) disclaim responsibility for any injury to people or property resulting from any ideas, methods, instructions or products referred to in the content.

Article

Combined Midportion Achilles and Plantaris Tendinopathy: A 1-Year Follow-Up Study after Ultrasound and Color-Doppler-Guided WALANT Surgery in a Private Setting in Southern Sweden

Håkan Alfredson [1,2,*], Markus Waldén [3,4], David Roberts [3] and Christoph Spang [5,6]

1 Department of Community Medicine and Rehabilitation, Sports Medicine, Umeå University, 90187 Umeå, Sweden
2 Alfredson Tendon Clinic, Capio Ortho Center Skåne, 21532 Malmö, Sweden
3 Capio Ortho Center Skåne, 21532 Malmö, Sweden
4 Department of Health, Medicine and Caring Sciences, Linköping University, 58183 Linköping, Sweden
5 Department of Sports Science, University of Würzburg, 97074 Sanderring, Germany
6 Integrative Medical Biology, Anatomy Section, Umeå University, 90187 Umeå, Sweden
* Correspondence: hakan.alfredson@umu.se

Abstract: *Background and Objectives*: Chronic painful midportion Achilles combined with plantaris tendinopathy can be a troublesome condition to treat. The objective was to prospectively follow patients subjected to ultrasound (US)- and color doppler (CD)-guided wide awake, local anesthetic, no-tourniquet (WALANT) surgery in a private setting. *Material and Methods*: Twenty-six Swedish patients (17 men and 9 women, mean age 50 years (range 29–62)) and eight international male patients (mean age of 38 years (range 25–71)) with combined midportion Achilles and plantaris tendinopathy in 45 tendons altogether were included. All patients had had >6 months of pain and had tried non-surgical treatment with eccentric training, without effect. US + CD-guided surgical scraping of the ventral Achilles tendon and plantaris removal under local anesthesia was performed on all patients. A 4–6-week rehabilitation protocol with an immediate full-weight-bearing tendon loading regime was used. The VISA-A score and a study-specific questionnaire evaluating physical activity level and subjective satisfaction with the treatment were used for evaluation. *Results*: At the 1-year follow-up, 32/34 patients (43 tendons) were satisfied with the treatment result and had returned to their pre-injury Achilles tendon loading activity. There were two dropouts (two tendons). For the Swedish patients, the mean VISA-A score increased from 34 (0–64) before surgery to 93 (61–100) after surgery ($p < 0.001$). There were two complications, one wound rupture and one superficial skin infection. *Conclusions*: For patients suffering from painful midportion Achilles tendinopathy and plantaris tendinopathy, US + CD-guided surgical Achilles tendon scraping and plantaris tendon removal showed a high satisfaction rate and good functional results 1 year after surgery.

Keywords: Achilles tendinopathy; plantaris tendinopathy; surgical treatment; follow-up

1. Introduction

Midportion Achilles tendinopathy is relatively common in the general population [1–4] and is known to be a problematic injury for runners [5–7]. The etiology is unknown, but overuse among active and non-actives is generally considered to be the main causative factor [5–7]. The condition has also been shown to be relatively common among individuals suffering from diagnoses involved in the metabolic syndrome with high blood lipids, type 2 diabetes, and hypertension [8]. Men and women are equally affected [1].

Treatment is known to be difficult, but painful eccentric calf muscle training has been shown to be an efficient non-surgical method [9–12]. Multiple different surgical methods have been described, but most of them are tendon invasive and require long rehabilitation [13–20]. Studies on surgical biopsies have shown nerves in close relation to blood vessels outside but not inside the tendons [21,22]. These findings have been used for the development of the ultrasound (US)- and color doppler (CD)-guided surgical scraping method outside the ventral side of the Achilles tendon [23,24]. More recently, the plantaris tendon has shown similar tendinopathic changes as in the Achilles tendon, but also sensory nerves inside and outside the plantaris tendon [25,26]. The plantaris tendon can also mechanically interfere with the Achilles tendon [27]. For patients with insufficient symptom relief from non-surgical treatment methods, US + CD-guided combined Achilles scraping targeting the regions with high blood flow and nerves outside the tendon and local plantaris tendon removal has been shown to be successful in many patients [28–30].

Midportion Achilles tendinopathy is a debilitating condition among individuals on multiple different activity levels, and there is an obvious need to find an appropriate treatment method. Avoiding intratendinous surgery has major advantages, and new research has opened the possibility of using methods focusing on the outside of the Achilles. The aim of this prospective study was to introduce the US + CD-guided wide awake, local anesthetic, no-tourniquet (WALANT) surgery for patients suffering from chronic painful midportion Achilles combined with plantaris tendinopathy in a private setting in southern Sweden and evaluate the 1-year functional outcome and subjective patient satisfaction with the treatment.

2. Materials and Methods

2.1. Patients and Clinical Examination

Informed written consent was obtained from all patients. Twenty-six consecutive Swedish patients (17 men and 9 women, mean age 50 years (range 29–62), were included (Table 1) between August 2020 and March 2022. The patients' activity levels were recreational athletes ($n = 12$); non-actives ($n = 5$); padel ($n = 4$); gym ($n = 1$); and elite athletes participating in soccer ($n = 2$), triathlon ($n = 1$), and orienteering ($n = 1$). In a separate group during the same study period, 8 international male patients (11 tendons) were also included and operated on. There were 6 professional athletes involved in soccer ($n = 4$), cross-country skiing ($n = 1$), and hurling ($n = 1$), as well as 2 high-level recreational athletes involved in marathon running ($n = 1$) and dancing ($n = 1$). There were no smokers among the patients, and 4 patients had treatment for hypertension.

Table 1. Patients' characteristics.

Values	Females	Males	Total
Age	51 (29–61)	49 (32–62)	50 (29–62)
Height	168 (164–173)	185 (179–191)	181 (164–191)
Weight	65 (58–78)	88 (80–104)	80 (58–104)

Inclusion criteria: adult patients ($\geq$18 years) with long duration (>6 months) of midportion Achilles tendon pain and eccentric training without effect, or inability to perform eccentric training because of back, hip, knee, ankle, or foot problems. Exclusion criteria: chronic systemic inflammatory conditions and previous surgery inside or close to the Achilles tendon.

Patients were examined and operated on at Capio Orthocenter Skåne in Malmö, Sweden. Clinical examination demonstrated a thickening of the Achilles midportion with tenderness located on both the ventral and the medial side of the tendon thickening in all cases. High resolution gray-scale US + CD (S-500, Siemens AG, Germany) using a linear multifrequency (8–13 MHz) probe showed a thickened Achilles midportion (>7 mm) with irregular tendon structure. On the medial side of the Achilles midportion, there was a wide or thick plantaris tendon (Figure 1). There was also a localized high blood flow outside and inside the regions with structural tendon changes.

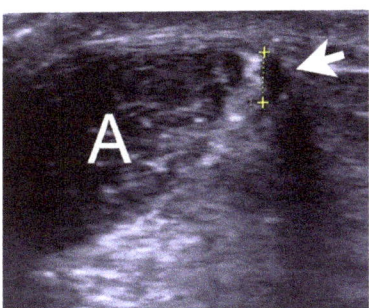

Figure 1. Gray-scale ultrasound picture of a patient suffering from midportion Achilles and plantaris tendinopathy showing a widened plantaris tendon (arrow/yellow scale) located close to the medial side of the Achilles tendon A.

2.2. Midportion Achilles Tendon Scraping and Local Plantaris Tendon Removal

Same-day pre-operative US + CD examination was carried out by the first author for verification and applying skin markers to map the **region** with maximum palpation tenderness, the localized high blood flow outside the deep side of the tendon, and where the plantaris tendon was positioned close to the medial side of the Achilles.

After disinfecting the skin with wet cloths of chlorhexidine cutaneous solution (Klorhexidionsprit 5 mg/mL, Fresenius Kabi, Germany), 4–7 mL of a local anesthetic (Xylocain + adrenalin 10 mg/mL + 5 µg/mL, Aspen, South Africa) was injected on the medial and ventral side (the mapped region) of the Achilles midportion. The skin was then scrubbed and draped with a sterile paper-cover exposing only the midportion of the Achilles tendon.

A longitudinal skin incision (1–2 cm) was placed on the medial side of the Achilles midportion. Following blunt dissection, the plantaris tendon was carefully identified (Figure 2), released, and followed distally and proximally from the skin incision. The plantaris was cut in both ends, resulting in 5–8 cm of the tendon being extirpated. Any vascularized fat tissue inter-positioned between the Achilles and the plantaris tendons was scraped. Then, the traditional Achilles scraping procedure was performed [23,24,28]. In the regions with US + CD-verified high blood flow outside the ventral and medial side of the tendon, the tendon was completely released from the ventral soft tissue. This scraping procedure was performed by sharp dissection using a scalpel, staying close to the ventral tendon. Following careful hemostasis using bi-polar diatermia, the skin was closed by single non-resorbable sutures, which were removed after 3 weeks.

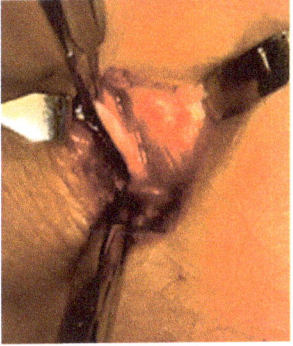

Figure 2. Surgery of a patient with midportion Achilles and plantaris tendinopathy. There is a thick and wide plantaris tendon located close to the medial side of a thickened Achilles midportion.

2.3. Postoperative Rehabilitation

There was clinical and US + CD follow-up 3 and 6 weeks after the operation. Then, extra follow-up only if there were complications.

Day 1: Surgery day: rest, elevated foot;
Day 2: ROM (range of movement) exercises and short, full-weight-bearing walks;
Day 3–7: Gradually increased walking activity, light seated stretching (bent knee);
Day 8–21: Start light bicycling; longer and faster walks;
Week 4: Free walking and biking;
Week 5: Introduce jogging: walk 50 m, jog 50 m; walk 50 m, jog 100 m; etc.;
Week 6: Jogging–running.

The described protocol was based on previous studies [23,24,28,29].

2.4. Outcome Measures

The self-administered Victorian Institute of Sports Assessment Achilles (VISA-A) functional score [30] and a study-specific questionnaire evaluating subjective satisfaction with treatment (satisfied or not satisfied), physical activity level, medication, sick leave, and complications were used for evaluation. The VISA-A score was completed by the patients on the day of surgery (pre-treatment) and after 1 year (post-treatment). The study-specific questionnaire was completed only at the 1-year follow-up. In the sub-group of international athletes, follow-up was restricted to mail contact evaluating subjective satisfaction with the treatment and return to their sport activity. It was not possible to get VISA-A scoring.

2.5. Ethical Consideration

Ethics approval was received from the Ethical Board in Uppsala-dnr 2022-02889-01. Informed written consent was obtained from all patients.

2.6. Statistical Methods

SPSS (Statistical Package of Social Science) that has been shown to be useful and reliable [30] was used to analyze the data (SPSS Inc., Chicago, IL, USA). All calculations were measured at the group level. Paired Student's t-test was selected to identify differences before and after surgery. The level of significance was set to $p < 0.05$.

3. Results

At the 1-year follow-up, 32/34 patients (43 tendons) were satisfied with the treatment. There was a significant ($p < 0.001$) increase in the mean VISA-A score from 34 (range 0–64) before surgery to 93 (range 61–100) after surgery (see also Table 2).

Table 2. Comparison of VISA-A baseline measure and follow-up comparison (mean (range)).

Baseline	Follow-Up	p
34 (0–64)	93 (61–100)	<0.001

There were two dropouts (two tendons). These patients did not answer the letter, telephone calls, or text messages. From the media, we know that one of these patients played professional soccer 2 months after the operation.

In the separate group with international athletes, all were satisfied and back in full activity in their sport.

There was one wound rupture that needed a re-operation, and one superficial skin infection successfully treated with antibiotics.

4. Discussion

This 1-year follow-up study on 34 patients suffering from combined midportion Achilles and plantaris tendinopathy in 45 tendons and undergoing WALANT surgery with US + CD-guided Achilles tendon scraping and local plantaris removal showed high satisfaction rates and good functional results.

4.1. Patients and Main Findings

The patients in the current study represent two different groups. The larger group containing 26 patients is from the general population in the most southern part of Sweden, referred from various insurance companies. The smaller group consisted of eight male international athletes referred directly from club/federation medical staff or via the athletes themselves. Altogether, it is a generally healthy group of patients who all had a long duration of tendon pain not responding to non-surgical treatment including eccentric training. The activity levels varied from mainly recreational actives in the Swedish group to elite athletes in the international group. The US + CD-guided surgical scraping procedure with local plantaris removal has in previous studies in northern Sweden been shown to be a successful treatment method [23,24,28–30]. In the current study, similar subjective satisfaction and good functional results were reproduced in a private setting involving patients referred from insurance companies in the very south of Sweden.

4.2. Plantaris Involvement

Treatment with eccentric training is generally efficient for patients suffering from chronic painful midportion Achilles tendinopathy [9–12]. In a minor group of patients, symptoms do not improve with gradual tendon loading regimes, and a possible reason to lack of effect of eccentric training could be mechanical interference from the plantaris tendon [26,27,31,32]. Our experiences over the years with the treatment of patients with midportion Achilles tendinopathy are that if the plantaris tendon is involved, there is often a paradoxical worsening with eccentric training with localized sharp pain on the medial side of the Achilles tendon.

Plantaris tendinopathy together with Achilles tendinopathy has been demonstrated in previous studies [25–27,31,33]. The plantaris tendon was found to be thickened, located close to, and seemingly interfering with the medial side of the Achilles tendon [28,31,34]. The findings from these initial studies led to the development of a surgical method where removal of the plantaris was performed routinely in cases where it was located close to the medial Achilles at the site of the symptoms. Histological examination of the excised thickened plantaris tendons showed similar tendinosis changes, as has been identified in Achilles tendinopathy [25,26,35]. In addition, the richly vascularized fat tissue between the Achilles and the plantaris tendons was found to be richly innervated, often by multiple sensory nerves [35].

4.3. Surgical Procedures

Traditional surgical treatment methods for midportion Achilles tendinopathy include different approaches for debridement with excision of tendinopathic regions inside the tendon [13–17], sometimes combined with flexor hallucis longus transfer procedures and multiple longitudinal splitting [18–20]. All these procedures are tendon invasive and require periods with low load or even immobilization after surgery with accompanying long rehabilitation periods before return to full Achilles-tendon-loading activities. The main advantage of the US + CD-guided surgical procedure used in this study is that the operation is performed outside the tendon, not directly affecting the Achilles tendon structure, allowing for immediate full weight bearing loading. This opens up the possibility for an accelerated rehabilitation and also minimizing the potential risks related to immobilization. Most patients in the current study were back in full Achilles tendon loading activities within 6–8 weeks, and only one patient (with the wound rupture) needed to be on sick leave after the operation. Another advantage is that the surgery is performed under local anesthesia (WALANT), thereby also avoiding risks related to general or spinal anesthesia. Finally, US + CD guidance localizes the exact target for the surgical procedure, making it possible to minimize the skin incision and the tissue trauma during the procedure.

4.4. Complications

There were two complications among the 45 operated Achilles and plantaris tendons. The most serious complication was a wound rupture occurring one week after suture removal (4 weeks after surgery). There was no infection involved and no direct trauma or heavy Achilles tendon loading, but for some unknown reason, there was slow skin healing. After healing, another **minor** operation in local anesthetics was needed to remove excessive scar tissue affecting the Achilles tendon movement. Wound healing was uncomplicated following this subsequent surgery, and the patient was back in full training after six months. Although there was only one wound rupture in this sample, the first author's experience from operating on a large number of individuals with this diagnosis in other settings is that delayed skin healing can sometimes occur. As a precaution, we therefore nowadays do not remove the sutures before three weeks and carefully inform the patients about proper wound care. In another patient, there was a superficial skin infection (staphylococcus) successfully treated with antibiotics without surgical debridement needed. Two patients had a prolonged rehabilitation period, and heavy Achilles tendon loading could not be started until 6 months after the operation. In these two patients, who were carefully followed with repeated US + CD examinations, there were no partial ruptures visible, but the Achilles tendon was swollen with a high blood flow in the whole tendon, and the Achilles tendon was sensitive to load. This is another experience from the first author that there can be a delayed healing response for unknown reasons before the patients are pain-free and can return to full Achilles tendon loading activities. Therefore, follow-up after surgery is essential. In a study by Maffulli et al., it was shown that the results after surgery were worse in a non-athletic population [20]. In the current study, there were no differences in the results between non-actives, recreationally actives, and elite level actives.

4.5. Limitations

A weakness in the current study is that it was only a 1-year follow up. The results could maybe have changed over time, but our experiences from other studies on this surgical method **are** that the failures tend to show up within the first six months, and longer-term follow-up studies have shown stable good results [28,29]. Another weakness is the use of only a questionnaire follow-up. It would have been ideal to also perform a clinical and ultrasound follow-up, but this was unfortunately not possible due to logistical reasons. It can be discussed as to whether randomized studies comparing the results after the US + CD method with other surgical methods are needed, but we believe it would have been an ethical dilemma to use tendon-invasive operations when operation outside the tendon in multiple studies have shown very high success rates [23,24,28,29].

5. Conclusions

For treatment of midportion Achilles tendinopathy, avoiding intratendinous surgery has major advantages, and new research has opened up the possibility of using surgical treatment methods targeting the outside of the Achilles. On the basis of research findings on innervation patterns for chronic painful midportion Achilles tendinopathy and plantaris tendon involvement, this 1-year follow-up study on insurance patients in the south of Sweden and international elite athletes showed good functional effects and allowed for a quick return to Achilles tendon loading activities after treatment with US + CD-guided surgical scraping outside the tendon combined with local plantaris tendon removal.

Author Contributions: Conceptualization, H.A., M.W., D.R. and C.S.; formal analysis, M.W. and D.R.; investigation, H.A.; writing—original draft preparation, H.A; writing—review and editing, M.W., D.R. and C.S.; visualization, H.A. and C.S.; supervision, H.A. All authors have read and agreed to the published version of the manuscript.

Funding: This research received no external funding.

Institutional Review Board Statement: The study was conducted in accordance with the Declaration of Helsinki and approved by the Institutional Ethics Committee of Ethical Board in Uppsala-dnr 2022-02889-01.

Informed Consent Statement: Informed consent was obtained from all subjects involved in the study.

Data Availability Statement: The data presented in this study are available on request from the corresponding author.

Acknowledgments: We would like to thank Gustav Dahlin for valuable help.

Conflicts of Interest: The authors declare no conflict of interest.

References

1. De Jonge, S.; Van den Berg, C.; De Vos, R.J.; Van der Heide, H.J.; Weir, A.; Verhaar, J.A.; Bierma-Zeinstra, S.M.; Tol, J.L. Incidence of midportion Achilles tendinopathy in the general population. *Br. J. Sport. Med.* **2011**, *45*, 1026–1028. [CrossRef]
2. Galloway, M.T.; Joki, P.; Dayton, O.W. Achilles tendon overuse injuries. *Clin. Sport. Med.* **1992**, *11*, 771–782. [CrossRef]
3. Jarvinen, T.A.H.; Kannus, P.; Paavola, M.; Jarvinen, T.L.N.; Jozsa, L.; Jarvinen, M. Achilles tendon injuries. *Curr. Opin. Rheumatol.* **2001**, *13*, 150–155. [CrossRef]
4. Schepsis, A.A.; Jones, H.; Haas, A.L. Achilles tendon disorders in athletes. *Am. J. Sport. Med.* **2002**, *30*, 287–305. [CrossRef]
5. Cosca, D.D.; Navazio, F. Common problems in endurance athletes. *Am. Fam. Physician* **2007**, *76*, 237–244.
6. Kvist, M. Achilles Tendon Injuries in Athletes. *Sport. Med.* **1994**, *18*, 173–201. [CrossRef]
7. Knobloch, K.; Yoon, U.; Vogt, P.M. Acute and overuse injuries correlated to hours of training in master running athletes. *Foot Ankle Int.* **2008**, *29*, 671–676. [CrossRef]
8. Gaida, J.E.; Alfredson, L.; Kiss, Z.S.; Wilson, A.M.; Alfredson, H.; Cook, J.L. Dyslipidemia in Achilles tendinopathy is characteristic of insuline resistance. *Med. Sci. Sport. Exerc.* **2009**, *41*, 1194–1197. [CrossRef]
9. Alfredson, H.; Pietilä, T.; Lorentzon, R. Heavy-load eccentric calf muscle training for the treatment of chronic Achilles tendinosis. *Am. J. Sport. Med.* **1998**, *26*, 360–366. [CrossRef]
10. Fahlström, M.; Jonsson, P.; Lorenzon, R.; Alfredson, H. Chronic Achilles tendon pain treated with eccentric calf-muscle training. *Knee Surg. Sport. Traumatol. Arthrosc.* **2003**, *11*, 327–333. [CrossRef]
11. Murtaugh, B.; Ihm, J. Eccentric training for the treatment of tendinopathies. *Curr. Sport. Med. Rep.* **2013**, *12*, 175–182. [CrossRef]
12. Roos, E.M.; Engström, M.; Lagerquist, A.; Söderberg, B. Clinical improvement after 6 weeks of eccentric exercise in patients with mid-portion Achilles tendinopathy—A randomized trial with 1-year follow up. *Scand. J. Med. Sci. Sport.* **2004**, *14*, 286–295. [CrossRef]
13. Nelen, G.; Martens, M.; Burssens, A. Surgical treatment of chronic Achilles tendinitis. *Am. J. Sport. Med.* **1989**, *17*, 754–759. [CrossRef]
14. Leadbetter, W.B.; Mooar, P.A.; Lane, G.J.; Lee, S.J. The surgical treatment of tendinitis. Clinical rationale and biologic basis. *Clin. Sport. Med.* **1992**, *11*, 679–712. [CrossRef]
15. Åström, M. On the Nature and Etiology of Chronic Achilles Tendinopathy. Ph.D. Thesis, Lund University, Lund, Sweden, 1997.
16. Rolf, C.; Movin, T. Etiology, histopathology, and outcome of surgery in achillodynia. *Foot Ankle Int.* **1997**, *18*, 565–569. [CrossRef]
17. Tallon, C.; Coleman, B.D.; Khan, K.M.; Maffulli, N. Outcome of surgery for chronic Achilles tendinopathy: A critical review. *Am. J. Sport. Med.* **2001**, *29*, 315–320. [CrossRef]
18. Maffulli, N.; Oliva, F.; Testa, V.; Capasso, G.; Del Buono, A. Multiple percutaneous longitudinal tenotomies for chronic Achilles tendinopathy in runners: A long-term study. *Am. J. Sport. Med.* **2013**, *41*, 2151–2157. [CrossRef]
19. Longo, U.G.; Ramamurthy, C.; Denaro, V.; Maffulli, N. Minimally invasive stripping for chronic Achilles tendinopathy. *Disabil. Rehabil.* **2008**, *30*, 1709–1713. [CrossRef]
20. Maffulli, N.; Testa, V.; Capasso, G.; Oliva, F.; Sullo, A.; Benazzo, F.; Regine, R.; King, J.B. Surgery for chronic Achilles tendinopathy yields worse results in nonathletic patients. *Clin. J. Sport. Med.* **2006**, *16*, 123–128. [CrossRef]
21. Alfredson, H.; Ohberg, L.; Forsgren, S. Is vasculo-neural ingrowth the cause of pain in chronic Achilles tendinosis? An investigation using ultrasonography and colour Doppler, immunohistochemistry, and diagnostic injections. *Knee Surg. Sport. Traumatol. Arthrosc.* **2003**, *11*, 334–338. [CrossRef]
22. Andersson, G.; Danielson, P.; Alfredson, H.; Forsgren, S. Nerve-related characteristics of ventral paratendinous tissue in chronic Achilles tendinosis. *Knee Surg. Sport. Traumatol. Arthrosc.* **2007**, *15*, 1272–1279. [CrossRef]
23. Alfredson, H. Ultrasound and Doppler-guided mini-surgery to treat midportion Achilles tendinosis: Results of a large material and a randomised study comparing two scraping techniques. *Br. J. Sport. Med.* **2011**, *45*, 407–410. [CrossRef]
24. Alfredson, H.; Öhberg, L.; Zeisig, E.; Lorentzon, R. Treatment of midportion Achilles tendinosis: Similar clinical results with US and CD-guided surgery outside the tendon and sclerosing polidocanol injections. *Knee Surg. Sport. Traumatol. Arthrosc.* **2007**, *15*, 1504–1509. [CrossRef]
25. Spang, C.; Alfredson, H.; Ferguson, M.; Roos, B.; Bagge, J.; Forsgren, S. The plantaris tendon in association with mid-portion Achilles tendinosis—Tendinosis-like morphological features and presence of a non-neuronal cholinergic system. *Histol. Histopathol.* **2013**, *28*, 623–632.

26. Spang, C.; Alfredson, H.; Docking, S.I.; Masci, L.; Andersson, G. The plantaris tendon. A narrative review focusing on anatomical features and clinical importance. *Bone Jt. J.* **2016**, *98*, 1312–1319. [CrossRef]
27. Smith, J.; Alfredson, H.; Masci, L.; Sellon, J.L.; Woods, C.D. Differential Plantaris-Achilles Tendon Motion: A Sonographic and Cadaveric Investigation. *PM&R* **2017**, *9*, 691–698.
28. Masci, L.; Neal, B.S.; Wynter Bee, W.; Spang, C.; Alfredson, H. Achilles scraping and plantaris tendon removal improves pain and tendon structure in patients with mid-portion Achilles tendinopathy—A two-year follow-up case series. *J. Clin. Med.* **2021**, *10*, 2695. [CrossRef]
29. Ruergård, A.; Spang, C.; Alfredson, H. Results of minimally invasive Achilles tendon scraping and plantaris tendon removal in patients with chronic midportion Achilles tendinopathy-a longer-term follow-up study. *SAGE Open Med.* **2019**, *7*, 2050312118822642. [CrossRef]
30. Korakakis, V.; Whiteley, R.; Kotsifaki, A.; Stefanakis, M.; Sotiralis, Y.; Thorborg, K. A systematic review evaluating the clinimetric properties of the Victorian Institute of Sport Assessment (VISA) questionnaires for lower limb tendinopathy shows moderate to high-quality evidence for sufficient reliability, validity and responsiveness-part II. *Knee Surg. Sport. Traumatol. Arthrosc.* **2021**, *29*, 2765–2788.
31. Alfredson, H. Midportion Achilles tendinosis and the plantaris tendon. *Br. J. Sport. Med.* **2011**, *45*, 1023–1025. [CrossRef]
32. Van Stekenburg, M.N.; Kerkhoffs, G.M.; Kleipool, R.P.; van Dijk, C.N. The plantaris tendon and a potential role in mid-portion Achilles tendinopathy: An observational anatomical study. *J. Anat.* **2011**, *218*, 336–341. [CrossRef]
33. Van Stekenburg, M.N.; Kerkhoffs, G.M.; van Dijk, C.N. Good outcome after stripping the plantaris tendon in patients with chronic mid-portion Achilles tendinopathy. *Knee Surg. Sport. Traumatol. Arthrosc.* **2011**, *19*, 1362–1366. [CrossRef]
34. Masci, L.; Spang, C.; van Schie, H.T.; Alfredson, H. How to diagnose plantaris tendon involvement in midportion Achilles tendinopathy - clinical and imaging findings. *BMC Musculoskelet. Disord.* **2016**, *17*, 97. [CrossRef]
35. Spang, C.; Harandi, V.M.; Alfredson, H.; Forsgren, S. Marked innervation but also signs of nerve degeneration between the Achilles and plantaris tendons and presence of innervation within the plantaris tendon in midportion Achilles tendinopthy. *J. Musculoskelet. Neuronal Interact.* **2015**, *15*, 197–206.

Disclaimer/Publisher's Note: The statements, opinions and data contained in all publications are solely those of the individual author(s) and contributor(s) and not of MDPI and/or the editor(s). MDPI and/or the editor(s) disclaim responsibility for any injury to people or property resulting from any ideas, methods, instructions or products referred to in the content.

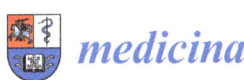

Case Report

Anatomical Augmentation Using Suture Tape for Acute Syndesmotic Injury in Maisonneuve Fracture: A Case Report

Sung-Joon Yoon [1,†], Ki-Jin Jung [1,†], Yong-Cheol Hong [1], Eui-Dong Yeo [2], Hong-Seop Lee [3], Sung-Hun Won [4], Byung-Ryul Lee [1], Jae-Young Ji [5], Dhong-Won Lee [6] and Woo-Jong Kim [1,*]

1. Department of Orthopaedic Surgery, Soonchunhyang University Hospital Cheonan, 31, Suncheonhyang 6-gil, Dongam-gu, Cheonan 31151, Republic of Korea
2. Department of Orthopaedic Surgery, Veterans Health Service Medical Center, Seoul 05368, Republic of Korea
3. Department of Foot and Ankle Surgery, Nowon Eulji Medical Center, Eulji University, 68, Hangeulbiseok-ro, Nowon-gu, Seoul 01830, Republic of Korea
4. Department of Orthopaedic Surgery, Soonchunhyang University Hospital Seoul, 59, Daesagwan-ro, Yongsan-gu, Seoul 04401, Republic of Korea
5. Department of Anesthesiology and Pain Medicine, Soonchunhyang University Hospital Cheonan, 31, Suncheonhyang 6-gil, Dongam-gu, Cheonan 31151, Republic of Korea
6. Department of Orthopaedic Surgery, Konkuk University Medical Center, 120-1, Neungdong-ro, Gwangjin-gu, Seoul 05030, Republic of Korea
* Correspondence: kwj9383@hanmail.net; Tel.: +82-41-570-2170
† These authors contributed equally to this work.

Abstract: Ankle syndesmosis is crucial to the integrity of the ankle joint and weight-bearing; an injury to this structure can lead to significant disability. The treatment methods for distal syndesmosis injuries are controversial. The representative treatment methods include transsyndesmotic screw fixation and suture-button fixation, and good results with suture tape augmentation have recently been reported. However, an augmentation using suture tape is only possible when the posterior inferior tibiofibular ligament (PITFL) is intact. This study describes the case of an unstable syndesmosis injury, accompanied by anterior inferior tibiofibular ligament (AITFL) and PITFL injuries, which were treated successfully using suture tape. A 39-year-old male patient sustained right ankle damage while skateboarding. His leg and ankle radiographs revealed a widening of the medial clear space, a posterior malleolus fracture, a reduced "syndesmosis overlap" compared with the contralateral side, and a proximal fibula fracture. The magnetic resonance imaging revealed ruptured deltoid ligaments, accompanied by AITFL, PITFL, and interosseous ligament injuries. A diagnosis of a Maisonneuve fracture with an unstable syndesmotic injury was made. The patient underwent an open syndesmotic joint reduction, along with an AITFL and PITFL augmentation. This anatomical reduction was confirmed using intraoperative arthroscopy and postoperative computed tomography (CT). An axial CT that was performed at the 6-month follow-up exam revealed a similar alignment of the syndesmosis between the injured and uninjured sides. There were no surgical complications and the patient did not complain of discomfort in his daily life. At the 12-month follow-up exam, a good clinical outcome was confirmed. As a treatment for unstable syndesmosis injury, ligament augmentation using suture tape shows satisfactory clinical outcomes and can be considered as a useful and reliable method for anatomical restoration and rapid rehabilitation.

Keywords: syndesmosis injury; instability; suture tape; anatomic augmentation

1. Introduction

The tibiofibular syndesmosis, a fibrous joint that stabilizes the fibula and tibia, consists of four lateral ligaments: the anterior inferior tibiofibular ligament (AITFL), interosseous ligament (IOL), transverse ligament (TL), and posterior inferior tibiofibular ligament (PITFL). These ligaments stabilize the syndesmosis and prevent the excessive motion of the fibula, such that an appropriate fibular position is maintained; they also play an important role in syndesmotic function and the talar position [1]. Within the syndesmotic ligament complex, the AITFL and PITFL play the most important roles in stabilizing the distal syndesmosis [2].

Distal tibiofibular syndesmotic injury is involved in 10% of all ankle fractures and up to 20% of rotational ankle fractures [3–5]. The distal tibiofibular syndesmosis is crucial for the congruity and integrity of the ankle joint, which, in turn, is critical for weight-bearing [6,7]. An injury to these critical structures can lead to significant disability [8–10]. According to a cadaveric study [11], in cases of syndesmosis injury, tibiotalar contact pressure can be reduced by 42% with only a 1 mm lateral shift of the talus. The stabilization of the syndesmosis is essential to achieving good long-term, functional outcomes for the ankle joint, and to preventing posttraumatic arthritis [5,12].

One traditional method for reducing the syndesmosis is a transosseous screw fixation. However, the position, diameter, number, and retrieval of the syndesmotic screws, as well as the method of cortical fixation, remain controversial [13–16]. Recently, several studies have reported the use of suture tape for a ligament augmentation in cases of syndesmosis injury [17–20]. In one study, this novel fixation method proved to be as effective as screw fixation [21], while, in a cadaver model, a minimally invasive anatomic augmentation of the anterior and posterior syndesmosis was achieved by using suture tape [22]. In this study, we report a case of unstable syndesmotic injury, in which the anatomical reduction of the syndesmosis was achieved by an augmentation of the AITFL and PITFL using suture tape.

2. Case Presentation

This case report was approved by the Institutional Review Board (IRB) of Soonchunhyang University Cheonan Hospital, Cheonan, South Korea (IRB No. 2023-01-007). The patient provided written informed consent for the publication of this report and the accompanying images.

A 39-year-old male presented to the emergency department of our hospital with severe pain and swelling in the right ankle. The patient stated that he fell off a skateboard and rotated his ankle. He had no history of illness, or of genetic or familial diseases. A physical examination revealed ankle swelling, extreme tenderness, and ecchymosis in the medial aspect of the ankle and the proximal fibula. There were no neurological deficits, and the dorsalis pedis and tibialis posterior arteries were palpable.

The anteroposterior, lateral, and mortise view right ankle radiographs revealed a widening of the medial clear space and a posterior malleolus fracture. Moreover, the "syndesmosis overlap" was reduced in comparison with the contralateral side. Additionally, a full-length radiograph of the lower leg revealed a proximal fibula fracture (Figure 1). Computed tomography (CT) scans were taken for an accurate evaluation of the syndesmosis. On the axial CT, the fibula was not located in the fibula notch; it was found to be displaced laterally and posteriorly at a point 1 cm above the tibial plafond (Figure 2). The magnetic resonance imaging (MRI) revealed that there were ruptured deltoid ligaments, along with AITFL, PITFL, and interosseous membrane (IOM) injuries (Figure 3). The final diagnosis was a Maisonneuve fracture with a proximal fibular fracture, a syndesmosis injury with an IOM rupture, and a medial deltoid ligament injury; these findings were confirmed during surgery. On day 2 after the injury, the patient underwent a syndesmosis reduction and fixation. The patient was placed on the operating table in the supine position, and arthroscopy was performed using standard anteromedial and anterolateral portals. We did not observe a cartilage injury, syndesmotic instability (lateral malleolus displacement > 5 mm), or PITFL rupture at the point of the tibia insertion (Figure 4). We planned to use suture tape for the syndesmosis joint reduction and fixation. InternalBrace (Arthrex, Naples, FL, USA), a nonabsorbable suture tape, was used for the fixation. First, the AITFL rupture was confirmed to be approximately 4 cm above the distal tibiofibular joint. We checked the distal tibial footprints and a 3.4 mm bone tunnel was created. A 2.7 mm drilling was performed on the footprints of the syndesmosis ligament in the distal fibula, from front to back, to create a bone tunnel. The suture tape was passed through and fixed with 3.5 mm interference screws (SwiveLock; Arthrex). After internally rotating the patient's leg, a longitudinal incision was made approximately 5 cm above the Volkmann tubercle. We palpated the Volkmann tubercle and passed the suture tape between the peroneus tendon and the bone. After reducing the syndesmosis joint, the free ends of the suture tape were fixed to the bone tunnel on the tibia side, which was prepared under C-arm guidance with 4.75 mm SwiveLock®anchors (Figure 5). Then, the medial clear space was reduced to within the normal range. A deltoid ligament repair was not performed and the proximal fibula fracture was treated conservatively. A plain X-ray and CT were performed immediately after the surgery had confirmed a successful syndesmotic reduction (Figure 6).

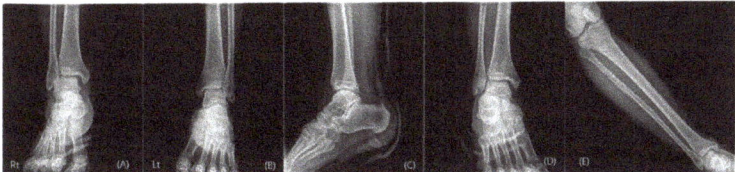

Figure 1. Preoperative plain radiographs showing widening of the medial clear space ((**A**) anteroposterior view of the site of injury, and (**B**) anteroposterior view), a posterior malleolar fracture ((**C**) lateral view), reduced syndesmosis overlap ((**D**) mortise view), and a proximal fibula fracture ((**E**) full-length radiograph of the lower leg; anteroposterior view).

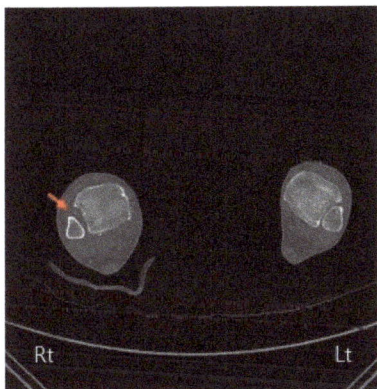

Figure 2. Preoperative axial computed tomography scan showing a syndesmotic injury in the right ankle. It can be seen that the fibula is dislocated from the fibula notch (red arrow).

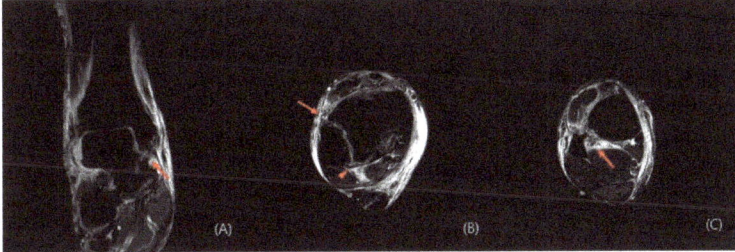

Figure 3. Coronal magnetic resonance imaging (MRI). An area of high signal intensity (red arrow) indicates a deltoid ligament injury (**A**). Axial MRI showing the anterior inferior tibiofibular ligament (red arrow) and posterior inferior tibiofibular ligament (red arrowhead) injuries (**B**). Axial MRI showing interosseous membrane rupture (red arrow) (**C**).

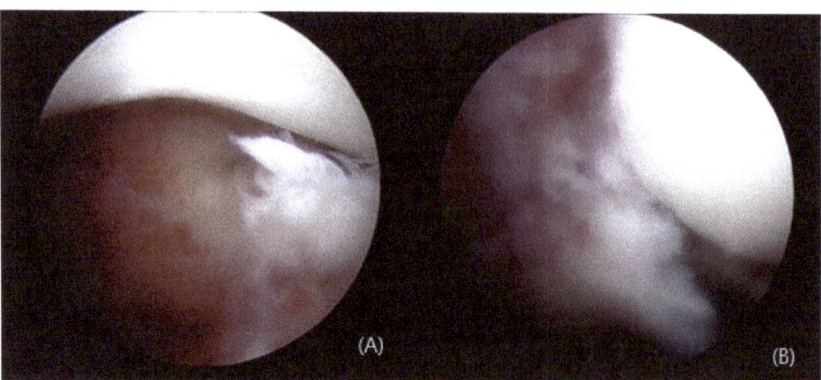

Figure 4. Intraoperative arthroscopic findings of syndesmotic injury with widening of the gap between the fibula and tibia (**A**), and posterior inferior tibiofibular ligament rupture at the point of tibial insertion (**B**).

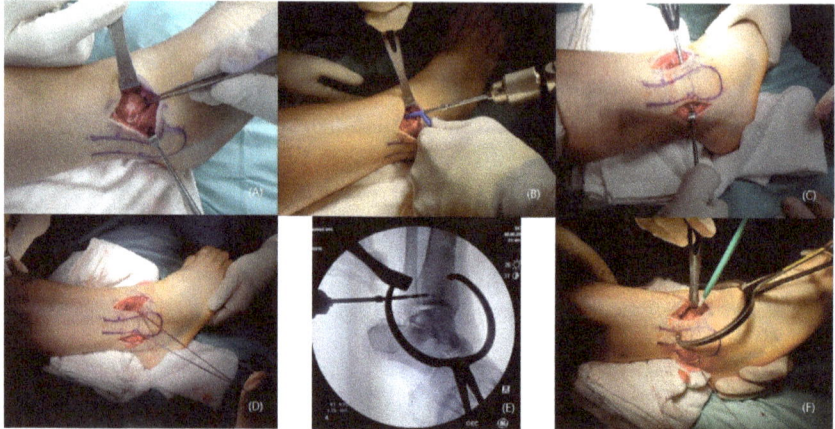

Figure 5. (**A**) Confirmation of anterior inferior tibiofibular ligament rupture. (**B**) Check of the distal tibial footprints and a 3.4 mm bone tunnel was created. (**C**) In the syndesmosis ligament in the distal fibula using a 2.7 mm drill. (**C**) A 2.7 mm drilling was performed on the footprints of the syndesmosis ligament in the distal fibula from front to back to create a bone tunnel. (**D**) Suture tape was passed through the bone tunnel and fixed with interference screws. (**E**) Under C-arm guidance, a bone tunnel was created in the posterior syndesmosis on the Volkmann tubercle side. (**F**) After reducing the syndesmosis joint, the free ends of the suture tape were fixed with 4.75 mm SwiveLock screws.

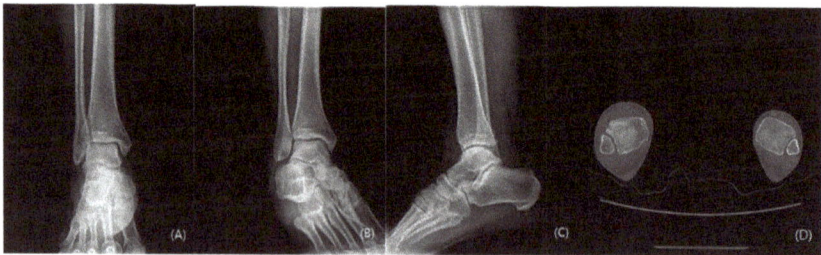

Figure 6. The syndesmosis joint was clearly reduced on the postoperative X-ray ((**A**) anteroposterior view, (**B**) lateral view, and (**C**) mortise view); this was confirmed by axial computed tomography (**D**).

Postoperatively, a short leg splint was worn for approximately 2 weeks. The patient was instructed to use an ankle brace for an additional 2 weeks. Active and passive ankle range of motion exercises were performed from 4 weeks postoperatively, and full weight-bearing walking was then allowed with braces. The braces were removed after 6 weeks. Then, a 3-month rehabilitation program consisting of ankle muscle strength, balance, and functional performance training was completed. An axial CT that was performed 6 months after the surgery revealed a similar alignment of the syndesmosis between the injured and uninjured sides (Figure 7). There were no complications and the patient did not complain of discomfort in daily life.

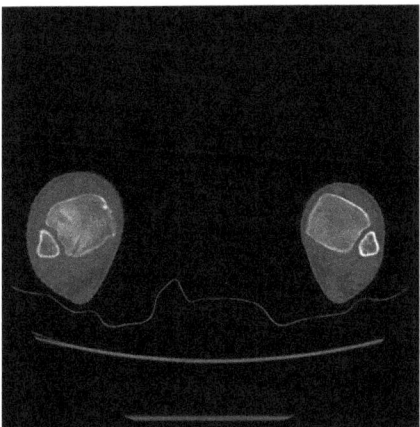

Figure 7. Axial computed tomography performed at the 6-month follow-up exam revealed similar alignment of the syndesmosis between the injured and uninjured sides.

At the 1-year postoperative follow-up exam, the Olerud–Molander Ankle Score and The American Orthodefic Foot and Ankle Society Ankle-Hindfoot scale were at 95 and 90 points, respectively, and the visual analog scale pain score was at 1 point. The range of motion of the ankle joint– injured° (uninjured°)was checked presenting an ankle dorsiflexion of 15° (20°), an ankle plantar flexion of 40° (40°), a varus of 20° (20°), and a valgus of 10° (10°), showing almost no limitations.

3. Discussion

Traumatic distal tibiofibular syndesmosis injuries commonly occur during contact sports. Syndesmotic injuries that are associated with ankle rotation account for approximately 10% of all ankle fractures, >20% of which are treated surgically [3,4]. A retrospective study found that the proportion of syndesmotic injuries that were sustained by athletes that could be classified as acute sprains was approximately 20% [23,24]. Missed or improperly treated syndesmosis injuries can result in unnecessary pain or functional impairment, which may ultimately progress to arthritis [25,26]. Achieving and maintaining an anatomical reduction is important for good long-term, complication-free outcomes in cases of syndesmotic injury [25].

The treatment methods for distal syndesmosis injuries are highly controversial [3,9,27]. The traditional fixation method for an unstable syndesmosis is transsyndesmotic screw fixation. Although the number of screws, the fixation period, and the removal time are debatable, this traditional fixation is still the most widely used technique. However, its disadvantages include screw breakage, malreduction, synostosis, the need for screw removal (and diastasis thereafter), delayed weight-bearing, and disuse osteoporosis [28–30]. Good outcomes of suture-button fixation have been reported by studies that applied this technique to overcome the drawbacks of the traditional fixation [8,27,29,31]. However, the potential complications of suture-button fixation include soft tissue complications, infections, osteolysis, and heterotopic ossification [32–34]. In a biomechanical study, suture-button fixation alone did not provide an adequate rotational stability [21,35]. Forsythe et al. reported that FiberWire-button (Arthrex) fixation was less effective for maintaining syndesmotic reduction in the immediate postoperative period, relative to a metallic screw [36]. Moreover, Teramoto et al. reported that neither single- nor double-suture-button fixation stabilized the syndesmosis in cases of inversion and external rotation, although the former was sufficient for physiologic stability [37].

Several studies have reported good results from using suture tape in conjunction with suture-button fixation for an AITFL augmentation [21,35]. Nonabsorbable suture tape that is designed for the treatment of ankle lateral instability has been widely applied, while the InternalBrace (Arthrex) was developed in 2012. This device uses SwiveLock screws for a knotless aperture fixation, and FiberTape (Arthrex) fixed to each ligament enhances the repair and augmentation.

Nelson proposed an open anatomic repair for AITFL injuries, and reported that this technique can restore the ankle's mortise stability and facilitate bone repair, in order to promote an early return to functional exercises and activities [38]. Moreover, there is no requirement for a syndesmotic screw fixation. Lee et al. introduced a repair technique for the AITFL by using suture tape under arthroscopic guidance [39]. Although their approach has a basic concept similar to that of Nelson, it also has distinct advantages in terms of weight-bearing and rehabilitation in the early stage after surgery, a lack of any requirements for screw removal, and no functional limitations [38,39]. Kwon et al. reported that the use of the InternalBrace for AITFL injuries was an effective and safe adjunctive strategy for addressing syndesmotic instability [19]. Lee et al. reported that open anterior syndesmotic repair using suture tape provided a torsional strength that was similar to screw fixation in cases of ankle syndesmotic injury, and suggested that it could serve as an alternative treatment option [21].

The suture tape techniques described above have a notable limitation: they can only be performed when the PITFL is intact. In a cadaver model, Regauer et al. introduced a minimally invasive anterior and posterior augmentation technique using the InternalBrace device [22]. When using such techniques in actual patients, an initial examination should be performed to determine whether the patient is a suitable candidate. If a PITFL rupture is confirmed by an ankle axial CT, an MRI, and arthroscopy, and if a reduction is also deemed to be required, the AITFL and PITFL augmentation can be performed using InternalBrace. To confirm a successful surgical outcome when using the InternalBrace fixation, the degree of syndesmosis reduction should be assessed by an axial CT immediately, through a comparison with the uninjured side.

4. Conclusions

As a treatment for unstable syndesmosis injury, a ligament augmentation using suture tape provides satisfactory clinical outcomes and can be considered to be a useful and reliable method for anatomical restoration and rapid rehabilitation. However, cadaveric biomechanical studies are needed for validation.

Author Contributions: Conceptualization, W.-J.K. and K.-J.J.; methodology, Y.-C.H.; software, E.-D.Y.; validation, S.-H.W. and B.-R.L.; formal analysis, J.-Y.J.; investigation, E.-D.Y.; resources, S.-J.Y.; data curation, Y.-C.H.; writing—original draft preparation, W.-J.K.; writing—review and editing, W.-J.K. and S.-J.Y.; visualization, H.-S.L.; supervision, J.-Y.J.; project administration, Y.-C.H.; and funding acquisition, D.-W.L. All authors have read and agreed to the published version of the manuscript.

Funding: The authors would like to thank the Soonchunhyang University Research Fund for supporting this work (2023-0002).

Institutional Review Board Statement: This study was conducted according to the guidelines of the Declaration of Helsinki, and was approved by the IRB and Human Research Ethics Committee of Soonchunhyang University Cheonan Hospital (IRB No. 2023-01-007).

Informed Consent Statement: Written informed consent has been obtained from the patient for the publication of this paper.

Data Availability Statement: Data sharing is not applicable to this article as no datasets were generated or analyzed during the current study.

Conflicts of Interest: All authors declare that they have no commercial associations (e.g., any consultancy, stock ownership, equity interest, or patent/licensing arrangement) that might pose a conflict of interest in connection with the submitted article.

Abbreviations

AITFL	anterior inferior tibiofibular ligament
IOL	interosseous ligament
TL	transverse ligament
PITFL	posterior inferior tibiofibular ligament
CT	computed tomography
MRI	magnetic resonance imaging

References

1. Jelinek, J.A.; Porter, D.A. Management of unstable ankle fractures and syndesmosis injuries in athletes. *Foot Ankle Clin.* **2009**, *14*, 277–298. [CrossRef]
2. Van Heest, T.J.; Lafferty, P.M. Injuries to the ankle syndesmosis. *J. Bone Jt. Surg. Am.* **2014**, *96*, 603–613. [CrossRef] [PubMed]
3. van den Bekerom, M.P.; Lamme, B.; Hogervorst, M.; Bolhuis, H.W. Which ankle fractures require syndesmotic stabilization? *J. Foot Ankle Surg.* **2007**, *46*, 456–463. [CrossRef] [PubMed]
4. Stark, E.; Tornetta, P., 3rd; Creevy, W.R. Syndesmotic instability in Weber B ankle fractures: A clinical evaluation. *J. Orthop. Trauma* **2007**, *21*, 643–646. [CrossRef] [PubMed]
5. Egol, K.A.; Pahk, B.; Walsh, M.; Tejwani, N.C.; Davidovitch, R.I.; Koval, K.J. Outcome after unstable ankle fracture: Effect of syndesmotic stabilization. *J. Orthop. Trauma* **2010**, *24*, 7–11. [CrossRef]
6. van Zuuren, W.J.; Schepers, T.; Beumer, A.; Sierevelt, I.; van Noort, A.; van den Bekerom, M.P.J. Acute syndesmotic instability in ankle fractures: A review. *Foot Ankle Surg.* **2017**, *23*, 135–141. [CrossRef]
7. Bartoníček, J. Anatomy of the tibiofibular syndesmosis and its clinical relevance. *Surg. Radiol. Anat.* **2003**, *25*, 379–386. [CrossRef]
8. Gan, K.; Xu, D.; Hu, K.; Wu, W.; Shen, Y. Dynamic fixation is superior in terms of clinical outcomes to static fixation in managing distal tibiofibular syndesmosis injury. *Knee Surg. Sports Traumatol. Arthrosc.* **2020**, *28*, 270–280. [CrossRef]
9. Tourné, Y.; Molinier, F.; Andrieu, M.; Porta, J.; Barbier, G. Diagnosis and treatment of tibiofibular syndesmosis lesions. *Orthop. Traumatol. Surg. Res.* **2019**, *105*, S275–S286. [CrossRef]
10. Cornu, O.; Manon, J.; Tribak, K.; Putineanu, D. Traumatic injuries of the distal tibiofibular syndesmosis. *Orthop. Traumatol. Surg. Res.* **2021**, *107*, 102778. [CrossRef]
11. Ramsey, P.L.; Hamilton, W. Changes in tibiotalar area of contact caused by lateral talar shift. *J. Bone Jt. Surg. Am.* **1976**, *58*, 356–357. [CrossRef]
12. Sagi, H.C.; Shah, A.R.; Sanders, R.W. The functional consequence of syndesmotic joint malreduction at a minimum 2-year follow-up. *J. Orthop. Trauma* **2012**, *26*, 439–443. [CrossRef] [PubMed]
13. Schepers, T.; van der Linden, H.; van Lieshout, E.M.; Niesten, D.D.; van der Elst, M. Technical aspects of the syndesmotic screw and their effect on functional outcome following acute distal tibiofibular syndesmosis injury. *Injury* **2014**, *45*, 775–779. [CrossRef] [PubMed]
14. Peek, A.C.; Fitzgerald, C.E.; Charalambides, C. Syndesmosis screws: How many, what diameter, where and should they be removed? A literature review. *Injury* **2014**, *45*, 1262–1267. [CrossRef] [PubMed]
15. Høiness, P.; Strømsøe, K. Tricortical versus quadricortical syndesmosis fixation in ankle fractures: A prospective, randomized study comparing two methods of syndesmosis fixation. *J. Orthop. Trauma* **2004**, *18*, 331–337. [CrossRef] [PubMed]
16. Walker, L.; Willis, N. Weber C ankle fractures: A retrospective audit of screw number, size, complications, and retrieval rates. *J. Foot Ankle Surg.* **2015**, *54*, 454–457. [CrossRef]
17. Jamieson, M.D.; Stake, I.K.; Brady, A.W.; Brown, J.; Tanghe, K.K.; Douglass, B.W.; Clanton, T.O. Anterior Inferior Tibiofibular Ligament Suture Tape Augmentation for Isolated Syndesmotic Injuries. *Foot Ankle Int.* **2022**, *43*, 994–1003. [CrossRef]
18. Harris, N.J.; Nicholson, G.; Pountos, I. Anatomical reconstruction of the anterior inferior tibiofibular ligament in elite athletes using InternalBrace suture tape. *Bone Jt. J.* **2022**, *104-b*, 68–75. [CrossRef]
19. Kwon, J.Y.; Stenquist, D.; Ye, M.; Williams, C.; Giza, E.; Kadakia, A.R.; Kreulen, C. Anterior Syndesmotic Augmentation Technique Using Nonabsorbable Suture-Tape for Acute and Chronic Syndesmotic Instability. *Foot Ankle Int.* **2020**, *41*, 1307–1315. [CrossRef]
20. Takahashi, K.; Teramoto, A.; Murahashi, Y.; Nabeki, S.; Shiwaku, K.; Kamiya, T.; Watanabe, K.; Yamashita, T. Comparison of Treatment Methods for Syndesmotic Injuries With Posterior Tibiofibular Ligament Ruptures: A Cadaveric Biomechanical Study. *Orthop. J. Sports Med.* **2022**, *10*, 23259671221122811. [CrossRef]

21. Lee, H.S.; Kim, W.J.; Young, K.W.; Jeong, G.M.; Yeo, E.D.; Lee, Y.K. Comparison of Open Anterior Syndesmotic Repair Augmented With Suture-Tape and Trans-syndesmotic Screw Fixation: A Biomechanical Study. *J. Foot Ankle Surg.* **2021**, *60*, 339–344. [CrossRef] [PubMed]
22. Regauer, M.; Mackay, G.; Lange, M.; Kammerlander, C.; Böcker, W. Syndesmotic InternalBrace(TM) for anatomic distal tibiofibular ligament augmentation. *World J. Orthop.* **2017**, *8*, 301–309. [CrossRef] [PubMed]
23. Roemer, F.W.; Jomaah, N.; Niu, J.; Almusa, E.; Roger, B.; D'Hooghe, P.; Geertsema, C.; Tol, J.L.; Khan, K.; Guermazi, A. Ligamentous Injuries and the Risk of Associated Tissue Damage in Acute Ankle Sprains in Athletes: A Cross-sectional MRI Study. *Am. J. Sports Med.* **2014**, *42*, 1549–1557. [CrossRef]
24. Gerber, J.P.; Williams, G.N.; Scoville, C.R.; Arciero, R.A.; Taylor, D.C. Persistent disability associated with ankle sprains: A prospective examination of an athletic population. *Foot Ankle Int.* **1998**, *19*, 653–660. [CrossRef] [PubMed]
25. Switaj, P.J.; Mendoza, M.; Kadakia, A.R. Acute and Chronic Injuries to the Syndesmosis. *Clin. Sports Med.* **2015**, *34*, 643–677. [CrossRef]
26. Kim, J.S.; Shin, H.S. Suture Anchor Augmentation for Acute Unstable Isolated Ankle Syndesmosis Disruption in Athletes. *Foot Ankle Int.* **2021**, *42*, 1130–1137. [CrossRef]
27. Xu, Y.; Kang, R.; Li, M.; Li, Z.; Ma, T.; Ren, C.; Wang, Q.; Lu, Y.; Zhang, K. The Clinical Efficacy of Suture-Button Fixation and Trans-Syndesmotic Screw Fixation in the Treatment of Ankle Fracture Combined With Distal Tibiofibular Syndesmosis Injury: A Retrospective Study. *J. Foot Ankle Surg.* **2022**, *61*, 143–148. [CrossRef]
28. Sanders, D.; Schneider, P.; Taylor, M.; Tieszer, C.; Lawendy, A.R. Improved Reduction of the Tibiofibular Syndesmosis With TightRope Compared With Screw Fixation: Results of a Randomized Controlled Study. *J. Orthop. Trauma* **2019**, *33*, 531–537.
29. Kim, J.H.; Gwak, H.C.; Lee, C.R.; Choo, H.J.; Kim, J.G.; Kim, D.Y. A Comparison of Screw Fixation and Suture-Button Fixation in a Syndesmosis Injury in an Ankle Fracture. *J. Foot Ankle Surg.* **2016**, *55*, 985–990. [CrossRef]
30. Ebraheim, N.A.; Mekhail, A.O.; Gargasz, S.S. Ankle fractures involving the fibula proximal to the distal tibiofibular syndesmosis. *Foot Ankle Int.* **1997**, *18*, 513–521. [CrossRef]
31. Xu, G.; Chen, W.; Zhang, Q.; Wang, J.; Su, Y.; Zhang, Y. Flexible fixation of syndesmotic diastasis using the assembled bolt-tightrope system. *Scand. J. Trauma Resusc. Emerg. Med.* **2013**, *21*, 71. [CrossRef]
32. Naqvi, G.A.; Shafqat, A.; Awan, N. Tightrope fixation of ankle syndesmosis injuries: Clinical outcome, complications and technique modification. *Injury* **2012**, *43*, 838–842. [CrossRef]
33. McMurray, D.; Hornung, B.; Venkateswaran, B.; Ali, Z. Walking on a tightrope: Our experience in the treatment of traumatic ankle syndesmosis rupture. *Injury Extra* **2008**, *39*, 182. [CrossRef]
34. Willmott, H.J.; Singh, B.; David, L.A. Outcome and complications of treatment of ankle diastasis with tightrope fixation. *Injury* **2009**, *40*, 1204–1206. [CrossRef]
35. Shoji, H.; Teramoto, A.; Suzuki, D.; Okada, Y.; Sakakibara, Y.; Matsumura, T.; Suzuki, T.; Watanabe, K.; Yamashita, T. Suture-button fixation and anterior inferior tibiofibular ligament augmentation with suture-tape for syndesmosis injury: A biomechanical cadaveric study. *Clin. Biomech.* **2018**, *60*, 121–126. [CrossRef] [PubMed]
36. Forsythe, K.; Freedman, K.B.; Stover, M.D.; Patwardhan, A.G. Comparison of a novel FiberWire-button construct versus metallic screw fixation in a syndesmotic injury model. *Foot Ankle Int.* **2008**, *29*, 49–54. [CrossRef] [PubMed]
37. Teramoto, A.; Suzuki, D.; Kamiya, T.; Chikenji, T.; Watanabe, K.; Yamashita, T. Comparison of different fixation methods of the suture-button implant for tibiofibular syndesmosis injuries. *Am. J. Sports Med.* **2011**, *39*, 2226–2232. [CrossRef] [PubMed]
38. Nelson, O.A. Examination and repair of the AITFL in transmalleolar fractures. *J. Orthop. Trauma* **2006**, *20*, 637–643. [CrossRef]
39. Lee, S.H.; Kim, E.S.; Lee, Y.K.; Yeo, E.D.; Oh, S.R. Arthroscopic syndesmotic repair: Technical tip. *Foot Ankle Int.* **2015**, *36*, 229–231. [CrossRef]

Disclaimer/Publisher's Note: The statements, opinions and data contained in all publications are solely those of the individual author(s) and contributor(s) and not of MDPI and/or the editor(s). MDPI and/or the editor(s) disclaim responsibility for any injury to people or property resulting from any ideas, methods, instructions or products referred to in the content.

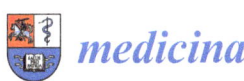

Article

Risk Factors Associated with Intraoperative Iatrogenic Fracture in Patients Undergoing Intramedullary Nailing for Atypical Femoral Fractures with Marked Anterior and Lateral Bowing

Yong Bum Joo [1], Yoo Sun Jeon [2], Woo Yong Lee [1] and Hyung Jin Chung [3],*

[1] Department of Orthopedic Surgery, Chungnam National University Hospital, Chungnam National University College of Medicine, Daejeon 35015, Republic of Korea
[2] Department of Orthopedic Surgery, Korea Worker's Compensation & Welfare Service Daejeon Hospital, 637, Gyejok-ro, Daedeok-gu, Daejeon 34384, Republic of Korea
[3] Department of Orthopedic Surgery, Chungnam National University Sejong Hospital, Chungnam National University College of Medicine, Sejong 30099, Republic of Korea
* Correspondence: leecomet@hanmail.net; Tel.: +82-44-995-4798

Abstract: *Background and objectives*: Iatrogenic fractures are potential complications during intramedullary (IM) nailing for atypical femoral fractures (AFFs). The risk factors associated with iatrogenic fractures remain unclear, although excessive femoral bowing and osteoporosis are hypothesized to be contributing factors. The present study aimed to determine the risk factors for the occurrence of iatrogenic fractures during IM nailing in patients with AFFs. *Materials and Methods*: This retrospective cross-sectional study evaluated 95 patients with AFF (all female; age range: 49–87 years) who underwent IM nailing between June 2008 and December 2017. The patients were divided into two groups: Group I (with iatrogenic fracture: *n* = 20) and Group II (without iatrogenic fracture: *n* = 75). Background characteristics were retrieved from medical records and radiographic measurements were obtained. Univariate and multivariate logistic regression analyses were performed to identify risk factors for the occurrence of intraoperative iatrogenic fractures. Receiver operating curve (ROC) analysis was conducted to determine a cut-off value for the prediction of iatrogenic fracture occurrence. *Results*: Iatrogenic fractures occurred in 20 (21.1%) patients. The two groups exhibited no significant differences regarding age and other background characteristics. Group I exhibited significantly lower mean femoral bone mineral density (BMD) and significantly greater mean lateral and anterior femoral bowing angles than Group II (all $p < 0.05$). There were no significant differences in AFF location, nonunion, and IM nail diameter, length, or nail entry point between the two groups. In the univariate analysis, femoral BMD and lateral bowing of the femur differed significantly between the two groups. On multivariate analysis, only lateral bowing of the femur remained significantly associated with iatrogenic fracture occurrence. The ROC analysis determined a cut-off value of 9.3° in lateral bowing of the femur for prediction of iatrogenic fracture occurrence during IM nailing for AFF treatment. *Conclusions*: The lateral bowing angle of the femur is an important predictive factor for intraoperative iatrogenic fracture occurrence in patients undergoing IM nailing for AFF treatment.

Keywords: diaphyseal atypical femoral fracture; intramedullary nail; iatrogenic fracture; femoral bowing angle; bone density

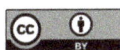

1. Introduction

In 2013, according to the revised criteria of the American Society for Bone and Mineral Research (ASMBR) task force report, atypical femoral fractures (AFFs) are defined as "fractures located along the femoral diaphysis from just distal to the lesser trochanter to just proximal to the supracondylar flare". In addition, at least four of the five major features must be present (Table 1) [1]. Recently, there has been increasing interest in AFFs, considered as a type of insufficiency fracture associated with long-term use of bisphosphonate (BP) [2]. BPs prevent osteoporotic fractures by inhibiting osteoclast-mediated bone resorption. However, the consequent decrease in bone turnover may compromise the mechanical and regenerative properties of the bone, resulting in fracture onset and delayed bone healing [2,3]. AFFs also occur in patients without exposure to BPs [1,4,5]. In the second report from the American Society of Bone and Mineral Research Task Force, the pathogenesis of AFFs was considered to involve stress or insufficiency [1]. Furthermore, lower limb geometry and Asian race may contribute to the risk of AFF occurrence [1,6].

Table 1. ASBMR Task Force 2013 revised case definition of AFFs.

Major Criteria
✓ The fracture is associated with minimal or no trauma, as in a fall from a standing height or less.
✓ The fracture line originates at the lateral cortex and is substantially transverse in its orientation, although it may become oblique as it progresses medially across the femur.
✓ Complete fractures extend through both cortices and may be associated with a medial spike; incomplete fractures involve only the lateral cortex.
✓ The fracture is noncomminuted or minimally.
✓ Localized periosteal or endosteal thickening of the lateral cortex is present at the fracture site ('beaking' or 'flaring').

Minor Criteria
✓ Generalized increase in cortical thickness of the femoral diaphyses
✓ Unilateral or bilateral prodromal symptoms such as dull or aching pain in the groin or thigh
✓ Bilateral incomplete or complete femoral diaphysis fractures
✓ Delayed fracture healing

The femur is one of the human bones that exhibits racial and sex differences [7]. Asian females have greater anterolateral bowing of the femur compared with White, African-American persons, and males, respectively [8]. With greater lateral bowing of the femur, AFFs are more likely to occur in the diaphyseal region than in the subtrochanteric region [9]. Moreover, in older patients, the occurrence of low energy diaphyseal femoral fracture can be attributed to an increased range of anterior and lateral bowing [10]. Therefore, curvature of the femur should be considered a potential contributor to AFF development.

Currently, intramedullary (IM) nailing is the preferred surgical method for AFF [1,11]. However, in cases with a mismatch between the bowing of the femur and the curvature of the IM nails, several problems can arise. Some challenges include iatrogenic fractures, straightening of the femur, medial gap opening, leg-length discrepancy, penetration of the distal anterior femoral cortex, delayed union, and nonunion [2,12–17]. Prasarn et al. [17] reported that the most frequent surgical complication in BP-associated AFFs was intraoperative cortical fracture during nail insertion. To overcome excessive bowing of the femur, some surgeons have examined the use of pre-bent nails according to the curvature of the femur or a nail for the opposite femur [15,16,18]. Park et al. [18] reported a new technique for IM nailing that relieves excessive bowing of the femur in AFFs by rotating the nail outward when the nail passes through the apex of the curve. Despite these methods, the possibility of an iatrogenic fracture during IM nailing remains a constant concern for surgeons [2,17–19]. When iatrogenic fracture occurs, it can cause instability of the inserted nail, which is one of the important problems for patients because it can affect bone healing. In addition, iatrogenic cortical fracture around the fracture site in complete AFFs was identified as an independent predictive factor for problematic healing [2].

To date, no studies have examined the risk factors associated with the occurrence of iatrogenic fractures during IM nailing in AFF treatment. The purpose of this study was to determine the risk factors that could lead to an iatrogenic fracture in patients undergoing

IM nailing for AFFs. It was hypothesized that in AFFs, iatrogenic fractures during IM nailing are more likely to occur with excessive bowing of the femur and osteoporosis.

2. Material and Methods

2.1. Study Population

This was a retrospective cross-sectional study of 136 patients with AFF who underwent IM nailing between June 2008 and December 2017. The study was approved by our Institutional Review Board (Approval No. 2020-02-075, 19 March 2020), and the need for informed consent from all patients was waived. AFF was defined according to the second report of the American Society for Bone and Mineral Research (ASMBR) Task Force (Table 1) [1]. We examined the X-ray and computed tomography (CT) images to see whether there was periosteal or endosteal reaction of the lateral cortex thickening. Endosteal cortical thickening is defined as the increased cortical thickness of the fracture line just distal to the fracture site and formation of an endosteal callus, seen as "beaking" or "flaring" (Figure 1).

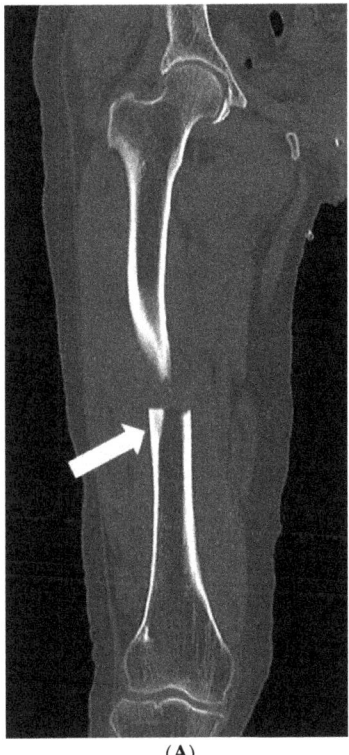
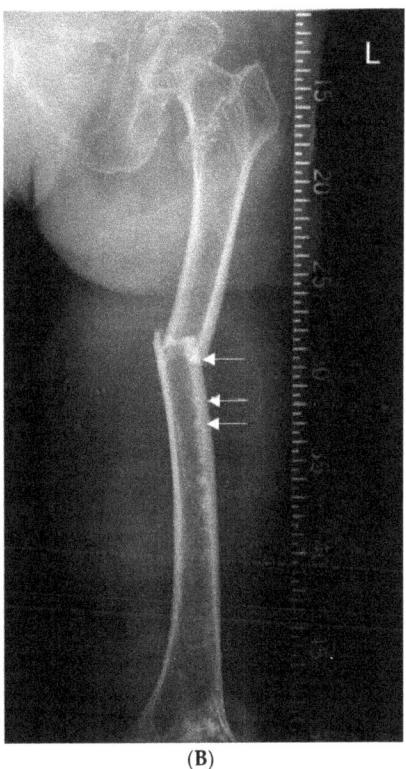

(A) (B)

Figure 1. (**A**) Atypical femur fracture in the right femur CT view. Lateral cortical thickening at the fracture site can be observed (depicted by block arrow). (**B**) Atypical femur fracture in the left femur scanogram. Endosteal cortical thickening can be observed at multiple sites near the fracture lesion (depicted by line arrows).

The following patients were excluded: (1) presence of comminuted fracture with high-energy trauma ($n = 10$); (2) bilateral AFFs ($n = 9$); (3) conservative treatment ($n = 3$); (4) internal fixation using proximal femoral nail antirotation or plate ($n = 5$); (5) use of glucocorticoid, proton pump inhibitor, or hormone ($n = 3$); (6) presence of metastatic bone tumor ($n = 1$); (7) unmeasurable bowing angle at the opposite intact femur ($n = 2$); and (8) no follow-up for more than 2 years after surgery ($n = 7$). Finally, 95 patients were included in the study. The patients were divided into two groups: Group I (with iatrogenic fracture; n = 20) and Group II (without iatrogenic fracture; n = 75) (Figure 2).

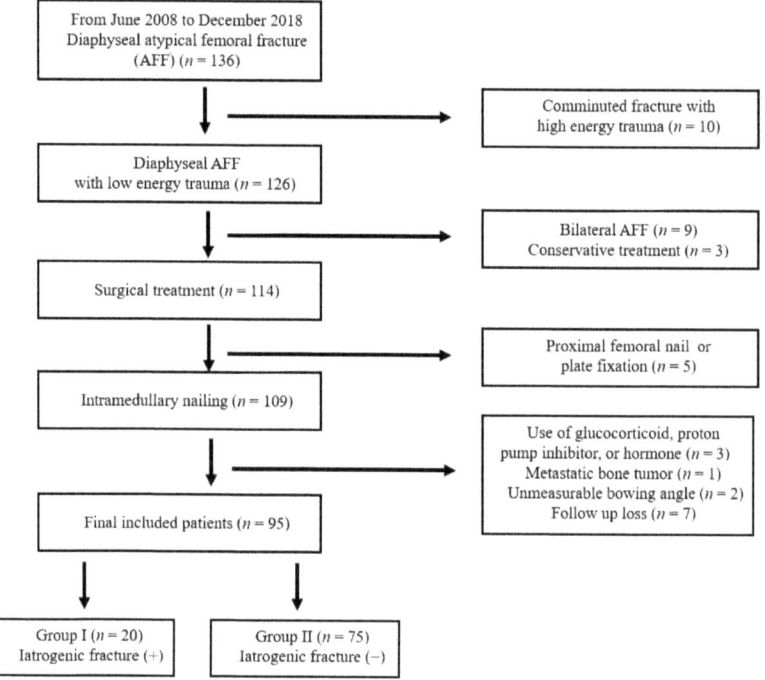

Figure 2. Flow chart of the patient selection.

2.2. Surgical Procedures & Postoperative Managements

All operations were performed under aseptic conditions according to established surgical procedures. All patients were positioned supine on the fracture table, and then closed reduction was performed under fluoroscopy. Patients underwent surgical treatment with antegrade IM nail insertion. From June 2008 to November 2012, an IM nail (T2 Femoral Nailing System; Stryker, Schönkirchen, Germany) with an entry point located in the piriformis fossa was used (n = 16; 16.8%). From December 2012 to December 2017, a different IM nail (Expert Asian Femoral Nail, A2FN; Synthes, Solothurn, Switzerland) with an entry point located lateral to the tip of the greater trochanter was used (n = 79; 83.2%). The medullary cavity was reamed at 1.5 mm larger than the intended nail diameter. All surgeries were performed by two senior surgeons. After surgery, patients did not apply a long leg splint or brace. They were allowed to sit on the first postoperative day while wheelchair and partial weight bearing was initiated between the third and seventh postoperative days depending on the degree of reduction, systemic condition, and pain. Weight bearing was gradually increased according to the extent of fracture union determined by radiography.

2.3. Clinical Assessment

The medical records of the enrolled patients were reviewed to evaluate the demographic data. Data for surgical complication, BP intake and duration, smoking history, prodromal symptoms, body mass index (BMI), bone mineral density (BMD), Charlson comorbidity index (CCI) [20], American Society of Anesthesiologist (ASA) classification [21], and Koval walking grade [22] were collected. Dual-energy X-ray absorptiometry was performed to measure BMD in the anteroposterior direction of the lumbar spine and hip.

In this way, we investigated the clinical differences between the two groups to identify the risk factors for iatrogenic fracture.

2.4. Radiographic Measurements

According to the fracture level, the AFFs were divided into proximal third, middle third, and distal third groups using the diaphyseal segment of the Arbeitsgemeinschaft für Osteosynthesefragen classification. An iatrogenic fracture was defined as an additional fracture lesion that newly occurred during surgery (Figure 3). Anteroposterior and lateral radiographs of the intact opposite femur were obtained to measure bowing of the femur. The bowing was defined as the angle between lines bisecting the femur at 0 and 5 cm below the lowest portion of the lesser trochanter and a line connecting points bisecting the femur at 5 and 10 cm above the distal articular surface [23] (Figure 4).

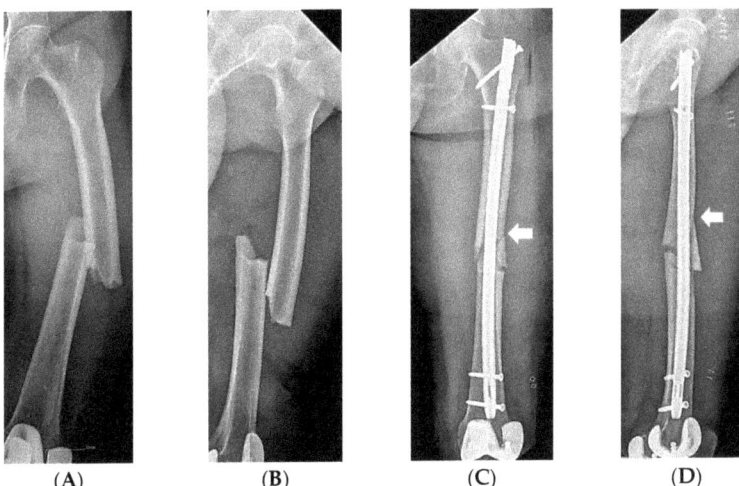

Figure 3. (**A**,**B**) X-rays of a 74-year-old woman showing a complete diaphyseal atypical femoral fracture. (**C**,**D**) Postoperative radiographs showing the intramedullary nail fixation and an iatrogenic fracture (arrows).

To investigate the effect of IM nail insertion on the occurrence of iatrogenic fracture, the entry points of the nails and the nail sizes were analyzed. The medullary cavity diameter of the fractured femur was measured at the narrowest shaft region on an anteroposterior radiograph of the femur. All patients were followed up for at least 2 years. At the last follow-up, fracture healing of the primary AFF and any iatrogenic fractures were evaluated. Fracture healing was defined as bridging of the fracture site by callus or bone at three cortices on plain radiographs [24]. All radiologic evaluations were conducted by two of the authors using plain radiographs of the femur with a picture archiving and communication system workstation (Maroview, version 5.4.10.52; Marotech, Seoul, Republic of Korea). Measurements were performed twice by both authors and the average values were used. To eliminate memory effects, the measurements were conducted 4 weeks apart. The authors performed the measurements independently without information about the patients. Intraclass correlation coefficients (ICCs) were assessed to determine inter- and intra-observer agreements for the radiologic measurements. The ICCs for agreement were interpreted as follows [25]: <0.5: poor; $\geq$0.5 but $\leq$0.9: good; and >0.9: excellent. The inter- and intra-observer reliabilities for all radiologic measurements were excellent (ICC > 0.90). As such, we identified secondary outcomes through radiologic measurement.

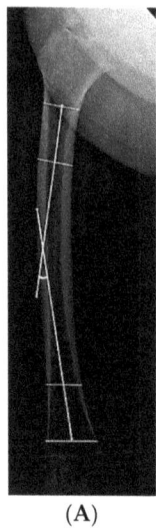 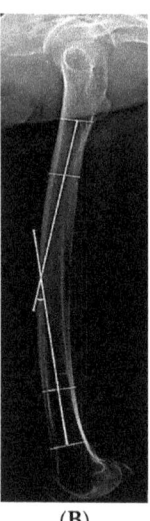

(A)   (B)

Figure 4. Measurement of femoral bowing in the opposite intact femur. (**A**) Lateral bowing on an anteroposterior X-ray. (**B**) Anterior bowing on a lateral X-ray.

2.5. Statistical Analysis

Statistical analyses were conducted using SPSS software (version 26.0; IBM Corporation, Armonk, NY, USA). Univariate analysis was used to identify significance between-group differences, defined as $p < 0.05$. Fisher's exact test was performed when the number of categorical variables was 2, and a chi-square test was performed when the number of categorical variables was ≥ 3. The frequency and percentage of the categorical variables were presented. Student's *t*-test was used to analyze continuous variables. When heterogeneity of variance was found in the distribution of the continuous variables using Levene's test, Welch's method was applied. Statistical data were presented as means ± standard deviations. Univariate and multivariate logistic regression analyses were performed to identify risk factors for an iatrogenic fracture as the primary outcome. Odds ratios (ORs) and 95% confidence intervals (CIs) were calculated for relative risks. In the multivariate analysis, a receiver operating characteristic (ROC) curve analysis was conducted for variables that were significantly related to predict iatrogenic fracture occurrence. The ROC curve analysis was also used to identify a cut-off value for lateral bowing angle of the femur to predict iatrogenic fracture. The cut-off point on the ROC curve is equivalent to the point at which the sensitivity and specificity were maximal as a secondary outcome.

3. Results

All 95 patients were female and iatrogenic fractures occurred in 20 (21.1%). There were no significant differences in age, affected femur (left and right sides), BMI, smoking habit, duration of BPs, CCI, ASA classification, Koval score, and prodromal symptoms between the two groups (Table 2).

Table 2. Comparison of demographic data between patients with and without iatrogenic fracture.

Variables	Group I (Iatrogenic Fracture, n = 20)	Group II (Non-Iatrogenic Fracture, n = 75)	p-Value
Age, years	73.5 ± 10.9 (50–87)	71.8 ± 9.0 (49–86)	0.472
Female sex	20 (100%)	75 (100%)	1.000
Affected side, Rt: Lt	11 (55.0%):9 (45.0%)	32 (42.7%):42 (57.3%)	0.449
Height, cm	150.3 ± 6.1 (138–160)	151.4 ± 7.2 (125–165)	0.550
Weight, kg	52.9 ± 8.6 (38–73)	53.8 ± 8.1 (35–75)	0.662
Body mass index, kg/m^2	23.4 ± 3.4 (18.1–32.9)	23.5 ± 3.3 (16.7–34.9)	0.893
Smoking, n	0 (0.0%)	4 (5.3%)	0.576
Bisphosphonate use	14 (70%)	61 (81%)	0.354
Duration of BPs, month	59.1 ± 7.1	66.5 ± 4.0	0.225
Charlson comorbidity index			0.739
1 or 2	1 (5.0%)	6 (8.0%)	
3 or 4	12 (60.0%)	46 (61.3%)	
≥5	7 (35.0%)	23 (30.7%)	
ASA [a] classification			0.158
I or II	19 (95.0%)	54 (72.0%)	
III or IV	1 (5.0%)	21 (28.0%)	
Koval score			0.359
1	19 (95.0%)	61 (81.3%)	
2 or 3	0 (0.0%)	11 (14.7%)	
4 or 5	0 (0.0%)	2 (2.7%)	
6 or 7	1 (5.0%)	1 (1.3%)	
Prodromal symptom	2 (10.0%)	16 (21.3%)	0.345

Data are expressed as mean ± standard deviation or number (percentage). [a], ASA American Society of Anesthesiologists.

The fracture characteristics are shown in Table 3. The mean femoral BMD in Group I (−2.9; range: −4.3 to −0.8) was significantly lower than that in Group II (−2.5; range: −4.5 to −0.3; $p = 0.046$). The mean lateral bowing angle in Group I (14.7° ± 5.9°; range: 2.4–24.8°) was significantly higher than that in Group II (7.9° ± 6.5°; range: 0.2–21.9°; $p < 0.001$). The mean anterior bowing angle in Group I (16.6° ± 4.2°; range: 9.7–25.1°) was also significantly higher than that in Group II (13.0° ± 7.8°; range: 1.0–29.5°; $p = 0.008$). However, no significant differences were observed in spinal BMD, diaphyseal AFF location, nail entry point, nail diameter, nail length, medullary cavity diameter and the difference (ΔD) in mm between the inner canal and IM nail diameter between the two groups. Nonunion occurred in 1 of 20 patients (5.0%) in Group I, and 5 patients (6.7%) in Group II ($p = 1.000$). All iatrogenic fracture sites were completely healed (Figure 5). The time to full weight bearing after surgery in Group I (24.4 ± 1.3 days; range: 20–28) was significantly longer than that in Group II (1.6 ± 0.3 day; range: 1–5; $p < 0.001$).

The results of univariate and multivariate logistic regression analyses are shown in Table 4. In the univariate analyses, femoral BMD and lateral bowing of the femur exhibited significant between-group differences ($p = 0.050$ and $p < 0.001$, respectively). In the multivariate analysis, a significant association was identified between lateral bowing of the femur and iatrogenic fracture (adjusted OR = 1.205; 95% CI: 1.046–1.389; $p = 0.010$), whereas femoral BMD was not identified as a significant risk factor.

In the ROC curve analysis, the area under the curve for lateral bowing of the femur and iatrogenic fracture was significant (0.786; $p = 0.010$) and the cut-off value for lateral bowing of the femur to predict iatrogenic fracture was 9.3° (Figure 6).

Table 3. Comparison of fracture- and surgery-related characteristics between patients with and without iatrogenic fracture.

Variables	Group I (Iatrogenic Fracture, n = 20)	Group II (Non-Iatrogenic Fracture, n = 75)	p-Value
Spinal BMD [a], T-score	−3.1 ± 1.1 (−5.2 to −1.1)	−2.8 ± 0.8 (−4.8 to −0.9)	0.204
Femoral BMD, T-score	−2.9 ± 1.0 (−4.3 to −0.8)	−2.5 ± 0.9 (−4.5 to −0.3)	0.046 [b]
AFF [c] location			0.803
Proximal third, n	6 (30.0%)	18 (24.0%)	
Middle third, n	13 (65.0%)	51 (68.0%)	
Distal third, n	1 (5.0%)	6 (8.0%)	
Lateral bowing, °	14.7 ± 5.9 (2.4–24.8)	7.9 ± 6.5 (0.2–21.9)	<0.001 [b]
Anterior bowing, °	16.6 ± 4.2 (9.7–25.1)	13.0 ± 7.8 (1.0–29.5)	0.008 [b]
Nail entry point			
Greater trochanter, n	17 (85.0%)	62 (82.7%)	1.000
Piriformis, n	3 (15.0%)	13 (17.3%)	1.000
Nail diameter, mm	11.9 ± 1.2 (9–13)	11.5 ± 1.4 (9–14)	0.185
Nail length, mm	334.0 ± 27.6 (280–380)	336.0 ± 23.5 (280–380)	0.745
Medullary cavity diameter, mm	13.3 ± 2.0 (9.6–16.6)	12.8 ± 2.3 (8.2–17.8)	0.328
Medullary cavity—Nail diameter, mm			0.125
<1 mm, n	8 (40.0%)	37 (49.3%)	
1–2 mm, n	8 (40.0%)	14 (18.7%)	
>2 mm, n	4 (20.0%)	24 (32.0%)	
Nonunion, n	1 (5.0%)	5 (6.7%)	1.000
Full-weight bearing after surgery, day	24.4 ± 1.3 (20–28)	1.6 ± 0.3 (1–5)	<0.001 [b]
Final follow up period, months	29.3 ± 8.3 (24–59)	31.9 ± 10.2 (24–73)	0.294

Data are expressed as mean ± standard deviation (range) or number (percentage). [a] BMD bone mineral density, [b] Statistically significant, [c] AFF Atypical femoral fracture.

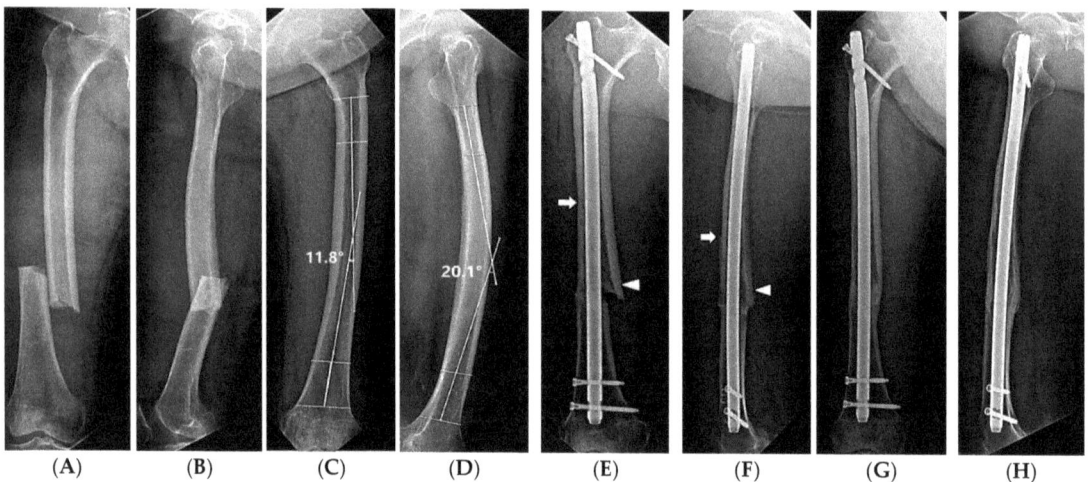

(A) (B) (C) (D) (E) (F) (G) (H)

Figure 5. A series of X-rays from a 79-year-old female patient who underwent intramedullary nailing under the diagnosis of AFF and experienced an iatrogenic diaphyseal fracture. (A,B) X-ray images of the AFF from the first visit to the emergency room. (C,D) X-ray images of the opposite intact femur. A lateral bowing angle of 11.8° and an anterior bowing angle of 20.1° were measured. (E,F) Medial gap opening (arrowheads) and iatrogenic diaphyseal fracture (arrows) occurred during intramedullary nailing. (G,H) Osseous union was obtained at 2 years after surgery.

Table 4. Univariate and multivariate analysis of variables associated with iatrogenic fracture.

Variables	Crude OR (95% CI)	p Value	Adjusted OR (95% CI)	p Value
Spine BMD [a]	0.701 (0.406–1.213)	0.205	1.185 (0.441–3.183)	0.737
Femoral BMD	0.546 (0.299–0.999)	0.050 [b]	0.577 (0.208–1.605)	0.292
Lateral bowing, °	1.154 (1.065–1.251)	<0.001 [b]	1.205 (1.046–1.389)	0.010 [b]
Anterior bowing, °	1.067 (0.997–1.141)	0.061	1.048 (0.915–1.199)	0.500

[a] BMD bone mineral density, [b] Statistically significant.

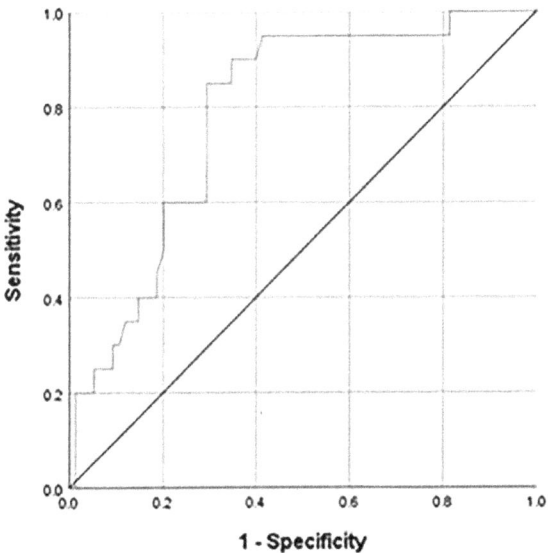

Figure 6. Receiver operating characteristic curve of the lateral bowing angle. The area under the curve, cut-off value, Youden's index, sensitivity, and specificity of the lateral bowing angle were 0.786 (0.684–0.888), 9.30, 0.557, 0.850, and 0.707, respectively ($p < 0.001$).

4. Discussion

In this study, we confirmed that greater lateral bowing of the femur is an important predictive factor for intraoperative iatrogenic fracture in patients undergoing IM nailing for AFFs.

AFFs are often associated with long-term use of BPs [26–30] but can also occur in patients without BP use, and increased femoral curvature may be an important causative factor for low-energy AFFs [1,9,10]. AFFs are stress fractures and that the geometry of the entire lower extremity can contribute to altered stress on the lateral cortex of the femur [1,6,9]. Anterolateral bowing of the femur is a risk factor for AFFs and the risk is five times higher in Asian populations compared with Caucasian populations [6,8,18]. In addition, lateral bowing of the femur was shown to determine the location of AFFs [3,9]. Yoo et al. [3] reported that the mean lateral bowing of the femur was 10.1° ± 3.79° in the diaphyseal AFF group and 3.3° ± 2.4° in the subtrochanteric AFF group. When the lateral bowing of the femur was greater than 5.2°, diaphyseal AFFs were more frequent than subtrochanteric AFFs. Kim et al. [9] also reported that the mean lateral bowing in the diaphyseal AFF group was significantly greater than that in the subtrochanteric AFF group (7.8° ± 4.8° versus 1.6° ± 1.8°). In other words, they found that as the lateral bowing of the femur increased, AFFs tended to occur more often in the diaphyseal region than in the subtrochanteric region. In the present study, the mean lateral bowing of the femur was 14.7° ± 5.9° in Group I (with iatrogenic fracture) and 7.9° ± 6.5° in Group II (without iatrogenic fracture). Similar to the findings in previous studies, all patients displayed large lateral bowing of the femur. In particular, the lateral bowing of the femur in Group I was twice as large as that in Group II, which was a meaningful finding related to iatrogenic fracture occurrence (Table 2).

Mismatching between the bowing of the femur and the curvature of the IM nail can produce an eccentric position of the distal nail tip and lead to an iatrogenic fracture due to straightening of the femur [13,14,17]. This complication can also lead to medial gap opening, leg-length discrepancy, and nonunion [2,16]. The incidence of iatrogenic fracture during IM nailing in AFFs currently remains unclear. Lim et al. [2] reported an incidence of 4.6% (5/109) whereas Prasarn et al. [17] reported 29.4% (5/17). The incidence in the present study was 21.1% (20/95), which is in agreement with those of previous studies. However, the incidence appears to vary from study to study because the participants are different and there are slight differences in surgical techniques. Therefore, more research is required to clarify the incidence. The present study focused on determining risk factors for iatrogenic fracture occurrence during IM nailing in AFFs. In our study, Group I displayed greater lateral and anterior bowing of the femur than Group II (Table 2). Therefore, because of the large curvature of the femur, there was considerable nail mismatching in Group I and iatrogenic fractures were more likely to occur. However, anterior bowing of the femur was excluded as a risk factor for iatrogenic fracture occurrence in the multivariate analysis (Table 3). Therefore, we confirmed that greater lateral bowing of the femur was a significant risk factor for iatrogenic fracture occurrence during IM nailing for AFFs.

Increased bowing of the femur is related to impaired fracture healing in AFFs, and lateral bowing of the femur exceeding $10°$ may contribute to the high rate of delayed union [2]. Meanwhile, iatrogenic cortical fracture around the primary fracture site displayed problematic healing with an adjusted OR of 19.7 in complete AFFs [2]. Therefore, if an iatrogenic fracture occurs during IM nailing in AFFs with excessive lateral bowing of the femur, the risk of complications such as nonunion or delayed union may be increased. In our cohort, there was no between-group difference in the healing rate, although Group I exhibited excessive lateral bowing ($14.7°$) and additional iatrogenic fractures. The difference in results compared to other studies may potentially be due to the different patient cohorts and surgical procedures. Our results further showed that even if an iatrogenic fracture occurred during IM nailing, there was no effect on final bone union. However, for patients with an iatrogenic fracture, weight-bearing may begin later or rehabilitation may take longer, even if there is no effect on fracture healing. This can lead to increased mortality and morbidity [31]. In the present study, the patients in Group II were allowed to undertake immediate postoperative full weight bearing, whereas the patients in Group I began full weight bearing at a mean of 24.4 days after surgery ($p < 0.001$) (Table 2). Therefore, for early rehabilitation, it is important to prevent iatrogenic fracture occurrence during surgery. Although we cannot completely overcome the risk of iatrogenic fracture occurrence during IM nailing in AFFs in patients with excessive bowing of the femur, we can predict its likelihood and carefully select an appropriate implant before performing the procedure.

AFFs represent a form of osteoporotic fracture [32]. AFFs may be related to age >65 years, more lateral bowing, Asian females, and lower BMD [8,9,33–35]. Unexpected iatrogenic fractures can occur during IM nailing in the diaphyseal region of the femur in patients with osteoporosis [36]. Therefore, as the severity of osteoporosis increases, the probability of developing an iatrogenic fracture during IM nailing in AFFs becomes higher. In the present study, the mean femoral BMD in Group I was significantly lower than that in Group II (Table 2). However, femoral BMD was not a significant risk factor in the multivariate analysis (Table 3). Nevertheless, decreased femoral BMD should not be completely ignored as a risk factor because osteoporotic bone is susceptible to fracture [37].

To our knowledge, this is the first study to determine the risk factors for intraoperative iatrogenic fracture occurrence during intramedullary nailing for AFFs. The strength of the study is that factors that can cause iatrogenic fractures were evaluated using univariate and multivariate logistic regression analyses. The univariate analyses revealed correlations with iatrogenic fractures for femoral BMD, as well as lateral and anterior bowing of the femur. The multivariate analysis confirmed that lateral bowing of the femur was a reliable risk factor associated with iatrogenic fracture occurrence. In addition, the cut-off value for lateral bowing of the femur with significant sensitivity and specificity for prediction of iatrogenic fracture occurrence was determined at 9.3°. In other words, iatrogenic femoral fracture occurrence is more frequent during IM nailing for AFFs when the lateral bowing of the femur is larger than 9.3°. Thus, when IM nailing is planned for AFF, measurement of the lateral bowing of the femur should be considered in the preoperative planning to provide a reference value for predicting iatrogenic fracture occurrence.

According to previous studies, various methods have been proposed to reduce the incidence of iatrogenic fractures during IM nailing. For example, the entry point of the nail was planned with caution in order to avoid anterior or external deviation. Proper reaming for bowing shape was also selected [38,39]. In 2017, Park et al. reported new grading systems for anterolateral femoral bowing [18]. Furthermore, they introduced the new intramedullary nailing technique by which the nail is rotated externally for femur bowing. Recently, three-dimensional (3D) technologies have been introduced to help prevent iatrogenic fractures by planning surgery in advance [40].

In this way, various methods have been introduced to prevent iatrogenic fracture during surgery, and we also contemplated means to prevent iatrogenic fractures based on these factors. By extension, we considered the risk factors for iatrogenic fractures and identified significant risk factors through the cut-off value of the lateral bowing angle. Based on this, surgeons may benefit from identifying the bowing angle of the femur before surgery to evaluate the predictability of perioperative iatrogenic fractures and make efforts to reduce iatrogenic fractures.

The present study has several limitations. First, because the study was retrospective, bone metabolic markers were not evaluated before the patients presented with fractures. Second, the study was not a randomized controlled trial. A larger, multicenter, prospective study is required to confirm our findings. Third, because the lateral and anterior bowing angles were measured on the opposite intact femur, these angles could be different from those of the fractured femur. Fourth, the study was limited to Asians. Therefore, various races need to be evaluated in prospective studies to confirm the present findings.

5. Conclusions

The present study analyzed the risk factors for intraoperative iatrogenic fracture during IM nailing for diaphyseal AFFs. Lateral bowing of the femur was identified as a significant risk factor and its cut-off value for prediction of an intraoperative iatrogenic fracture was 9.3°. Surgeons should evaluate the lateral bowing of the femur during preoperative planning for diaphyseal AFFs, and if patients exhibit large lateral bowing of the femur, care should be taken to prevent the occurrence of iatrogenic fractures during surgery.

Author Contributions: Conceptualization, H.J.C.; data curation, Y.S.J. and H.J.C.; writing—original draft, Y.B.J. and H.J.C.; Writing—review and editing, Y.B.J.; supervision, W.Y.L.; statistical analysis, Y.S.J. All authors have read and agreed to the published version of the manuscript.

Funding: This work was supported by research fund of Chungnam National University.

Institutional Review Board Statement: Internal review board approval was obtained—Chungnam National University Hospital, No. CNUH 2020-02-075.

Informed Consent Statement: Not required.

Data Availability Statement: The data presented in this study are available on request from the corresponding author.

Conflicts of Interest: The authors declare that have no conflict of interest.

References

1. Shane, E.; Burr, D.; Abrahamsen, B.; Adler, R.A.; Brown, T.D.; Cheung, A.M.; Cosman, F.; Curtis, J.R.; Dell, R.; Dempster, D.W.; et al. Atypical Subtrochanteric and Diaphyseal Femoral Fractures: Second Report of a Task Force of the American Society for Bone and Mineral Research. *J. Bone Miner. Res.* **2013**, *29*, 1–23. [CrossRef]
2. Lim, H.-S.; Kim, C.-K.; Park, Y.-S.; Moon, Y.-W.; Lim, S.-J.; Kim, S.-M. Factors Associated with Increased Healing Time in Complete Femoral Fractures After Long-Term Bisphosphonate Therapy. *J. Bone Jt. Surg.* **2016**, *98*, 1978–1987. [CrossRef]
3. Yoo, H.; Cho, Y.; Park, Y.; Ha, S. Lateral Femoral Bowing and the Location of Atypical Femoral Fractures. *Hip Pelvis* **2017**, *29*, 127–132. [CrossRef] [PubMed]
4. Yoon, R.S.; Hwang, J.S.; Beebe, K.S. Long-term bisphosphonate usage and subtrochanteric insufficiency fractures: A cause for concern? *J. Bone Jt. Surg.* **2011**, *93*, 1289–1295. [CrossRef]
5. Tan, S.C.; Koh, S.B.J.; Goh, S.K.; Howe, T.S. Atypical femoral stress fractures in bisphosphonate-free patients. *Osteoporos. Int.* **2011**, *22*, 2211–2212. [CrossRef] [PubMed]
6. Marcano, A.; Taormina, D.; Egol, K.A.; Peck, V.; Tejwani, N.C. Are Race and Sex Associated With the Occurrence of Atypical Femoral Fractures? *Clin. Orthop. Relat. Res.* **2013**, *472*, 1020–1027. [CrossRef] [PubMed]
7. Harma, A.; Germen, B.; Karakas, H.; Elmali, N.; Inan, M. The comparison of femoral curves and curves of contemporary intramedullary nails. *Surg. Radiol. Anat.* **2005**, *27*, 502–506. [CrossRef]
8. Maratt, J.; Schilling, P.L.; Holcombe, S.; Dougherty, R.; Murphy, R.; Wang, S.C.; Goulet, J.A. Variation in the Femoral Bow: A novel high-throughput analysis of 3922 femurs on cross-sectional imaging. *J. Orthop. Trauma* **2014**, *28*, 6–9. [CrossRef]
9. Kim, J.W.; Kim, J.J.; Byun, Y.-S.; Shon, O.-J.; Oh, H.K.; Park, K.C.; Kim, J.-W.; Oh, C.-W. Factors affecting fracture location in atypical femoral fractures: A cross-sectional study with 147 patients. *Injury* **2017**, *48*, 1570–1574. [CrossRef] [PubMed]
10. Sasaki, S.; Miyakoshi, N.; Hongo, M.; Kasukawa, Y.; Shimada, Y. Low-energy diaphyseal femoral fractures associated with bisphosphonate use and severe curved femur: A case series. *J. Bone Miner. Metab.* **2012**, *30*, 561–567. [CrossRef]
11. Unnanuntana, A.; Saleh, A.; Mensah, K.A.; Kleimeyer, J.P.; Lane, J.M. Atypical Femoral Fractures: What Do We Know about Them? AAOS Exhibit Selection. *J. Bone Jt. Surg.* **2013**, *95*, e8.1–e8.13. [CrossRef]
12. Gausepohl, T.; Pennig, D.; Koebke, J.; Harnoss, S. Antegrade femoral nailing: An anatomical determination of the correct entry point. *Injury* **2002**, *33*, 701–705. [CrossRef] [PubMed]
13. Leung, K.S.; Procter, P.; Robioneck, B.; Behrens, K. Geometric Mismatch of the Gamma Nail to the Chinese Femur. *Clin. Orthop. Relat. Res.* **1996**, *323*, 42–48. [CrossRef] [PubMed]
14. Egol, K.A.; Chang, E.Y.; Cvitkovic, J.; Kummer, F.J.; Koval, K.J. Mismatch of Current Intramedullary Nails With the Anterior Bow of the Femur. *J. Orthop. Trauma* **2004**, *18*, 410–415. [CrossRef] [PubMed]
15. Park, J.H.; Lee, Y.; Shon, O.-J.; Shon, H.C.; Kim, J.W. Surgical tips of intramedullary nailing in severely bowed femurs in atypical femur fractures: Simulation with 3D printed model. *Injury* **2016**, *47*, 1318–1324. [CrossRef] [PubMed]
16. Lee, K.-J.; Min, B.-W. Surgical Treatment of the Atypical Femoral Fracture: Overcoming Femoral Bowing. *Hip Pelvis* **2018**, *30*, 202–209. [CrossRef] [PubMed]
17. Prasarn, M.L.; Ahn, J.; Helfet, D.L.; Lane, J.M.; Lorich, D.G. Bisphosphonate-associated Femur Fractures Have High Complication Rates with Operative Fixation. *Clin. Orthop. Relat. Res.* **2012**, *470*, 2295–2301. [CrossRef]
18. Park, Y.-C.; Song, H.-K.; Zheng, X.-L.; Yang, K.-H. Intramedullary Nailing for Atypical Femoral Fracture with Excessive Anterolateral Bowing. *J. Bone Jt. Surg.* **2017**, *99*, 726–735. [CrossRef]
19. Castellanos, J.; Garcia-Nuño, L.; Cavanilles-Walker, J.M.; Roca, J. Iatrogenic femoral neck fracture during closed nailing of the femoral shaft fracture. *Eur. J. Trauma Emerg. Surg.* **2009**, *35*, 479–481. [CrossRef]
20. Charlson, M.E.; Pompei, P.; Ales, K.L.; MacKenzie, C.R. A new method of classifying prognostic comorbidity in longitudinal studies: Development and validation. *J. Chronic Dis.* **1987**, *40*, 373–383. [CrossRef] [PubMed]
21. Owens, M.W.D.; Felts, M.J.A.; Spitznagel, E.L. ASA Physical Status Classifications: A study of consistency of ratings. *Anesthesiology* **1978**, *49*, 239–243. [CrossRef] [PubMed]
22. Koval, K.J.; Aharonoff, G.B.; Rosenberg, A.D.; Bernstein, R.L.; Zuckerman, J.D. Functional outcome after hip fracture. Effect of general versus regional anesthesia. *Clin. Orthop. Relat. Res.* **1998**, 37–41, 9553531.
23. Kim, J.-M.; Hong, S.-H.; Lee, B.-S.; Kim, D.-E.; Kim, K.-A.; Bin, S.-I. Femoral shaft bowing in the coronal plane has more significant effect on the coronal alignment of TKA than proximal or distal variations of femoral shape. *Knee Surg. Sport. Traumatol. Arthrosc.* **2014**, *23*, 1936–1942. [CrossRef] [PubMed]
24. Corrales, L.A.; Morshed, S.; Bhandari, M.; Miclau, T. Variability in the Assessment of Fracture-Healing in Orthopaedic Trauma Studies. *J. Bone Jt. Surg.* **2008**, *90*, 1862–1868. [CrossRef]
25. Koo, T.K.; Li, M.Y. A Guideline of Selecting and Reporting Intraclass Correlation Coefficients for Reliability Research. *J. Chiropr. Med.* **2016**, *15*, 155–163. [CrossRef]
26. Capeci, C.M.; Tejwani, N.C. Bilateral Low-Energy Simultaneous or Sequential Femoral Fractures in Patients on Long-Term Alendronate Therapy. *J. Bone Jt. Surg.* **2009**, *91*, 2556–2561. [CrossRef] [PubMed]
27. Rosenberg, Z.S.; Vieira, R.L.R.; Chan, S.S.; Babb, J.; Akyol, Y.; Rybak, L.D.; Moore, S.; Bencardino, J.T.; Peck, V.; Tejwani, N.C.; et al. Bisphosphonate-Related Complete Atypical Subtrochanteric Femoral Fractures: Diagnostic Utility of Radiography. *Am. J. Roentgenol.* **2011**, *197*, 954–960. [CrossRef]

28. Shane, E.; Burr, D.; Ebeling, P.R.; Abrahamsen, B.; Adler, R.A.; Brown, T.D.; Cheung, A.M.; Cosman, F.; Curtis, J.R.; Dell, R.; et al. Atypical subtrochanteric and diaphyseal femoral fractures: Report of a task force of the american society for bone and mineral Research. *J. Bone Miner. Res.* **2010**, *25*, 2267–2294. [CrossRef]
29. Meier, R.P.H.; Perneger, T.V.; Stern, R.; Rizzoli, R.; Peter, R.E. Increasing Occurrence of Atypical Femoral Fractures Associated with Bisphosphonate Use. *Arch. Intern. Med.* **2012**, *172*, 930–936. [CrossRef]
30. Schilcher, J.; Koeppen, V.; Aspenberg, P.; Michaëlsson, K. Risk of atypical femoral fracture during and after bisphosphonate use. *Acta Orthop.* **2015**, *86*, 100–107. [CrossRef]
31. Bouchard, J.A.; Barei, D.; Cayer, D.; O'Neil, J. Outcome of Femoral Shaft Fractures in the Elderly. *Clin. Orthop. Relat. Res.* **1996**, *332*, 105–109. [CrossRef] [PubMed]
32. Abrahamsen, B.; Eiken, P.; Eastell, R. Cumulative Alendronate Dose and the Long-Term Absolute Risk of Subtrochanteric and Diaphyseal Femur Fractures: A Register-Based National Cohort Analysis. *J. Clin. Endocrinol. Metab.* **2010**, *95*, 5258–5265. [CrossRef] [PubMed]
33. Karakaş, H.M.; Harma, A. Femoral shaft bowing with age: A digital radiological study of Anatolian Caucasian adults. *Diagn. Interv. Radiol.* **2008**, *14*, 29–32.
34. Koeppen, V.A.; Schilcher, J.; Aspenberg, P. Atypical fractures do not have a thicker cortex. *Osteoporos. Int.* **2012**, *23*, 2893–2896. [CrossRef] [PubMed]
35. Saita, Y.; Ishijima, M.; Mogami, A.; Kubota, M.; Baba, T.; Kaketa, T.; Nagao, M.; Sakamoto, Y.; Sakai, K.; Kato, R.; et al. The fracture sites of atypical femoral fractures are associated with the weight-bearing lower limb alignment. *Bone* **2014**, *66*, 105–110. [CrossRef] [PubMed]
36. Elbarbary, A.N.; Hassen, S.; Badr, I.T. Outcome of intramedullary nail for fixation of osteoporotic femoral shaft fractures in the elderly above 60. *Injury* **2021**, *52*, 602–605. [CrossRef]
37. Unnanuntana, A.; Gladnick, B.P.; Donnelly, E.; Lane, J.M. The Assessment of Fracture Risk. *J. Bone Jt. Surg.* **2010**, *92*, 743–753. [CrossRef] [PubMed]
38. Carr, J.B.; Williams, D.; Richards, M. Lateral Decubitus Positioning for Intramedullary Nailing of the Femur Without the Use of a Fracture Table. *Orthopedics* **2009**, *32*, 721. [CrossRef]
39. Kim, J.W.; Byun, S.-E.; Oh, W.-H.; Kim, J.J. Bursting Fracture of the Proximal Femur during Insertion of Unreamed Femoral Nail for Femur Shaft Fracture—A Case Report. *J. Korean Fract. Soc.* **2010**, *23*, 227–231. [CrossRef]
40. Moldovan, F.; Gligor, A.; Bataga, T. Structured Integration and Alignment Algorithm: A Tool for Personalized Surgical Treatment of Tibial Plateau Fractures. *J. Pers. Med.* **2021**, *11*, 190. [CrossRef]

Disclaimer/Publisher's Note: The statements, opinions and data contained in all publications are solely those of the individual author(s) and contributor(s) and not of MDPI and/or the editor(s). MDPI and/or the editor(s) disclaim responsibility for any injury to people or property resulting from any ideas, methods, instructions or products referred to in the content.

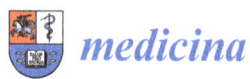 medicina

Article

The Efficacy of Low-Dose Risperidone Treatment for Post-Surgical Delirium in Elderly Orthopedic Patients

Lotan Raphael, Epstein Edna, Kaykov Irina and Hershkovich Oded *

Department of Orthopedic Surgery, Wolfson Medical Center, Sackler School of Medicine, Tel Aviv 5822012, Israel
* Correspondence: oded.hershkovich@gmail.com; Tel.: +972-3-5028383; Fax: +972-3-5028774

Abstract: *Background*: Delirium is an acute and typically reversible failure of essential cognitive and attentional functions and is a growing public health concern, with an incidence of 20–50% in patients older than 65 after major surgery and 61% in patients undergoing hip fracture surgery. Numerous treatment strategies have been examined with no conclusive results. The purpose of this study is to assess the efficacy of a three-day low-dose risperidone treatment protocol, 0.5 mg BID, in treating delirium in elderly hospitalized orthopedic surgery department patients. *Methods*: This study is a prospective non-randomized study involving the senior patient population, older than 65, in an Orthopedic Surgery Department in 2019 and 2020. Delirium was diagnosed by a confusion assessment method (CAM) questionnaire. A three-day 0.5 mg risperidone BID treatment protocol was initiated following diagnosis. Patient data collected included age, gender, chronic diseases, type of surgery and anesthesia and delirium characteristics. *Results*: The delirium study group included 47 patients with an average age of 84.4 years (±8.6), of whom 53.2% were females. Delirium incidence was 3.7% in all patients older than 65 (1759 patients) and 9.3% in the proximal femoral fracture group. We did not correlate electrolyte imbalance, anemia, polypharmacy and chronic diseases to delirium onset characteristics. Following the three-day low-dose risperidone treatment protocol, 0.5 mg BID, 14.9% of the patients showed CAM score normalization after one day of treatment, and 93.6% within two days. *Conclusions*: We found our rigid three-day low-dose risperidone treatment protocol, 0.5 mg BID, efficacious in fast delirium resolution, without side effects.

Keywords: delirium; risperidone; post-surgical; elderly; protocol

Citation: Raphael, L.; Edna, E.; Irina, K.; Oded, H. The Efficacy of Low-Dose Risperidone Treatment for Post-Surgical Delirium in Elderly Orthopedic Patients. *Medicina* **2023**, *59*, 1052. https://doi.org/10.3390/medicina59061052

Academic Editor: Woo Jong Kim

Received: 2 March 2023
Revised: 20 May 2023
Accepted: 28 May 2023
Published: 30 May 2023

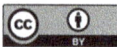

Copyright: © 2023 by the authors. Licensee MDPI, Basel, Switzerland. This article is an open access article distributed under the terms and conditions of the Creative Commons Attribution (CC BY) license (https://creativecommons.org/licenses/by/4.0/).

1. Introduction

Delirium is an acute and typically reversible failure of essential cognitive and attentional functions. Delirium is usually associated with an altered fluctuating level of consciousness. It can manifest as agitation (hyperactive type), lethargy (hypoactive type), or alternating between these (mixed type). With the increase in life expectancy and the ageing population, many frail elderly patients require surgery, such as osteoporotic proximal femur fractures. Postoperative delirium is a growing public health concern, with an incidence of 20–50% in patients older than 65 after major surgery and 61% in patients undergoing hip fracture surgery [1,2]. Postoperative delirium can become the most deleterious element of the perioperative experience, both for the patient and the family, and is associated with increased mortality [1], cognitive and functional decline [2], increased hospital length of stay, and healthcare costs. The pathophysiology of delirium remains obscure, and the diagnosis is clinical.

Delirium is currently diagnosed according to the Diagnostic and Statistical Manual of Mental Disorders (DSM-V) or the 10th revision of the International Statistical Classification of Diseases and Related Health Problems (ICD-10). Faster and simpler delirium screening tools were described, including the confusion assessment method (CAM) [3–5], the delirium observation screening scale, delirium symptom interview, and the NEECHAM confusion scale [6], with low sensitivity (about 30%) compared with an expert delirium assessment (that is, by a psychiatrist, geriatrician, or neurologist) [7,8]. However, diagnostic disagreement may be typical among experts and disciplines. Whatever tool is used to diagnose delirium, a reassessment should be repeated every 6 h for three to five days following surgery.

Postoperative delirium risk factors include age greater than 65 years, preoperative cognitive impairment, visual or hearing impairment, presence of infection, inadequate or exaggerated pain control, impaired left ventricular function, electrolyte disorders, depression, alcoholism, smoking, high perioperative transfusion requirements, intraoperative pressure fluctuation [9], sleep deprivation, urinary retention or constipation, renal insufficiency, poor nutrition, dehydration, immobilization [10] or poor mobility, use of anticholinergic medications, sedative-hypnotics, and meperidine. Polypharmacy (five drugs or more) is another risk factor for delirium.

Although postoperative delirium is quite a common diagnosis, treatment is lacking. Delirium management starts with prevention, is multidisciplinary, and deals with 10 aspects: cerebral oxygenation, fluid, and electrolyte homeostasis, pain control, reduction of psychoactive drugs, bowel and urinary function optimization, nutritional support, early out-of-bed practice, prevention of postoperative complications, keeping adequate environmental stimuli, and treatment of delirium symptoms. Delirium management can be non-pharmacological or pharmacological [3,11–13].

Non-pharmacological delirium management focuses on mediating a calm and quiet patient environment, clock and calendar patient orientation, including familiar relatives, reducing treating staff rotation, "education about early mobilization", reducing noise and lighting during night hours and opening windows and curtains during daylight hours, as well as improving patient communication by using hearing and visual aids. Mindful breathing also showed a 15–50% decrease in delirium incidence [14].

Intraoperative measures include light instead of heavy sedation and bispectral index (BIS) anesthesia guidance [15]. The role of regional versus general anesthesia in delirium remains unknown [16–18]. Postoperative pain control uses non-opiate alternatives instead of opiate-only regimens or combining regional anesthesia [13,19]. Gabapentin has been used in postoperative pain control but was found to be highly deliriogenic [20]. Postoperative measures include reviewing pain control and medications, physical examination with urinary catheter insertion if needed, and searching for an infection (pneumonia, sepsis, line sepsis, surgical site infection), and metabolic derangement.

Use of preventive antipsychotic medications and cholinesterase inhibitors is inconclusive. Some RCT studies showed that antipsychotic drugs, such as haloperidol, are efficacious in treating existing delirium, with side effects such as extrapyramidal manifestations and QT-interval elongation on ECG [21,22]. Their use is limited in patients suffering from hepatic insufficiency neuroleptic malignant syndrome. Another treatment option is atypical antipsychotic medications, such as risperidone or olanzapine, with the same side effects [23]. Risperidone stands out due to its notable affinity with serotonin and dopamine receptors. By exerting antagonistic effects on serotonin receptors, it can alleviate dopamine antagonism associated with extrapyramidal symptoms. As a result, risperidone exhibits superior advantages in terms of side effects compared to traditional antipsychotics, making it a preferred first-line treatment option for delirium [24,25]. Regardless of the treatment, the lowest effective dose for the shortest possible duration should be used to treat severely agitated or distressed patients that threaten themselves or their surroundings.

While numerous treatment strategies were examined with no conclusive results, this study aims to assess the efficacy of a three-day low-dose risperidone treatment protocol, 0.5 mg BID, in treating delirium in elderly hospitalized orthopedic surgery department patients.

2. Methods

This study is a prospective observational non-randomized study involving the senior patient population in an Orthopedic Surgery Department in 2019 and 2020. The study included patients older than 65 who suffered from delirium. A confusion assessment method (CAM) questionnaire diagnosed the patient's delirium as evident from the presence or absence of the following four features: 1. mental status alteration from baseline (acute onset or fluctuating), 2. inattention, 3. disorganized thinking, and 4. altered level of consciousness. Delirium was identified only if there was evidence of the first essential features (1 + 2) and either of the following features (3 or 4, or both). Delirium was treated by cessation of opiates and psychoactive drugs and received a three-day BID treatment of 0.5 mg risperidone. This treatment protocol was chosen due to its simplicity, low dosage and short treatment period. Exclusion criteria included patients younger than 65 or patients who did not meet the CAM criteria for delirium or did not complete the three-day treatment protocol.

Patient data collected included age, gender, chronic diseases, type of surgery, type of anesthesia, type of anesthetic agents used during surgery, the timing of the delirium onset, delirium duration, and CAM scores at the protocol completion.

Statistical analysis included the Shapiro–Wilk test of normal distribution and students t-test for numerical parameters, and the Chi-square test for categorical parameters. In addition, Pearson and Spearman's correlation coefficients measured the influence of gender, drugs, type of surgery, and anesthesia on delirium onset and duration. To counteract the multiple comparisons issue and the increase in probability of observing a rare event under multiple hypotheses, a Bonferroni correction was used as required.

3. Results

A total of 47 patients 65 years old or older out of the 1759 patients admitted to the Orthopedic Surgery Department between March 2019 and December 2020 suffered from perioperative delirium, in other words, 3.7% of the patients. The number of patients suffering proximal femoral fractures during the same period was 698; thus, there was 9.3% of delirium in this group of patients. The average age was 84.4 years (±8.6), and 53.2% were females. The average body mass index (BMI) was 25.4 (±6.4) (Table 1).

Some 80% of the patients in this study had proximal femoral fractures, which could be divided into subcapital (37.1%) and intertrochanteric fractures (44.7%). Three patients suffered pelvic fractures, pubic rami fractures that did not require surgery and were treated with physiotherapy, and deep vein thrombosis prevention and pain control. Six patients developed delirium following other surgeries; one case of open reduction internal fixation (ORIF) of a humeral fracture, one case of ORIF of a distal femoral fracture, one case of lumbar decompression laminectomy, one case of ORIF of an olecranon fracture and two cases of late femoral surgical site infection (SSI) debridement. General anesthesia accounted for 61.4% of surgeries, and regional anesthesia with sedation accounted for 38.6%.

Delirium assessment was carried out once in a nursing shift, i.e., three times a day. The average CAM score at delirium onset was 3 ± 1, and patients tended to develop perioperative delirium during the evening (18:00–24:00 p.m.), but it did not reach statistical significance. A total of 63.8% of delirium onset occurred during the first three days of hospitalization and 76.6% during the first four days (Figure 1). In addition, 75% of the delirium occurred within the first two days following surgery and 81.8% during the first three postoperative days. In our study, females tended to develop delirium earlier during hospitalization (2.45 days ± 1.68) compared to males (5.16 days ± 7.41) ($p = 0.05$).

Examining factors influencing delirium onset, duration and severity, gender but not age, correlates with an earlier development of perioperative delirium ($p = 0.046$) and a tendency to prolonged delirium ($p = 0.058$). Unfortunately, the study sample size did not allow statistical significance for the correlation between gender and the duration of delirium.

Table 1. Patients' characteristics.

Parameter	Number (%)
Study group	47
Males	22 (46.8)
Females	25 (53.2)
Age (years)	84.4 ± 8.6
BMI	25.4 ± 6.4
Type of Surgery	
Pertrochanteric Fracture Fixation	21 (44.7)
Femoral Arthroplasty	12 (25.5)
Subcapital Femoral Fracture Fixation	5 (10.6)
Conservative Treatment	3 (6.4)
Other Surgeries	6 (12.8)
Surgery Duration (mins)	56.3 ± 30.8
Anaesthesia	
General	27 (61.4)
Regional with Sedation	17 (38.6)
Delirium	
Delirium Onset from Hospitalization (days)	4 ± 6
Delirium Onset by Postoperative Day	2 ± 2
Initial CAM Score	3 ± 1
Days to Delirium Resolution	1.98 ± 0.68
CAM Score at the End of Treatment	0.11 ± 0.31

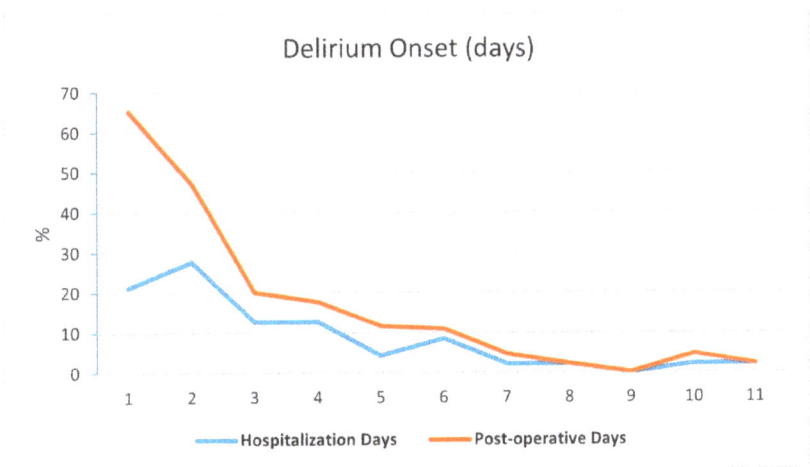

Figure 1. Delirium onset by days from hospitalization and postoperative time.

Opiates, benzodiazepine, anxiolytics and antidepressant treatments were not found to influence the rate of development of perioperative delirium in our study group or the effect of the treatment protocol. A history of malignancy, CVA, depression, and dementia did not change the course of the perioperative delirium either. Smoking did not correlate to the study group's delirium characteristics. Common chronic diseases, such as diabetes, ischemic heart disease, and hypercholesterolemia, did not correlate to delirium onset or duration. Chronic renal failure, even when requiring dialysis, did not alter the delirium manifestation (Figure 2).

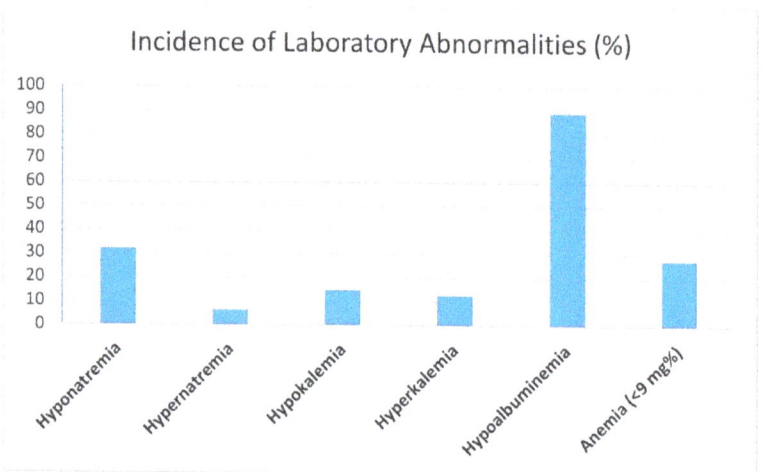

Figure 2. Incidence of laboratory abnormalities (%).

Sensual impairments, visual and auditory, did not correlate to delirium duration, severity or onset. Blood electrolyte disturbances, such as hypo- and hyper-natremia and kalemia (Figure 3), did not influence perioperative delirium. Constipation and urinary retention did not correlate to the study group's delirium onset, severity, and duration measured by Pearson and Spearman's correlation coefficients.

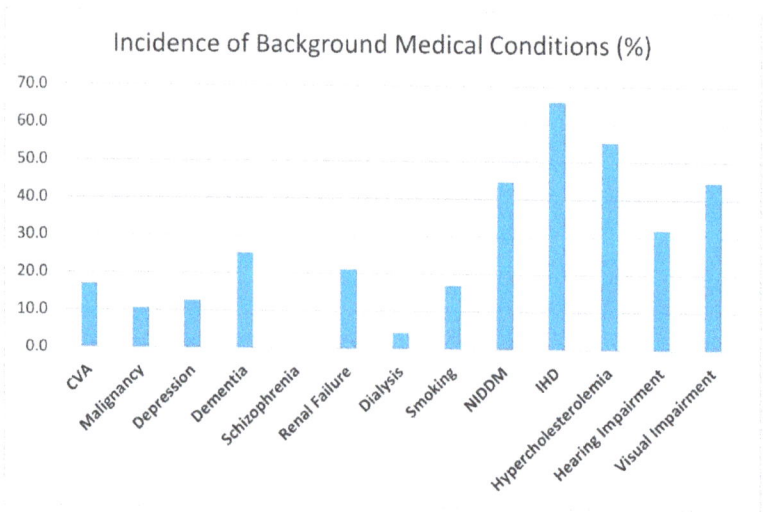

Figure 3. Incidence of background medical conditions.

Polypharmacy (more than five drugs) in the study group showed a low correlation to the duration of the perioperative delirium (r = 0.16), while higher blood albumin levels (r = −0.17) and younger age (p = 0.03) shortened the delirium period.

When we examined the effect of the type of anesthesia on postoperative delirium, we found that patients tended to develop delirium earlier following regional anesthesia with sedation (1.75 ± 2.41 days) as compared to general anesthesia (2.69 days ± 2.41 days) ($p = 0.02$). However, delirium following general anesthesia tended to last longer (2.15 ± 0.77 days) compared to regional anesthesia (1.24 ± 2.17 days) ($p = 0.05$).

Duration of surgery in the study group did not correlate to the onset, severity and duration of postoperative delirium. We found a trend towards earlier delirium onset in the arthroplasty group than the fracture fixation, but it did not reach statistical significance due to the sample size. There was no difference between hip arthroplasty and femoral fracture fixation groups regarding the duration of postoperative delirium. In this study, surgeries other than proximal femoral fractures developed more extended delirium periods than those of femoral fractures (2.71 ± 1.25 days vs. 1.87 ± 0.43 days, respectively) ($p = 0.01$).

The time between surgery and the first physiotherapy treatment correlated to delirium development ($r = 0.34$, $p = 0.01$). A possible bias that can explain this correlation is the patient's post-surgical status; patients with lower vital signs or postoperative hemoglobin levels are not treated by physiotherapists until considered stable.

Following the three-day low-dose risperidone treatment protocol, 0.5 mg BID, 14.9% of the patients showed a CAM score normalization after one day of treatment, and 93.6% within two days (Figure 4). However, 6.3% of the patients needed up to five days to normalize their CAM scores. None of the study's patients suffered delirium for more than a five-day total following the three-day low-dose risperidone treatment protocol.

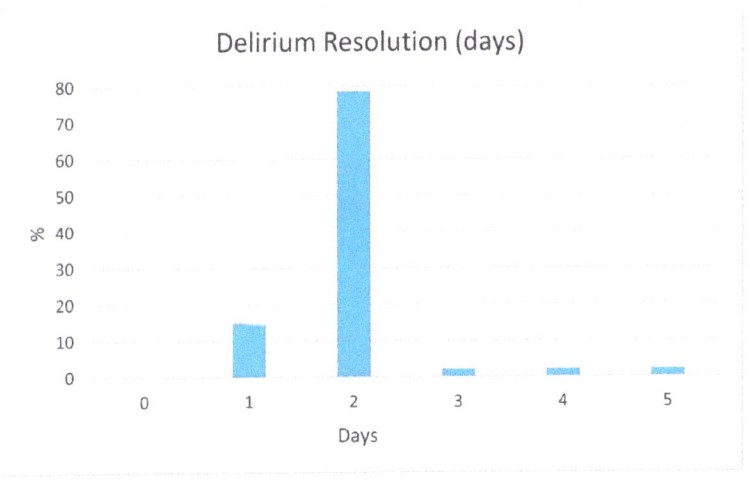

Figure 4. Time to delirium resolution (days).

None of the delirium study group's patients ceased the three-day low-dose respiridone protocol due to delirium escalation requiring a higher respiridone dose or a different medication. The only excluded patients not described in this study were a few requiring hospitalizations in another department due to acute medical conditions such as post-resuscitation, upper gastrointestinal bleeding, or rapid atrial fibrillation.

Study group patients were monitored for low dose risperidone treatment protocol adverse effects, such as nausea, vomiting, diarrhea or constipation, heartburn, dry mouth, increased salivation, stomach pain, anxiety, agitation, restlessness, vision impairment, muscle or joint pain, dry or discolored skin, difficulty urinating, confusion, tachycardia or arrhythmias, seizures, rash and difficulty breathing or swallowing. No adverse effects were registered.

4. Discussion

Delirium, characterized by acute cognitive and attentional dysfunction, poses a significant concern in healthcare. Its association with fluctuating consciousness levels and varied manifestations of agitation, lethargy, or mixed symptoms makes it particularly challenging. The aging population and increased life expectancy have led to a rise in postoperative delirium cases, including those following major surgeries or hip fractures [1,2]. Postoperative delirium adversely affects patient outcomes, leading to higher mortality rates [1], cognitive and functional decline [2], prolonged hospital stays, and increased healthcare costs. Despite clinical diagnosis using established manuals such as the DSM-V and ICD-10, there is a need for simpler and faster screening tools such as the CAM and delirium observation screening scales, albeit with lower sensitivity compared to expert assessments [3–8]. Various risk factors, including age, cognitive impairment, comorbidities, and medication use, contribute to postoperative delirium [9,10].

Effective management involves a multidisciplinary approach, encompassing preventive and therapeutic measures [11–13]. Non-pharmacological interventions emphasize creating a calm environment, patient orientation, early mobilization, optimizing physiological functions, and mindful breathing [14]. Intraoperative strategies involve lighter sedation and appropriate pain control, while postoperative care includes pain and medication reviews, infection monitoring, and metabolic assessment. The use of antipsychotics such as haloperidol and atypical agents such as risperidone has shown efficacy in treating delirium, though they carry side effects [21–23]. Risperidone, with its affinity for serotonin and dopamine receptors, offers advantages over traditional antipsychotics, making it a preferred first-line treatment [24,25]. Treatment decisions should prioritize using the minimum effective dose for the shortest necessary duration, particularly in severely agitated patients who threaten themselves or others.

Perioperative delirium is an important entity that affects senior patients. Although perioperative delirium was quite common in some studies, the incidence was relatively low in this study, with 3.7% of all patients older than 65 and 9.3% in the proximal femoral fracture group. Nevertheless, since perioperative delirium involves almost a tenth of the orthopedic surgery department's patients and concerns the patient, family, and treating personnel, awareness and screening should be routine.

Delirium pathogenesis is still unknown, but a systemic review of the patient's risk factors is warranted, recognizing past medical issues, electrolyte imbalance, drug treatment and sensual impairment. Although this practice makes sense, in this study we did not recognize physiological factors as affecting perioperative delirium development or duration. We found that the type of anesthesia influenced the timing and length of delirium. Regional anesthesia is related to earlier and shorter delirium, while general anesthesia is related to later and prolonged delirium. These findings suggest that perioperative delirium usually is not the consequence of a significant physiological impairment but instead due to an abrupt environmental change or the stress caused by the proximal femoral fracture and surgery performed. Further support for this theory is the lower delirium incidence in the elective surgery group, probably due to their being better prepared mentally for hospitalization. In this study, delirium tended to appear during the evening, 18:00 to 24:00, adding to the environmental aspect of delirium.

We found that younger age correlates to a shorter delirium period, as expected, but did not influence delirium incidence. Higher blood albumin levels are also correlated to shorter delirium periods, maybe due to their role in buffering serum drug levels.

There is no well-defined treatment protocol for postoperative delirium. Several drugs were used for treatment but with inconclusive results regarding efficiency. Our proposed rigid three-day low-dose risperidone treatment protocol, 0.5 mg BID, achieved 93.6% of delirium resolution within two days, as measured by CAM score normalization. A limitation of our study is the relatively small study group. We did not find that background diseases, medications and hemodialysis affect the development of postoperative delirium; the effect may be lower than expected and thus unnoticed in our study. Other limitations include the lack of delirium severity quantification and the lack of a control group. Although this is a relatively small observational and non-randomized study group, our low-dose risperidone treatment protocol suggests a clinical benefit and had no significant adverse effects. Earlier delirium resolution allows better physiotherapy adherence, earlier discharge and a better patient-family experience.

5. Conclusions

Postoperative delirium in elderly patients suffering proximal femoral fractures is common. Treatment protocols are varied, inconclusive and conflicting. We recommend routine delirium screening, risk factor assessment and early management. We found in our observational study that the rigid three-day low-dose risperidone treatment protocol, 0.5 mg BID, was efficacious in delirium resolution, without side effects. Our treatment protocol showed promising results and should be further studied with a larger-scale RCT.

Author Contributions: L.R.: Concept and design, acquisition of subjects and data, analysis and interpretation of data, and preparation of manuscript. E.E.: Concept and design, acquisition of subjects and data, analysis and interpretation of data, and preparation of manuscript. K.I.: Concept and design, acquisition of subjects and data, analysis and interpretation of data, and preparation of manuscript. H.O.: Concept and design, acquisition of subjects and data, analysis and interpretation of data, and preparation of manuscript. All authors have read and agreed to the published version of the manuscript.

Funding: This research received no external funding.

Institutional Review Board Statement: The study was conducted in accordance with the Declaration of Helsinki, and approved by the Edith Wolfson Medical Center (WOMC-0236-20-WOMC, 22 September 2020), Holon, affiliated with the Sackler School of Medicine, Tel Aviv, Israel.

Informed Consent Statement: No informed consent was required for this study.

Data Availability Statement: The complete data are available under a confidentiality restriction.

Conflicts of Interest: The authors declare no conflict of interest.

References

1. Gottschalk, A.; Hubbs, J.; Vikani, A.R.; Gottschalk, L.B.; Sieber, F.E. The impact of incident postoperative delirium on survival of elderly patients after surgery for hip fracture repair. *Anesth. Analg.* **2015**, *121*, 1336. [CrossRef] [PubMed]
2. Sprung, J.; Roberts, R.; Weingarten, T.; Nunes Cavalcante, A.; Knopman, D.; Petersen, R.; Hanson, A.; Schroeder, D.; Warner, D.O. Postoperative delirium in elderly patients is associated with subsequent cognitive impairment. *BJA Br. J. Anaesth.* **2017**, *119*, 316–323. [CrossRef] [PubMed]
3. Robinson, T.N.; Eiseman, B. Postoperative delirium in the elderly: Diagnosis and management. *Clin. Interv. Aging* **2008**, *3*, 351. [CrossRef] [PubMed]
4. Whitlock, E.L.; Vannucci, A.; Avidan, M.S. Postoperative delirium. *Minerva Anestesiol.* **2011**, *77*, 448. [PubMed]
5. Aya, A.G.; Pouchain, P.-H.; Thomas, H.; Ripart, J.; Cuvillon, P. Incidence of postoperative delirium in elderly ambulatory patients: A prospective evaluation using the FAM-CAM instrument. *J. Clin. Anesth.* **2019**, *53*, 35–38. [CrossRef]
6. Hattori, H.; Kamiya, J.; Shimada, H.; Akiyama, H.; Yasui, A.; Kuroiwa, K.; Oda, K.; Ando, M.; Kawamura, T.; Harada, A. Assessment of the risk of postoperative delirium in elderly patients using E-PASS and the NEECHAM Confusion Scale. *Int. J. Geriatr. Psychiatry* **2009**, *24*, 1304–1310. [CrossRef]
7. Kratz, T.; Heinrich, M.; Schlauß, E.; Diefenbacher, A. Preventing postoperative delirium: A prospective intervention with psychogeriatric liaison on surgical wards in a general hospital. *Dtsch. Ärzteblatt Int.* **2015**, *112*, 289.
8. Yamamoto, M.; Yamasaki, M.; Sugimoto, K.; Maekawa, Y.; Miyazaki, Y.; Makino, T.; Takahashi, T.; Kurokawa, Y.; Nakajima, K.; Takiguchi, S. Risk evaluation of postoperative delirium using comprehensive geriatric assessment in elderly patients with esophageal cancer. *World J. Surg.* **2016**, *40*, 2705–2712. [CrossRef]
9. Radinovic, K.; Denic, L.M.; Milan, Z.; Cirkovic, A.; Baralic, M.; Bumbasirevic, V. Impact of intraoperative blood pressure, blood pressure fluctuation, and pulse pressure on postoperative delirium in elderly patients with hip fracture: A prospective cohort study. *Injury* **2019**, *50*, 1558–1564. [CrossRef]
10. Brouquet, A.; Cudennec, T.; Benoist, S.; Moulias, S.; Beauchet, A.; Penna, C.; Teillet, L.; Nordlinger, B. Impaired mobility, ASA status and administration of tramadol are risk factors for postoperative delirium in patients aged 75 years or more after major abdominal surgery. *Ann. Surg.* **2010**, *251*, 759–765. [CrossRef]

11. Aakerlund, L.; Rosenberg, J. Postoperative delirium: Treatment with supplementary oxygen. *BJA Br. J. Anaesth.* **1994**, *72*, 286–290. [CrossRef]
12. Popp, J.; Arlt, S. Prevention and treatment options for postoperative delirium in the elderly. *Curr. Opin. Psychiatry* **2012**, *25*, 515–521. [CrossRef] [PubMed]
13. Song, K.-J.; Ko, J.-H.; Kwon, T.-Y.; Choi, B.-W. Etiology and related factors of postoperative delirium in orthopedic surgery. *Clin. Orthop. Surg.* **2019**, *11*, 297. [CrossRef] [PubMed]
14. Lisann-Goldman, L.R.; Pagnini, F.; Deiner, S.G.; Langer, E.J. Reducing Delirium and Improving Patient Satisfaction With a Perioperative Mindfulness Intervention: A Mixed-Methods Pilot Study. *Holist. Nurs. Pract.* **2019**, *33*, 163–176. [CrossRef]
15. Chan, M.T.; Cheng, B.C.; Lee, T.M.; Gin, T.; Group, C.T. BIS-guided anesthesia decreases postoperative delirium and cognitive decline. *J. Neurosurg. Anesthesiol.* **2013**, *25*, 33–42. [CrossRef]
16. Sieber, F.E.; Zakriya, K.J.; Gottschalk, A.; Blute, M.-R.; Lee, H.B.; Rosenberg, P.B.; Mears, S.C. Sedation depth during spinal anesthesia and the development of postoperative delirium in elderly patients undergoing hip fracture repair. *Mayo Clin. Proc.* **2020**, *85*, 18–26. [CrossRef]
17. Ishii, K.; Makita, T.; Yamashita, H.; Matsunaga, S.; Akiyama, D.; Toba, K.; Hara, K.; Sumikawa, K.; Hara, T. Total intravenous anesthesia with propofol is associated with a lower rate of postoperative delirium in comparison with sevoflurane anesthesia in elderly patients. *J. Clin. Anesth.* **2016**, *33*, 428–431. [CrossRef] [PubMed]
18. Sieber, F.; Neufeld, K.J.; Gottschalk, A.; Bigelow, G.E.; Oh, E.S.; Rosenberg, P.B.; Mears, S.C.; Stewart, K.J.; Ouanes, J.-P.P.; Jaberi, M. Depth of sedation as an interventional target to reduce postoperative delirium: Mortality and functional outcomes of the Strategy to Reduce the Incidence of Postoperative Delirium in Elderly Patients randomised clinical trial. *Br. J. Anaesth.* **2019**, *122*, 480–489. [CrossRef]
19. Vaurio, L.E.; Sands, L.P.; Wang, Y.; Mullen, E.A.; Leung, J.M. Postoperative delirium: The importance of pain and pain management. *Anesth. Analg.* **2006**, *102*, 1267–1273. [CrossRef]
20. Jin, Z.; Lee, C.; Zhang, K.; Gan, T.J.; Bergese, S.D. Safety of treatment options available for postoperative pain. *Expert Opin. Drug Saf.* **2021**, *20*, 549–559. [CrossRef]
21. Schrader, S.L.; Wellik, K.E.; Demaerschalk, B.M.; Caselli, R.J.; Woodruff, B.K.; Wingerchuk, D.M. Adjunctive haloperidol prophylaxis reduces postoperative delirium severity and duration in at-risk elderly patients. *Neurologist* **2008**, *14*, 134–137. [CrossRef] [PubMed]
22. Fukata, S.; Kawabata, Y.; Fujisiro, K.; Katagawa, Y.; Kuroiwa, K.; Akiyama, H.; Terabe, Y.; Ando, M.; Kawamura, T.; Hattori, H. Haloperidol prophylaxis does not prevent postoperative delirium in elderly patients: A randomized, open-label prospective trial. *Surg. Today* **2014**, *44*, 2305–2313. [CrossRef] [PubMed]
23. Han, C.-S.; Kim, Y.-K. A double-blind trial of Risperidone and Haloperidol for the treatment of delirium. *Psychosomatics* **2004**, *45*, 297–301. [CrossRef]
24. Leysen, J.E.; Gommeren, W.; Eens, A.; De Courcelles, D.D.C.; Stoof, J.C.; Janssen, P.A. Biochemical profile of risperidone, a new antipsychotic. *J. Pharmacol. Exp. Ther.* **2014**, *247*, 661–670.
25. Torres, R.; Mittal, D.; Kennedy, R. Use of quetiapine in delirium. *Psychosomatics* **2001**, *42*, 347–349. [CrossRef] [PubMed]

Disclaimer/Publisher's Note: The statements, opinions and data contained in all publications are solely those of the individual author(s) and contributor(s) and not of MDPI and/or the editor(s). MDPI and/or the editor(s) disclaim responsibility for any injury to people or property resulting from any ideas, methods, instructions or products referred to in the content.

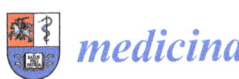

Case Report

Taekwondo Athlete's Bilateral Achilles Tendon Rupture: A Case Report

Jun Young Lee [1,†], Sung Hwan Kim [2,†], Joo Young Cha [2] and Young Koo Lee [2,*]

1 Department of Orthopaedic Surgery, Chosun University Hospital, 365, Pilmundae-ro, Dong-gu, Gwangju 61453, Republic of Korea
2 Department of Orthopaedic Surgery, Soonchunhyang University Hospital Bucheon, 170, Jomaru-ro, Wonmi-gu, Gyeonggi-do, Bucheon-si 14584, Republic of Korea; shk9528@naver.com (S.H.K.)
* Correspondence: brain0808@hanmail.net
† These authors contributed equally to this work.

Abstract: (1) *Background*: Achilles tendon rupture is a common sports injury that may result in severe disability. The overall incidence of Achilles tendon rupture is increasing as a result of growing sports participation. However, cases of spontaneous bilateral Achilles tendon rupture with no underlying disease or risk factors, such as systemic inflammatory disease, steroid or (fluoro)quinolone antibiotics use, are rare. (2) *Objective*: Here, we report a case of a Taekwondo athlete's bilateral Achilles tendon rupture after kicking and landing. By sharing the experience of treatment and the patient's course, we suggest one of the possible treatment options and the need to establish a treatment method. (3) *Procedure*: A 23-year-old male Taekwondo athlete visited the hospital, presenting foot plantar flexion failure and severe pain in both tarsal joints, which had occurred upon kicking and landing on both feet earlier that day. During surgery, no degenerative changes or denaturation were observed in the ruptured areas of the Achilles tendons. Bilateral surgery was performed using the modified Bunnel method on the right side and minimum-section suturing on the left side was performed using the Achillon system, followed by lower limb casting. (4) *Result*: Good outcomes were observed on both sides at 19 months postoperatively. (5) *Conclusion*: The possibility of bilateral Achilles tendon rupture during exercise in young subjects with no risk factors should be acknowledged, especially in association with landing. In addition, in athletes, even if there is a possibility of complications, surgical treatment should be considered for functional recovery.

Keywords: bilateral Achilles tendon rupture; Taekwondo athlete; young athlete

1. Introduction

The Achilles tendon (AT) is the largest and thickest tendon in the human body and contributes to foot plantar flexion, hind foot inversion, and even knee flexion [1]. AT rupture is a common sports injury that may result in severe disability. The most common age of AT injury is 30–50 years and it is much more common in men [2]. The overall incidence of AT rupture is increasing as a result of growing sports participation. Spontaneous AT rupture can occur for various reasons and is often reported in patients with systemic inflammatory disease and in those undergoing corticosteroid or (fluoro)quinolone antibiotic treatment or blood dialysis [3]. In patients with peripheral sensory neurological disorders, AT rupture is caused by negative feedback from the physical receptor when the ankle joint is overloaded [4–6]. An imbalance between the damage and recovery of the tendon and chronic tendon disease due to degenerative changes can induce AT rupture. Systemic disease and factors like dehydration, secondary hyperparathyroidism, and a reduced blood supply to the tendon in patients on blood dialysis can induce tendon damage via hypoxia and inappropriate metabolism in the tendon [7,8].

AT ruptures are diagnosed by physical examination and imaging studies, which provide additional clinical information [9]. On physical examination, diffuse swelling and

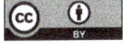

bruising are common. When the swelling is severe, a gap may be palpable 2–6 cm proximal to the tendon insertion [10]. Other disease-specific tests are used to confirm the diagnosis, such as the Thompson and Copeland tests [11]. Imaging modalities such as ultrasound and magnetic resonance imaging (MRI) facilitate the diagnosis and monitoring of AT rupture and are used to rule out other injuries [12].

Bilateral spontaneous AT ruptures are uncommon, with an overall incidence of <1% [13]. Most previously reported cases involved risk factors, and there were few papers on the case where there are no risk factors of AT ruptures such as a history of corticosteroid injection or using (fluoro)quinolone [3,14]. To our knowledge, there are no reports in English about bilateral AT rupture in young, healthy Taekwondo athletes with no underlying disease or risk factors. Here, we report the case of a 23-year-old male Taekwondo athlete in whom bilateral AT rupture occurred spontaneously. By sharing our experience of treatment and the patient's course, we suggest one of the possible treatment options and the need to establish a treatment method.

2. Case Presentation

2.1. Preoperative Evaluation

A 23-year-old male Taekwondo athlete visited the hospital due to foot plantar flexion failure and severe pain in both tarsal joints, which had occurred upon kicking and landing on both feet earlier that day (Figure 1). The patient had no direct injury, no risk factors for spontaneous AT rupture, and no history of steroid treatment. He had begun to practice Taekwondo when he was in kindergarten and was a university Taekwondo athlete at the time of presentation. He reported no previous experience of pain in the bilateral ATs for 16 years from the start of exercise.

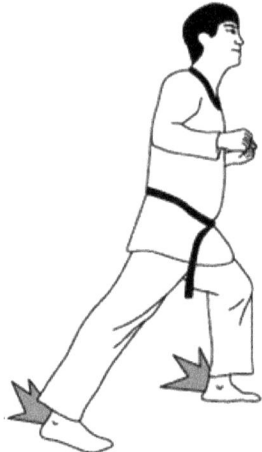

Figure 1. Schematic illustration of the mechanism of injury in a young Taekwondo athlete after kicking and landing on both feet simultaneously.

At the time of admission, the Thompson squeeze test was positive in both ankles, and digital exploration revealed dimpling 6 cm superior to the calcaneal tendon attachment site. Preoperative ankle radiographs showed no abnormality in the bone or surrounding soft tissue, other than the loss of Kager's triangle (Figure 2). MRI confirmed the diagnosis of bilateral AT rupture (Figure 3).

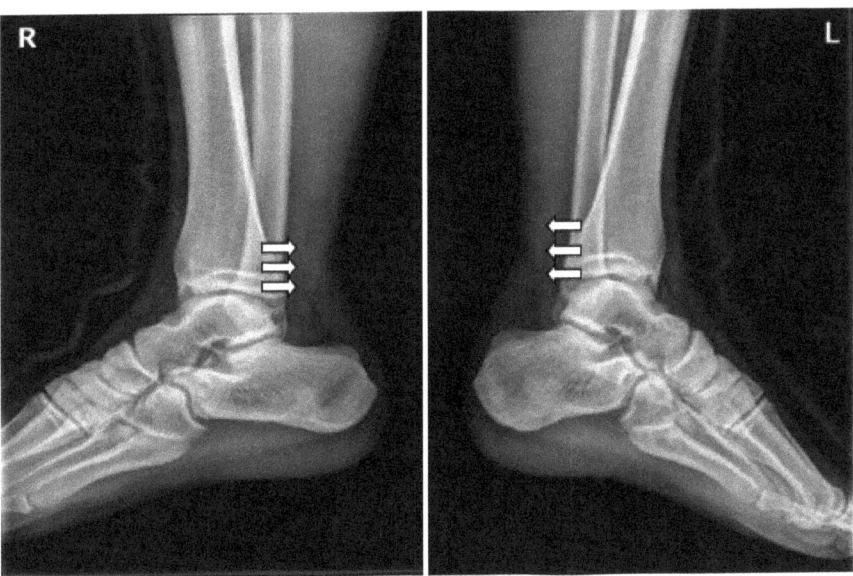

Figure 2. Lateral conventional radiographs of both ankles following bilateral Achilles tendon rupture show marked thickening of the Achilles tendons, loss of the normal sharp anterior borders (white arrows), and effacement of the pre-Achilles/Kager's fat pad.

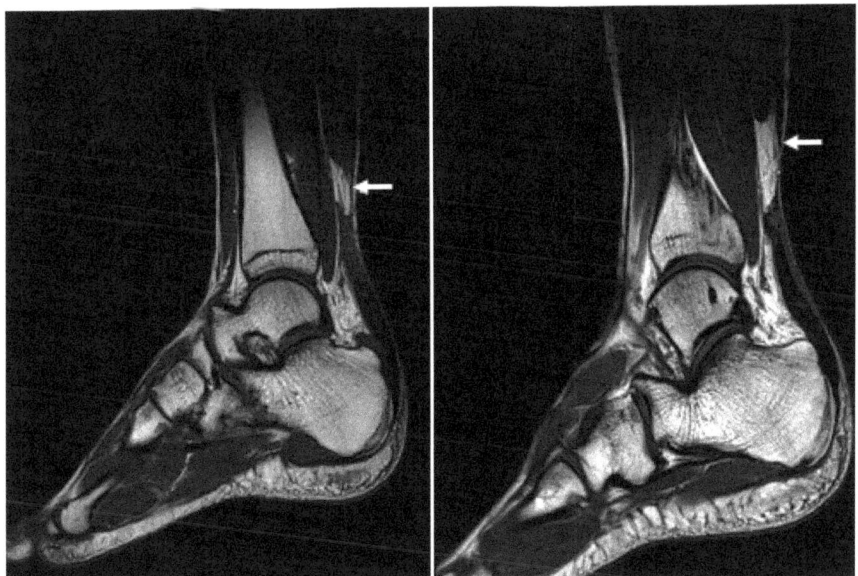

Figure 3. Preoperative sagittal magnetic resonance images of both ankles show rupture of the Achilles tendons (white arrow).

2.2. Surgical Procedure

Surgery was performed with the patient under general anesthesia and in the prone position. We decided to do surgery on the right side first. The ruptured ATs were exposed via posteromedial skin incisions, and invasive tendinosuture was performed (Figure 4). After incising the paratenons, the ATs were sutured securely using the modified Bunnel method. The peritenon tissues surrounding the ATs were also sutured sufficiently to maintain blood circulation to the greatest degree possible. During surgery, complete oblique rupture of the ATs was observed approximately 6 cm superior to the calcaneal tendon attachment sites, with no additional findings. On the left side, the area of AT rupture was explored digitally, and an approximately 3 cm skin incision was made (Figure 5a). Minimally invasive suturing was performed by passing an ETHIBOND no. 2 suture in parallel from the medial to the lateral side using the Achillon tendon suture system (The Achillon Technique Guide, No. 2 FiberWire; Arthrex, Naples, FL, USA), and then crossing it over to pass approximately 1 cm distal to the ruptured area. The same procedure was performed proximal to the ruptured area, and the suture was passed to the distal site after plantar flexion of the ankle to enable passage into the interior, followed by strain knotting (Figure 5b). Then, the left side, including the peritenon, was sutured anatomically, followed by suturing of the surgical wound. Casts were applied to both feet in complete plantar flexion, and the wounds were sterilized by opening windows in the casts.

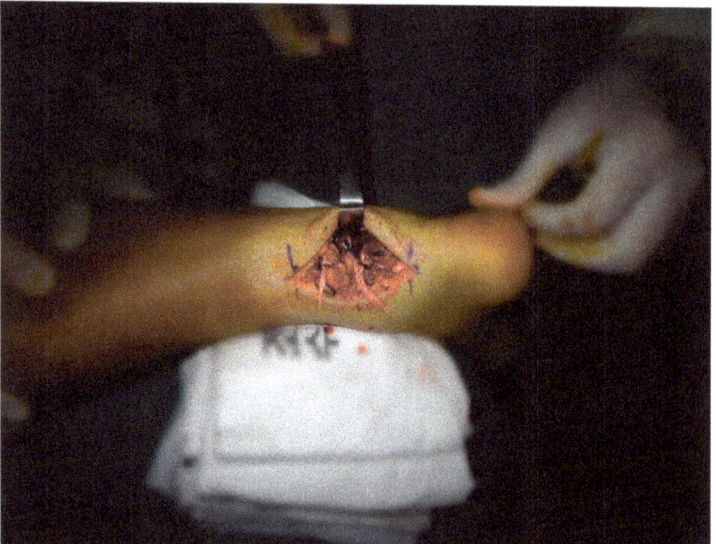

Figure 4. Intraoperative finding of Achilles tendon rupture in the right ankle.

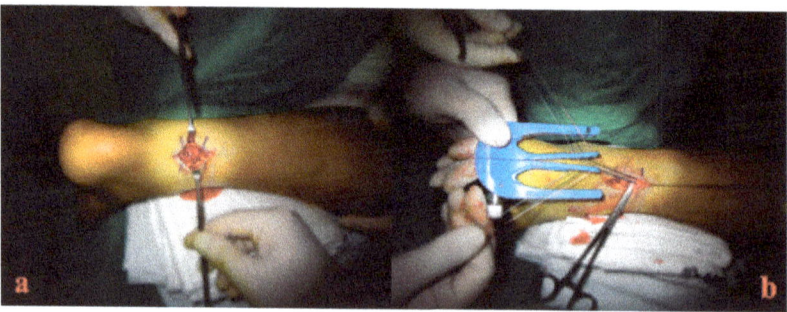

Figure 5. (a) Intraoperative finding of Achilles tendon rupture in the left ankle. (b) The Achillon® instrument was introduced proximally under the paratenon, and three needles were passed.

2.3. Postoperative Care

The patient's hospitalization was uneventful. The sutures on both sides were removed, short lower limb casts were applied 2 weeks postoperatively, and the patient was discharged. The patient underwent a 6-week course of physical therapy with assisted 90° movement of the ankle joint. At 3 months after the operation, clinical evaluation was done using the American Orthopedic Foot and Ankle Society (AOFAS) ankle-hindfoot functional score, the Achilles Tendon total Rupture Score (ATRS), and Visual Analog Scale (VAS) scores. His AOFAS ankle-hindfoot functional score, ATRS, and VAS scores were 85, 77, and 3 points, respectively. He began jogging and one-heel squatting at 3 months postoperatively and resumed Taekwondo practice approximately 8 months postoperatively. He had regained normal range of motion at 19 months after the operation (Figure 6). At the final follow-up, the scoring methods performed at 3 months were investigated once more. The AOFAS ankle-hindfoot functional score, ATRS, and VAS were 100, 97, and 1, respectively. Other complications such as infection, rerupture, and nerve damage did not occur and MRI of the ankle joints, which was performed 19 months after the operation, confirmed that both ATs were well maintained (Figure 7).

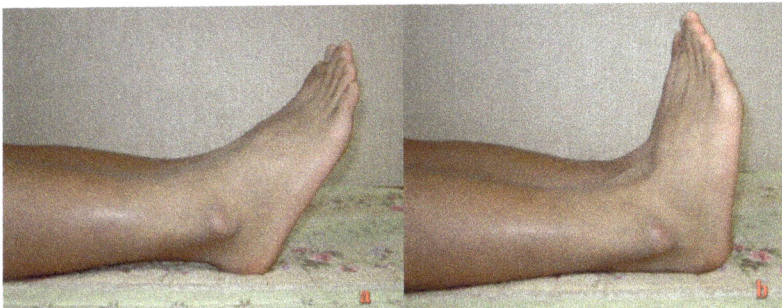

Figure 6. Postoperative clinical outcome (19 months after operation): (**a**) plantar flexion and (**b**) dorsiflexion.

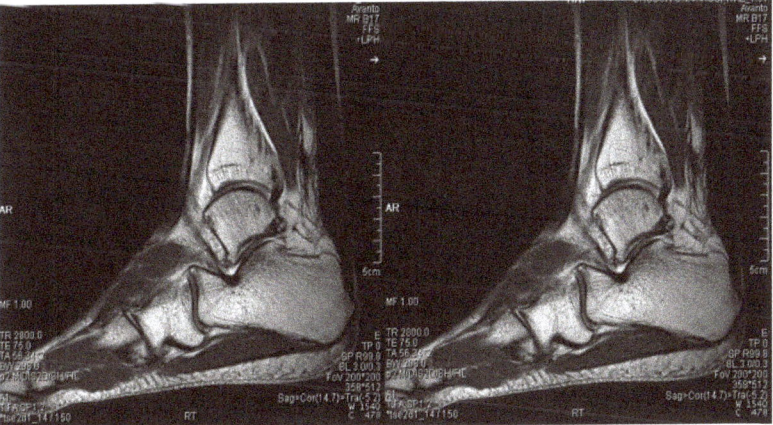

Figure 7. Postoperative (19 months after operation) sagittal magnetic resonance images of both ankles showing good continuity of the Achilles tendons.

3. Discussion

Our patient was a healthy 23-year-old male with no previous symptoms or lesions of the AT; thus, general degenerative changes were unlikely to be present. He was very healthy with no underlying disease and had no risk factors for AT rupture, such as a history of corticosteroid injection or using (fluoro)quinolone, as mentioned above. This bilateral AT rupture was likely caused by a high-energy bilateral load upon landing. We study and report a fairly rare case, and it is hard to find articles that treated both sides in different ways. We suggest one of the possible treatment options and the need to establish a treatment method in cases similar to this one.

Taekwondo is the national martial art of the Republic of Korea and an official Olympic sport. It involves a combination of movements, with "Poomsae", emphasizing mental concentration and defense-orientated movements using the whole body, and "Gyorugi", being more offensively orientated; the fists and feet are used to hit and stomp, respectively [15]. The sport is normally done bare-footed. As a result, Taekwondo athletes tend to have injuries involving the lower extremities and ankles [16,17]. As with many other martial arts where little to no protective gear is allowed on the legs and ankles, the forces acting on the foot and ankle can be great [18]. Excessive loading can cause the rupture of a healthy AT [5]; this can occur during abrupt plantar flexion. Habusta reported bilateral AT rupture in a gymnast caused by simultaneously raising both feet from a lowered position [19].

The treatment options for AT rupture include various invasive and percutaneous surgical procedures and conservative treatment. Surgical treatment has more complications but reduces the likelihood of rerupture [20]. Since our patient was an athlete, it was important to reduce the possibility of rerupture, have early motion, and have rehabilitation. Thus, even though there was a possibility of complications, surgical treatment was selected on the bilateral side at the same time. According to some studies, complications associated with invasive suturing can be reduced by percutaneous surgery [8,21,22]. In this case, as the patient is right-footed, he requested definite repair under direct vision using open technique on the right side. So, invasive suturing was performed on the right side and minimal suturing was performed on the left side. The patient recovered a normal range of movement in both ankles, and there were no wound-related problems. This case demonstrates that the clinical outcomes of invasive tendon suturing and minimum section suturing to treat the same injury do not differ markedly.

This study has several limitations. First, there was no follow-up after the patient returned to Taekwondo matches. Therefore, return to sport could not be evaluated. Second, no specific rehabilitation protocol was applied; unlike unilateral AT rupture, there is no specific rehabilitation protocol for bilateral AT rupture because the frequency is low. Since bilateral AT rupture is expected to increase with the frequency of AT rupture, it is necessary to establish a specific protocol by studying many cases through a multi-institutional study.

4. Conclusions

In summary, the possibility of bilateral AT rupture during exercise in young subjects with no risk factors should be acknowledged, especially in association with landing. In addition, in athletes, even if there is a possibility of complications, surgical treatment should be considered for functional recovery.

Author Contributions: Conceptualization, S.H.K.; methodology, J.Y.C.; validation, J.Y.L.; investigation, J.Y.C.; resources, J.Y.L.; data curation, Y.K.L.; writing—original draft preparation, S.H.K.; writing—review and editing, Y.K.L.; visualization, J.Y.L.; supervision, J.Y.L.; project administration, Y.K.L.; funding acquisition, S.H.K. All authors have read and agreed to the published version of the manuscript.

Funding: The authors would like to thank the Soonchunhyang University Research Fund for financial support. (No. 2023-0008).

Institutional Review Board Statement: The study was conducted in accordance with the Declaration of Helsinki, and approved by the Institutional Review Board and Human Research Ethics Committee of Soonchunhyang University Bucheon Hospital (IRB No. 2023-02-014, 21 February 2023).

Informed Consent Statement: All of informed consent has been obtained from the patient to publish this paper.

Data Availability Statement: Data sharing is not applicable to this article because any datasets were made or analyzed during this study.

Conflicts of Interest: The authors declare no conflict of interest.

Abbreviations

AT   Achilles tendon
MRI Magnetic resonance imaging

References

1. Thomopoulos, S.; Parks, W.C.; Rifkin, D.B.; Derwin, K.A. Mechanisms of tendon injury and repair. *J. Orthop. Res.* **2015**, *33*, 832–839. [CrossRef] [PubMed]
2. Fox, G.; Gabbe, B.; Richardson, M.; Oppy, A.; Page, R.; Edwards, E.; Hau, R.; Ekegren, C.L. Twelve-month outcomes following surgical repair of the Achilles tendon. *Injury* **2016**, *47*, 2370–2374. [CrossRef]
3. Cruz, C.A.; Wake, J.L.; Bickley, R.J.; Morin, L.; Mannino, B.J.; Krul, K.P.; Ryan, P. Bilateral Achilles Tendon Rupture: A Case Report and Review of the Literature. *Osteology* **2022**, *2*, 70–76. [CrossRef]
4. Inglis, A.E.; Sculco, T.P. Surgical repair of ruptures of the tendo Achillis. *Clin. Orthop. Relat. Res.* **1981**, *156*, 160–169. [CrossRef]
5. Leppilahti, J.; Orava, S. Total Achilles tendon rupture: A review. *Sport. Med.* **1998**, *25*, 79–100. [CrossRef]
6. Simoneau, G.G.; Derr, J.A.; Ulbrecht, J.S.; Becker, M.B.; Cavanagh, P.R. Diabetic sensory neuropathy effect on ankle joint movement perception. *Arch. Phys. Med. Rehabil.* **1996**, *77*, 453–460. [CrossRef]
7. Krackow, K.A.; Thomas, S.C.; Jones, L.C. A new stitch for ligament-tendon fixation. *J. Bone Jt. Surg. Am.* **1986**, *68*, 764–765. [CrossRef]
8. Metz, R.; Verleisdonk, E.-J.M.; van der Heijden, G.J.-M.-G.; Clevers, G.-J.; Hammacher, E.R.; Verhofstad, M.H.; van der Werken, C. Acute Achilles tendon rupture: Minimally invasive surgery versus nonoperative treatment with immediate full weightbearing—A randomized controlled trial. *Am. J. Sport. Med.* **2008**, *36*, 1688–1694. [CrossRef]
9. Egger, A.C.; Berkowitz, M.J. Achilles tendon injuries. *Curr. Rev. Musculoskelet. Med.* **2017**, *10*, 72–80. [CrossRef]
10. Tarantino, D.; Palermi, S.; Sirico, F.; Corrado, B. Achilles tendon rupture: Mechanisms of injury, principles of rehabilitation and return to play. *J. Funct. Morphol. Kinesiol.* **2020**, *5*, 95. [CrossRef]
11. Longo, U.G.; Petrillo, S.; Maffulli, N.; Denaro, V. Acute achilles tendon rupture in athletes. *Foot Ankle Clin.* **2013**, *18*, 319–338. [CrossRef] [PubMed]
12. Dams, O.C.; Reininga, I.H.; Gielen, J.L.; van den Akker-Scheek, I.; Zwerver, J. Imaging modalities in the diagnosis and monitoring of Achilles tendon ruptures: A systematic review. *Injury* **2017**, *48*, 2383–2399. [CrossRef] [PubMed]
13. Rao, S.; Navadgi, B.; Vasdev, A. Bilateral spontaneous rupture of Achilles tendons: A case report. *J. Orthop. Surg.* **2005**, *13*, 178–180. [CrossRef] [PubMed]
14. Chopra, A.; Parekh, A.S.; Ramanathan, D.; Parekh, S.G. Bilateral Achilles Tendon Ruptures in the NFL. *Foot Ankle Spec.* **2022**, 19386400221108400.
15. Lee, K.T.; Choi, Y.S.; Lee, Y.K.; Lee, J.P.; Young, K.W.; Park, S.Y. Extensor hallucis longus tendon injury in taekwondo athletes. *Phys. Ther. Sport* **2009**, *10*, 101–104. [CrossRef]
16. Stricevic, M.V.; Patel, M.R.; Okazaki, T.; Swain, B.K. Karate: Historical perspective and injuries sustained in national and international tournament competitions. *Am. J. Sport. Med.* **1983**, *11*, 320–324. [CrossRef]
17. Zemper, E.; Pieter, W. Injury rates during the 1988 US Olympic Team Trials for taekwondo. *Br. J. Sport. Med.* **1989**, *23*, 161–164. [CrossRef] [PubMed]
18. Schwartz, M.L.; Hudson, A.R.; Fernie, G.R.; Hayashi, K.; Coleclough, A.A. Biomechanical study of full-contact karate contrasted with boxing. *J. Neurosurg.* **1986**, *64*, 248–252. [CrossRef]
19. Habusta, S.F. Bilateral simultaneous rupture of the Achilles tendon: A rare traumatic injury. *Clin. Orthop. Relat. Res.* **1995**, *320*, 231–234. [CrossRef]
20. Ochen, Y.; Beks, R.B.; van Heijl, M.; Hietbrink, F.; Leenen, L.P.; van der Velde, D.; Heng, M.; van der Meijden, O.; Groenwold, R.H.H.; Houwert, R.M. Operative treatment versus nonoperative treatment of Achilles tendon ruptures: Systematic review and meta-analysis. *BMJ* **2019**, *364*, k5120. [CrossRef]
21. Calder, J.; Saxby, T. Independent evaluation of a recently described Achilles tendon repair technique. *Foot Ankle Int.* **2006**, *27*, 93–96. [CrossRef] [PubMed]
22. Khan, R.J.; Smith, R.L.C. Surgical interventions for treating acute Achilles tendon ruptures. *Cochrane Database Syst. Rev.* **2010**, CD003674. [CrossRef] [PubMed]

Disclaimer/Publisher's Note: The statements, opinions and data contained in all publications are solely those of the individual author(s) and contributor(s) and not of MDPI and/or the editor(s). MDPI and/or the editor(s) disclaim responsibility for any injury to people or property resulting from any ideas, methods, instructions or products referred to in the content.

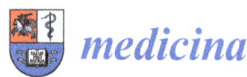

Article

Is the Direct Anterior Approach for Total Hip Arthroplasty Effective in Obese Patients? Early Clinical and Radiographic Results from a Retrospective Comparative Study

Alberto Di Martino [1,2,*], Niccolò Stefanini [1,2], Matteo Brunello [1,2], Barbara Bordini [3], Federico Pilla [1,2], Giuseppe Geraci [1,2], Claudio D'Agostino [1,2], Federico Ruta [1,2] and Cesare Faldini [1,2]

1. I Orthopedic and Traumatology Clinic, IRCCS Istituto Ortopedico Rizzoli, 40136 Bologna, Italy
2. Department of Biomedical and Neuromotor Science-DIBINEM, University of Bologna, 40136 Bologna, Italy
3. Medical Technology Laboratory, IRCCS Istituto Ortopedico Rizzoli, 40136 Bologna, Italy
* Correspondence: albertocorrado.dimartino@ior.it; Tel.: +39 3497880236

Abstract: *Background and objectives:* Total hip arthroplasty (THA) in obese patients (BMI > 30) is considered technically demanding, and it is associated with higher rates of general and specific complications including infections, component malpositioning, dislocation, and periprosthetic fractures. Classically, the Direct Anterior Approach (DAA) has been considered less suitable for performing THA surgery in the obese patient, but recent evidence produced by high-volume DAA THA surgeons suggests that DAA is suitable and effective in obese patients. At the authors' institution, DAA is currently the preferred approach for primary and revision THA surgery, accounting for over 90% of hip surgeries without specific patient selection. Therefore, the aim of the current study is to evaluate any difference in early clinical outcomes, perioperative complications, and implant positioning after primary THAs performed via DAA in patients who were divided according to BMI. *Material and methods:* This study is a retrospective review of 293 THA implants in 277 patients that were performed via DAA from 1 January 2016 to 20 May 2020. Patients were further divided according to BMI: 96 patients were normal weight (NW), 115 were overweight (OW), and 82 were obese (OB). All the procedures were performed by three expert surgeons. The mean follow-up was 6 months. Patients' data, American Society of Anesthesiologists (ASA) score, surgical time, days in rehab unit, pain at the second post-operative day recorded by using a Numerical Rating Scale (NRS), and number of blood transfusions were recorded from clinical charts and compared. Radiological evaluation of cup inclination and stem alignment was conducted on post-operative radiographs; intra- and post-operative complications at latest follow-up were recorded. *Results:* The average age at surgery of OB patients was significantly lower compared to NW and OW patients. The ASA score was significantly higher in OB patients compared to NW patients. Surgical time was slightly but significantly higher in OB patients (85 ± 21 min) compared to NW (79 ± 20 min, $p = 0.05$) and OW patients (79 ± 20 min, $p = 0.029$). Rehab unit discharge occurred significantly later for OB patients, averaging 8 ± 2 days compared to NW patients (7 ± 2 days, $p = 0.012$) and OW patients (7 ± 2 days; $p = 0.032$). No differences in the rate of early infections, number of blood transfusions, NRS pain at the second post-operative day, and day of post-operative stair climbing were found among the three groups. Acetabular cup inclination and stem alignment were similar among the three groups. The perioperative complication rate was 2.3%; that is, perioperative complication occurred in 7 out of 293 patients, with a significantly higher incidence of surgical revisions required in obese patients compared to the others. In fact, OB patients showed a higher revision rate (4.87%) compared to other groups, with 1.04% for NW and 0% for OW ($p = 0.028$, Chi-square test). Causes for revision in obese patients were aseptic loosening (2), dislocation (1), and clinically significant post-operative leg length discrepancy (1), with a revision rate of 4/82 (4.87%) during follow-up. *Conclusions:* THA performed via DAA in obese patients could be a solid choice of treatment, given the relatively low rate of complications and the satisfying clinical outcomes. However, surgical expertise on DAA and adequate instrumentation for this approach are required to optimise the outcomes.

Citation: Di Martino, A.; Stefanini, N.; Brunello, M.; Bordini, B.; Pilla, F.; Geraci, G.; D'Agostino, C.; Ruta, F.; Faldini, C. Is the Direct Anterior Approach for Total Hip Arthroplasty Effective in Obese Patients? Early Clinical and Radiographic Results from a Retrospective Comparative Study. *Medicina* **2023**, *59*, 769. https://doi.org/10.3390/medicina59040769

Academic Editor: Woo Jong Kim

Received: 21 March 2023
Revised: 12 April 2023
Accepted: 13 April 2023
Published: 16 April 2023

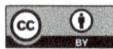

Copyright: © 2023 by the authors. Licensee MDPI, Basel, Switzerland. This article is an open access article distributed under the terms and conditions of the Creative Commons Attribution (CC BY) license (https://creativecommons.org/licenses/by/4.0/).

Keywords: Total hip arthroplasty; Direct Anterior Approach; obese; overweight; outcomes

1. Introduction

Obesity is defined as a Body Mass Index (BMI) higher than 30 kg/m^2 [1]. This condition has exponentially increased in the last decade in developed countries, predisposing patients to multiple pathologies, including diabetes, dyslipidaemia, and heart attack [2–4]. Among orthopaedic conditions, obese people are at a high risk of developing osteoarthritis, which generally occurs at a younger age when compared to non-obese patients, due to the mechanical overload of the lower limbs caused by excessive weight [5,6]. In end-stage osteoarthritis, joint replacement surgery is associated with acceptable risks and a good chance of recovery of function.

Total hip arthroplasty (THA) is regularly carried out in obese patients, with more than one third of implants performed in this patient population [5,7]. However, it is well known that obesity-associated comorbidities may hamper the operability of patients and that THA in obese patients is associated with an overall increase in intra- and peri-operative complications; among these, the most severe include infections, component malpositioning leading to implant instability and dislocation, and periprosthetic femur fractures [8].

The optimal surgical approach to minimise intra- and post-operative complications in obese patients is still under debate [9,10]. Reconstructive orthopaedic surgeons all over the world generally favour posterolateral and direct lateral approaches, mainly because these are considered easier to extend to better expose the acetabulum and femur in case of intraoperative complications. The Direct Anterior Approach (DAA) is used in THA to reduce the invasiveness of surgery and to promote a faster post-operative recovery [11–13]. However, the use of DAA to perform THA in obese patients is greatly debated in the literature. Although according to several authors [14–17], DAA in the obese patient is contraindicated because of the worse outcomes when compared to other surgical approaches, more recent studies [18–20] performed in institutions with high-volume DAA THAs show that obese patients could significantly benefit from the reduced invasiveness of DAA in terms of blood loss, operating time, and functional recovery [19].

At the authors' institution, DAA is currently the preferred surgical approach for primary and revision THA surgery, accounting for over 90% of the procedures, and it is performed without a specific restriction with respect to body weight. Therefore, the aim of the current study is to evaluate any potential difference in early clinical outcomes, perioperative complications, and implant positioning after primary THAs performed via DAA, in patients divided according to BMI.

2. Materials and Methods

The current study and all the case collections were approved by the Local Ethical Committee (CE-AVEC) with the code 021 ANT-HIP, 347/2021/Oss/IOR. Patients were considered for inclusion retrospectively if they were operated on for primary THA from 1 January 2016 to 20 May 2020 at the authors' institution (Figure 1). Inclusion criteria were as follows: patients affected by primary osteoarthritis and treated with THA through DAA, and a follow-up of at least 6 months. Exclusion criteria were patients treated with approaches other than DAA and patients operated on for secondary osteoarthritis to avoid possible bias given by pre-existing clinical conditions including hip deformity, trauma, and infection that could hamper THA outcomes. All the procedures were performed by three expert senior surgeons of the unit. The average follow-up was 6 months. At the acetabular level, all the patients were implanted with a VERSAFIT-Cup or MPACT-Cup (Medacta International, Castel San Pietro, Switzerland); at the femur site, implants were AMIStem (Medacta International, Castel San Pietro, Switzerland).

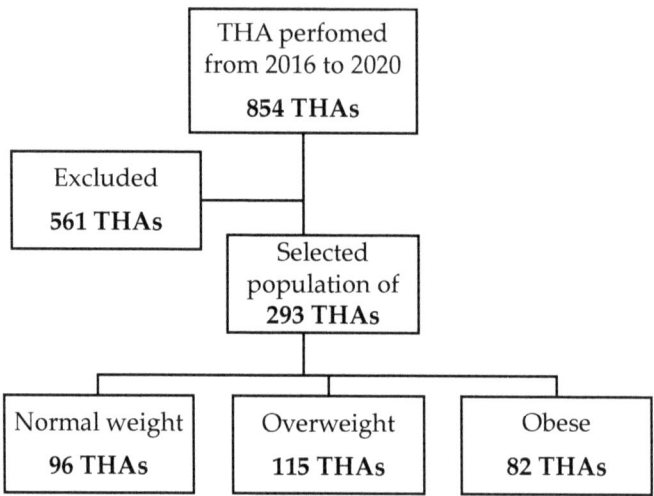

Figure 1. Flow-chart of the study.

Patients were subsequently divided into 3 groups according to their BMI: normal weight (BMI < 25 kg/m^2, NW), overweight (25 kg/m^2 ≤ BMI ≤ 30 kg/m^2, OW), and obese (BMI > 30 kg/m^2, OB). Demographic and clinical parameters were retrospectively collected from the medical records of the hospital: age at surgery, American Society of Anesthesiologists (ASA) score, surgical time (from surgical incision to end of suture), in-hospital length of stay, pain at the second post-operative day recorded by using a Numerical Rating Scale (NRS), day of post-operative stair climbing, and number of blood transfusions were recorded and compared. Any intra- and post-operative complications were recorded while the patients were in hospital and at outpatient evaluations performed at 1, 3, and 6 months post-operatively.

2.1. Surgical Technique

The surgical technique for THA performance through DAA was the same for each patient independently of the body habitus. All patients received prophylactic antibiotic therapy with 2 g of intravenous cefazolin. Patients were positioned supine with the foot of the operated leg secured by a boot on a specific traction table managed by a non-scrubbed assistant, which allows for the control of traction, rotation, and adduction or abduction (Figure 1). The patient's lower limb was positioned with the leg at 30° of flexion, with neutral abduction and rotation (Figure 2). In obese patients, the adipose tissue at the abdomen is generally placed anteriorly and above the inguinal ligament [21], as it represents an obstacle for the surgical incision; it is displaced towards the contralateral side, being anchored by using an adhesive drape to improve the exposure at the surgical site (Figure 2A,B).

The surgical incision was performed 2 cm distally and 2 cm laterally from the anterior superior iliac spine averaging 7–9 cm (Figure 3). After subcutaneous tissue dissection, fascia was cut over the belly of the tensor fascia lata muscle to minimise the risk of injury to the lateral femoral cutaneous nerve. Subsequently, the intermuscular and interneural space was dissected by blunt dislocation of the muscles: the tensor fascia lata muscle was retracted laterally, and the sartorius and the rectus femoris were retracted medially. Branches of the lateral circumflex artery can be ligated or coagulated. The capsula was completely exposed and carefully opened, creating a thick flap reflected proximally, and it was sutured at the end of surgery. Osteotomy of the femoral neck was performed with the head in situ by using an oscillating saw. The head was then removed by using a corkscrew, with the leg in slight traction and external rotation to widen the space of the osteotomy.

Acetabular and femoral bones were prepared for implant positioning by using dedicated instrumentation; handles of the reamer and of the broaches should be curved and off-set to ease bone preparation and to avoid impingement against the soft tissues. Iliofemoral and pubofemoral ligaments were incised to improve proximal femur exposure. Accurate posterior–medial capsular release at the proximal femur was performed before femoral broaching, which requires the patient's leg to be positioned in external rotation, extension, and adduction. After the positioning of cup and femur implants, a reduction manoeuvre was performed, and a suture was started.

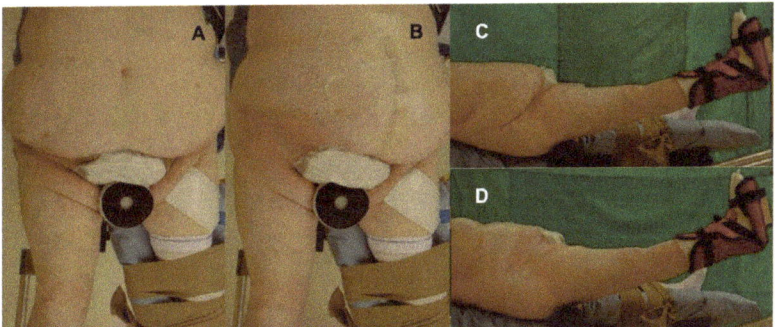

Figure 2. (A) Coronal view of patient positioning on the traction table to perform THA via DAA. (B) Coronal view, in which adipose tissue is displaced from the point of incision with an adhesive drape. (C) Sagittal view of patient positioning on the traction table; the leg is placed in a boot and is positioned with the leg at 30° of flexion, with neutral abduction and rotation. The belly fat is placed over the incision site. (D) Sagittal view, in which the incision site is free; adipose tissue is moved on contralateral side with adhesive drape.

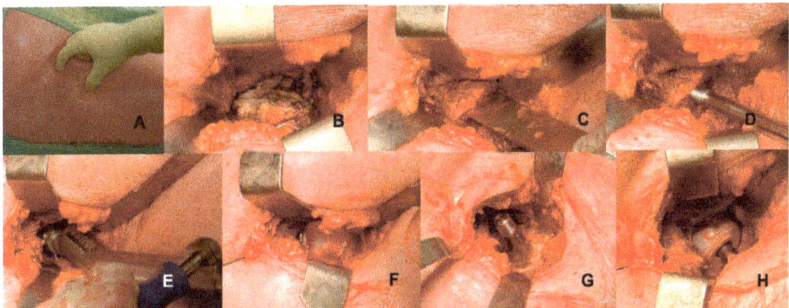

Figure 3. (A) DAA incision is performed 2 cm distally and 2 cm laterally from the anterior superior iliac spine; (B) through the intermuscular space between the tensor fascia latae and sartorious and rectus femoris muscles, the capsula is completely exposed. (C) Neck osteotomy is performed with the head in situ; it is performed with an oscillating saw, and it is completed via an osteotome, which allows mobilisation of the head of the femur. (D) The femoral head is removed with a corkscrew, with the leg in increased traction and external rotation. (E) Reaming of the acetabulum is performed with increasing reamers; in the anterior approach, the use of off-setted handles and instrument is required to improve accuracy and to decrease the impingement against the soft tissues. (F) The exposure of the acetabular cup via the anterior approach is optimal and allows a full view of the cup and ceramic liner. (G) Femur is exposed in full extension, external rotation, and adduction; after femoral broaching, the definitive stem implant is inserted at the femoral shaft. (H) Ceramic head is impacted, and joint reduction is performed via limb abduction, flexion, and internal rotation.

2.2. Post-Operative Care

After surgery, pain medications were administered according to hospital protocols to promote a faster recovery. Weight-bearing is allowed at patients' tolerance with the aid of crutches. At the authors' institution, patients remained in-hospital after surgery to begin rehabilitation, which was assisted by the physical therapists. It started on the same day of the surgery, or the day after if THA was performed in the afternoon. Patients were encouraged to sit as soon as the epidural analgesia wore off, and they were helped to stand upright as soon as they felt comfortable to do so. Isometric exercises with active knee extension were promoted, together with flexion–extension of the ankle, both to be independently performed in bed. The patient was educated on the prevention of movements that could promote dislocation, namely, adduction combined with hyperextension and external rotation. Stair climbing was allowed as soon as the patient gained walking autonomy, and it was set as a goal from the second day after surgery. As soon as the patient was clinically stable and able to walk autonomously with crutches, to climb stairs with aids, to get dressed, and to access the bathroom independently, they were discharged home or were moved to another facility.

2.3. Radiological Evaluation

Radiological evaluation was performed on standard post-operative radiographs to evaluate cup inclination and stem alignment (Figure 4). Cup inclination (Figure 4a) was compared to Lewinnek's safe zone, which is $40° \pm 10°$ [22]. Stem alignment (Figure 4b) was considered good when the angle between the axis of the stem and that of the femur was $0° \pm 5°$; above or below the range, the implant alignment was considered in varus or valgus, respectively [23].

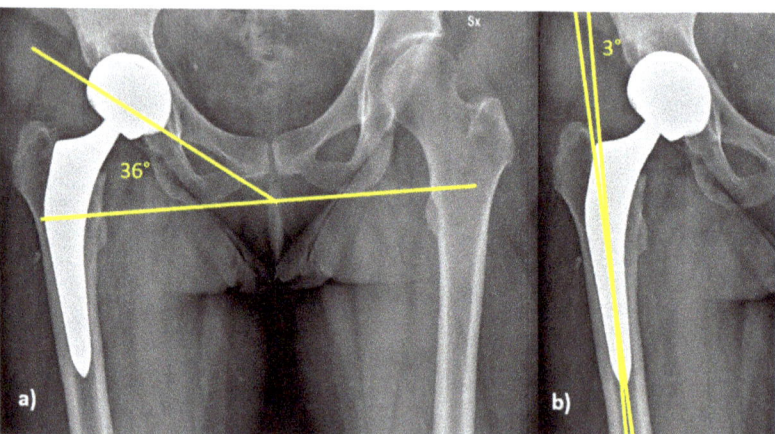

Figure 4. (**a**) Cup inclination is measured as the angle between the line tangent to the border of the acetabular cup and a line parallel to the horizontal plane. (**b**) Stem alignment is the angle between the axis of the stem and of the femur.

2.4. Statistical Analysis

Study variables were analysed and compared among groups. Comparison among the groups was performed by using Kruskal–Wallis and Chi-square tests (SPSS 14.0, version 14.0.1; SPSS Inc, Chicago, IL, USA). Significance was set at p-value < 0.05.

3. Results

From a total of 549 primary THAs performed from 1 January 2016 to 20 May 2020, 293 implants in 277 patients (145 males and 132 females; 52% M and 48% F) matched the inclusion criteria and were retrieved for analysis; according to BMI, 96 out of 293 implants were allocated in the NW group (41 males and 55 females; 43% M and 57% F), 115 were allocated in the OW group (69 males and 46 females; 60% M and 40% F), and 82 were allocated in the OB group (56% males and 44% females).

3.1. Patients' Demographics and Characteristics

Age at surgery was significantly different between groups ($p = 0.005$, Kruskal–Wallis test) (Table 1). In particular, OB patients were significantly younger at surgery, averaging 58.6 years (range 36–83) when compared to OW patients (63.9 yo; range 34–86; $p = 0.006$, Kruskal–Wallis test) and NW patients (63.3 yo; range 34–86; $p = 0.028$, Kruskal–Wallis test). OB patients had significantly worse ASA scores at surgery compared to NW and OW patients ($p = 0.009$, Chi-square test). Sex distribution in different groups did not show significative differences.

Table 1. Surgery-related parameters.

Patients Characteristics	NW (n = 96)	OW (n = 115)	OB (n = 82)
Age (Years)	63.3 (34–86 years)	63.9 (34–86 years)	58.6 (36–83 years)
Sex (M/F)	43% M/57% F (41 M 55 F)	60% M/40% F (69 M 46 F)	56% M/44% F (46 M 36 F)
ASA I	39% (37)	23% (26)	16% (13)
ASA II	47% (45)	62% (71)	63% (52)
ASA III	14% (14)	15% (18)	21% (17)

Surgical time was slightly but significantly higher in OB patients (86 ± 21 min) compared to NW (79 ± 20 min, $p = 0.05$) and OW patients (80 ± 20 min) ($p = 0.029$; Kruskal–Wallis test). The overall incidence of perioperative complications was 2.3%, occurring in 7 out of 293 patients (Table 2). No difference in the overall rate of surgery-related complications was found among groups ($p = 0.1868$, Chi-square test), with an incidence of 4.87%, compared to 2.08% in NW and 0.87% in OW patients; the incidence of infections did not show difference in complication rate ($p = 0.27540$, Chi-square test). The two intra-operative femur fractures occurred in one NW and one OW patient, and these were intra-operatively managed by wiring cerclages. OB patients showed a higher revision rate (4.87%) compared to other groups, with 1.04% for NW and 0% for OW ($p = 0.028$, Chi-square test). Two OB patients experienced recurrent early dislocations in the first month after surgery; in both cases, the first episode occurred after a fall. One patient was managed via stem revision to correct anteversion, and the other via cup repositioning to correct inclination and anteversion of the implant. Two patients showed aseptic loosening of the femur, which was managed via stem revision. One OB patient experienced early wound dehiscence, which was managed via surgical revision and targeted antibiotic therapy (Table 2).

Table 2. Complications that occurred in the study group.

Complications	NW	OW	OB	Total
Wound dehiscence	-	-	1/82 (1.22%)	1/293 (0.34%)
Intra-operative femur fracture	1/96 (1.04%)	1/115 (0.87%)	-	2/293 (0.68%)
Dislocation	-	-	2/82 (2.43%)	2/293 (0.68%)
Aseptic loosening	1/96 (1.04%)	-	1/82 (1.22%)	2/293 (0.68%)
Total	2/96 (2.08%)	1/115 (0.87%)	4/82 (4.87%)	7/293 (2.3%)

The time of in-hospital stay of the patients was significantly longer for OB patients, averaging 8 ± 2.4 days, compared to 7 ± 1.8 days for NW patients ($p = 0.021$, Kruskal–Wallis test) and 7 ± 2.2 days for OW patients ($p = 0.032$, Kruskal–Wallis test).

No differences in the number of blood transfusions were observed when the three groups were compared (*p*= 0.28), with NW patients requiring transfusions in 22% (23/96), OW requiring transfusions in 15% (13/115), and OB patients requiring transfusions in 22% (26/82). No differences in the rate of early infections were found among the three groups ($p = 0.27$, Chi-square test). No other significant differences were found when comparing the three groups in terms of pain at the second post-operative day recorded by using Numerical Rating Scale (NRS) and day of post-operative stair climbing (Table 3).

Table 3. Secondary clinical parameters.

	NW	OW	OB	
NRS at 2nd post-operative day	1.2 ± 1.0	1.3 ± 1.1	1.5 ± 1.0	*p* = 0.346
Day of post-operative stair climbing	3.4 ± 1.7	3.5 ± 1.9	3.7 ± 1.7	*p* = 0.456

3.2. Radiographic Analysis

The analysis on cup inclination showed no significant differences among groups; in particular, cup inclination in the three groups had the same average value (34°), with standard deviations of 6.2° in NW, 7.2° in OW and 7.9° in OB patients ($p = 0.571$, Kruskal–Wallis, test). Acetabular cup inclination was within the safe zone in 222 patients (75.8%): 74/96 (77.1%) in NW group, 86/115 (74.8%) in the OW group, and 62/82 (75.8%) in OB patients. No significant differences were found comparing the distributions of acetabular cup inclination according to Lewinnek ($p = 0.927$, Chi-square test); 71/293 (24.2%) patients had acetabular cup inclination outside the safe zone, being below in 67/71, and above in 4/71; 3 out of these 4 patients were in the OB group (Table 4).

Table 4. Distribution of acetabular cup inclination.

	NW	OW	OB	Total
Within Lewinnek's safe zone	74 (77.1%)	86 (74.8%)	62 (75.6%)	222 (75.8%)
Out of Lewinnek's safe zone	22 (22.9%)	29 (25.2%)	20 (24.4%)	71 (24.2%)
Total	96	115	82	293

The three groups showed the median value for stem alignment of 0°, with standard deviations of 2.2° in NW, 2.2° in OW, and 2.0° in OB. In the NW group, all the stems (96 patients) were positioned in the range of tolerance. In the OW group, 113/115 stems were positioned in the range, and 2/115 stems were above the tolerance value, with 1 being in valgus of 9.4° and 1 being in varus of 5.4°. In OB patients, 80/82 stems were implanted in the range. In total, 2 out of 82 stems in the OB patients were beyond the range, both being aligned in valgus of 5.4° and 7°, respectively. No significant difference in the distribution among the groups was observed for stem alignment ($p = 0.943$, Chi-square test).

4. Discussion

Our study retrospectively evaluated the early outcomes and complications of THAs performed through DAA in 277 consecutive patients divided into 3 groups according to their BMI: normal weight (NW), overweight (OW), and obese (OB). OB patients had a lower age at surgery and higher ASA score, together with a slightly but significantly longer surgical time and in-hospital stay. A significantly higher number of revision surgeries was observed in patients in the OB group, which were due to dislocation (n = 2), wound dehiscence (n = 1), and aseptic mobilisation (n = 1) ($p = 0.028$); interestingly, no significant differences ($p = 0.27$) in the incidence of infections was found when comparing obese and non-obese patients.

Patients in the OB group were significantly younger compared to NW and OW patients (59.47 vs. 64.02 and 63.59, respectively). These data are in accordance with the observations of Haynes [24] and Clement and Deehan [25], who found that patients with a BMI > 30 kg/m^2 were subjected to primary THA in their early sixties compared to non-obese patients that were closer to their seventies, supporting the role of obesity in the development of early hip arthritis. OB patients in our study also showed higher ASA scores compared to non-obese patients, in agreement with data from the literature [26].

Surgical time for THA implant in OB patients was significantly longer (86 ± 21 min) compared to NW (79 ± 20 min) and OW (80 ± 20 min) patients; this finding is in line with others available in the literature [27–29], in which surgical time for DAA in obese patients is, on average, 10.9 min above the average time for non-obese patients (104.0 vs. 115.9 min). However, the slight increase in surgical time in our OB patients, which is less than 10 min compared to NW and OW, has a low impact from a clinical point of view, as mirrored by the absence of difference in the rate of post-operative infections and blood transfusion requirements among the three groups. Sang et al. [28] reported a significant increase in blood loss in obese patients undergoing THA, often requiring allogeneic blood transfusions; DAA in the OB patients might be of advantage in this scenario since, according to our findings, no difference in blood transfusions between obese and non-obese patients was found in patients operated on via this minimally invasive approach.

In our study, the in-hospital stay was slightly but significantly longer in OB patients, in disagreement with the findings by Hartford et al. [29], who reported similar results in NW and OB patients (2.7 vs. 2.81 days). In the current study, however, patients were not discharged until they gained functional autonomy; the average 1-day-longer hospital stay for OB patients could be related to the increase in the overall comorbidities in this patient population, and not just to the surgery itself.

Several authors reported a higher rate of surgery-related complications in obese patients operated on for THA. DeMik et al. [8] investigated a pool of 64,648 patients that had THA, 37.48% of whom were obese. They found that OB patients having THA had higher rates of complications compared to the non-obese, including wound complications (1.53% vs. 0.72%), deep infections (0.58% vs. 0.24%), and reoperations (2.11% vs. 1.59%). When patients are operated on through DAA, intra-operative femoral fractures and implant malpositioning could occur because of the impingement of the surgical instruments against the adipose tissue [14,16,30]. In order to reduce periprosthetic fracture, specific short stems seem to reduce the risk; in addition, dedicated off-set instrumentation is required to permit a suitable placement of implants without force [31]. Russo et al. [14] reported an increased rate of infectious complications in patients with BMI over 30 kg/m^2. In our study, we found a higher overall number of complications requiring revision surgery but no statistically significant differences in the rate of infections comparing the 3 groups: only 1 out of 72 patients had a wound infection requiring revision surgery, an incidence lower than previously reported [14]. In addition, Avinash et al. reported a low rate of infection, specifically, of 0.58%, in a study of more than 800 THAs in a population with an average BMI of 28 [32]. These data could support the protective role of minimally invasive DAA against infections, even in high-risk OB patients [33]. However, considering the restricted number of patients of the examined cohort, there is the risk of underestimating the rate of complications. We could not find any difference in terms of blood loss, implant positioning, and intra- and post-operative complications; our data are in agreement with the findings of Argyrou et al. [19], who, in a population of 82 OB patients compared to 172 NW patients undergoing THA surgery, did not find significant differences in blood loss, intra- and post-operative complications, or implant positioning and alignment. Intra-operative femur fracture is traditionally reported as the main complication of DAA in OB patients, with a reported incidence of up to 8.4% of cases [34–36]; however, in our patient population, no perioperative femur fractures occurred in the OB group.

The radiological evaluation of implant positioning in the current study focused on cup inclination and stem alignment. Cup inclination was analysed with respect to Lewinnek's safe zone of 40° ± 10° [22]. The relevance of Lewinnek's safe zone as an outcome measurement of THA has been recently discussed [37]. The results of the current study seem to support this issue: in fact, even with a non-negligible number of patients (see Table 2) with cup inclination outside the "safe zone", a low incidence (2/293, 0.68%) of implant dislocations was found. Measured cup inclination was comparable among the three groups, showing that DAA allows a consistent implant positioning, independently of the body habitus. This is in line with the findings of Davidovitch et al. [38], who, in a study on 509 fluoroscopy-assisted DAA THAs divided into 3 groups according to BMI, Group I (<30 kg/m^2), Group II (≥30 to <35 kg/m^2), and Group III (≥35 kg/m^2), did not find significant differences in acetabular component positioning when obese and non-obese patients were compared. Good stem positioning (range −5°/+5°) was observed in most patients, with a prevalence of mild varus stems (167/293; 57%); the data are in agreement with the findings of Haversath et al. [39], who reported the same prevalence of mild varus (+2.2°) stem alignment when THA was performed via DAA.

This study has some limitations. The first is associated with its retrospective nature, which is associated with a selection bias. Moreover, collected patients were operated on in a surgical unit with great expertise on DAA, which is currently used in over 90% of THAs for both primary and revision surgeries. The follow-up was short and focused only on early results, reaching up to 6 months; however, since the purpose of the study was to evaluate the feasibility and safety of DAA in OB compared to non-obese patients, follow-up was no longer deemed necessary to support the study questions. Moreover, surgery-related complications, including dislocations, occur in over 50% of cases in the first 3 months after surgery [40].

5. Conclusions

In conclusion, the results of the current study support the performance of minimally invasive DAA for THA in obese patients by surgeons experienced in this approach, because it can improve the outcomes of THA surgery in this patient population [27,41,42]. Thanks to its low invasiveness, THA performed via DAA is associated with good early functional outcomes and with an acceptable rate of complications. For those reasons, this approach should be taken into account by the hip surgeon when treating an obese patient.

Author Contributions: Conceptualisation, A.D.M. and C.F.; methodology, M.B., F.P. and B.B.; validation A.D.M.; formal analysis, B.B.; writing—original draft preparation, M.B., N.S. and F.R.; writing—review and editing, C.D. and G.G.; supervision, A.D.M.; project administration, C.F. All authors have read and agreed to the published version of the manuscript.

Funding: This research received no external funding.

Institutional Review Board Statement: The study was conducted in accordance with the Declaration of Helsinki and approved by the Institutional Ethics Committee for studies involving humans. Ethical Committee "Area Vasta Emilia Centro", Approval Code: CE-AVEC 347/2021/Oss/IOR on 7 May 2021.

Informed Consent Statement: Informed consent was obtained from all subjects involved in the study.

Data Availability Statement: Not applicable.

Conflicts of Interest: The authors declare no conflict of interest.

Abbreviation

THA	Total hip arthroplasty
DAA	Direct Anterior Approach
BMI	Body Mass Index
NW	Normal weight patients
OW	Overweight patients
OB	Obese patients
ASA	American Society of Anesthesiologists
NRS	Numerical Rating Scale

References

1. Yumuk, V.; Tsigos, C.; Fried, M.; Schindler, K.; Busetto, L.; Micic, D.; Toplak, H. European Guidelines for Obesity Management in Adults. *Obes. Facts* **2015**, *8*, 402–424. [CrossRef]
2. Caroline, M.; Apovian, M.D. Obesity: Definition, Comorbidities, Causes, and Burden. *Am. J. Manag. Care.* **2016**, *22*, S176–S185.
3. Andolfi, C.; Fisichella, P.M. Epidemiology of Obesity and Associated Comorbidities. *J. Laparoendosc. Adv. Surg. Tech.* **2018**, *28*, 919–924. [CrossRef] [PubMed]
4. Khaodhiar, L.; McCowen, K.C.; Blackburn, G.L. Obesity and its comorbid conditions. *Clin. Cornerstone* **1999**, *2*, 17–31. [CrossRef] [PubMed]
5. Obesity and Total Joint Arthroplasty. *J. Arthroplast.* **2013**, *28*, 714–721. [CrossRef]
6. Runhaar, J.; Koes, B.W.; Clockaerts, S.; Bierma-Zeinstra, S.M.A. A systematic review on changed biomechanics of lower extremities in obese individuals: A possible role in development of osteoarthritis. *Obes. Rev.* **2011**, *12*, 1071–1082. [CrossRef] [PubMed]
7. de Guia, N.; Zhu, N.; Keresteci, M.; Shi, J.E. Obesity and joint replacement surgery in Canada: Findings from the Canadian Joint Replacement Registry (CJRR). *Healthc. PolicyPolit. De Sante* **2006**, *1*, 36–43. [CrossRef]
8. DeMik, D.E.; Bedard, N.A.; Dowdle, S.B.; Elkins, J.M.; Brown, T.S.; Gao, Y.; Callaghan, J.J. Complications and Obesity in Arthroplasty—A Hip is Not a Knee. *J. Arthroplast.* **2018**, *33*, 3281–3287. [CrossRef]
9. Petis, S.; Howard, J.L.; Lanting, B.L.; Vasarhelyi, E.M. Surgical approach in primary total hip arthroplasty: Anatomy, technique and clinical outcomes. *Can. J. Surg.* **2015**, *58*, 128–139. [CrossRef] [PubMed]
10. Pincus, D.; Jenkinson, R.; Paterson, M.; Leroux, T.; Ravi, B. Association Between Surgical Approach and Major Surgical Complications in Patients Undergoing Total Hip Arthroplasty. *JAMA* **2020**, *323*, 1070–1076. [CrossRef]
11. Post, Z.D.; Orozco, F.; Diaz-Ledezma, C.; Hozack, W.J.; Ong, A. Direct anterior approach for total hip arthroplasty: Indications, technique, and results. *J. Am. Acad. Orthop. Surg.* **2014**, *22*, 595–603. [CrossRef] [PubMed]
12. Faldini, C.; Perna, F.; Mazzotti, A.; Stefanini, N.; Panciera, A.; Geraci, G.; Mora, P.; Traina, F. Direct anterior approach versus posterolateral approach in total hip arthroplasty: Effects on early post-operative rehabilitation period. *J. Biol. Regul. Homeost. Agents* **2017**, *31*, 75–81.
13. Faldini, C.; Perna, F.; Pilla, F.; Stefanini, N.; Pungetti, C.; Persiani, V.; Traina, F. Is a minimally invasive anterior approach effective in old patients? A pilot study. *J. Biol. Regul. Homeost. Agents* **2016**, *30*, 193–199. [PubMed]
14. Russo, M.W.; Macdonell, J.R.; Paulus, M.C.; Keller, J.M.; Zawadsky, M.W. Increased Complications in Obese Patients Undergoing Direct Anterior Total Hip Arthroplasty. *J. Arthroplast.* **2015**, *30*, 1384–1387. [CrossRef] [PubMed]
15. Shah, N.V.; Huddleston, H.P.; Wolff, D.T.; Newman, J.M.; Pivec, R.; Naziri, Q.; Shah, V.R.; Maheshwari, A.V. Does Surgical Approach for Total Hip Arthroplasty Impact Infection Risk in the Obese Patient? A Systematic Review. *Orthopedics* **2022**, *45*, e67–e72. [CrossRef]
16. Watts, C.; Houdek, M.T.; Wagner, E.R.; Sculco, P.; Chalmers, B.P.; Taunton, M. High Risk of Wound Complications Following Direct Anterior Total Hip Arthroplasty in Obese Patients. *J. Arthroplast.* **2015**, *30*, 2296–2298. [CrossRef] [PubMed]
17. Rhind, J.-H.; Baker, C.; Roberts, P.J. Total Hip Arthroplasty in the Obese Patient: Tips and Tricks and Review of the Literature. *Indian J. Orthop.* **2020**, *54*, 776–783. [CrossRef] [PubMed]
18. Nizam, I.; Dabirrahmani, D.; Alva, A.; Choudary, D. Bikini anterior hip replacements in obese patients are not associated with an increased risk of complication. *Arch. Orthop. Trauma Surg.* **2021**, *142*, 2919–2926. [CrossRef]
19. Argyrou, C.; Tzefronis, D.; Sarantis, M.; Kateros, K.; Poultsides, L.; Macheras, G.A. Total hip arthroplasty through the direct anterior approach in morbidly obese patients. *Bone Jt. Open* **2022**, *3*, 4–11. [CrossRef]
20. Macheras, G.; Stasi, S.; Sarantis, M.; Triantafyllou, A.; Tzefronis, D.; A Papadakis, S. Direct anterior approach vs Hardinge in obese and nonobese osteoarthritic patients: A randomized controlled trial. *World J. Orthop.* **2021**, *12*, 877–890. [CrossRef] [PubMed]
21. Johnston, F.E.; Wadden, T.A.; Stunkard, A.J.; Peña, M.; Wang, J.; Pierson, R.N.; Van Itallie, T.B. Body fat deposition in adult obese women. I Patterns of fat distribution. *Am. J. Clin. Nutr.* **1988**, *47*, 225–228. [CrossRef]
22. Lewinnek, G.E.; Lewis, J.L.; Tarr, R.; Compere, C.L.; Zimmerman, J.R. Dislocations after total hip-replacement arthroplasties. *J. Bone Joint. Surg. Am.* **1978**, *60*, 217–220. [CrossRef]
23. Khalily, C.; Lester, D. Results of a tapered cementless femoral stem implanted in varus. *J. Arthroplast.* **2002**, *17*, 463–466. [CrossRef]
24. Haynes, J.; Nam, D.; Barrack, R.L. Obesity in total hip arthroplasty: Does it make a difference? *Bone Jt. J.* **2017**, *99*, 31–36. [CrossRef]
25. Clement, N.D.; Deehan, D.J. Overweight and Obese Patients Require Total Hip and Total Knee Arthroplasty at a Younger Age. *J. Orthop. Res.* **2019**, *38*, 348–355. [CrossRef] [PubMed]
26. Gurunathan, U.; Anderson, C.; Berry, K.E.; Whitehouse, S.L.; Crawford, R.W. Body mass index and in-hospital postoperative complications following primary total hip arthroplasty. *HIP Int.* **2018**, *28*, 613–621. [CrossRef] [PubMed]
27. Antoniadis, A.; Dimitriou, D.; Flury, A.; Wiedmer, G.; Hasler, J.; Helmy, N. Is Direct Anterior Approach a Credible Option for Severely Obese Patients Undergoing Total Hip Arthroplasty? A Matched-Control, Retrospective, Clinical Study. *J. Arthroplast.* **2018**, *33*, 2535–2540. [CrossRef]
28. Sang, W.; Zhu, L.; Ma, J.; Lu, H.; Wang, C. The Influence of Body Mass Index and Hip Anatomy on Direct Anterior Approach Total Hip Replacement. *Med. Princ. Pract. Int. J. Kuwait. Univ. Health Sci. Cent.* **2016**, *25*, 555–560. [CrossRef] [PubMed]
29. Hartford, J.M.; Graw, B.P.; Frosch, D.L. Perioperative Complications Stratified by Body Mass Index for the Direct Anterior Approach to Total Hip Arthroplasty. *J. Arthroplast.* **2020**, *35*, 2652–2657. [CrossRef]

30. Purcell, R.L.; Parks, N.L.; Gargiulo, J.M.; Hamilton, W.G. Severely Obese Patients Have a Higher Risk of Infection After Direct Anterior Approach Total Hip Arthroplasty. *J. Arthroplast.* **2016**, *31*, 162–165. [CrossRef]
31. Luger, M.; Hipmair, G.; Schopper, C.; Schauer, B.; Hochgatterer, R.; Allerstorfer, J.; Gotterbarm, T.; Klasan, A. Low rate of early periprosthetic fractures in cementless short-stem total hip arthroplasty using a minimally invasive anterolateral approach. *J. Orthop. Traumatol.* **2021**, *22*, 1–9. [CrossRef]
32. Alva, A.; Nizam, I.; Gogos, S. Minimizing complications in bikini incision direct anterior approach total hip arthroplasty: A single surgeon series of 865 cases. *J. Exp. Orthop.* **2021**, *8*, 1–9. [CrossRef] [PubMed]
33. Sprowls, G.R.; Allen, B.C.; Lundquist, K.F.; Sager, L.N.; Barnett, C.D. Incision site fat thickness and 90-day complications for direct anterior and posterior approach total hip arthroplasty. *HIP Int.* **2020**, *32*, 431–437. [CrossRef] [PubMed]
34. Aggarwal, V.K.; Elbuluk, A.; Dundon, J.; Herrero, C.; Hernandez, C.; Vigdorchik, J.M.; Schwarzkopf, R.; Iorio, R.; Long, W.J. Surgical approach significantly affects the complication rates associated with total hip arthroplasty. *Bone Jt. J.* **2019**, *101*, 646–651. [CrossRef]
35. Griffiths, S.Z.; Post, Z.D.; Buxbaum, E.J.; Paziuk, T.M.; Orozco, F.R.; Ong, A.C.; Ponzio, D.Y. Predictors of Perioperative Vancouver B Periprosthetic Femoral Fractures Associated With the Direct Anterior Approach to Total Hip Arthroplasty. *J. Arthroplast.* **2019**, *35*, 1407–1411. [CrossRef] [PubMed]
36. Stringer, M.R.; Hooper, G.J.; Frampton, C.; Kieser, D.C.; Deng, Y. Periprosthetic fractures of the femur in primary total hip arthroplasty: A New Zealand Joint Registry analysis. *ANZ J. Surg.* **2021**, *91*, 404–408. [CrossRef]
37. Sadhu, A.; Nam, D.; Coobs, B.R.; Barrack, T.N.; Nunley, R.M.; Barrack, R.L. Acetabular Component Position and the Risk of Dislocation Following Primary and Revision Total Hip Arthroplasty: A Matched Cohort Analysis. *J. Arthroplast.* **2017**, *32*, 987–991. [CrossRef]
38. Davidovitch, R.; Riesgo, A.; Bolz, N.; Murphy, H.; Anoushiravani, A.A.; Snir, N. The Effect of Obesity on Fluoroscopy-Assisted Direct Anterior Approach Total Hip Arthroplasty. *Bull. NYU Hosp. Jt. Dis.* **2020**, *78*, 187–194.
39. Haversath, M.; Lichetzki, M.; Serong, S.; Busch, A.; Landgraeber, S.; Jäger, M.; Tassemeier, T. The direct anterior approach provokes varus stem alignment when using a collarless straight tapered stem. *Arch. Orthop. Trauma Surg.* **2020**, *141*, 891–897. [CrossRef]
40. Gillinov, S.M.; Joo, P.Y.; Zhu, J.R.; Moran, J.; Rubin, L.E.; Grauer, J.N. Incidence, Timing, and Predictors of Hip Dislocation After Primary Total Hip Arthroplasty for Osteoarthritis. *J. Am. Acad. Orthop. Surg.* **2022**, *30*, 1047–1053. [CrossRef]
41. Manrique, J.; Paskey, T.; Tarabichi, M.; Restrepo, C.; Foltz, C.; Hozack, W.J. Total Hip Arthroplasty Through the Direct Anterior Approach Using a Bikini Incision Can Be Safely Performed in Obese Patients. *J. Arthroplast.* **2019**, *34*, 1723–1730. [CrossRef] [PubMed]
42. Dienstknecht, T.; Lüring, C.; Tingart, M.; Grifka, J.; Sendtner, E. A minimally invasive approach for total hip arthroplasty does not diminish early post-operative outcome in obese patients: A prospective, randomised trial. *Int. Orthop.* **2013**, *37*, 1013–1018. [CrossRef] [PubMed]

Disclaimer/Publisher's Note: The statements, opinions and data contained in all publications are solely those of the individual author(s) and contributor(s) and not of MDPI and/or the editor(s). MDPI and/or the editor(s) disclaim responsibility for any injury to people or property resulting from any ideas, methods, instructions or products referred to in the content.

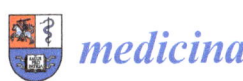 *medicina*

Article

Correlations of Sesamoid Bone Subluxation with the Radiologic Measures of Hallux Valgus and Its Clinical Implications

Sung Hwan Kim [†], Young Hwan Kim [†], Joo Young Cha and Young Koo Lee *

Department of Orthopaedic Surgery, Soonchunhyang University Bucheon Hospital, 170, Jomaru-ro, Wonmi-gu, Bucheon-si 14584, Gyeonggi-do, Republic of Korea; shk9528@naver.com (S.H.K.); remedios@schmc.ac.kr (Y.H.K.); cacarito@hanmail.net (J.Y.C.)
* Correspondence: brain0808@hanmail.net
† These authors contributed equally to this work.

Abstract: *Background and Objectives*: Hallux valgus is one of the most common chronic foot complaints, with prevalences of over 23% in adults and up to 35.7% in older adults. However, the prevalence is only 3.5% in adolescents. The pathological causes and pathophysiology of hallux valgus are well-known in various studies and reports. A change in the position of the sesamoid bone under the metatarsal bone of the first toe is known to be the cause of the initial pathophysiology. *Purpose*: The relationships between the changes in the location of the sesamoid bone and each radiologically measured angle and joint congruency in the hallux valgus remain as yet unknown. Therefore, this study investigated the relationships of sesamoid bone subluxation with the hallux valgus angle, intermetatarsal angle, and metatarsophalangeal joint congruency in hallux valgus patients. The goal is to know the hallux valgus angle, the intermetatarsal angle, and metatarsophalangeal joint congruency's correlation with hallux valgus severity and prognosis by revealing the relationship between each measured value and sesamoid bone subluxation. *Materials and Methods*: We reviewed 205 hallux valgus patients who underwent radiographic evaluation and subsequent hallux valgus correction surgery in our orthopedic clinic between March 2015 and February 2020. Sesamoid subluxation was assessed using a new five-grade scale on foot radiographs, and other radiologic measurements were assessed, such as hallux valgus angle, the intermetatarsal angle, distal metatarsal articular angle, joint congruency, etc. *Conclusions*: Measurements of the hallux valgus angle, interphalangeal angle, and joint congruency exhibited high interobserver and intraobserver reliabilities in this study. They also showed correlations with sesamoid subluxation grade.

Keywords: hallux valgus; hallux valgus angle; intermetatarsal angle; joint congruency; sesamoid bone; sesamoid bone subluxation

Citation: Kim, S.H.; Kim, Y.H.; Cha, J.Y.; Lee, Y.K. Correlations of Sesamoid Bone Subluxation with the Radiologic Measures of Hallux Valgus and Its Clinical Implications. *Medicina* **2023**, *59*, 876. https://doi.org/10.3390/medicina59050876

Academic Editor: Cory Xian

Received: 22 March 2023
Revised: 21 April 2023
Accepted: 28 April 2023
Published: 2 May 2023

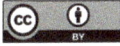

Copyright: © 2023 by the authors. Licensee MDPI, Basel, Switzerland. This article is an open access article distributed under the terms and conditions of the Creative Commons Attribution (CC BY) license (https://creativecommons.org/licenses/by/4.0/).

1. Introduction

Hallux valgus is one of the most common chronic foot complaints, with reported prevalences of over 23% in adults, 35.7% in older adults, and only 3.5% in adolescents [1,2]. Hallux valgus recurrence after corrective surgery is a well-known phenomenon; the long-term recurrence rate can reach up to 50%. The causes of recurrence are thought to be multifactorial, including surgical factors such as choice of the appropriate procedure and technical competency and patient-related factors such as anatomic predisposition, medical comorbidities, and compliance with post-correction instructions [3]. The etiology of hallux valgus is multifactorial; both intrinsic and extrinsic factors may be involved, and the condition tends to be inherited [2]. Hypermobility of the first ray began to be considered as an etiologic factor and related as a primary cause of hallux valgus [4]. Hallux valgus can make it difficult for patients to wear fashionable shoes; it may also impair their quality of life by restricting daily and recreational activities [3]. Difficulties associated with hallux valgus include foot pain, impaired balance, awkward gait pattern, and fall down, especially in older adults [5]. Flat foot and navicular bone drop are typical symptoms of hallux valgus. Patients may experience gradual changes in the alignment and shape of the forefoot and midfoot, and the changes frequently occur in the medial direction [6]. Medial deviation of the first metatarsal bone is common, along with lateral deviation of the first phalange, deformity of the phalangeal bone and interphalangeal joint, and pronation of the big toe in conjunction with sesamoid subluxation [7]. Radiologic studies showed that the metatarsophalangeal joint changes into a curved shape in hallux valgus patients. The first metatarsal bone's length also increases. Abnormal alignment and structure of the first metatarsophalangeal joint would contribute to the collapse of the medial longitudinal arch of the foot in hallux valgus patients [8]. Intense plantar pressure below the hallux and first metatarsal area are well-known biomechanical characteristics of hallux valgus [9]. Zhang et al. found that the metatarsal areas exhibited more stress in the hallux valgus patients, especially the first metatarsal area, in a finite element study that dealt with the subject of metatarsal stress and metatarsophalangeal loadings between hallux valgus patients and a healthy control group. Moreover, foot kinematics analyzed in a multi-segmental study resulted in differences between hallux valgus patients and the healthy control group [10]. Treatment options for hallux valgus deformity comprise surgical treatment and conservative treatment [11]. Although more than 100 open surgical methods are available, there is no clear consensus regarding which is the most effective option [12]. To name just a few examples, in surgical treatments, Akin osteotomy, the first metatarsal osteotomy, the McBride procedure and the Lapidus procedure are widely used surgical options for moderate or severe hallux valgus patients with discomfort [13]. Percutaneous approaches and minimally invasive surgery are increasingly used because these approaches can achieve results that are at least equivalent to the results of conventional open surgery and have lower complications [14,15]. Conservative treatment is also recommended for specific patient groups. In previous studies, it was proven that foot orthosis could lower peak pressure loadings of the hallux valgus patients' feet [16,17]. Lee et al. *. and Karabicak et al. found that kinesiology tape for the foot could relieve foot pain and decrease the hallux valgus angle [18,19]. Less frequent jogging and the avoidance of shoes can be beneficial for the intrinsic muscles of the foot, thus promoting healthy foot arch development and gait [20].

Evaluation of hallux valgus deformity via conventional radiography provides surgeons with the necessary information to choose the correct treatment option and appropriate surgical procedure if the patient needs surgery. Considering those facts, systematic radiographic evaluation of hallux valgus deformity is important for the achievement of good surgical outcomes [21]. However, most radiographic measurements focus on the angular deformities in the transverse plane, which are measured on dorsoplantar foot radiographs [5]. Rotational deformities in the coronal plane have attracted less attention, although they are likely to affect those in the coronal plane [22]. Radiological measurements, including the hallux valgus angle, the intermetatarsal angle, the distal metatarsal articular angle, and the first metatarsophalangeal joint congruency, are used to determine deformity etiology, grade, and extent. Almost all of these radiographic measurements are used to identify etiology, grade the extent of deformity, and decide the treatment plan and its surgical method if needed [23]. The value of hallux valgus angle, intermetatarsal angle and extent of sesamoid displacement are used to classify hallux valgus deformity and help to derive treatment algorithms [9,24]. The value of the hallux valgus angle on plain foot X-rays is an important predictor of the outcome of hallux valgus correction surgery [25]. Hallux valgus deformity is usually indicated by sesamoid subluxation beginning in the first metatarsal head [26]. In a study by Ryuhei et al., it was demonstrated that the sesamoid bone's lateral displacement is strongly associated with the severity of hallux valgus [27]. Okuda et al. demonstrated whether reduction of the sesamoid bone to the first metatarsal head is completed or not would be an important component in the correction surgery of hallux valgus because the incomplete reduction of the sesamoid bone may cause the deformity to recur postoperatively [28]. Considering that knowledge, precise and detailed assessment of the sesamoid bone is important to ensure that the most appropriate treatment option for hallux valgus deformity is selected. The sesamoid bone of the first metatarsophalangeal joint has several functions. For example, it absorbs most weight on the first ray; this protects the flexor hallucis longus tendon, which courses over the first plantar surface of the metatarsal head and enhances the mechanical function of the intrinsic muscles of the first ray [9]. The intersesamoid ligament, which is under the first metatarsal head, contributes to the intrinsic stability of the sesamoid complex.

Foot weight-bearing computer tomography (CT) has become an accurate and highly valuable radiological method to assess several foot and ankle diseases [29–31]. Collan et al. were the first to use weight-bearing CT for the assessment of hallux valgus patients [32]. Hallux valgus measurements obtained via weight-bearing CT are highly reliable. In particular, the distal metatarsal articular angle can be measured with high accuracy. However, Zhong et al. do not recommend foot weight-bearing CT for all hallux valgus patients because not every hallux valgus patients need to take a foot weight-bearing CT scan [8]. In fact, it is not easy for clinicians to use such a method because not many hospitals have foot-weight-bearing CT equipment. Considering issues such as cost, ease of inspection, and radiation exposure, a plain radiograph is still an attractive option that cannot be ignored. Even considering the diagnostic aspect, except for the distal metatarsal articular angle, some parameters (hallux valgus angle, intermetatarsal angle, proximal phalangeal articular angle, and sesamoid subluxation) measured by plain radiographic are comparable to weight-bearing CT [6].

So far, there are many studies that report the reliability of various radiographic measurements evaluating a hallux valgus deformity with a plain radiograph [33–35]. However, to our knowledge, the correlation between sesamoid bone subluxation and hallux valgus angle, the intermetatarsal angle, and metatarsophalangeal joint congruency in hallux valgus patients with foot plain radiograph have not been described in English-language medical literature. We hypothesized that the degree of subluxation of sesamoid bone might have a relationship with radiologic measurement and severity of the hallux valgus. The purpose of our study is to establish the reliability of eight radiologic measurements and to determine the relationship of sesamoid subluxation with other radiologic measurements with a plain foot radiograph.

2. Materials and Methods

We retrospectively reviewed 205 hallux valgus patients who underwent radiographic evaluation and subsequent hallux valgus correction surgery in our orthopedic clinic between March 2015 and February 2020. The radiographic evaluation included weight-bearing dorsoplantar and lateral foot radiographs. We excluded 25 patients, including 10 who only had non-weight-bearing scans, four with brachymetatarsia, three with cavus foot deformity, three with Charcot arthritis, two with claw toe deformity, one with bunionette deformity, one with gouty arthritis, and one with crushing injury (Figure 1). These patients were excluded because non-weight-bearing radiographs cannot clearly show hallux valgus deformity, and combined diseases like inflammatory arthritis, trauma, and other toe deformities can influence the hallux valgus condition. In total, images of both feet of 180 patients were included in the final analysis. The mean patient age was 52.78 years (range: 15–78 years; 18 men and 162 women) (Table 1). The study was conducted in accordance with the Declaration of Helsinki, and approved by the Institutional Review Board and Human Research Ethics Committee of Soonchunhyang University Bucheon Hospital (IRB No. 2023-02-015-001, 20 March 2023).

Foot radiographs were acquired using the Innovision-SH instrument (DK Medical Systems, Seoul, Republic of Korea; 50 kVp, 5 mAs) at a distance of 100 cm and with each patient standing upright. We retrieved the radiographic images using a picture archiving and communication system (PACS; DEJA-VIEW; Dongeun Information Technology, Bucheon, Republic of Korea). Radiographic measurements were performed using PACS 1.42 software.

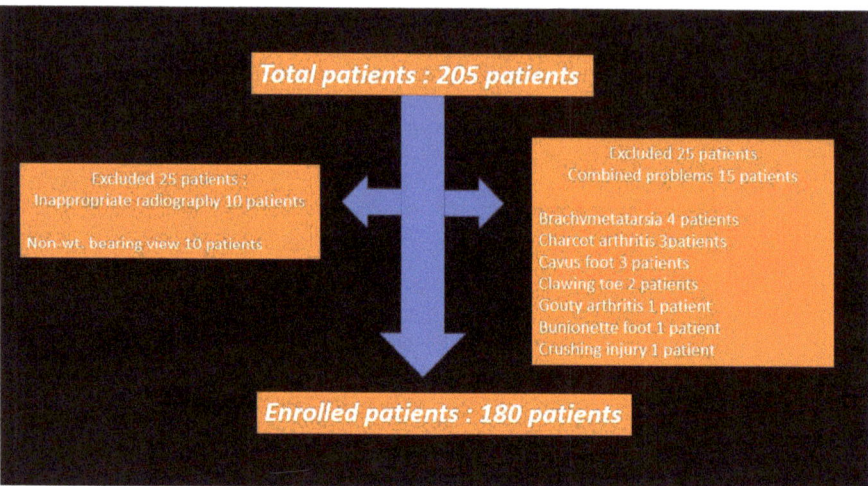

Figure 1. Summary of Enrolled patients: Total patients (n = 205)/10 patients excluded because of lack of weight-bearing scan/15 patients excluded because of: Brachymetatarsia (n = 4)/Charcot arthritis (n = 3)/Cavus foot deformity (n = 3)/Claw toe deformity (n = 2)/Gouty arthritis (n = 1)/Bunionette deformity (n = 1)/Crushing injury (n = 1)/Enrolled patients (n = 180).

Table 1. Patient clinical and demographic characteristics.

Total	205
Excluded patients	25
Patient number	180
Age	52.78
Male:Female	18:162
Operated feet	240
Operated sided Right:Left:Bilateral	54:66:60

Eight radiological measurements were made, including seven on dorsoplantar foot radiographs (hallux valgus angle, intermetatarsal angle, distal metatarsal articular angle, proximal phalangeal articular angle, hallux interphalangeal angle, sesamoid subluxation, and congruency) and one on lateral view radiographs (tarso-first metatarsal angle [i.e., Meary's angle]). On foot weight-bearing plain radiographs, the hallux valgus angle is the angle between the longitudinal axis of the first metatarsal bone and the longitudinal axis of the proximal phalanx bone; the intermetatarsal angle is the angle between the longitudinal axis of the first and second metatarsal bones; the distal metatarsal articular angle is the angle between a line perpendicular to the longitudinal axis of the first metatarsal bone and a line delineating the orientation of the articular surface of the metatarsal bone's head; the proximal phalangeal articular angle is the angle between a line delineating the orientation of the base of the proximal phalangeal articular surface and a line delineating the orientation of the proximal phalangeal distal articular surface; and the hallux interphalangeal angle is the angle between the longitudinal axis of the proximal phalanx bone and the longitudinal axis of the distal phalanx of the hallux.

Sesamoid subluxation was assessed using a new five-grade scale, which can also describe the relationship between the tibial sesamoid and the longitudinal axis of the first metatarsal bone. A sesamoid, which had no lateral displacement relative to the bisection line, was deemed as grade 0. Grade 1 occurred when there was an overlap of less than 25% of the sesamoid to the bisection. Grade 2 was when the overlap of the sesamoid became greater than 25% and less than 50% of the bisection. Grade 3 was when the overlap of the sesamoid became greater than 50% and less than 75% of the bisection. Grade 4 was when the overlap of the sesamoid became greater than 75% (Table 2). The congruency of the metatarsophalangeal joint was determined based on the relationship between the articular surface of the base of the proximal phalangeal bone and the first metatarsal bone's head (Figure 2). Tarso-first metatarsal angle (Meary angle) assessed the longitudinal arch of the medial column of the foot and was measured between the long axis of the talus drawn from the midpoint of the talar body through the mid-diameter of the talonavicular joint and the long axis of the first metatarsal bone (Figure 3).

Table 2. Sesamoid subluxation grade.

Grade	
0	No sesamoid lateral displacement
1	Sesamoid overlap < 25%
2	25% < Sesamoid overlap < 50%
3	50% < Sesamoid overlap < 75%
4	75% < Sesamoid overlap

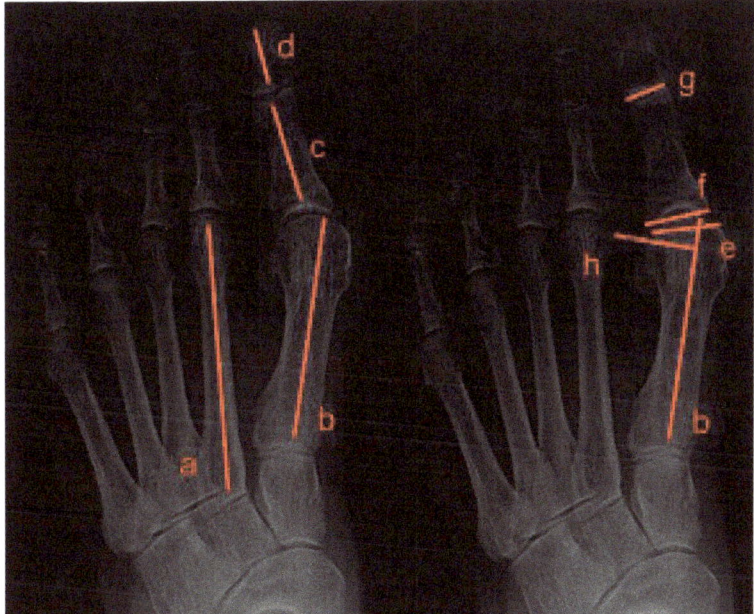

Figure 2. Angles between lines were measured on weight-bearing dorsoplantar foot radiographs. Line a is the longitudinal axis of the second metatarsal, line b is the longitudinal axis of the first metatarsal, line c is the longitudinal axis of the proximal phalanx, line d is the longitudinal axis of the distal phalanx, line e is the orientation of the first metatarsal distal articular surface, line f is the orientation of the proximal phalangeal base articular surface, line g is the orientation of the proximal phalangeal distal articular surface, and line h is the perpendicular axis of the longitudinal axis of the first metatarsal. The hallux valgus angle is the angle between b and c, and the intermetatarsal angle is the angle between a and b, the hallux interphalangeal angle is the angle between c and d, the proximal phalangeal articular angle is the angle between f and g, and the distal metatarsal articular angle is the angle between h and f.

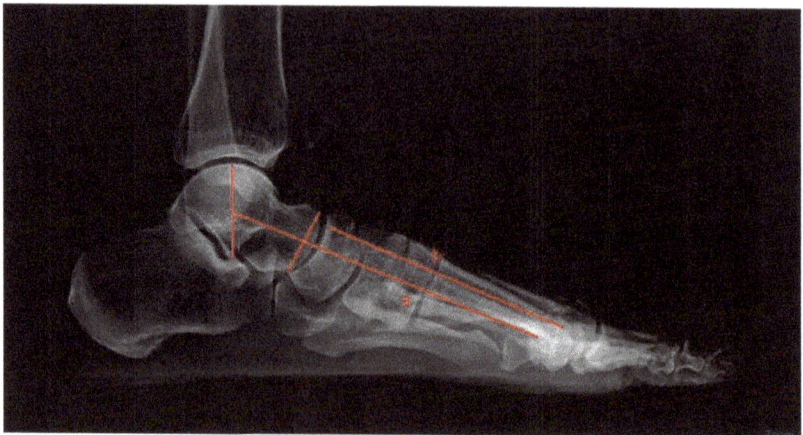

Figure 3. Angles between lines were measured on weight-bearing lateral foot radiographs. Line a is the lateral central axis of the talus, and line b is the longitudinal axis of the first metatarsal. The tarso-first metatarsal angle (Meary's angle) is the angle between a and b.

Three orthopedic surgeons (a first-year resident, third-year resident, and foot and ankle fellow) independently performed the radiographic measurements. They were each blinded to the patients' clinical information and measurements by the other surgeons. To determine intraobserver reliability, the three surgeons repeated measurements of 240 radiographs after an interval of two weeks. We assessed interobserver and intraobserver reliabilities using intraclass correlation coefficients (ICCs); 95% confidence intervals were also calculated using a two-way random effects model. Continuous variables were assessed for normality using the Shapiro–Wilk test. All data were normally distributed; thus, parametric tests were performed. Continuous variables are presented as means ± standard deviations. Analysis of variance and Fisher's exact test were used to compare independent groups. All comparative analyses were two-tailed, and p-values < 0.05 were considered statistically significant. All analyses were conducted using SPSS software (version 26.0; IBM Corp., Armonk, NY, USA). All analyses were conducted by statistician Eun Ae Jung (Soonchunhyang University, Gyeonggi-do, Republic of Korea)

3. Results

With respect to intraobserver reliability, all ICC values for Observers 1 and 2 were at least moderate according to the classification established by Koo et al. [36]. However, for Observer 3, the ICC values of the distal metatarsal articular angle and proximal phalangeal articular angle were < 0.5 on both sides. For all observers, the right and left distal metatarsal articular angles had the lowest ICC values. All sesamoid subluxation kappa values were above the threshold for good observer agreement (0.60) suggested by Landis et al. [37]. In terms of joint congruency, Observers 2 and 3 had kappa values exceeding the threshold for good agreement, whereas Observer 1 did not (Table 3).

In terms of interobserver reliability, most measurements showed ICC values that were at least moderate. However, the ICCs of the intermetatarsal and distal metatarsal articular angles were <0.5 for both the first and second measurements. ICCs were similar for the first proximal phalangeal articular angle measurement. Among all measurements, the right and left distal metatarsal articular angles had the lowest ICC values for both the first and second measurements. With respect to the sesamoid subluxation grade, all kappa values were >0.8, indicating substantial concordance. Finally, all kappa values for joint congruency were <0.5 (Table 4).

Table 3. Intraobserver reliability data of Observers 1–3.

	Observer1			Observer2			Observer3		
	CCC	95% CI		CCC	95% CI		CCC	95% CI	
R HVA	0.890	(0.844	0.923)	0.989	(0.984	0.992)	0.649	(0.530	0.743)
R IMA	0.810	(0.736	0.865)	0.909	(0.872	0.936)	0.756	(0.669	0.823)
R DMAA	0.650	(0.535	0.741)	0.842	(0.779	0.888)	0.306	(0.135	0.460)
R T-MA	0.875	(0.824	0.913)	0.974	(0.962	0.982)	0.541	(0.411	0.650)
R Ppa	0.734	(0.637	0.808)	0.922	(0.889	0.945)	0.396	(0.238	0.533)
R HIA	0.804	(0.731	0.859)	0.924	(0.892	0.947)	0.734	(0.638	0.807)
L HVA	0.964	(0.950	0.975)	0.986	(0.981	0.990)	0.945	(0.922	0.961)
L IMA	0.154	(0.052	0.253)	0.950	(0.930	0.964)	0.704	(0.605	0.782)
L DMAA	0.611	(0.494	0.706)	0.860	(0.806	0.899)	0.335	(0.177	0.476)
L T-Ma	0.864	(0.813	0.902)	0.979	(0.970	0.985)	0.554	(0.435	0.653)
L Ppa	0.827	(0.764	0.874)	0.908	(0.873	0.935)	0.395	(0.266	0.510)
L HIA	0.754	(0.671	0.819)	0.932	(0.904	0.951)	0.503	(0.361	0.623)

CCC: Concordance correlation coefficient

	Observer1			Observer2			Observer3		
	Weighted Kappa	95% CI		Weighted Kappa	95% CI		Weighted Kappa	95% CI	
R Sesa	0.647	(0.515	0.778)	0.924	(0.874	0.974)	1.000	(1.000	1.000)
L Sesa	0.692	(0.583	0.800)	0.966	(0.932	1.000)	0.994	(0.982	1.000)

	Observer1			Observer2			Observer3		
	Kappa	95% CI		Kappa	95% CI		Kappa	95% CI	
R Cong	0.581	(0.378	0.784)	0.936	(0.864	1.000)	0.939	(0.856	1.000)
L Cong	0.468	(0.285	0.651)	0.937	(0.866	1.000)	1.000	(1.000	1.000)

CI, confidence interval; CCC, concordance correlation coefficient; R, right side; L, left side; HVA, hallux valgus angle; IMA, intermetatarsal angle; DMAA, distal metatarsal articular angle; T-MA, tarso-first metatarsal angle; PPAA, proximal phalangeal articular angle; HIA, hallux interphalangeal; SSG, sesamoid subluxation grade.

Table 4. Interobserver reliability of Observers 1–3 for the first and second measurements.

	First			Second		
	CCC	95% CI		CCC	95% CI	
R HVA	0.747	(0.591	0.843)	0.867	(0.810	0.907)
R IMA	0.377	(0.271	0.481)	0.407	(0.318	0.507)
R DMAA	0.285	(0.183	0.411)	0.189	(0.099	0.320)
R T-MA	0.640	(0.552	0.718)	0.611	(0.528	0.690)
R Ppa	0.531	(0.393	0.634)	0.644	(0.521	0.727)
R HIA	0.656	(0.551	0.774)	0.773	(0.692	0.843)
L HVA	0.861	(0.785	0.898)	0.866	(0.802	0.903)
L IMA	0.131	(0.020	0.542)	0.539	(0.424	0.623)
L DMAA	0.322	(0.237	0.424)	0.206	(0.101	0.320)
L T-Ma	0.667	(0.588	0.740)	0.575	(0.485	0.663)
L Ppa	0.489	(0.369	0.660)	0.752	(0.664	0.853)
L HIA	0.591	(0.500	0.674)	0.675	(0.599	0.753)

CCC: Concordance correlation coefficient

	first		second	
	Kendall's Coefficient	p-value	Kendall's Coefficient	p-value
R Sesa	0.890	<0.0001	0.846	<0.0001
L Sesa	0.817	<0.0001	0.819	<0.0001

	1st			2nd		
	Kappa	95% CI		Kappa	95% CI	
R Cong	0.412	(0.306	0.519)	0.393	(0.286	0.499)
L Cong	0.501	(0.400	0.602)	0.483	(0.382	0.584)

CI, confidence interval; CCC, concordance correlation coefficient; R, right side; L, left side; HVA, hallux valgus angle; IMA, intermetatarsal angle; DMAA, distal metatarsal articular angle; T-MA, tarso-first metatarsal angle; PPAA, proximal phalangeal articular angle; HIA, hallux interphalangeal; SSG, sesamoid subluxation grade.

We hypothesized whether there is a correlation between sesamoid subluxation grade and the value of each other angle. We also attempted to find out whether there is a correlation between sesamoid subluxation and whether or not there is joint congruency. As a result, sesamoid subluxation grade was shown to have a correlation with hallux valgus angle, intermatatarsal angle and joint congruency (Tables 5 and 6).

Table 5. Correlations of sesamoid subluxation with radiological angles and joint congruency for Observer 1.

	Sesamoid Subluxation									p-Value †
	0		1		2		3		4	
Patients, n	1		5		18		19		70	
HVA	16.40		20.40	±4.62	24.49	±6.37	23.36	±5.45	33.39	±9.40	<0.0001
IMA	4.40		10.22	±1.97	11.14	±2.24	11.24	±1.81	14.52	±2.61	<0.0001
DMAA	8.00		15.36	±9.78	11.90	±6.13	10.91	±5.13	12.81	±5.80	0.4906
T-MA	5.90		5.92	±10.69	4.74	±4.81	0.90	±6.51	0.72	±6.96	0.1122
Ppa	14.20		5.02	±3.53	7.56	±4.01	8.24	±4.29	6.80	±4.27	0.2065
HIA	19.20		11.24	±4.90	10.83	±4.18	9.78	±3.46	7.19	±4.74	0.0009
Cong											<0.0001
C	1	(100.0%)	4	(80.0%)	4	(22.2%)	7	(36.8%)	5	(7.1%)	
N	0	(0.0%)	1	(20.0%)	14	(77.8%)	12	(63.2%)	65	(92.9%)	

† Analysis of variance or Fisher's exact test.

Table 6. Correlations of sesamoid subluxation with radiological angles and joint congruency for Observer 2.

	Sesamoid Subluxation									p-Value †
	0		1		2		3		4	
Patients, n	1		5		18		20		70	
HVA	15.30		15.44	±7.15	22.91	±6.86	23.07	±4.18	32.59	±8.94	<0.0001
IMA	5.60		9.14	±3.43	10.60	±1.92	11.04	±2.12	14.82	±2.53	<0.0001
DMAA	0.90		10.02	±7.11	8.83	±7.05	9.85	±4.91	11.42	±5.83	0.2089
T-MA	16.80		5.08	±6.17	3.64	±7.11	1.41	±6.25	0.56	±7.29	0.0710
Ppa	6.40		9.80	±3.40	7.16	±4.27	8.74	±3.97	6.85	±4.35	0.3061
HIA	15.10		13.82	±4.99	11.24	±4.92	11.12	±3.01	8.48	±4.96	0.0107
Cong											<0.0001
C	1	(100.0%)	5	(100.0%)	10	(55.6%)	13	(65.0%)	5	(7.1%)	
N	0	(0.0%)	0	(0.0%)	8	(44.4%)	7	(35.0%)	65	(92.9%)	

† Analysis of variance or Fisher's exact test. HVA, hallux valgus angle; IMA, intermetatarsal angle; DMAA, distal metatarsal articular angle; T-MA, tarso-first metatarsal angle; PPAA, proximal phalangeal articular angle; HIA, hallux interphalangeal.

4. Discussion

In this study, the hallux valgus angle had the highest ICC, and most of the radiographic measurements had high ICC values on interobserver and intraobserver reliability testing. It means that most of the hallux valgus angle measurements show concordance and seem to have reliability. However, some of the items show low ICC values and less concordance. Specifically, the distal metatarsal angle had lower ICC values in the intraobserver reliability test and interobserver reliability test and much lower ICC values compared with previous study results [35,38]. Additionally, sesamoid subluxation grade has a correlation with the hallux valgus angle, the intermetatarsal angle and joint congruency.

Various radiographic measurements have been developed for the evaluation of hallux valgus. Multiple radiographic angles are used to assess the extent of deformity, determine whether the patient requires surgical or conservative treatment, select the type of surgery surgical intervention, and assess postoperative outcomes. In terms of surgical treatment, more than 100 procedures have been used for hallux valgus correction; no single operation can treat all hallux valgus deformities [6]. In addition, more recently, a minimally invasive procedure using an intramedullary nail device (MIIND) has been used for hallux valgus deformity correction, and Carlo Biz et al. reported that the intermetatarsal angle and hallux valgus angle significantly decreased after operative intervention using MIIND [39]. The surgical procedure should be carefully selected based on symptoms and preoperative radiological measurements. The use of those radiologic angle measurements in various areas is based on the reliance that they have reproducibility and reliability and provide a constant value for comparison. It is a major issue if those measurements are accurate, reliable, and repeatable or not [40]. The most widely performed measurements are the hallux valgus angle, the intermetatarsal angle, the proximal phalangeal metatarsal angle and the distal metatarsal articular angle. To date, using standardized weight-bearing plain radiographic images is considered the gold standard for the assessment of hallux valgus foot [41]. The traditional measuring methods of angles in plain radiographs include using a marking pen, pointing to the reference area, identifying each bone's axis, and, finally, measuring angles with the goniometer. However, this approach is associated with intraobserver and interobserver errors, particularly with respect to the distal metatarsal articular angle. Moreover, it can be difficult to identify the articular surface [22,42]. Robinson et al. reported that the distal metatarsal articular angle considerably varied with the axial rotation of the first metatarsal bone, suggesting that measurements of the distal metatarsal angle on foot plain radiographs are susceptible to error [42]. It seems that such technical and structural limitations of plain radiographs are also related to the fact that distal metatarsal articular angle's ICC has exceptionally low value in our study. So, in order to solve such limitations, the opinion to use foot weight-bearing CT for the diagnosis of hallux valgus was first reported in 2013 [32]. Many subsequent studies have described the use of weight-bearing CT to diagnose hallux valgus and facilitate treatment decision-making. However, in reality, it is difficult for clinicians to use foot-weight-bearing CT because of various limitations. First of all, hospitals equipped with equipment and facilities for foot weight-bearing CT are rare, the cost is relatively expensive when implemented, and there are issues regarding radiation exposure. Above all, it is not easy to know before the examination whether a hallux valgus patients are severe enough to operate. Therefore, weight-bearing CT is not recommended for routine examination of the hallux valgus foot. In addition, a foot plain radiograph is not only worth screening in terms of cost-effectiveness but also can be the only alternative in determining a treatment direction and a surgical treatment method in an environment where foot weight-bearing CT is not present. The errors that may occur with conventional radiographic measurements could be avoided by standardizing the technique used for the acquisition of weight-bearing plain radiographs and using specific reference points [43]. For example, the American Orthopaedic Foot and Ankle Society reference points for the metaphyseal–diaphyseal junction of the first and second metatarsal bones, as well as the proximal phalanx bone, are commonly used.

Talbot et al. reported that sesamoid subluxation beginning at the first metatarsal head is indicative of hallux valgus deformity [44]. The fact that during the progression of hallux valgus deformity, the head of the first metatarsal bone drifts away to the medial side from the sesamoids is widely understood, whereas the sesamoid bone maintains its anatomical relationship with the second metatarsal bone [45,46]. The adductor hallucis tendon, which has an insertion site in the base of the proximal phalanx and lateral sesamoid bones, stabilizes the sesamoid complex. The distance between the lateral sesamoid bone and the second metatarsal bone tends to remain constant, regardless of hallux valgus deformity [44,47]. Attempts have been made to analyze the relationship between the degree of medial subluxation of the sesamoid bone and the severity of hallux valgus deformity [9,48]. Traditionally, a foot tangential or axial sesamoid view radiograph has been suggested to be obtained to assess the amount of sesamoid subluxation. Particularly in cases of congruent hallux valgus feet, the sesamoid bone can seem subluxated on the weight-bearing plain radiograph yet be anatomically reduced in its facets. Kuwano et al. compared the rotation angle of the sesamoid bone between tangential sesamoid and plain radiographs; they found that plain radiographs were not appropriate for efforts to determine the grade of sesamoid subluxation [49]. Yildrim et al. demonstrated that the severity of sesamoid subluxation was inversely related to the degree of metatarsophalangeal joint dorsiflexion; they also found that measurements made on tangential sesamoid images were unreliable [50]. The recently reported study showed little difference between the two different radiograph views and also showed a significant correlation in the sesamoid bone position [26]. Based on these results, standard weight-bearing plain radiographs were used in the present study.

To date, there have been several articles that have studied how to measure each angle or what those angles mean. However, some may not be necessary, and their relationships have not been well established. We, therefore, investigated the reliabilities of radiographic measurements and correlations of sesamoid subluxation with the hallux valgus angle, the intermetatarsal angle and joint congruency to determine which radiographic measurements predicted the severity and prognosis of hallux valgus. The correlation of the sesamoid subluxation with the intermetatarsal angle was shown in this study. Lee et al*. reported that the intermetatarsal angle correlated with the sesamoid rotation angle [51]. From this correlation between radiographic measurements, we assumed valgus and pronation occur concurrently at the first tarsometatarsal joint. If this is true, the proximal metatarsal osteotomy should include a rotational component and reduce the intermetatarsal angle [22]. Okutda et al. argued postoperative sesamoid positions were important in the surgical outcome [28]. It is important to determine the sesamoid subluxation in preoperative evaluation. According to our study, the sesamoid subluxation grade will be helpful for the preoperative evaluation of a hallux valgus deformity.

This study has several limitations. Although several observers conducted this study, there was only one radiographic program, leading to some bias in measurements, and the results may lack generalizability. Although the number of patients involved in this study is quite large, the patient group is limited to only one institution. In the future, it is considered that a study to prove the results of this study is needed, using various imaging programs targeting patients in various institutions.

5. Conclusions

Measurements of the hallux valgus angle, interphalangeal angle, and joint congruency exhibited high interobserver and intraobserver reliabilities in this study; they also showed correlations with sesamoid subluxation grade. These measurements are important in cases of hallux valgus deformity, particularly because the sesamoid subluxation grade reflects the severity and prognosis of hallux valgus.

Author Contributions: Conceptualization, S.H.K.; methodology, J.Y.C.; validation, Y.H.K.; investigation, J.Y.C.; resources, S.H.K.; data curation, Y.K.L.; writing—original draft preparation, S.H.K.; writing—review and editing, Y.K.L.; visualization, Y.H.K.; supervision, Y.H.K.; project administration, S.H.K.; funding acquisition, S.H.K. All authors have read and agreed to the published version of the manuscript.

Funding: The authors would like to thank the Soonchunhyang University Research Fund for financial support. (No. 2023-0006).

Institutional Review Board Statement: The study was conducted in accordance with the Declaration of Helsinki and approved by the Institutional Review Board and Human Research Ethics Committee of Soonchunhyang University Bucheon Hospital (IRB No. 2023-02-015-001, 20 March 2023).

Informed Consent Statement: All informed consent has been obtained from the patients to publish this paper.

Data Availability Statement: Data sharing is not applicable to this article because no datasets were made or analyzed during this study.

Conflicts of Interest: The authors declare no conflict of interest.

References

1. Nix, S.; Smith, M.; Vicenzino, B. Prevalence of hallux valgus in the general population: A systematic review and meta-analysis. *J. Foot Ankle Res.* **2010**, *3*, 1–9. [CrossRef] [PubMed]
2. Mahmoud, K.; Metikala, S.; Mehta, S.D.; Fryhofer, G.W.; Farber, D.C.; Prat, D. The role of weightbearing computed tomography scan in hallux valgus. *Foot Ankle Int.* **2021**, *42*, 287–293. [CrossRef] [PubMed]
3. Campbell, J.T. Hallux valgus: Adult and juvenile. In *Orthopaedic Knowledge Update: Foot and Ankle*; American Academy of Orthopaedic Surgeons: Rosemont, IL, USA, 2004.
4. Biz, C.; Maso, G.; Malgarini, E.; Tagliapietra, J.; Ruggieri, P. Hypermobility of the First Ray: The Cinderella of the measurements conventionally assessed for correction of Hallux Valgus. *Acta Bio Med. Atenei Parm.* **2020**, *91*, 47.
5. Zhong, Z.; Zhang, P.; Duan, H.; Yang, H.; Li, Q.; He, F. A Comparison between x-ray imaging and an innovative computer-aided design method based on weightbearing CT scan images for assessing hallux valgus. *J. Foot Ankle Surg.* **2021**, *60*, 6–10. [CrossRef] [PubMed]
6. Grande-del-Arco, J.; Becerro-de-Bengoa-Vallejo, R.; Palomo-López, P.; López-López, D.; Calvo-Lobo, C.; Pérez-Boal, E.; Losa-Iglesias, M.E.; Martin-Villa, C.; Rodriguez-Sanz, D. Radiographic analysis on the distortion of the anatomy of first metatarsal head in dorsoplantar projection. *Diagnostics* **2020**, *10*, 552. [CrossRef] [PubMed]
7. Coughlin, M.J.; Mann, R.A.; Saltzman, C.L. Surgery of the foot and ankle. *Rev. Rev.* **2007**, *26*, 1.
8. Steinberg, N.; Finestone, A.; Noff, M.; Zeev, A.; Dar, G. Relationship between lower extremity alignment and hallux valgus in women. *Foot Ankle Int.* **2013**, *34*, 824–831. [CrossRef] [PubMed]
9. Yavuz, M.; Hetherington, V.J.; Botek, G.; Hirschman, G.B.; Bardsley, L.; Davis, B.L. Forefoot plantar shear stress distribution in hallux valgus patients. *Gait Posture* **2009**, *30*, 257–259. [CrossRef]
10. Zhang, Y.; Awrejcewicz, J.; Szymanowska, O.; Shen, S.; Zhao, X.; Baker, J.S.; Gu, Y. Effects of severe hallux valgus on metatarsal stress and the metatarsophalangeal loading during balanced standing: A finite element analysis. *Comput. Biol. Med.* **2018**, *97*, 1–7. [CrossRef]
11. Wülker, N.; Mittag, F. The treatment of hallux valgus. *Dtsch. Ärztebl. Int.* **2012**, *109*, 857. [CrossRef]
12. Malagelada, F.; Sahirad, C.; Dalmau-Pastor, M.; Vega, J.; Bhumbra, R.; Manzanares-Céspedes, M.C.; Laffenêtre, O. Minimally invasive surgery for hallux valgus: A systematic review of current surgical techniques. *Int. Orthop.* **2019**, *43*, 625–637. [CrossRef] [PubMed]
13. Chopra, S.; Moerenhout, K.; Crevoisier, X. Subjective versus objective assessment in early clinical outcome of modified Lapidus procedure for hallux valgus deformity. *Clin. Biomech.* **2016**, *32*, 187–193. [CrossRef] [PubMed]
14. Biz, C.; Fosser, M.; Dalmau-Pastor, M.; Corradin, M.; Rodà, M.G.; Aldegheri, R.; Ruggieri, P. Functional and radiographic outcomes of hallux valgus correction by mini-invasive surgery with Reverdin-Isham and Akin percutaneous osteotomies: A longitudinal prospective study with a 48-month follow-up. *J. Orthop. Surg. Res.* **2016**, *11*, 157. [CrossRef] [PubMed]
15. Kaufmann, G.; Dammerer, D.; Heyenbrock, F.; Braito, M.; Moertlbauer, L.; Liebensteiner, M. Minimally invasive versus open chevron osteotomy for hallux valgus correction: A randomized controlled trial. *Int. Orthop.* **2019**, *43*, 343–350. [CrossRef]
16. Doty, J.F.; Alvarez, R.G.; Ervin, T.B.; Heard, A.; Gilbreath, J.; Richardson, N.S. Biomechanical evaluation of custom foot orthoses for hallux valgus deformity. *J. Foot Ankle Surg.* **2015**, *54*, 852–855. [CrossRef]
17. Farzadi, M.; Safaeepour, Z.; Mousavi, M.E.; Saeedi, H. Effect of medial arch support foot orthosis on plantar pressure distribution in females with mild-to-moderate hallux valgus after one month of follow-up. *Prosthet. Orthot. Int.* **2015**, *39*, 134–139. [CrossRef]
18. Lee, S.-M.; Lee, J.-H. Effects of balance taping using kinesiology tape in a patient with moderate hallux valgus: A case report. *Medicine* **2016**, *95*, e5357. [CrossRef]
19. Karabicak, G.O.; Bek, N.; Tiftikci, U. Short-term effects of kinesiotaping on pain and joint alignment in conservative treatment of hallux valgus. *J. Manip. Physiol. Ther.* **2015**, *38*, 564–571. [CrossRef]
20. Holowka, N.B.; Wallace, I.J.; Lieberman, D.E. Foot strength and stiffness are related to footwear use in a comparison of minimally- vs. conventionally-shod populations. *Sci. Rep.* **2018**, *8*, 3679. [CrossRef]
21. Chhaya, S.A.; Brawner, M.; Hobbs, P.; Chhaya, N.; Garcia, G.; Loredo, R. Understanding hallux valgus deformity: What the surgeon wants to know from the conventional radiograph. *Curr. Probl. Diagn. Radiol.* **2008**, *37*, 127–137. [CrossRef]
22. Lee, K.M.; Ahn, S.; Chung, C.Y.; Sung, K.H.; Park, M.S. Reliability and relationship of radiographic measurements in hallux valgus. *Clin. Orthop. Relat. Res.* **2012**, *470*, 2613–2621. [CrossRef] [PubMed]
23. Perera, A.; Mason, L.; Stephens, M. The pathogenesis of hallux valgus. *J. Bone Jt. Surg.* **2011**, *93*, 1650–1661. [CrossRef] [PubMed]
24. Shi, G.G.; Whalen, J.L.; Turner, N.S., III; Kitaoka, H.B. Operative approach to adult hallux valgus deformity: Principles and techniques. *JAAOS J. Am. Acad. Orthop. Surg.* **2020**, *28*, 410–418. [CrossRef]
25. Okuda, R.; Kinoshita, M.; Yasuda, T.; Jotoku, T.; Shima, H.; Takamura, M. Hallux valgus angle as a predictor of recurrence following proximal metatarsal osteotomy. *J. Orthop. Sci.* **2011**, *16*, 760–764. [CrossRef]
26. Agrawal, Y.; Desai, A.; Mehta, J. Lateral sesamoid position in hallux valgus: Correlation with the conventional radiological assessment. *Foot Ankle Surg.* **2011**, *17*, 308–311. [CrossRef]
27. Katsui, R.; Samoto, N.; Taniguchi, A.; Akahane, M.; Isomoto, S.; Sugimoto, K.; Tanaka, Y. Relationship between displacement and degenerative changes of the sesamoids in hallux valgus. *Foot Ankle Int.* **2016**, *37*, 1303–1309. [CrossRef]
28. Okuda, R.; Kinoshita, M.; Yasuda, T.; Jotoku, T.; Kitano, N.; Shima, H. Postoperative incomplete reduction of the sesamoids as a risk factor for recurrence of hallux valgus. *J. Bone Jt. Surg.* **2009**, *91*, 1637–1645. [CrossRef] [PubMed]

29. De Cesar Netto, C.; Saito, G.H.; Roney, A.; Day, J.; Greditzer, H.; Sofka, C.; Ellis, S.J.; Weight Bearing CT Society; Richter, M.; Barg, A.; et al. Combined weightbearing CT and MRI assessment of flexible progressive collapsing foot deformity. *Foot Ankle Surg.* 2021, 27, 884–891. [CrossRef]
30. Netto, C.d.C.; Li, S.; Vivtcharenko, V.; Auch, E.; Lintz, F.; Ellis, S.J.; Femino, J.E.; de Cesar Netto, C. Three-Dimensional Distance and Coverage Maps in the Assessment of Peritalar Subluxation in Progressive Collapsing Foot Deformity. *Foot Ankle Orthop.* 2022, 7, 2473011421S00177. [CrossRef]
31. Bakshi, N.; Steadman, J.; Philippi, M.; Arena, C.; Leake, R.; Saltzman, C.L.; Barg, A. Association between hindfoot alignment and first metatarsal rotation. *Foot Ankle Int.* 2022, 43, 105–112. [CrossRef]
32. Collan, L.; Kankare, J.A.; Mattila, K. The biomechanics of the first metatarsal bone in hallux valgus: A preliminary study utilizing a weight bearing extremity CT. *Foot Ankle Surg.* 2013, 19, 155–161. [CrossRef] [PubMed]
33. Bryant, A.; Tinley, P.; Singer, K. A comparison of radiographic measurements in normal, hallux valgus, and hallux limitus feet. *J. Foot Ankle Surg.* 2000, 39, 39–43. [CrossRef]
34. D'Arcangelo, P.R.; Landorf, K.B.; Munteanu, S.E.; Zammit, G.V.; Menz, H.B. Radiographic correlates of hallux valgus severity in older people. *J. Foot Ankle Res.* 2011, 4, 1. [CrossRef]
35. Menz, H.B.; Munteanu, S.E. Radiographic validation of the Manchester scale for the classification of hallux valgus deformity. *Rheumatology* 2005, 44, 1061–1066. [CrossRef] [PubMed]
36. Koo, T.K.; Li, M.Y. A guideline of selecting and reporting intraclass correlation coefficients for reliability research. *J. Chiropr. Med.* 2016, 15, 155–163. [CrossRef]
37. Landis, J.R.; Koch, G.G. The measurement of observer agreement for categorical data. *Biometrics* 1977, 33, 159–174. [CrossRef]
38. Srivastava, S.; Chockalingam, N.; El Fakhri, T. Radiographic angles in hallux valgus: Comparison between manual and computer-assisted measurements. *J. Foot Ankle Surg.* 2010, 49, 523–528. [CrossRef]
39. Biz, C.; Crimì, A.; Fantoni, I.; Tagliapietra, J.; Ruggieri, P. Functional and radiographic outcomes of minimally invasive intramedullary nail device (MIIND) for moderate to severe hallux valgus. *Foot Ankle Int.* 2021, 42, 409–424. [CrossRef]
40. Xiang, L.; Mei, Q.; Wang, A.; Shim, V.; Fernandez, J.; Gu, Y. Evaluating function in the hallux valgus foot following a 12-week minimalist footwear intervention: A pilot computational analysis. *J. Biomech.* 2022, 132, 110941. [CrossRef]
41. Janssen, D.M.; Sanders, A.P.; Guldemond, N.A.; Hermus, J.; Walenkamp, G.H.; Van Rhijn, L.W. A comparison of hallux valgus angles assessed with computerised plantar pressure measurements, clinical examination and radiography in patients with diabetes. *J. Foot Ankle Res.* 2014, 7, 1–9. [CrossRef]
42. Cullen, N.; Robinson, A.; Chayya, N.; Kes, J. Variation of the distal metatarsal articular angle with axial rotation of the first metatarsal. In *Orthopaedic Proceedings*; The British Editorial Society of Bone & Joint Surgery: London, UK, 2008; p. 228.
43. Chi, T.D.; Davitt, J.; Younger, A.; Holt, S.; Sangeorzan, B.J. Intra-and inter-observer reliability of the distal metatarsal articular angle in adult hallux valgus. *Foot Ankle Int.* 2002, 23, 722–726. [CrossRef] [PubMed]
44. Talbot, K.D.; Saltzman, C.L. Assessing sesamoid subluxation: How good is the AP radiograph? *Foot Ankle Int.* 1998, 19, 547–554. [CrossRef] [PubMed]
45. Mann, R.A.; Coughlin, M.J. Hallux valgus—Etiology, anatomy, treatment and surgical considerations. *Clin. Orthop. Relat. Res.* 1981, 157, 31–41. [CrossRef]
46. Silver, D. The operative treatment of hallux valgus. *J. Bone Jt. Surg.* 1923, 5, 225–232.
47. Saragas, N.P.; Becker, P.J. Comparative radiographic analysis of parameters in feet with and without hallux valgus. *Foot Ankle Int.* 1995, 16, 139–143. [CrossRef]
48. Hardy, R.; Clapham, J. Observations on hallux valgus. *J. Bone Jt. Surg. Br. Vol.* 1951, 33, 376–391. [CrossRef] [PubMed]
49. Kuwano, T.; Nagamine, R.; Sakaki, K.; Urabe, K.; Iwamoto, Y. New radiographic analysis of sesamoid rotation in hallux valgus: Comparison with conventional evaluation methods. *Foot Ankle Int.* 2002, 23, 811–817. [CrossRef]
50. Yildirim, Y.; Cabukoglu, C.; Erol, B.; Esemenli, T. Effect of metatarsophalangeal joint position on the reliability of the tangential sesamoid view in determining sesamoid position. *Foot Ankle Int.* 2005, 26, 247–250. [CrossRef]
51. Lee, K.; Cho, N.; Park, H.; Seon, J.; Lee, S. A comparison of proximal and distal Chevron osteotomy, both with lateral soft-tissue release, for moderate to severe hallux valgus in patients undergoing simultaneous bilateral correction: A prospective randomised controlled trial. *Bone Jt. J.* 2015, 97, 202–207. [CrossRef]

Disclaimer/Publisher's Note: The statements, opinions and data contained in all publications are solely those of the individual author(s) and contributor(s) and not of MDPI and/or the editor(s). MDPI and/or the editor(s) disclaim responsibility for any injury to people or property resulting from any ideas, methods, instructions or products referred to in the content.

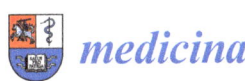 *medicina*

Review

Various Flexible Fixation Techniques Using Suture Button for Ligamentous Lisfranc Injuries: A Review of Surgical Options

Young Yi [1,*] and Sagar Chaudhari [2]

[1] Department of Orthopedic Surgery, Seoul Foot and Ankle Center, Inje University Seoul Paik Hospital, 85, 2-ga, Jeo-dong, Jung-gu, Seoul 04551, Republic of Korea
[2] Department of Orthopedic Surgery, K. B. Bhabha Hospital, Bandra, Mumbai 400050, Maharashtra, India; drsagarchaudhari@yahoo.com
* Correspondence: 20vvin@naver.com; Tel.: +82-2-2270-0028; Fax: +82-2-2270-0023

Abstract: Contrary to Lisfranc joint fracture-dislocation, ligamentous Lisfranc injury can lead to additional instability and arthritis and is difficult to diagnose. Appropriate procedure selection is necessary for a better prognosis. Several surgical methods have recently been introduced. Here, we present three distinct surgical techniques for treating ligamentous Lisfranc employing flexible fixation. First is the "Single Tightrope procedure", which involves reduction and fixation between the second metatarsal base and the medial cuneiform via making a bone tunnel and inserting Tightrope. Second is the "Dual Tightrope Technique", which is similar to the "Single Tightrope technique", with additional fixation of an intercuneiform joint using one MiniLok Quick Anchor Plus. Last but not least, the "internal brace approach" uses the SwiveLock anchor, particularly when intercueniform instability is seen. Each approach has its own advantages and disadvantages in terms of surgical complexity and stability. These flexible fixation methods, on the other hand, are more physiologic and have the potential to lessen the difficulties that have been linked to the use of conventional screws in the past.

Keywords: Lisfranc joint injury; flexible fixation technique; suture button; TightRope

1. Introduction

Only around 0.20% of all orthopedic injuries are Lisfranc joint injuries, which are an exceptionally uncommon trauma [1]. The severity of the injury is typically described as ranging from a little nondisplaced sprain to an apparent fracture dislocation of the midfoot. Ligamentous Lisfranc injury is typically produced by low energy trauma, making it challenging to identify and treat, in contrast to Lisfranc joint fracture-dislocation, which is typically caused by high energy trauma. If not properly and promptly treated, it may result in instability and post-traumatic arthritis in the patient [2]. Unfortunately, the prevalence of ligamentous Lisfranc injuries is rising as sports and professional athletes become more and more prominent (Figure 1). Numerous activities, including football, gymnastics, horseback riding, and jogging, have been linked to ligamentous Lisfranc injuries [3,4]. However, unlike high intensity injuries, indicators of ligamentous Lisfranc damage might not be as visible. The actual frequency of these injuries may thus be overestimated. Therefore, to diagnose ligamentous Lisfranc injuries, a proper physical examination and radiographs are needed.

After low intensity trauma, any patient who complains of midfoot discomfort should be examined, and Lisfranc damage should be ruled out. The injury mechanism is known to entail an axial stress applied to the forefoot being forcedly abducted or the foot being in a plantar flexed posture [5]. Physical findings that are favorable may include midfoot edema, plantar ecchymosis, difficulty bearing weight, a positive piano key stress test, and the dorsal drawer test of the medial column. Diastasis of the intermetatarsal gap between the first and second metatarsals, enlargement of the space between the medial cuneiform and second metatarsal base, the presence of a second metatarsal base fleck, and dorsal subluxation of the metatarsal base on a lateral view are all significant radiographic findings [6]. Patients with a strong clinical suspicion of Lisfranc injury and ambiguous radiographic results may undergo computerized tomography (CT) or magnetic resonance imaging (MRI).

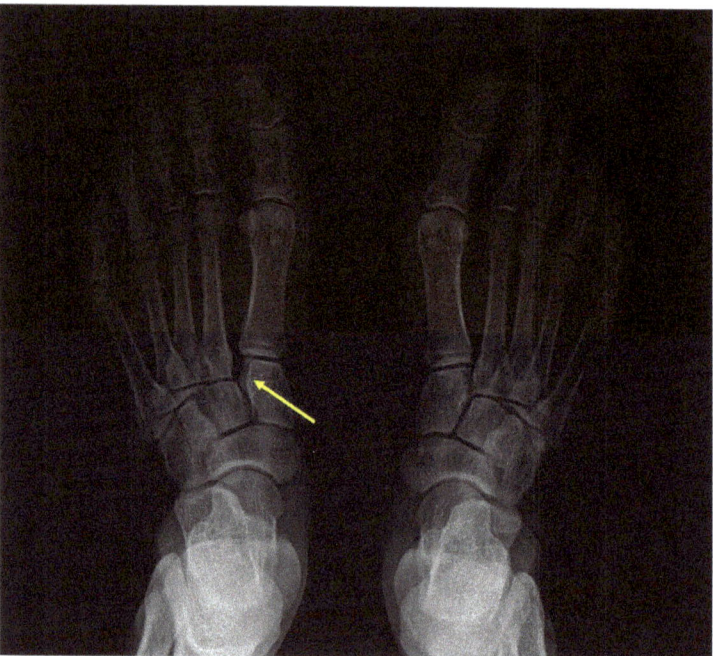

Figure 1. Standing plain radiographic image of bilateral foot. Diastasis between medial cuneiform and 2nd metatarsal base is observed on left foot (yellow arrow).

Computerized tomography (CT) is utilized to more precisely assess the congruity of the TMT joint because it can detect an avulsion fracture that would otherwise go undetected on conventional radiographs (Shim et al.) [7]. According to reports, examining and contrasting the affected and uninjured feet can aid in the diagnosis and treatment of Lisfranc ligament injuries. However, if there is no visible diastasis, subluxation, or dislocation, a minor Lisfranc injury could be overlooked on a typical CT scan. In their study, Kennelly et al. [8] contended that a typical CT scan only sometimes finds further injuries and does not offer any more information for individuals who have a positive weight-bearing film. Because it is a static modality of imaging, the traditional CT scan has a limited function in the diagnosis of mild Lisfranc injuries. A recent study found that a bilateral weight-bearing computed tomography is a good diagnostic tool for identifying Lisfranc injuries under physiological stress and provides a comparison with the unaffected side [8,9]. Patients may have a weight-bearing CT under an ankle block or may be sent to an orthopedic out-patient clinic for a few days following the accident if weight-bearing CT is not possible due to discomfort [8,10].

Dorsal, interosseous, and plantar Lisfranc ligaments are the three types of mild ligamentous injury that may be evaluated by magnetic resonance imaging (MRI). The first and most crucial step in treating a ligamentous Lisfranc injury is an accurate assessment of physical findings and radiography.

2. Classifications

Building on the work of earlier categorization methods, including those of Quenu, Kuss, and Hardcastle [11,12], Myerson developed the most well-known classification scheme in 1986. This method tries to group injuries based on the alignment of the joints, the location of the involvement, and the direction of instability. It is not predictive but it does shed light on different damage patterns and probable energy loss mechanisms that give rise to such patterns. This classification approach was found to have a good intra- and interobserver reliability [13]. Myerson recently modified his original categorization approach to include moderate, nondisplaced lesions [14]. He categorized these injuries as type D injuries and further separated them into D1 and D2 injuries. D1 injuries do not require surgical stabilization, in contrast to D2 injuries, which necessitate surgery if the medial cuneiform-second metatarsal gap increases by more than 2 mm. D2L injuries were exclusively ligamentous but D2B injuries were bone avulsions.

Nunley and Vertullo [15] developed a categorization system for sports Lisfranc sprains, which is shown in Table 1. This technique attempted to grade sprains using clinical information, weight-bearing radiographs, and bone scintigram findings. The ability to discriminate between injuries with and without longitudinal arch height collapse, as well as very mild nondisplaced injuries, is a benefit of this categorization system. However, due to the widespread use of magnetic resonance imaging (MRI) as an extra modality to detect moderate injuries, this categorization approach is not usually used. There are no categorization systems in use right now that can both direct care and predict results.

Table 1. Nunley and Vertullo classification of athletic Lisfranc injuries [15].

Type	Radiographic Diastasis	Radiographic Loss of Arch Length	Description
Stage I	None	None	- Ligament sprain. - Patients are unable to play sports. - Positive bone scintigram.
Stage II	1–5 mm	None	- Injury of the Lisfranc ligament accompanied with elongation or rupture.
Stage III	>5 mm	Decrease in distance between plantar base of the fifth metatarsal and plantar medial cuneiform.	- Progression of stage II accompanied by damaged plantar tarsometatarsal ligament and joints and potential fracture

Prior categories, however, had certain drawbacks in that choosing a surgical technique was not made any easier. Therefore, a new categorization for modest Lisfranc injury based on anatomical configuration is required. Medial cuneiform (C1)—second metatarsal bone (M2) ligament damage with diastasis is one possible variation of isolated Lisfranc ligament damage. Other variations include medial cuneiform (C1)—intermediate cuneiform (C2) instability, medial cuneiform (C1)—first metatarsal bone (M1) instability, and intermediate cuneiform (C2)—second metatarsal bone (M2) (Table 2 and Figure 2) [16].

Table 2. Classification of isolated ligamentous Lisfranc injuries based on anatomical configuration [16].

Type	Description
C1–M2	Medial cuneiform—second metatarsal bone damage with diastasis
C1–C2	Medial cuneiform—intermediate cuneiform instability
C1–M1	Medial cuneiform—first metatarsal bone instability
C2–M2	Intermediate cuneiform—second metatarsal bone instability

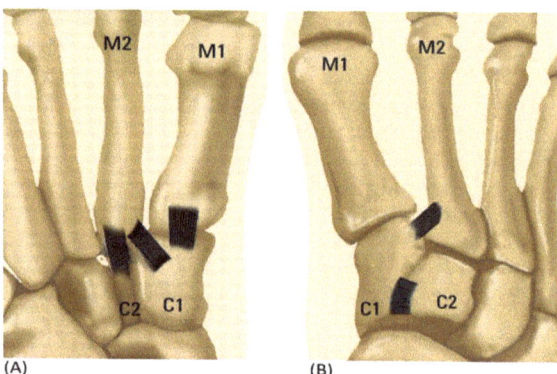

Figure 2. (**A**) A simplified illustration showing the anatomy of plantar sided ligamentous instability. (**B**) Isolated Ligamentous Lisfranc injuries reveal ligamentous instability in the dorsum.

According to the aforementioned types, a single tightrope may be preferred for C1-M2 injuries limited to diastasis [17], where damage with diastasis and the isolated Ligamentous Lisfranc injury are present. If C1–C2 instability is added [18] between medial cuneiform and intermediate cuneiform, a dual tightrope or internal brace may be preferred. Additionally, screw or plate fixation and reconstruction might be taken into consideration when there is joint instability. As a result, when considering flexible fixation surgery for ligamentous Lisfranc damage, surgeons must carefully assess the severity of the injury and the level of joint instability using adequate diagnostic skills, and they must then decide on the most suitable surgical strategy.

3. Previous Technical Overview

Over time, the operational method for Lisfranc injuries has evolved. For the best results, anatomic reduction should be performed regardless of the surgical technique [19]. There are several surgical methods available to treat Lisfranc injuries. The primary surgical options are K-wire fixation, screw fixation, adjustable suture button fixation, plate fixation, and arthrodesis [20,21]. When K-wires were used alone, high rates of fixation failure were seen [12]. Although the gold standard of therapy is screw fixation, complications include cartilage injury, screw loosening, head fracture, and the requirement for hardware removal continue to be a few of its issues [19,22–24] (Figure 3).

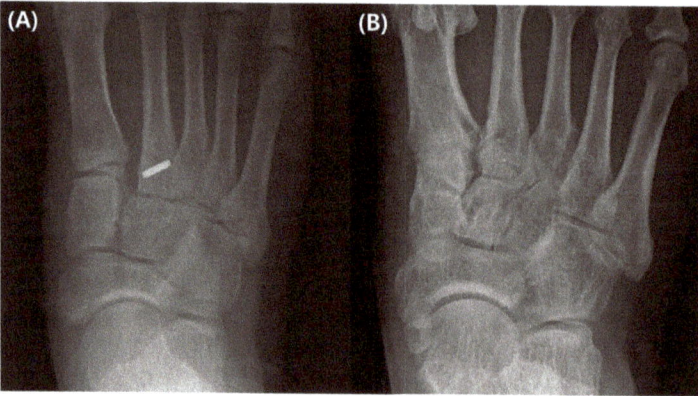

Figure 3. (**A**) A ligamentous Lisfranc injury has been treated with a conventional screw fixation. (**B**) A follow-up fluoroscopic picture taken following implant removal reveals decreased diastasis but arthritic change.

The orthopedic foot and ankle society has seen an increase in the use of suture buttons for ligamentous Lisfranc injuries in order to prevent these problems, which have positive clinical outcomes by better recreating normal architecture and providing greater physiological fixation [25,26].

Three flexible attachment methods will be covered in this article: Three different fixation methods are available: (1) Single TightRope (Arthrex, Naples, FL, USA), (2) Dual TightRope (MiniLok QuickAnchor Plus (DePuy, Mitek, Raynham, MA, USA), and (3) InternalBrace (Arthrex, Naples, FL, USA). Each surgical method will be briefly discussed and accompanied by a case study.

4. Operative Technique—Single TightRope

A pneumatic tourniquet was applied to the thigh during the procedure while the patient was in the supine position and under general or spinal anesthesia. Under fluoroscopy, the diastasis between the medial cuneiform and second metatarsal base was assessed. Just lateral to the second metatarsal base, a longitudinal dorsal skin incision was made, allowing for the identification and medial retraction of the extensor hallucis brevis. This was performed to safeguard the underlying neurovascular bundle. A medial skin incision was made over the center of medial cuneiform. A bone-reduction clamp was then used to reduce the damaged Lisfranc joint following this incision. The decrease achieved was then verified and documented using fluoroscopy. To properly reduce the Lisfranc joint, it is crucial to hold the clamp in the right vector. Under the supervision of fluoroscopy, a guide wire was then inserted along the Lisfranc ligament's length, beginning at the mid-coronal plane of the medial cuneiform and ending just distal to the insertion of the tibialis anterior to the base of the second metatarsal bone.

To avoid damaging the Lisfranc joint, a 3.5 mm reamer was utilized to ream along the guide wire from medial to lateral. Then, a passing pin was used to insert TightRope into the bone tunnel. An oblong button was then placed with the proper tension on the periosteum of the medial cuneiform after the leading button had been placed on the lateral cortex of the second metatarsal base (Figure 4).

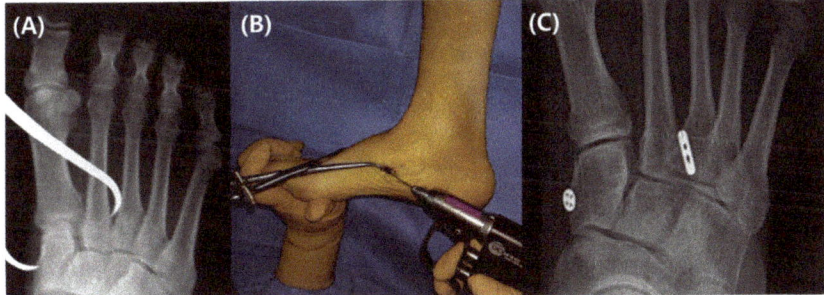

Figure 4. (**A**) A reduction clamp operated under a fluoroscopic image intensifier was used to diminish the diastasis between the medial cuneiform and second metatarsal base. (**B**) The Lisfranc joint was traversed using a guide wire. (**C**) An oblong button was positioned medial to the center of the medial cuneiform and an endobutton was positioned at the lateral cortex of the second metatarsal base.

Patients with poor bone mineral density, however, run the risk of experiencing suture button migration since the TightRope procedure necessitates reaming a bone tunnel (Figure 5). The Lisfranc joint might be lost or reduced as a result of further issues. Consequently, it is important to choose patients carefully, and extensive bone reaming should be avoided.

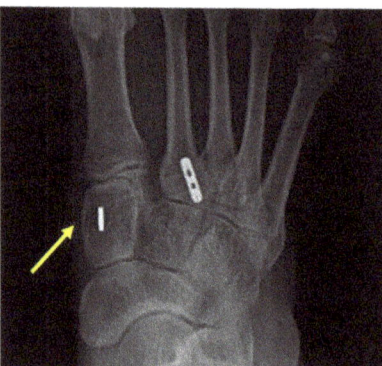

Figure 5. Recurrent diastasis of Lisfranc joint is observed due to internal migration of oblong button (yellow arrow).

5. Operative Technique—Dual TightRope

One Mini TightRope and one MiniLok QuickAnchor Plus were used for the Lisfranc fixation procedure employing dual TightRope. A medial skin incision was made across the center of the medial cuneiform and a similar longitudinal dorsal skin incision was performed just lateral to the second metatarsal base. Under the direction of fluoroscopy, a bone-reduction clamp was used to reduce the damaged Lisfranc joint. Surgeons must exercise caution to safeguard the neurovascular bundle dorsally and the anterior tibialis medially, which is equivalent to the single TightRope approach. After using the bone clamp to reduce the Lisfranc joint, the guide wire was initially positioned immediately distal to the second and third metatarsal articulations, from the medial cuneiform to the lateral cortex of the second metatarsal base. After reaming, a passing pin was used to introduce the Mini TightRope into the bone tunnel, making sure the lateral button was securely situated at the lateral cortex of the second metatarsal base. After ensuring that the medial button was firmly positioned at the medial cuneiform, the Mini TightRope was then tightened. Beginning proximally and dorsally to the first inserted Mini TightRope, the guide wire for the MiniLok QuickAnchor Plus crossed the intercuneiform joint between the medial and intermediate cuneiform. The middle of the intermediate cuneiform was reamed using a reamer. After using a bone clamp to narrow the gap between the medial and intermediate cuneiforms, a second anchor was subsequently placed. Pulling the connecting fiber wire gently confirms augmentation (Figure 6).

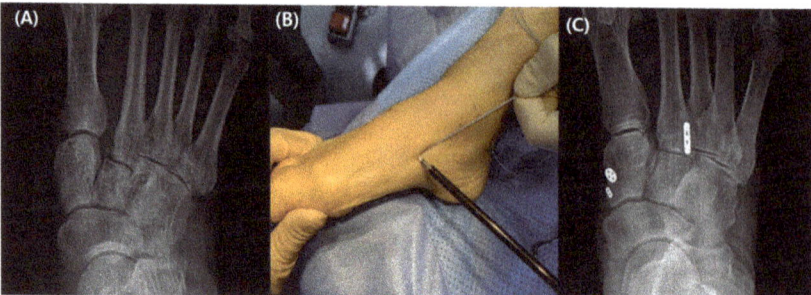

Figure 6. (**A**) A plain radiograph taken prior to surgery demonstrating diastasis of the Lisfranc joint (**B**) Mini TightRope put into the medial cuneiform (**C**) MiniLok QuickAnchor Plus anchor implanted more proximally than Mini TightRope.

6. Operative Technique—InternalBrace

InternalBrace Lisfranc fixation is advantageous, particularly when intercuneiform instability is noted following a Lisfranc joint fixed. Using a Freer elevator, the stability of the intercuneiform joint was assessed, and an unrestricted passage of the Freer between the medial and intermediate cuneiform verified the instability of the joint. After achieving the proper reduction of the Lisfranc joint, the guide wire was placed similarly to the previous two procedures from the base of the second metatarsal to the medial cuneiform. A 4.75 mm SwiveLock Anchor was then fixed to the center of the medial cuneiform while the proper tension was given, after which the button was inserted at the lateral cortex of the second metatarsal base. The remaining FiberTape suture was then moved over to the intermediate cuneiform through the dorsal incision using a pair of mosquito forceps. The remaining FiberTape was then passed through the hole from the dorsum to the plantar side, starting at the dorsum of the intermediate cuneiform and drilling perpendicularly. A 3.5 mm SwiveLock Anchor was secured to the intermediate cuneiform after the proper amount of tension had been verified via fluoroscopy (Figure 7).

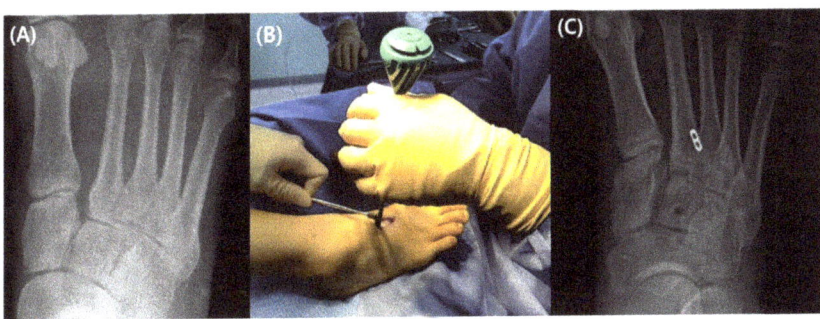

Figure 7. (**A**) A preoperative fluoroscopic image demonstrating the diastasis of the Lisfranc joint and the intercuneiform joint (**B**) A postoperative fluoroscopic image demonstrating the reduced Lisfranc joint and intercuneiform joint (**C**).

7. Other Surgical Technique (Ligament Reconstructions)

Flexible fixation of a Lisfranc injury may be achievable with ligamentous repair as a treatment option. Chronic Lisfranc instability, which is characterized as clinical impairments (pain, instability, or deformity in the tarsometatarsal region) due to post-traumatic symptoms that last longer than six weeks, has historically been treated with this technique [27–29]. However, Lisfranc joint arthrodesis is more recommended than ligamentous repair if there is an arthritic alteration in the tarsometatarsal joint [17,29,30].

There have been reports of several surgical procedures for ligamentous reconstruction. A third extensor digitorum longus tendon-based anatomical three bone tunnel reconstruction approach was developed by Nery et al. [31]. The Lisfranc joint has three layers: the dorsal, interosseous, and plantar parts. Biologically, the "Y" plantar ligament between the medial cuneiform and the second to third metatarsals and the Lisfranc ligament between the medial cuneiform and the second metatarsal are the two strongest ligaments [32]. The preparation of three bone tunnels is carried out in a similar manner. Between medial, intermediate, and lateral cuneiform, the first tunnel was created. A second tunnel was created between the second metatarsal and medial cuneiform. The third tunnel was then created between the third metatarsal and medial cuneiform.

Following that, Miyamoto et al. [17] reported a technique for ligamentous restoration using two bundles of the gracilis tendon. The strongest interosseous Lisfranc ligament can be stabilized by creating a bone tunnel between the medial cuneiform and the second metatarsal. The dorsal ligament and interosseous (Lisfranc) ligament, which has been reported as the strongest of these ligaments, were reconstructed, but the plantar ligament between the medial cuneiform and the second metatarsal bone could not be reconstructed due to technical difficulties. As a result, the technique does not achieve true anatomical reconstruction.

The gracilis tendon was used in a four-bundle repair procedure that was presented by De Los Santos-Real et al. [28]. The intermetatarsal joint initially consists of a bone tunnel between the medial cuneiform and second metatarsal, but additional bundles are subsequently produced on the dorsal and plantar portions of the joint. This method is advantageous in that it can recreate the dorsal, interosseous, and plantar layers of the Lisfranc joint to its original shape (Figure 8) [17,28,31]; nevertheless, it has drawbacks such as morbidity at the donor graft location and the need for precise technical skill to remove and deliver sufficient length graft to replicate the three ligament complex bundles.

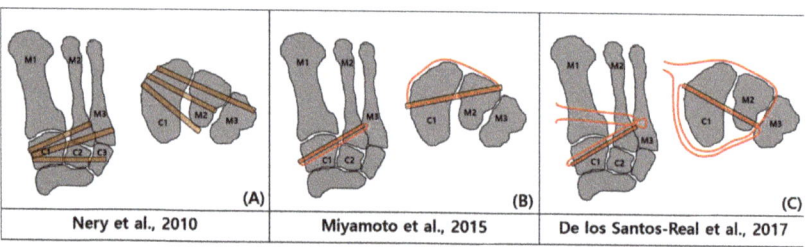

Figure 8. (**A**) third extensor digitorum longus tendon was employed in a triple bone tunnel by Nery et al. [31] to repair the Lisfranc ligament in patients with chronic Lisfranc injury who did not develop arthritis. (**B**) Gracilis tendon was used in a 2-bundled method by Miyamoto et al. [17] (**C**) De los Santos-Real et al. [28] built a 4-bundled repaired ligament using gracilis tendon.

Depending on the surgeon's experience, these Lisfranc ligamentous restoration approaches might be taken into consideration for revision surgery if the flexible fixation technique failed when using the same bone tunnel.

8. Postoperative Management

On postoperative day 3, a brief leg cast is put on the operated foot if there is no skin issue. Patients are kept off their feet for four weeks. At the fourth week following surgery, the cast is removed, and the patient is given a boot. At this point, gradual weight bearing and range of motion activities are started under the guidance of a medical professional. Patients are encouraged to wear regular shoes, receive physical therapy at two months, and are permitted to completely bear weight with an arch support. Three months after surgery, weight-bearing workouts and athletic endeavors can be started. To ensure the technique's best possible results, competitive sports can be resumed six months after surgery.

This technique has a benefit over others that use K-wire, screws, or plates since there is no need to remove hardware, theoretically. As a result, early rehabilitation may be started without worrying about late diastasis from poor ligament integrity following metal removal [33].

9. Discussion

The metatarsal joint is made up of the medial column, middle column, and lateral column, which together make up a substantial structural component of the mid-foot. It preserves the lateral stability of the joint by forming a characteristic "arch" structure in the cross section between the metatarsal and tarsal bones. The second metatarsal bone is placed between the medial cuneiform and the lateral bone to produce a mortise and tenon structure that acts as a "wedge stone" for the longitudinal stability of the tarsometatarsal joint [34,35]. A number of various sorts of injuries can affect the tarsometatarsal joint, ranging from low-energy ones with minimal subluxations or instability to high-energy ones with a very unstable mid-foot. Low energy injuries occur most commonly and are usually accompanied by ligamentous Lisfranc injuries as a result of axial, rotational, or twisting injuries, especially during movements such as sprinting, leaping, and twisting the weight-bearing foot [36–39]. The Lisfranc ligament, a strong tissue that joins the medial column to the middle column, is the most important interosseous ligament. Seventy-three percent of feet have a single bundle, while 27% have a double bundle [40].

The severity of a Lisfranc injury can range from ligamentous damage to tarsometatarsal joint fracture-dislocations. Ligamentous Lisfranc injuries are becoming more common as a result of people's increased involvement in sports. No matter the damage pattern, a sufficient decrease must be attained for the best results.

The best way to repair a Lisfranc injury is still up for debate [41]. Treatment options for Lisfranc injuries range from K-wire fixation to screw fixation to plate fixation to fixation employing different suture buttons [20,23,25,42]. Fixation has traditionally relied on hard fixation methods such as screw fixation or K-wire fixation. Screw fixation has been demonstrated to offer more biomechanical stability than K-wire fixation [41]. The higher risk of arthritis brought on by articular injury and the probable necessity for hardware removal are drawbacks of transarticular screw fixation [22,23,42]. In actuality, all stiff type fixations restrict mobility in the damaged foot's medial column, leading to discomfort or screw breakage during demanding exercises. Additionally, if a patient's fixation duration was very brief, it may have contributed to Lisfranc joint dissociation when the screw was removed [42].

For ligamentous, lower-energy injuries, the authors favor maintaining the midfoot articulations. When using various suture button procedures to treat ligamentous Lisfranc injury, authors have seen good clinical and radiological results. By using biological replacements, a notion of non-rigid fixation in Lisfranc joint damage has been put forth. The same idea is used in Fiberwire devices, which avoid sacrificing the autologous tendons and their associated morbidities [43,44].

Single mini-TightRope Lisfranc fixations have had positive clinical outcomes [25,45]. While reducing the Lisfranc joint's anatomical and physiological dimensions, mobility is preserved. Comparative to the other two suture button procedures, this one is rather straightforward. However, it is possible to see subsidence and the displacement of the buttons into the brand-new tunnel.

Additionally, research on cadavers demonstrates that a single TightRope does not offer enough stability in comparison to screw fixation [46]. The intercuneiform joint between the medial and intermediate cuneiform benefits from the insertion of a second TightRope because it offers more rotational and compressive stability, which prevents Lisfranc joint diastasis from occurring again [18]. The Lisfranc and intercuneiform joints may suffer articular injury with this dual TightRope method, which is more difficult to execute than a single TightRope approach.

Using a 1.6 mm K-wire instead of a 3.5 mm drill bit, InternalBrace has the benefit of reducing articular injury when compared to the suture button procedure. Additionally, it stabilizes the intercuneiform joint as well as the Lisfranc joint, similar to the dual TightRope approach. The dorsal cortex of the medial and intermediate cuneiform, however, may become irritated by Fiberwire. It should be highlighted that InternalBrace Lisfranc fixation is a relatively new procedure, and further research will be required to evaluate its clinical efficacy and failure rate [47] (Table 3).

Skin issues, infections, loss of reduction, neurovascular damage, and post-traumatic arthritis, which may be a possible source of persistent pain, are possible complications of these procedures after surgical therapy. In order to avoid the "N" wrinkle of the implanted suture and reduce friction between the suture and the bone tunnel during foot movement, which ultimately prevents the disruption of the suture, it is also important to prevent the alteration of the bone tunnel between the medial cuneiform bone and the second metatarsal bone. Additionally, while knotting in the medial surface of the medial cuneiform bone, great care should be given to ensuring that the knot is not too big as this might quickly result in a subcutaneous foreign body response and inflammation. Patients with underlying infections, considerable soft tissue edema, medical conditions, peripheral vascular disease, severe bone comminution, and Charcot neuropathy are also often contraindicated for these treatments.

Table 3. Advantages and disadvantages of three flexible fixation technique.

Surgical Technique	Advantages	Disadvantages
Single TightRope Technique	- Preservation of mobility on Lisfranc joint - Relatively simple procedure [45]	- Relatively weak stability [17]
Dual TightRope Technique	- Higher resistance to rotational force [18]	- Relatively challenging procedure [18]
Internal brace Technique	- Minimal articular damage on Lisfranc joint [48]	- Irritation on dorsal cortex of cuneiforms [49]

10. Conclusions

For the treatment of ligamentous Lisfranc injuries, various flexible fixation methods can be utilized as an alternative to the screw fixation approach. With early rehabilitation and range-of-motion, fixation utilizing a tightrope and internal brace better preserves the natural anatomy and is therefore more physiological. Additionally, it avoids subsequent surgery for hardware removal and lessens the possibility of articular injury brought on by screw fixation.

Author Contributions: The study was designed and supervised by Y.Y.; Y.Y. and S.C. wrote the initial draft of the manuscript and analyzed the data; Y.Y. wrote the manuscript; S.C. performed the statistical analysis; Y.Y. revised the manuscript and was the guarantor of this work and had full access to all the data used in the study and takes responsibility for the integrity of the data and the accuracy of the data analysis. All authors have read and agreed to the published version of the manuscript.

Funding: This research received no external funding.

Institutional Review Board Statement: Not applicable.

Informed Consent Statement: Not applicable.

Data Availability Statement: Not applicable.

Conflicts of Interest: The authors have no conflict of interest.

References

1. Shapiro, M.S.; Wascher, D.C.; Finerman, G.A. Rupture of Lisfranc's ligament in athletes. *Am. J. Sport. Med.* **1994**, *22*, 687–691. [CrossRef] [PubMed]
2. Garríguez-Pérez, D.; Puerto-Vázquez, M.; Tomé Delgado, J.L.; Galeote, E.; Marco, F. Impact of the Subtle Lisfranc Injury on Foot Structure and Function. *Foot Ankle Int.* **2021**, *42*, 1303–1310. [CrossRef] [PubMed]
3. Kalia, V.; Fishman, E.K.; Carrino, J.A.; Fayad, L.M. Epidemiology, imaging, and treatment of Lisfranc fracture-dislocations revisited. *Skelet. Radiol.* **2012**, *41*, 129–136. [CrossRef]
4. De Orio, M.; Erickson, M.; Usuelli, F.G.; Easley, M. Lisfranc injuries in sport. *Foot Ankle Clin.* **2009**, *14*, 169–186. [CrossRef]
5. Curtis, M.J.; Myerson, M.; Szura, B. Tarsometatarsal joint injuries in the athlete. *Am. J. Sport. Med.* **1993**, *21*, 497–502. [CrossRef] [PubMed]
6. Gupta, R.T.; Wadhwa, R.P.; Learch, T.J.; Herwick, S.M. Lisfranc injury: Imaging findings for this important but often-missed diagnosis. *Curr. Probl. Diagn. Radiol.* **2008**, *37*, 115–126. [CrossRef]
7. Shim, D.W.; Choi, E.; Park, Y.-C.; Shin, S.C.; Lee, J.W.; Sung, S.-Y. Comparing bilateral feet computed tomography scans can improve surgical decision making for subtle Lisfranc injury. *Arch. Orthop. Trauma Surg.* **2022**, *142*, 3705–3714. [CrossRef]
8. Kennelly, H.; Klaassen, K.; Heitman, D.; Youngberg, R.; Platt, S.R. Utility of weight-bearing radiographs compared to computed tomography scan for the diagnosis of subtle Lisfranc injuries in the emergency setting. *Emerg. Med. Australas.* **2019**, *31*, 741–744. [CrossRef]
9. Bhimani, R.; Ashkani-Esfahani, S.; Lubberts, B.; Guss, D.; Hagemeijer, N.C.; Waryasz, G.; DiGiovanni, C.W. Utility of volumetric measurement via weight-bearing computed tomography scan to diagnose syndesmotic instability. *Foot Ankle Int.* **2020**, *41*, 859–865. [CrossRef]
10. Ponkilainen, V.T.; Laine, H.-J.; Mäenpää, H.M.; Mattila, V.M.; Haapasalo, H.H. Incidence and characteristics of midfoot injuries. *Foot Ankle Int.* **2019**, *40*, 105–112. [CrossRef]

11. Quénu, E. Etude sur les luxations du metatarse (luxations metatarsotarsiennes) du diastasis entre 1er et le 2e metatarsien. *Rev. Chir.* **1909**, *39*, 1093–1134.
12. Hardcastle, P.; Reschauer, R.; Kutscha-Lissberg, E.; Schoffmann, W. Injuries to the tarsometatarsal joint. Incidence, classification and treatment. *J. Bone Jt. Surgery. Br. Vol.* **1982**, *64*, 349–356. [CrossRef] [PubMed]
13. Mahmoud, S.; Hamad, F.; Riaz, M.; Ahmed, G.; Al Ateeq, M.; Ibrahim, T. Reliability of the Lisfranc injury radiological classification (Myerson-modified Hardcastle classification system). *Int. Orthop.* **2015**, *39*, 2215–2218. [CrossRef] [PubMed]
14. Sivakumar, B.S.; An, V.V.; Oitment, C.; Myerson, M. Subtle Lisfranc injuries: A topical review and modification of the classification system. *Orthopedics* **2018**, *41*, e168–e175. [CrossRef] [PubMed]
15. Data from Nunley, J.A.; Vertullo, C.J. Classification, investigation, and management of midfoot sprains: Lisfranc injuries in the athlete. *Am. J. Sport. Med.* **2002**, *30*, 871–878. [CrossRef]
16. Sripanich, Y.; Steadman, J.; Kraehenbuehl, N.; Rungprai, C.; Saltzman, C.L.; Lenz, A.L.; Barg, A. Anatomy and biomechanics of the Lisfranc ligamentous complex: A systematic literature review. *J. Biomech.* **2021**, *119*, 110287. [CrossRef]
17. Miyamoto, W.; Takao, M.; Innami, K.; Miki, S.; Matsushita, T. Ligament reconstruction with single bone tunnel technique for chronic symptomatic subtle injury of the Lisfranc joint in athletes. *Arch. Orthop. Trauma Surg.* **2015**, *135*, 1063–1070. [CrossRef]
18. Crates, J.M.; Barber, F.A. Dual tightrope fixation for subtle lisfranc injuries. *Tech. Foot Ankle Surg.* **2012**, *11*, 163–167. [CrossRef]
19. Kuo, R.; Tejwani, N.; Digiovanni, C.; Holt, S.; Benirschke, S.; Hansen, S., Jr.; Sangeorzan, B. Outcome after open reduction and internal fixation of Lisfranc joint injuries. *JBJS* **2000**, *82*, 1609. [CrossRef]
20. Ly, T.V.; Coetzee, J.C. Treatment of primarily ligamentous Lisfranc joint injuries: Primary arthrodesis compared with open reduction and internal fixation: A prospective, randomized study. *J. Bone Jt. Surg.* **2006**, *88*, 514–520.
21. Stavlas, P.; Roberts, C.S.; Xypnitos, F.N.; Giannoudis, P.V. The role of reduction and internal fixation of Lisfranc fracture–dislocations: A systematic review of the literature. *Int. Orthop.* **2010**, *34*, 1083–1091. [CrossRef] [PubMed]
22. Panchbhavi, V.K.; Vallurupalli, S.; Yang, J.; Andersen, C.R. Screw fixation compared with suture-button fixation of isolated Lisfranc ligament injuries. *JBJS* **2009**, *91*, 1143–1148. [CrossRef] [PubMed]
23. Cho, J.; Kim, J.; Min, T.-H.; Chun, D.-I.; Won, S.H.; Park, S.; Yi, Y. Suture Button vs. Conventional Screw Fixation for Isolated Lisfranc Ligament Injuries. *Foot Ankle Int.* **2021**, *42*, 598–608. [CrossRef]
24. Chun, D.-I.; Kim, J.; Min, T.-H.; Cho, J.; Won, S.H.; Lee, M.; Yi, Y. Fixation of isolated Lisfranc ligament injury with the TightRope™: A technical report. *Orthop. Traumatol. Surg. Res.* **2021**, *107*, 102940. [CrossRef]
25. Brin, Y.S.; Nyska, M.; Kish, B. Lisfranc injury repair with the TightRope™ device: A short-term case series. *Foot Ankle Int.* **2010**, *31*, 624–627. [CrossRef]
26. Cottom, J.M.; Hyer, C.F.; Berlet, G.C. Treatment of Lisfranc fracture dislocations with an interosseous suture button technique: A review of 3 cases. *J. Foot Ankle Surg.* **2008**, *47*, 250–258. [CrossRef]
27. Charlton, T.; Boe, C.; Thordarson, D.B. Suture button fixation treatment of chronic Lisfranc injury in professional dancers and high-level athletes. *J. Danc. Med. Sci.* **2015**, *19*, 135–139. [CrossRef] [PubMed]
28. De los Santos-Real, R.; Canillas, F.; Varas-Navas, J.; Morales-Muñoz, P.; Barrio-Sanz, P.; Medina-Santos, M. Lisfranc joint ligament complex reconstruction: A promising solution for missed, delayed, or chronic Lisfranc injury without arthritis. *J. Foot Ankle Surg.* **2017**, *56*, 1350–1356. [CrossRef]
29. Sripanich, Y.; Weinberg, M.W.; Krähenbühl, N.; Rungprai, C.; Haller, J.; Saltzman, C.L.; Barg, A. Surgical outcome of chronic Lisfranc injury without secondary degenerative arthritis: A systematic literature review. *Injury* **2020**, *51*, 1258–1265. [CrossRef]
30. Zwipp, H.; Rammelt, S. Anatomical reconstruction of chronically instable Lisfranc's ligaments. *Der Unf.* **2014**, *117*, 791–797.
31. Data from Nery, C.; Réssio, C.; Alloza, J.F.M. Subtle Lisfranc joint ligament lesions: Surgical neoligamentplasty technique. *Foot Ankle Clin.* **2012**, *17*, 407–416. [CrossRef]
32. Hirano, T.; Niki, H.; Beppu, M. Anatomical considerations for reconstruction of the Lisfranc ligament. *J. Orthop. Sci.* **2013**, *18*, 720–726. [CrossRef]
33. VanPelt, M.D.; Athey, A.; Yao, J.; Ennin, K.; Kassem, L.; Mulligan, E.; Lalli, T.; Liu, G.T. Is routine hardware removal following open reduction internal fixation of tarsometatarsal joint fracture/dislocation necessary? *J. Foot Ankle Surg.* **2019**, *58*, 226–230. [CrossRef]
34. Cenatiempo, M.; Buzzi, R.; Bianco, S.; Iapalucci, G.; Campanacci, D.A. Tarsometatarsal joint complex injuries: A study of injury pattern in complete homolateral lesions. *Injury* **2019**, *50* (Suppl. 2), S8–S11. [CrossRef]
35. Moracia-Ochagavía, I.; Rodríguez-Merchán, E.C. Lisfranc fracture-dislocations: Current management. *EFORT Open Rev.* **2019**, *4*, 430–444. [CrossRef]
36. Pourmorteza, M.; Vosoughi, A.R. Lisfranc fleck sign: Characteristics and clinical outcomes following fixation using a percutaneous position Lisfranc screw. *Eur. J. Trauma Emerg. Surg.* **2022**, *48*, 471–479. [CrossRef] [PubMed]
37. Nery, C.; Baumfeld, D.; Baumfeld, T.; Prado, M.; Giza, E.; Wagner, P.; Wagner, E. Comparison of Suture-Augmented Ligamentplasty to Transarticular Screws in a Lisfranc Cadaveric Model. *Foot Ankle Int.* **2020**, *41*, 735–743. [CrossRef] [PubMed]
38. Porter, D.A.; Barnes, A.F.; Rund, A.; Walrod, M.T. Injury Pattern in Ligamentous Lisfranc Injuries in Competitive Athletes. *Foot Ankle Int.* **2019**, *40*, 185–194. [CrossRef]
39. Park, Y.H.; Ahn, J.H.; Choi, G.W.; Kim, H.J. Percutaneous Reduction and 2.7-mm Cortical Screw Fixation for Low-Energy Lisfranc Injuries. *J. Foot Ankle Surg.* **2020**, *59*, 914–918. [CrossRef] [PubMed]

40. Panchbhavi, V.K.; Molina, D., IV; Villarreal, J.; Curry, M.C.; Andersen, C.R. Three-dimensional, digital, and gross anatomy of the Lisfranc ligament. *Foot Ankle Int.* **2013**, *34*, 876–880. [CrossRef]
41. Lee, C.A.; Birkedal, J.P.; Dickerson, E.A.; Vieta, P.A.; Webb, L.X.; Teasdall, R.D. Stabilization of Lisfranc joint injuries: A biomechanical study. *Foot Ankle Int.* **2004**, *25*, 365–370. [CrossRef] [PubMed]
42. Alberta, F.G.; Aronow, M.S.; Barrero, M.; Diaz-Doran, V.; Sullivan, R.J.; Adams, D.J. Ligamentous Lisfranc joint injuries: A biomechanical comparison of dorsal plate and transarticular screw fixation. *Foot Ankle Int.* **2005**, *26*, 462–473. [CrossRef] [PubMed]
43. Grass, R.; Rammelt, S.; Biewener, A.; Zwipp, H. Peroneus longus ligamentoplasty for chronic instability of the distal tibiofibular syndesmosis. *Foot Ankle Int.* **2003**, *24*, 392–397. [CrossRef]
44. Baravarian, B.; Geffen, D. Lisfranc tightrope. *Foot Ankle Spec.* **2009**, *2*, 249–250. [CrossRef] [PubMed]
45. Yongfei, F.; Chaoyu, L.; Wenqiang, X.; Xiulin, M.; Jian, X.; Wei, W. Clinical outcomes of Tightrope system in the treatment of purely ligamentous Lisfranc injuries. *BMC Surg.* **2021**, *21*, 395. [CrossRef]
46. Ahmed, S.; Bolt, B.; McBryde, A. Comparison of standard screw fixation versus suture button fixation in Lisfranc ligament injuries. *Foot Ankle Int.* **2020**, *31*, 892–896. [CrossRef]
47. Delman, C.; Patel, M.; Campbell, M.; Kreulen, C.; Giza, E. Flexible fixation technique for Lisfranc injuries. *Foot Ankle Int.* **2019**, *40*, 1338–1345. [CrossRef]
48. Gentchos, C. Lisfranc Injuries. *Tech. Foot Ankle Surg.* **2021**, *20*, 66–74. [CrossRef]
49. Briceno, J.; Leucht, A.-K.; Younger, A.; Veljkovic, A. Subtle Lisfranc injuries: Fix it, fuse it, or bridge it? *Foot Ankle Clin.* **2020**, *25*, 711–726. [CrossRef]

Disclaimer/Publisher's Note: The statements, opinions and data contained in all publications are solely those of the individual author(s) and contributor(s) and not of MDPI and/or the editor(s). MDPI and/or the editor(s) disclaim responsibility for any injury to people or property resulting from any ideas, methods, instructions or products referred to in the content.

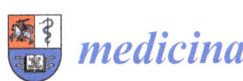

Article

The Superficial Peroneal Nerve Is at Risk during the "All Inside" Arthroscopic Broström Procedure: A Cadaveric Study

Sung Hwan Kim [1], Jae Hyuck Choi [2], Sang Heon Lee [1] and Young Koo Lee [1,*]

[1] Department of Orthopaedic Surgery, Soonchunhyang University Hospital Bucheon, 170, Jomaru-ro, Wonmi-gu, Bucheon-si 14584, Republic of Korea; shk9528@naver.com (S.H.K.); worldking70@naver.com (S.H.L.)
[2] Department of Orthopedics, Manjok Clinic, 178, Jibeom-ro, Suseong-gu, Daegu 42208, Republic of Korea; manjokclinic@naver.com
* Correspondence: brain0808@hanmail.net

Abstract: *Background*: The arthroscopic Broström procedure is a promising treatment for chronic ankle instability. However, little is known regarding the location of the intermediate superficial peroneal nerve at the level of the inferior extensor retinaculum; knowledge about this location is important for procedural safety. The purpose of this cadaveric study was to clarify the anatomical relationship between the intermediate superficial peroneal nerve and the sural nerve at the level of the inferior extensor retinaculum. *Methods*: Eleven dissections of cadaveric lower extremities were performed. The origin of the experimental three-dimensional axis was defined as the location of the anterolateral portal during ankle arthroscopy. The distances from the standard anterolateral portal to the inferior extensor retinaculum, sural nerve, and intermediate superficial peroneal nerve were measured using an electronic digital caliper. The location of inferior extensor retinaculum, the tract of sural nerve, and intermediate superficial peroneal nerve were checked using average and standard deviations. For the statistical analyses, data are presented as average ± standard deviation, and then they are reported as means and standard deviations. Fisher's exact test was used to identify statistically significant differences. *Results*: At the level of the inferior extensor retinaculum, the mean distances from the anterolateral portal to the proximal and distal intermediate superficial peroneal nerve were 15.9 ± 4.1 (range, 11.3–23.0) mm and 30.1 ± 5.5 (range, 20.8–37.9) mm, respectively. The mean distances from the anterolateral portal to the proximal and distal sural nerve were 47.6 ± 5.7 (range, 37.4–57.2) mm and 47.2 ± 4.1 (range, 41.0–51.8) mm, respectively. *Conclusions*: During the arthroscopic Broström procedure, the intermediate superficial peroneal nerve may be damaged by the anterolateral portal; the proximal and distal parts of the intermediate superficial peroneal nerve were located within 15.9 and 30.1 mm, respectively, at the level of the inferior extensor retinaculum in cadavers. These areas should be considered danger zones during the arthroscopic Broström procedure.

Keywords: arthroscopic modified Broström procedure; ankle anterolateral portal; cadaver; intermediate superficial peroneal nerve

1. Introduction

Ankle sprains, particularly lateral inversion sprains, are the most common ankle injuries; they constitute 85% of all cases [1]. The lateral ligament complex is typically involved in these injuries, which can vary from a microscopic tear to a complete tear [2]. In cases of inversion sprain, the most commonly injured ligament is the anterior talofibular ligament (ATFL), which stabilizes the ankle in plantar flexion during inversion stress. Acute injuries typically respond to conservative treatment, including immobilization and functional rehabilitation. However, up to 34% of patients experience repeated ankle sprains, leading to chronic ankle instability in 5–20% of cases [3,4]. The presence of pain and subjective sense of instability may result in additional ankle injuries. Chronic ankle instability may alter the ankle joint biomechanics, leading to cartilage degeneration and secondary osteoarthritis, which require surgical intervention [5]. In particular, varus ankle instability caused by medially shifting contact pressure can cause osteochondral lesions of the talus in the medial talar dome. The lateral ligament complex of the ankle consists of the ATFL, calcaneofibular ligament (CFL), and posterior talofibular ligament (PTFL). The ATFL and CFL are mainly responsible for ankle instability. The ATFL originates at the inferior segment of the anterior border of the distal fibula and inserts on the body of the talus, anterior to the lateral articular surface. The CFL originates immediately distal to the inferior band of the ATFL and inserts on the lateral calcaneal surface [6]. The ATFL prevents inversion and anterior displacement of the talus and the CFL stabilizes the subtalar joint. The lateral ligament complex is most commonly injured by inversion and plantar flexion. Although isolated ATFL ruptures are common, moderate to severe injuries may involve both the ATFL and CFL. Isolated CFL ruptures are uncommon and have rarely been reported [7].

There have been many studies and reports on effective surgical methodologies for correction of chronic ankle instability, including the Broström technique, with or without Gould modification, as well as the Watson-Jones, Evans, Larsen, Chrisman-Snook, and Pisani. Open surgery and arthroscopy are associated with good outcomes. Recently, there has been increasing implementation of minimally invasive surgery using arthroscopy, including anatomical repair and reconstruction by means of arthroscopy and percutaneous or mini-open techniques that do not require the use of an arthroscope. In 1966, Broström described an anatomical surgical procedure, which directly repairs the injured ligament in relation to using ATFL remnants to avoid muscle imbalance. In 1980, Gould modified this procedure by reinforcing the inferior extensor retinaculum to improve mechanical strength and to overcome the limitations of previous procedures, including procedural complexity, prolonged immobilization requirement, and ankle degeneration risk. The main advantages of the Gould modification are its simplicity, ability to preserve subtalar joint mobility and restore the physiological joint anatomy and kinematics, and association with fewer intraoperative and postoperative complications relative to conventional techniques [8]. Additionally, the Gould modification does not require loss of other tendons, thus preventing ankle degeneration related to non-anatomical forces. Currently, the Gould modification of the Broström procedure is regarded as the standard treatment for chronic ankle instability [9,10]. This procedure entails augmented Broström repair with additional reinforcements of the inferior extensor retinaculum, calcaneofibular ligament, and the lateral talocalcaneal ligament.

Arthroscopic ligament repair is increasingly utilized because it allows assessments of intra-articular pathology; it also leads to rapid recovery and low morbidity. The arthroscopic Broström procedure involves reinforcing the inferior extensor retinaculum with an anchor suture through the insertion of conventional anteromedial and anterolateral portals for diagnostic arthroscopy, as well as an accessory anterolateral portal that is inserted near the fibula tip. The suture anchor and instruments are passed through the anterolateral portal for ligament repair. This portal is inserted lateral to the peroneus tertius or the extensor digitorum longus tendon at the anterior joint line. Although this technique is associated with acceptable outcomes and is minimally invasive, complications may occur in 14–17% of cases [11]. Frekel published a review of complications of foot and ankle arthroscopy in 2001 [12]. They reported 612 cases of ankle arthroscopic procedures and found that complications occurred in 9% of patients undergoing ankle arthroscopy; half of the complications were neurological injuries, and 27% were iatrogenic superficial peroneal nerve injuries. Neurovascular complications are more common after ankle arthroscopy than after arthroscopy, involving other joints, such as the knees and shoulders. Ankle arthroscopic surgery can cause not only nerve damage, but also vascular damage. As the branches of the intermediate superficial peroneal nerve reported the most commonly damaged nerve, anterior tibial arteries and their branches showed their vulnerability in ankle arthroscopic surgery. Pseudoaneurysm of the anterior tibial artery after ankle arthroscopic surgery was reported by several studies [13,14]. Son et al. [14] reported anatomic analysis of the anterior tibial artery by using magnetic resonance imaging. In 6.2% of the 258 cases, the anterior tibial artery and its branches were located near the anterolateral portal, which introduces the risk of vascular damage during ankle arthroscopic surgery. In addition, the mean distance between the anterior tibial artery and the joint capsule was only 2.3 mm, which was very close to the anterior working space of the ankle joint. Ankle plantarflexion during portal placement significantly increases the distance between the malleolar artery and portal, thus diminishing the potential for injuries to the malleolar arteries [15].

Branches of the intermediate superficial peroneal nerve or sural nerve may be damaged by the anterolateral portal [16,17]. The superficial peroneal nerve provides motor innervation to the peroneus longus and brevis muscles. It passes through the lateral intermuscular septum, pierces the crural fascia, and provides the sensory supply to most of the dorsal foot. After piercing the fascia, it divides into two terminal branches: the medial dorsal cutaneous nerve and the intermediate dorsal cutaneous nerve [18]. Anatomic variations of the superficial peroneal nerve make it easier for neurological complications to occur in ankle arthroscopic surgery. Prakash et al. [19] reported a cadaver study associated with anatomic variations, including the course and the distribution of the superficial peroneal nerve. As we often know, the superficial peroneal nerve is located in the lateral compartment of the leg. However, according to their study, the superficial peroneal nerve was located in the anterior compartment of the leg in 28% of specimens. Additionally, in 20% of specimens, the superficial peroneal nerve did not divide into terminal branches after it had pierced the deep fascia. The superficial peroneal nerve branched before piercing the peroneus longus and extensor digitorum longus muscles, or it branched after piercing these two muscles and before piercing the deep fascia. In 33% of specimens, there was an additional branch from the sensory division of superficial peroneal nerve, which may be called the accessory deep peroneal nerve. It courses in the anterior compartment of the leg and supplies the ankle and the dorsum of foot. Other studies have reported similar proportions of anatomical variations of superficial peroneal nerve to this study [20–22].

There is a need to identify the locations of the inferior extensor retinaculum, intermediate superficial peroneal nerve, and sural nerve to prevent damage to these structures. The "nick and spread" technique is commonly used to prevent nerve damage by arthroscopic portals. However, the nerves are easily injured at the level of the inferior extensor retinaculum during ankle arthroscopy [23]. Previous studies have shown that the most common complication of the arthroscopic Broström procedure is damage to the intermediate superficial peroneal nerve [24]. Multiple studies have explored the course and distribution of the superficial peroneal nerve [25,26]. However, little is known regarding the location of the intermediate superficial peroneal nerve at the level of the inferior extensor retinaculum, where the intermediate superficial peroneal nerve may be injured during the arthroscopic Broström procedure. Although nerve damage after ankle arthroscopy is uncommon, such damage leads to severe patient discomfort and may be irreversible in severe cases. Additionally, it may negate the advantages of minimally invasive arthroscopic surgery. As a result, neural complications of ankle arthroscopy should not be overlooked. Masato et al. [27] reported a case of superficial peroneal nerve injury during ankle arthroscopy in a 20-year-old woman. She developed pain in the dorsum of the foot, which radiated from the insertion site of the anterolateral portal to the dorsomedial aspect of the foot. Because conservative treatment was ineffective, the patient underwent additional surgery, which revealed a neuroma in the intermediate superficial peroneal nerve.

It is important to develop strategies that can prevent nerve damage during the arthroscopic Broström procedure. Here, we evaluated the anatomical relationships of anterolateral portal sites with the intermediate superficial peroneal nerve and the sural nerve at the level of the inferior extensor retinaculum to identify the safest portal insertion sites for the arthroscopic Broström procedure.

2. Materials and Methods

This study was conducted using human cadavers. Therefore, research ethics review, such as IRB approval or the consent process of the subjects, were not conducted. In total, 11 embalmed frozen foot specimens without visible deformity or pathology were obtained from four male and two female cadavers with a mean foot size of 230.2 (range, 225–250) mm. The ankles were fixed at 90° with fixing plates. No limbs showed evidence of previous surgeries. The anterolateral portal site was immediately lateral to the peroneus tertius at the level of the ankle joint. After removal of the skin, the ankle was sequentially dissected; the distances from anterolateral portal point to the inferior extensor retinaculum, intermediate superficial peroneal nerve, and sural nerve were measured using an electronic digital caliper (CD-15CP; Mitutoyo Corp., Tokyo, Japan). Measurements (mm) were obtained to the nearest 0.1 mm.

Kirschner wires (K-wires) with an electric drill were used to mark each point. For the pointing to standard anterolateral portal, a K-wire was fixed directly anteriorly to posteriorly as x-axis. The x-axis runs anteriorly to posteriorly, the y-axis runs laterally to medially, and the z-axis runs runs superiorly to inferiorly. Each angle, verified by goniometry, is exactly 90-degrees (Figure 1).

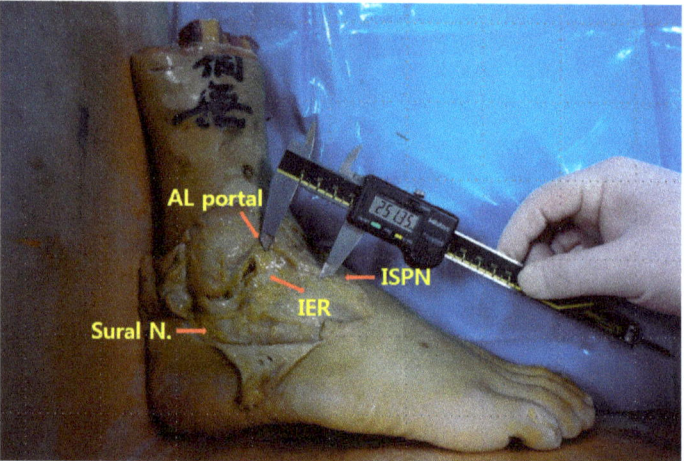

Figure 1. Distances from the insertion point of the anterolateral portal to the inferior extensor retinaculum), intermediate superficial peroneal nerve, and sural nerve were measured using an electronic digital caliper (CD-15CP; Mitutoyo Corp., Tokyo, Japan). That figure shows the measurement of the distance from the anterolateral portal to the farthest inferior extensor retinaculum.

The inferior extensor retinaculum was located along the labeled x-axis at the vertical right angle. The proximal and distal parts of the inferior extensor retinaculum were labeled as A1 and A2, respectively. The distances between anterolateral portal sites and A1 and A2 were measured. The sural nerve passes through the inferior extensor retinaculum, curves around the lateral malleolus, and divides into medial and lateral branches at the base of the fifth metatarsal. The proximal and distal contact points of the sural nerve and inferior extensor retinaculum are designated B1 and B2, respectively. The A1, A2, B1, and B2 points were joined to form an imaginary quadrangle on the inferior extensor retinaculum edge. The proximal and distal points of intersection of intermediate superficial peroneal nerve and inferior extensor retinaculum were designated D1 and D2, respectively.

We measured the distances between the nearest inferior extensor retinaculum edges in front of A1 and the anterolateral portal (O), between the farthest inferior extensor retinaculum edges in front of A2 and O, between the nearest intermediate superficial peroneal nerve branch locations at D1 and O, between the farthest intermediate superficial peroneal nerve locations at D2 and O, between the nearest sural nerve locations at B1 and O; between the farthest sural nerve locations at B2 and O, and between A1–B1, B1–B2, A2–B2, A1–A2, A1–D1, A2–D2, B1–D1, and B2–D2. The distances from the anterolateral portal to various points were measured using an electronic digital caliper.

A1 (blue), A2 (purple), B1 (yellow), B2 (brown), D1 (aqua), and D2 (red) are presented as mean ± standard deviation (range, min–max). Maya software was used for 3D rendering and mapping of our results (Figure 2).

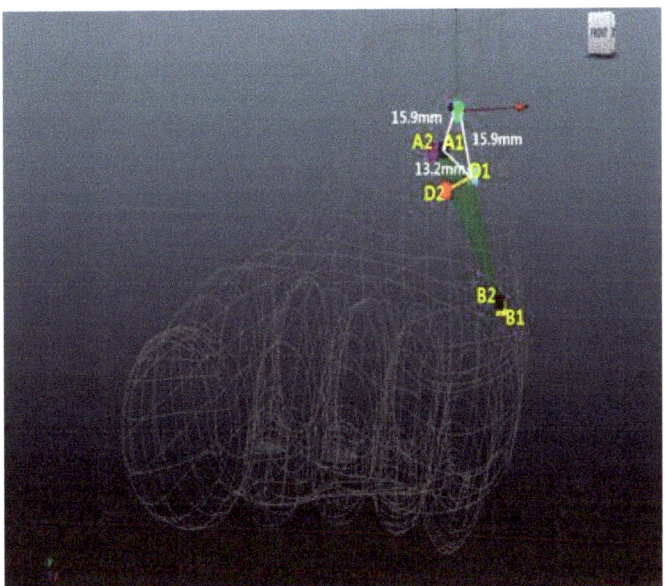

Figure 2. Mean distances from the anterolateral portal to *O* (AL portal sites), *A1* (blue; nearest edge of inferior extensor retinaculum), *A2* (purple; farthest inferior extensor retinaculum edge), *B1* (yellow; nearest sural nerve location on inferior extensor retinaculum), *B2* (brown; farthest sural nerve location on inferior extensor retinaculum), *D1* (aqua; nearest intermediate superficial peroneal nerve branch on inferior extensor retinaculum), and *D2* (red; farthest intermediate superficial peroneal nerve branch on inferior extensor retinaculum). The dark green quadrangle is the imaginary quadrangle, which is formed by A1, A2, B1, and B2 on the inferior extensor retinaculum.

Data were analyzed using Excel (Microsoft Corp., Redmond, WA, USA). Data are presented as means ± standard deviations. Fisher's exact test was used to identify statistically significant differences. To estimate the risk to each nerve from the anterolateral portal, we assumed that the nerves would be located within two standard deviations of the mean distance from anterolateral portal in 95% of cases; this was regarded as the minimum safe distance.

3. Results

The mean O–A1, O–A2, D1–O, D2–O, B1–O, B2–O, A1–B1, B1–B2, A2–B2, A1–A2, A1–D1, A2–D2, B1–D1, and B2–D2 distances were 15.9 ± 11 (range, 2.6–42.6) mm, 30.1 ± 9.8 (range, 16.8–46.4) mm, 15.9 ± 4.1 (range, 11.3–23.0) mm, 30.1 ± 5.5 (range, 20.8–37.9) mm, 47.6 ± 5.7 (range, 37.4–57.2) mm, 47.2 ± 4.1 (range, 41.0–51.8) mm, 52.1 ± 10.8 (range, 40.2–76.5) mm, 28 ± 12.5 (range, 11.2–55.9) mm, 41.6 ± 10.6 (range, 24–58.9) mm, 21.5 ± 10.6 (range, 9.8–42.7) mm, 13.2 ± 4.1 (range, 0–31.2) mm, 12.3 ± 10.8 (range, 0–30.6) mm, 40.3 ± 14 (range, 15.6–60.1) mm, and 32.1 ± 13.8 (range, 17.7–61.4) mm, respectively (Table 1).

Table 1. Average distances of O–A1, O–A2, D1–O, D2–O, B1–O, B2–O, A1–B1, B1–B2, A2–B2, A1–A2, A1–D1, A2–D2, B1–D1, and B2–D2. O (AL portal sites), A1 (nearest edge of inferior extensor retinaculum), A2 (farthest inferior extensor retinaculum edge), B1 (nearest sural nerve location on inferior extensor retinaculum), B2 (farthest sural nerve location on inferior extensor retinaculum), D1 (nearest intermediate superficial peroneal nerve branch on inferior extensor retinaculum), and D2 (farthest intermediate superficial peroneal nerve branch on inferior extensor retinaculum).

Point-Point	Mean Distance
O–A1	15.9 mm
O–A2	30.1 mm
D1–O	15.9 mm
D2–O	30.1 mm
B1–O	47.6 mm
B2–O	47.2 mm
A1–B1	52.1 mm
B1–B2	28.0 mm
A2–B2	41.6 mm
A1–A2	21.5 mm
A1–D1	13.2 mm
A2–D2	12.3 mm
B1–D1	40.3 mm
B2–D2	32.1 mm

4. Discussion

Care is needed to avoid nerve damage, particularly to the intermediate superficial peroneal nerve, during the insertion of an accessory anterolateral portal for the modified arthroscopic Broström procedure. Our results suggest that nerve damage can be prevented by avoiding an area of 15.9 mm around the anterolateral portal.

Surgical treatment of chronic ankle instability, first described in 1932, originally involved suturing the ruptured ligament and fortifying it by means of the peroneus brevis tendon [28]. Surgical treatment options have advanced over the past 30 years; they currently include direct anatomical repair, anatomical reconstruction, and non-anatomical reconstruction. The non-anatomical procedures include the Watson-Jones and Chrisman-Snook procedures, which involve the peroneus brevis tenodesis. These procedures are usually associated with good short-term outcomes; however, some patients may experience persistent pain, stiffness, wound complications, and impaired ankle and subtalar joint function [29,30]. Therefore, the use of non-anatomical reconstruction has decreased over time. The first-line surgical treatment of chronic ankle instability is direct anatomical repair by the Broström procedure with the Gould modification. Anatomical ATFL reconstruction using an autograft or allograft can be performed in patients with generalized laxity, insufficient remnant tissue, or failed prior stabilization procedures [31].

Recent arthroscopic advancements have enabled stabilization of the lateral ankle ligament complex, repair of lateral ankle instability, and early detection of intra-articular pathology (e.g., chondral lesions and loose bodies) with minimal incisions. This minimally invasive procedure involves the placement of a suture anchor in the fibula to repair the ATFL. A cadaveric study showed no differences in strength or stiffness between conventional open repair and arthroscopic direct anatomical repair [32]. Along with the standard anteromedial and anterolateral portals, an additional lateral working portal is needed to augment the inferior extensor retinaculum during ankle arthroscopy [17,24]. Although arthroscopy has excellent outcomes, the overall complication rates are similar to or higher than the rates for open procedures [33,34]. Wang et al. [34] demonstrated that 31 of 179 patients undergoing arthroscopic ATFL repair with the suture anchor technique developed complications, including portal site irritation, delayed wound healing, and nerve complications. Nerve complications were comprised of intermediate dorsal cutaneous nerve neuritis, superficial peroneal nerve numbness, and sural nerve neuritis.

Superficial peroneal nerve injury, sural neuritis, and knot prominence can occur after arthroscopy [35]. Although wound complications are more common after open surgery, superficial peroneal nerve damage is more common after arthroscopy [36]. The high rate of sensory nerve damage during arthroscopy is explained by the presence of a communicating branch between the superficial peroneal and sural nerves inferior to the fibula [37,38]. The most common complication of arthroscopy is superficial peroneal injury, with an incidence of 3–11% [11,24]. Intermediate superficial peroneal nerve entrapment, a major complication of arthroscopic ATFL repair, is the result of insufficient knowledge regarding the course of the intermediate superficial peroneal nerve. Superficial peroneal nerve entrapment leads to pain and paresthesia over the lateral aspect of the calf and dorsum of the foot.

The superficial peroneal nerve is the only nerve in the human body that is visible from the skin surface. Combined ankle plantar flexion and inversion can cause the superficial peroneal nerve to become more prominent. Because the anterior portals for ankle arthroscopy are inserted with the ankle in the neutral or slightly dorsiflexed position, the course of the superficial peroneal nerve should be identified preoperatively by ankle plantar flexion and inversion to avoid iatrogenic nerve injury. Multiple strategies have been suggested to avoid damage to the superficial peroneal nerve [35,36]; these strategies require the operator to have good anatomical knowledge. Nerve injury may be avoided by making vertical skin incisions parallel to the tendons and nerve, performing blunt dissection up to the level of the joint, and using minimal distraction and tourniquet inflation. Prolonged distraction can lead to various complications [12]. Acevedo et al. [24] suggested a "safe zone" 1.5 cm from the fibula tip. The "nick and spread" technique can help to avoid superficial peroneal nerve damage around the portal. This technique involves the use of a hemostat to spread soft tissues down to the joint capsule. Stephens and Kelly [39] demonstrated that the superficial peroneal nerve can be identified via direct inspection and palpation near the skin surface during ankle inversion and fourth toe flexion. However, the intermediate superficial peroneal nerve was visualized in only 30% of patients during ankle plantar flexion and inversion [18]. Ucerler et al. [40] demonstrated that the nearest superficial peroneal nerve branches were located 2.2–16.2 mm from the lateral border of the peroneus tertius tendon. Although multiple studies have evaluated the complications of ankle arthroscopy, particularly nerve damage, and corresponding preventive strategies, few studies have determined the distance between the intermediate superficial peroneal nerve and the accessory anterolateral portal. Woo et al. [41] demonstrated that, at the level of the ankle joint, the distance between the anterolateral portal and the intermediate superficial peroneal nerve was short (mean distance: 5.5 [range, 0.4–14.4] mm), so it was an anatomic hazard. Charles et al. [35] found that the mean distance from the portal to the superficial peroneal nerve was 13.11 (range, 2–24) mm; they suggested that the accessory lateral working portal was a safe access point because the major at-risk structures (superficial peroneal nerve branches, sural nerve branches, and peroneal tendons) were located > 1 cm from the anterolateral portal. Our results differ from the findings in previous studies because we used intermediate superficial peroneal nerve locations nearest and farthest from the inferior extensor retinaculum for measurements. We selected the inferior extensor retinaculum because it is an important anatomical landmark during the modified arthroscopic Broström procedure. Additionally, the location of the anterolateral portal can affect the distance to the intermediate superficial peroneal nerve. We created an anterolateral portal immediately lateral to the peroneus tertius tendon, whereas Charles et al. [35] created an anterolateral portal 1.5 cm anterior to the distal tip of the fibula.

In our study, the mean distance from the anterolateral portal to the intermediate superficial peroneal nerve at the level of the inferior extensor retinaculum was 15.9 (range, 11.3–23.0) mm. The intermediate superficial peroneal nerve passes through the quadrangle space formed by the inferior extensor retinaculum. The distances from the origin to the proximal (A1) and distal (A2) inferior extensor retinaculum were 15.9 and 30.1 mm, respectively. Intermediate superficial peroneal nerve (D) was located lateral to the inferior extensor retinaculum at A1 and A2. The A1–D1 and A2–D2 mean distances were 13.2 and 12.3 mm, respectively. The A1 and A2 points were located parallel to the anterolateral portal on the x-axis. The danger zone was located 13.2 mm lateral to A1 and 15.9 mm from the anterolateral portal. Therefore, caution is required when approaching the inferior extensor retinaculum during the arthroscopic Broström procedure.

In the present study, we determined the anatomical relationships between the portals and the neurovascular structures surrounding the inferior extensor retinaculum. However, this study had some limitations. First, only 11 embalmed frozen foot specimens were evaluated to determine the course of the intermediate superficial peroneal nerve. Further studies with larger sample sizes are needed to generalize our results and to identify anatomical variations. Although the superficial peroneal nerve typically divides into the medial dorsal cutaneous nerve and the intermediate dorsal cutaneous nerve after it has pierced the fascia, some patients may have up to five divisions of the superficial peroneal nerve [42]. Additionally, as we mentioned earlier, there are several anatomic variations of the superficial peroneal nerve, as reported in other cadaver studies. However, we only identified the two terminal branches of the superficial peroneal nerve, and we did not consider the anatomic variations of superficial peroneal nerve, as there were no specific anatomic variations in our specimens. Second, although ankles with visible deformity, pathology, or previous surgery were excluded, concomitant conditions (e.g., soft tissue stiffness and Achilles tendon tightness) were not evaluated. Chronic ankle instability may be caused by a lack of soft tissue stiffness, which can also lead to ankle structure displacement. Third, we did not evaluate the symptoms or effects of nerve damage because this was a cadaveric dissection study. Multicenter studies with large sample sizes and the inclusion of living patients are needed to characterize the anatomical relationships of ankle arthroscopy portals with major neurovascular structures and tendons. Despite these study limitations, our results may facilitate the development of strategies to prevent iatrogenic damage to the superficial peroneal nerve and its branches during arthroscopic Broström repair. In particular, an understanding of the anatomical relationships between the inferior extensor retinaculum and the surrounding nerves can facilitate the establishment of a safe zone for the arthroscopic Broström procedure.

5. Conclusions

When an anchor suture is placed during the arthroscopic Broström procedure for lateral ankle instability, the inferior extensor retinaculum is located 15.9–30.1 mm from the anterolateral portal on the x-axis. At the level of the inferior extensor retinaculum, the shortest distance between the intermediate superficial peroneal nerve and the anterolateral portal is 15.9 mm. As a result, surgeons should place the anterolateral portal away from this danger area to prevent the injury of intermediate superficial peroneal nerve, as long as it does not interfere with surgery, and care must be taken around this danger area.

Author Contributions: Conceptualization, S.H.K.; methodology, Y.K.L.; validation, J.H.C.; investigation, Y.K.L.; resources, J.H.C.; data curation, J.H.C.; writing—original draft preparation, S.H.K.; writing—review and editing, S.H.L.; visualization, Y.K.L.; supervision, S.H.L.; project administration, J.H.C.; funding acquisition, J.H.C. All authors have read and agreed to the published version of the manuscript.

Funding: The authors wish to thank the Soonchunhyang University Research Fund for financial support. (No. 2023-0039).

Institutional Review Board Statement: Not applicable.

Informed Consent Statement: Not applicable.

Data Availability Statement: Data sharing is not applicable to this article because no datasets were made or analyzed during this study.

Conflicts of Interest: The authors declare no conflict of interest.

References

1. Rigby, R.B.; Cottom, J.M. A comparison of the "all-inside" arthroscopic Broström procedure with the traditional open modified Broström-Gould technique: A review of 62 patients. *Foot Ankle Surg.* **2019**, *25*, 31–36. [CrossRef] [PubMed]
2. Guelfi, M.; Zamperetti, M.; Pantalone, A.; Usuelli, F.G.; Salini, V.; Oliva, X.M. Open and arthroscopic lateral ligament repair for treatment of chronic ankle instability: A systematic review. *Foot Ankle Surg.* **2018**, *24*, 11–18. [CrossRef] [PubMed]
3. van Rijn, R.M.; Van Os, A.G.; Bernsen, R.M.; Luijsterburg, P.A.; Koes, B.W.; Bierma-Zeinstra, S.M. What is the clinical course of acute ankle sprains? A systematic literature review. *Am. J. Med.* **2008**, *121*, 324–331.e7. [CrossRef] [PubMed]
4. DiGiovanni, B.F.; Partal, G.; Baumhauer, J.F. Acute ankle injury and chronic lateral instability in the athlete. *Clin. Sport. Med.* **2004**, *23*, 1–19. [CrossRef]
5. Bischof, J.E.; Spritzer, C.E.; Caputo, A.M.; Easley, M.E.; DeOrio, J.K.; Nunley, J.A., II; DeFrate, L.E. In vivo cartilage contact strains in patients with lateral ankle instability. *J. Biomech.* **2010**, *43*, 2561–2566. [CrossRef]
6. Matsui, K.; Takao, M.; Tochigi, Y.; Ozeki, S.; Glazebrook, M. Anatomy of anterior talofibular ligament and calcaneofibular ligament for minimally invasive surgery: A systematic review. *Knee Surg. Sport. Traumatol. Arthrosc.* **2017**, *25*, 1892–1902. [CrossRef]
7. Rigby, R.; Cottom, J.M.; Rozin, R. Isolated calcaneofibular ligament injury: A report of two cases. *J. Foot Ankle Surg.* **2015**, *54*, 487–489. [CrossRef]
8. Brostrom, L., VI. Surgical treatment of chronic ligament ruptures. *Acta Chir. Scand.* **1966**, *61*, 354–361.
9. Cao, Y.; Hong, Y.; Xu, Y.; Zhu, Y.; Xu, X. Surgical management of chronic lateral ankle instability: A meta-analysis. *J. Orthop. Surg. Res.* **2018**, *13*, 159. [CrossRef]
10. Gould, N.; Seligson, D.; Gassman, J. Early and late repair of lateral ligament of the ankle. *Foot Ankle* **1980**, *1*, 84–89. [CrossRef]
11. Deng, D.F.; Hamilton, G.A.; Lee, M.; Rush, S.; Ford, L.A.; Patel, S. Complications associated with foot and ankle arthroscopy. *J. Foot Ankle Surg.* **2012**, *51*, 281–284. [CrossRef] [PubMed]
12. Ferkel, R.D.; Small, H.N.; Gittins, J.E. Complications in foot and ankle arthroscopy. *Clin. Orthop. Relat. Res.* **2001**, *391*, 89–104. [CrossRef]
13. Darwish, A.; Ehsan, O.; Marynissen, H.; Al-Khaffaf, H. Pseudoaneurysm of the anterior tibial artery after ankle arthroscopy. *Arthrosc. J. Arthrosc. Relat. Surg.* **2004**, *20*, e63–e64. [CrossRef]
14. Son, K.-H.; Cho, J.H.; Lee, J.W.; Kwack, K.-S.; Han, S.H. Is the anterior tibial artery safe during ankle arthroscopy? Anatomic analysis of the anterior tibial artery at the ankle joint by magnetic resonance imaging. *Am. J. Sport. Med.* **2011**, *39*, 2452–2456. [CrossRef] [PubMed]
15. Başarır, K.; Esmer, A.F.; Tuccar, E.; Binnet, M.; Güçlü, B. Medial and lateral malleolar arteries in ankle arthroscopy: A cadaver study. *J. Foot Ankle Surg.* **2007**, *46*, 181–184. [CrossRef]
16. Shakked, R.J.; Karnovsky, S.; Drakos, M.C. Operative treatment of lateral ligament instability. *Curr. Rev. Musculoskelet. Med.* **2017**, *10*, 113–121. [CrossRef] [PubMed]
17. Cottom, J.M.; Rigby, R.B. The "all inside" arthroscopic Broström procedure: A prospective study of 40 consecutive patients. *J. Foot Ankle Surg.* **2013**, *52*, 568–574. [CrossRef]
18. De Leeuw, P.A.; Golanó, P.; Sierevelt, I.N.; Van Dijk, C.N. The course of the superficial peroneal nerve in relation to the ankle position: Anatomical study with ankle arthroscopic implications. *Knee Surg. Sport. Traumatol. Arthrosc.* **2010**, *18*, 612–617. [CrossRef]
19. Jayanthi, V.; Rajini, T.; Deepak Kumar Singh, A.K.B. Anatomic variations of superficial peroneal nerve: Clinical implications of a cadaver study. *Ital. J. Anat. Embryol.* **2010**, *115*, 223–228.
20. Canella, C.; Demondion, X.; Guillin, R.; Boutry, N.; Peltier, J.; Cotten, A. Anatomic study of the superficial peroneal nerve using sonography. *Am. J. Roentgenol.* **2009**, *193*, 174–179. [CrossRef]
21. Zhou, Q.; Tan, D.-Y.; Dai, Z.-S. The location of the superficial peroneal nerve in the leg and its relation to the surgical approach of the fibula. *Zhongguo Gu Shang China J. Orthop. Traumatol.* **2008**, *21*, 95–96.
22. Agthong, S.; Huanmanop, T.; Sasivongsbhakdi, T.; Ruenkhwan, K.; Piyawacharapun, A.; Chentanez, V. Anatomy of the superficial peroneal nerve related to the harvesting for nerve graft. *Surg. Radiol. Anat.* **2008**, *30*, 145–148. [CrossRef] [PubMed]
23. Vega, J.G.; Pellegrino, A. All-inside arthroscopic lateral collateral ligament repair for ankle instability with a knotless suture anchor technique. *Foot Ankle Int.* **2013**, *34*, 1701–1709. [CrossRef] [PubMed]
24. Acevedo, J.I.; Mangone, P. Arthroscopic brostrom technique. *Foot Ankle Int.* **2015**, *36*, 465–473. [CrossRef]
25. Ribak, S.; Fonseca, J.R.; Tietzmann, A.; Gama, S.A.; Hirata, H.H. The anatomy and morphology of the superficial peroneal nerve. *J. Reconstr. Microsurg.* **2016**, *32*, 271–275.
26. Klammer, G.; Schlewitz, G.; Stauffer, C.; Vich, M.; Espinosa, N. Percutaneous lateral ankle stabilization: An anatomical investigation. *Foot Ankle Int.* **2011**, *32*, 66–70. [CrossRef]
27. Takao, M.; Ochi, M.; Shu, N.; Uchio, Y.; Naito, K.; Tobita, M.; Matsusaki, M.; Kawasaki, K. A case of superficial peroneal nerve injury during ankle arthroscopy. *Arthrosc. J. Arthrosc. Relat. Surg.* **2001**, *17*, 403–404. [CrossRef]

28. Nilsonne, H. Making a new ligament in ankle sprain. *JBJS* **1932**, *14*, 380–381.
29. Rosenbaum, D.; Bertsch, C.; Claes, L. Tenodeses do not fully restore ankle joint loading characteristics: A biomechanical in vitro investigation in the hind foot. *Clin. Biomech.* **1997**, *12*, 202–209. [CrossRef]
30. Sammarco, V.J. Complications of lateral ankle ligament reconstruction. *Clin. Orthop. Relat. Res.* **2001**, *391*, 123–132. [CrossRef]
31. Dierckman, B.D.; Ferkel, R.D. Anatomic reconstruction with a semitendinosus allograft for chronic lateral ankle instability. *Am. J. Sport Med.* **2015**, *43*, 1941–1950. [CrossRef] [PubMed]
32. Giza, E.; Shin, E.C.; Wong, S.E.; Acevedo, J.I.; Mangone, P.G.; Olson, K.; Anderson, M.J. Arthroscopic suture anchor repair of the lateral ligament ankle complex: A cadaveric study. *Am. J. Sport. Med.* **2013**, *41*, 2567–2572. [CrossRef]
33. Moorthy, V.; Sayampanathan, A.A.; Yeo, N.E.M.; Tay, K.S. Clinical outcomes of open versus arthroscopic Broström procedure for lateral ankle instability: A meta-analysis. *J. Foot Ankle Surg.* **2021**, *60*, 577–584. [CrossRef] [PubMed]
34. Wang, J.; Hua, Y.; Chen, S.; Li, H.; Zhang, J.; Li, Y. Arthroscopic repair of lateral ankle ligament complex by suture anchor. *Arthrosc. J. Arthrosc. Relat. Surg.* **2014**, *30*, 766–773. [CrossRef]
35. Pitts, C.C.; McKissack, H.M.; Anderson, M.C.; Buddemeyer, K.M.; Bassetty, C.; Naranje, S.M.; Shah, A. Anatomical structures at risk in the arthroscopic Broström-Gould procedure: A cadaver study. *Foot Ankle Surg.* **2020**, *26*, 343–346. [CrossRef] [PubMed]
36. Attia, A.K.; Taha, T.; Mahmoud, K.; Hunt, K.J.; Labib, S.A.; d'Hooghe, P. Outcomes of open versus arthroscopic Broström surgery for chronic lateral ankle instability: A systematic review and meta-analysis of comparative studies. *Orthop. J. Sport. Med.* **2021**, *9*, 23259671211015207. [CrossRef] [PubMed]
37. Yasui, Y.; Shimozono, Y.; Kennedy, J.G. Surgical procedures for chronic lateral ankle instability. *JAAOS-J. Am. Ademy Orthop. Surg.* **2018**, *26*, 223–230. [CrossRef]
38. Drizenko, A.; Demondion, X.; Luyckx, F.; Mestdagh, H.; Cassagnaud, X. The communicating branches between the sural and superficial peroneal nerves in the foot: A review of 55 cases. *Surg. Radiol. Anat.* **2004**, *26*, 447–452. [CrossRef]
39. Stephens, M.; Kelly, P.M. Fourth toe flexion sign: A new clinical sign for identification of the superficial peroneal nerve. *Foot Ankle Int.* **2000**, *21*, 860–863. [CrossRef]
40. Ucerler, H.; Ikiz, Z.A.A.; Uygur, M. A cadaver study on preserving peroneal nerves during ankle arthroscopy. *Foot Ankle Int.* **2007**, *28*, 1172–1178. [CrossRef]
41. Woo, S.-B.; Wong, T.-M.; Chan, W.-L.; Yen, C.-H.; Wong, W.-C.; Mak, K.-L. Anatomic variations of neurovascular structures of the ankle in relation to arthroscopic portals: A cadaveric study of Chinese subjects. *J. Orthop. Surg.* **2010**, *18*, 71–75. [CrossRef] [PubMed]
42. Takao, M.; Uchio, Y.; Shu, N.; Ochi, M. Anatomic bases of ankle arthroscopy: Study of superficial and deep peroneal nerves around anterolateral and anterocentral approach. *Surg. Radiol. Anat.* **1999**, *20*, 317–320. [CrossRef]

Disclaimer/Publisher's Note: The statements, opinions and data contained in all publications are solely those of the individual author(s) and contributor(s) and not of MDPI and/or the editor(s). MDPI and/or the editor(s) disclaim responsibility for any injury to people or property resulting from any ideas, methods, instructions or products referred to in the content.

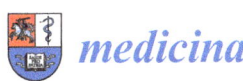

Case Report

Type V Tibial Tubercle Avulsion Fracture with Suspected Complication of Anterior Cruciate Ligament Injury: A Case Report

Hiroki Okamura [1,*], Hiroki Ishikawa [1], Takuya Ohno [1], Shogo Fujita [1], Kei Nagasaki [1], Katsunori Inagaki [2] and Yoshifumi Kudo [2]

1. Department of Orthopedic Surgery, Nihon Koukan Hospital, 1-2-1 Koukandori, Kawasaki 210-0852, Japan; hiroki.f.marinos@gmail.com (H.I.); shinenow44@yahoo.jp (T.O.); fala500104@yahoo.co.jp (S.F.); keppoko@hotmail.com (K.N.)
2. Department of Orthopedic Surgery, Showa University School of Medicine, 1-5-8 Hatanodai, Tokyo 142-8666, Japan; katsu@med.showa-u.ac.jp (K.I.); kudo_4423@yahoo.co.jp (Y.K.)
* Correspondence: 99okamu99@gmail.com; Tel.: +81-44-333-5591

Abstract: *Background and Objectives*: Type V tibial tubercle avulsion fractures are extremely rare; therefore, information on them remains limited. Furthermore, although these fractures are intra-articular, to the best of our knowledge, there are no reports on their assessment via magnetic resonance imaging (MRI) or arthroscopy. Accordingly, this is the first report to describe the case of a patient undergoing detailed evaluation via MRI and arthroscopy. *Case Presentation*: A 13-year-old male adolescent athlete jumped while playing basketball, experienced discomfort and pain at the front of his knee, and fell down. He was transported to the emergency room by ambulance after he was unable to walk. The radiographic examination revealed a Type V tibial tubercle avulsion fracture that was displaced. In addition, an MRI scan revealed a fracture line extending to the attachment of the anterior cruciate ligament (ACL); moreover, high MRI intensity and swelling due to ACL were observed, suggesting an ACL injury. On day 4 of the injury, open reduction and internal fixation were performed. Furthermore, 4 months after surgery, bone fusion was confirmed, and metal removal was performed. Simultaneously, an MRI scan obtained at the time of injury revealed findings suggestive of ACL injury; therefore, an arthroscopy was performed. Notably, no parenchymal ACL injury was observed, and the meniscus was intact. The patient returned to sports 6 months postoperatively. *Conclusion*: Type V tibial tubercle avulsion fractures are known to be extremely rare. Based on our report, we suggest that MRI should be performed without hesitation if intra-articular injury is suspected.

Keywords: tibial tubercle avulsion fractures; anterior cruciate ligament; knee; sports injury

1. Introduction

Tibial tubercle avulsion fractures are known to be relatively rare in adolescents, accounting for 0.4–2.7% of all pediatric fractures and <1% of all epiphysis injuries [1,2].

In 1955, Watson–Jones first reported the fracture morphology of tibial tubercle avulsion fractures and classified them from Type I to Type III. In 1980, Ogden et al. refined the classification to include subtypes according to the degree of displacement and comminution, and this classification has been widely used to date. Subsequently, in 1985, Ryu and Debenhum added Type IV, and in 2003, Mackoy added Type V to the classification [3,4]. According to a previous study, conservative treatment should be considered for Types I and II, and surgery is preferable for Type III and above if a dislocation is present [5]. In particular, Type V fracture involves the posterior bone cortex as well as the articular surface, and this fracture requires accurate repositioning, firm fixation, and careful postoperative therapy. Moreover, Type V fracture morphology is very rare and combines the morphology of Ogden Type IIIB with Salter–Haris Type IV [4]. Notably, there are very few reports of Ogden Type V fractures, with only five cases reported to date; hence, information on these fractures is limited [4,6,7]. Furthermore, although these fractures are intra-articular, to the best of our knowledge, there have been no reports of them being assessed via magnetic resonance imaging (MRI) or arthroscopy.

Here, we report our experience with a very rare case of Ogden Type V fracture, along with a literature review.

2. Case Report

A 13-year-old male adolescent athlete presented to our hospital's emergency room with right knee pain. He reported that he jumped while playing basketball, felt discomfort and pain at the front of his knee, and fell down. Furthermore, he had become unable to walk and was transported to the emergency room by ambulance. Notably, he presented with no past medical history.

An orthopedic physical examination of the right knee revealed tenderness from the patella tendon to the tibial tuberosity. Moreover, swelling was noted around the knee and proximal leg. In addition, knee joint effusion was noted. Notably, active flexion of the right knee was not possible, and the knee had a limited range of motion (ROM). Furthermore, the ligament stability test could not be performed because of pain. Nonetheless, the neurovascular status was intact.

Radiographic examination revealed a displaced Type V tibial tubercle avulsion fracture (Figure 1). Furthermore, the patient was hospitalized with splint immobilization, and his condition was carefully monitored until surgery. CT scan revealed a Type V tibial tubercle avulsion fracture (Figure 2a). In addition, an MRI scan revealed that the fracture line reached the attachment of the ACL, and high MRI intensity and swelling due to the ACL were observed, suggesting an ACL injury (Figure 2b). No meniscus or other ligament damage was noted. Fortunately, compartment syndrome was not developed, and open reduction and internal fixation were performed on day 4 of the injury. However, periosteum disruption and patella tendon rupture were observed (Figure 3). The fracture was fixed with a cannulated cancellous screw (CCS), and the disrupted periosteum and patella tendon were repaired (Figure 4).

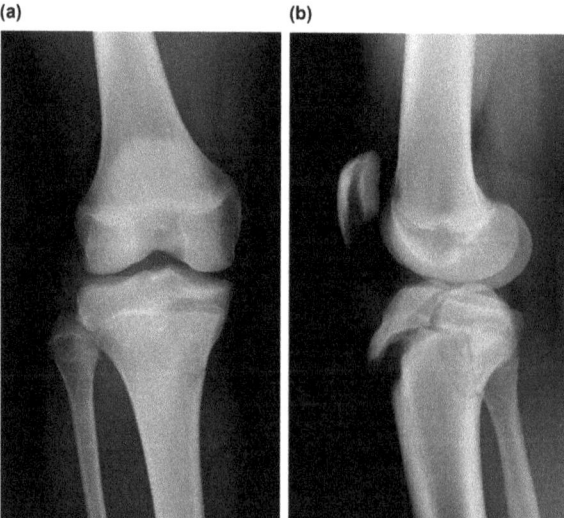

Figure 1. (a) Frontal view and (b) lateral view of plain radiographs obtained at the time of injury indicated Type V tibial tubercle avulsion fracture.

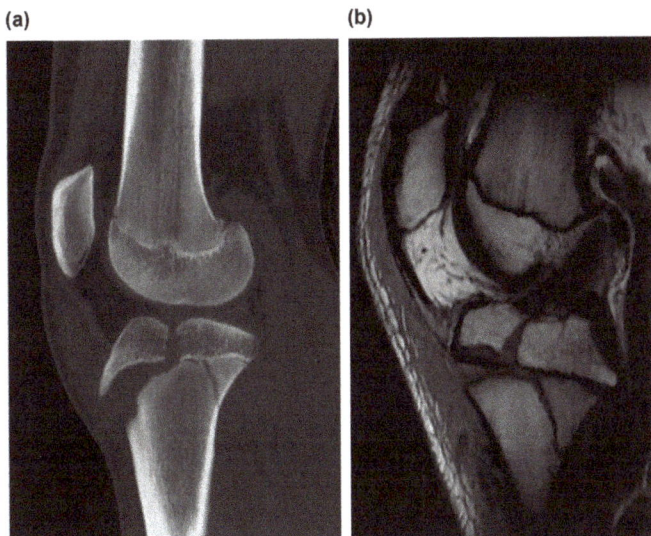

Figure 2. (a) CT and (b) MRI scans of the right knee, sagittal view. (a) CT scan revealed tibial tubercle fracture of Ogden Type IIIB and Salter–Harris Type IV, indicating tibial tubercle fracture of Ogden Type V. (b) MRI scan revealed that the fracture line reached the attachment of ACL, and high MRI intensity and swelling due to ACL were observed, suggesting an ACL injury. CT, computed tomography; MRI, magnetic resonance image; and ACL, anterior cruciate ligament.

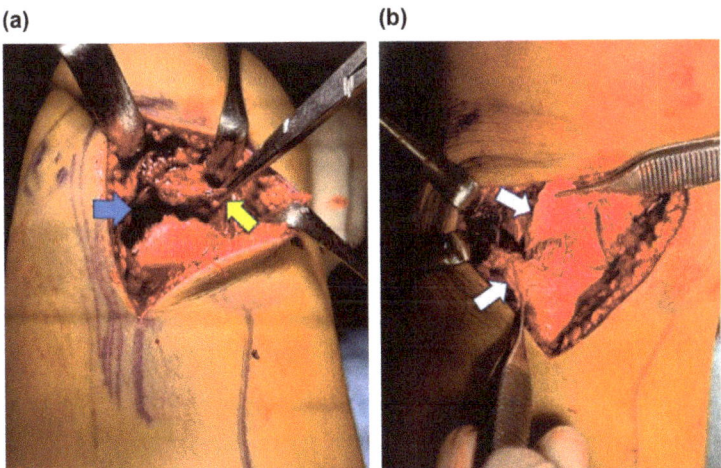

Figure 3. Intraoperative image of the right knee fracture area. (a) Disruption of the periosteum (yellow arrow) embedded in the fracture site (blue arrow). (b) Partial rupture of the patellar tendon (white arrow) was noted.

The patient was non-weight bearing, 1/3-weight bearing, 1/2-weight bearing, 2/3-weight bearing, and full-weight bearing 6, 6, 8, 10, and 12 weeks after surgery, respectively. Furthermore, postoperatively, after 3 weeks of splint immobilization, the patient started ROM exercises. Furthermore, full ROM was achieved 8 weeks after surgery, and the patient was able to sit upright. Anterior drawer and Lachman tests were negative. Four months after surgery, bone fusion was confirmed, and the patient underwent metal removal (Figure 5).

Meanwhile, an MRI scan obtained at the time of injury revealed findings that indicated ACL injury, and based on the wishes of the patient's family, arthroscopy was performed after obtaining consent from the patient (Figure 6). Notably, no parenchymal ACL injury was observed, and the meniscus was intact. The patient returned to sports at 6 months postoperatively. His knee injury and osteoarthritis outcome score at 6 months postoperatively was 100, and there was no evidence of premature closure of the proximal tibial epiphysis or growth retardation at this time.

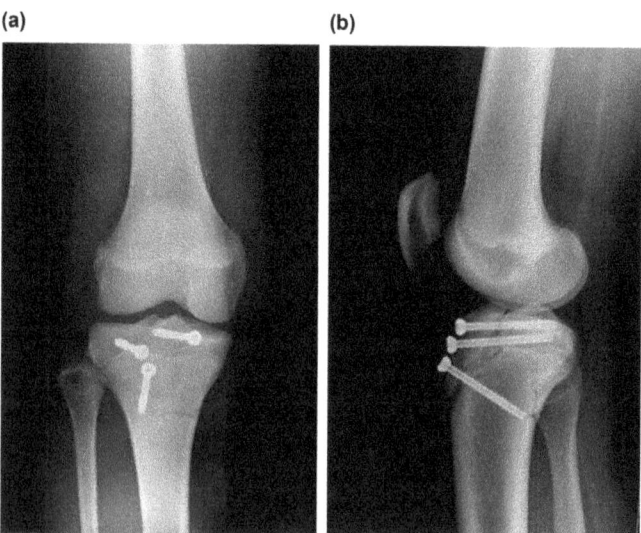

Figure 4. (a) Frontal view and (b) lateral view of postoperative plain radiographs revealed good fixation by repositioning.

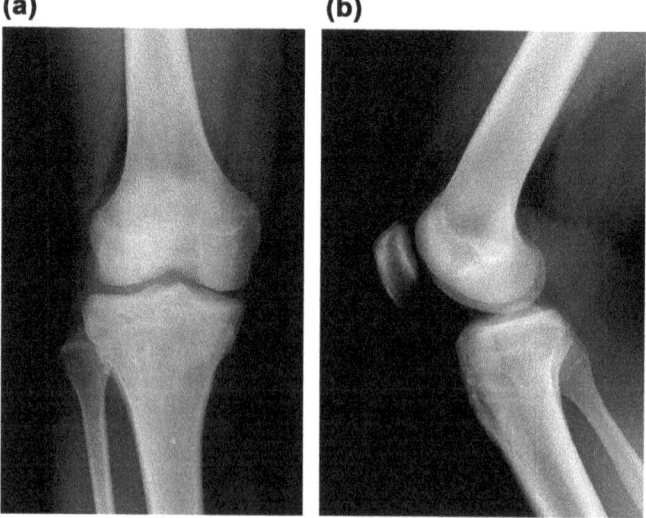

Figure 5. (a) Frontal view and (b) lateral view of plain radiographs obtained after metal removal revealed good bone union.

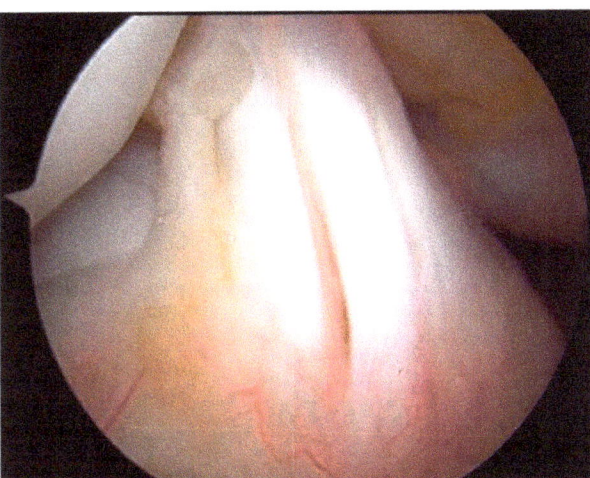

Figure 6. Arthroscopic image of the ACL in the right knee. ACL was segmented with no synovial coverage, but there was no obvious tearing. ACL, anterior cruciate ligament.

3. Discussion

In adolescents, tibial tubercle avulsion fractures are relatively rare and account for 0.4–2.7% of all pediatric fractures and <1% of all epiphysis injuries [1,2]. At present, the fracture morphology of tibial tubercle avulsion fractures has been widely reported and used to classify fractures into Types I–V [8]. Notably, the morphology of Ogden Type V fracture is characterized by the morphology of Ogden Type IIIB fracture combined with that of Salter–Haris Type IV fracture, and this is a very rare fracture morphology [4]. However, the information on Ogden Type V fracture remains limited because of the scarcity of reports on this fracture, with only five cases reported to date [4,6,7]. Furthermore, despite the fact that this is an intra-articular fracture, there have been no reports of its evaluation using MRI or arthroscopy. To the best of our knowledge, this is the first detailed case report of a patient with Ogden Type V fracture evaluated via MRI and arthroscopic findings.

The ossification of tibial tuberosity can be classified into four stages: the cartilaginous, apophyseal, epiphyseal, and osseous stages [9]. In particular, during the epiphyseal stage, traction-sensitive physeal hypertrophic columnar cartilage replaces fibrocartilage [9]. This osseous pattern and apophyseal stage can create a mechanically weak area, facilitating the avulsion of the tibial tuberosity [4,10]. The epiphyseal stage is typically observed in girls aged 10–15 years and boys aged 11–17 years. Notably, tubercle avulsion fracture usually occurs during 8–15 years of age, and men are 10 times more likely to be injured than women [11–13]. In the present case, tibial tuberosity injury was noted at the epiphyseal stage when the patient was aged 13 years, and the tuberosity was vulnerable to traction forces.

X-ray imaging has been used for diagnostic evaluation and classification of fractures. However, Pace et al. reported that further evaluation with CT or MRI is necessary owing to the possibility of complications such as quadriceps rupture, patella tendon rupture, and intra-articular tissue damage [7]. Moreover, MRI is recommended for similar intra-articular fractures, such as avulsion fracture of tibia eminence and fracture of tibia plateau, to examine the damage to the intra-articular tissues, including ACL [14,15]. Conversely, to the best of our knowledge, no studies on Ogden Type V fractures have evaluated the intra-articular region using MRI or arthroscopy to date. In our patient, an MRI scan revealed that the fracture line had reached the ACL attachment area, indicating the possibility of an ACL injury. Arthroscopy findings revealed no damage to the intra-articular ligaments or meniscus at the time of metal removal. In the future, MRI should be performed for patients exhibiting fracture lines on the articular surface.

It has been reported that treatment for Type I and II fractures should be conservative; conversely, surgery is preferred for Type III and above fractures if a dislocation is present [5]. Notably, CCS fixation is the most common surgical fixation method, although some studies have reported that plate fixation may be necessary [4,7]. However, in one of these studies, plate fixation was also found to be associated with early closure of the proximal tibial epiphysis [7]. In the present case, CCS provided good fixation force and outcomes. Furthermore, it has been reported that postoperative treatment should include the following: 4 weeks of immobilization, 2 weeks of knee brace application, and initiation of extensor mechanism strengthening after the removal of the knee brace. However, only a few standardized protocols are available for postoperative treatment [16]. In particular, Type V fracture involves both the posterior bone cortex and articular surface, and it requires cautious loading. In the present case, we applied a knee brace after 3 weeks of immobilization, started partial weight bearing at 6 weeks postoperatively, and achieved full-weight bearing and full flexion at 12 weeks postoperatively. Furthermore, after confirming that the muscles had regained their strength, the patient was allowed to return to sports in approximately 6 months. The present study reports novel findings with a detailed examination and treatment outcome of a very rare case of Ogden Type V fracture. To the best of our knowledge, no studies have reported on MRI-based evaluation of Ogden Type V fractures. In the present case, we found that the fracture line to the articular surface had reached the attachment of the ACL on an MRI scan; moreover, high MRI intensity and swelling due to ACL were observed, potentially causing parenchymal ACL injury. Finally, an arthroscopic evaluation was performed to assess intra-articular damage, including parenchymal damage to ACL, and this enabled our patient to successfully return to sports.

Previous studies have reported that perioperative complications of tibial tubercle fractures include bursitis and tenderness, refractures, wound infection, leg length differences associated with early closure of the proximal tibial epiphysis, and compartment syndrome [2,7,17–20]. Of these, the most common complication is bursitis, accounting for 56% of all complications, and it requires metal removal [18,20]. Notably, the complications specific to the adolescent age group include early closure of the proximal tibial epiphysis and the associated limb length difference and angular deformity [18]. According to Gautier et al., these complications are caused by growth acceleration or retardation at the proximal tibial epiphysis [18]. Moreover, Pace et al. reported early closure of the proximal tibial epiphysis in a patient for whom plate fixation was used [7]. In particular, compartment syndrome is a serious complication [2,8,19] caused by the disruption of branches of the anterior recurrent tibial artery, and it is reported to occur in 20% of cases of tibial tubercle fractures, especially in adolescents [8,19]. Burkhart et al. reported a case of a patient with compartment syndrome requiring below-knee amputation, a complication of particular concern [17]. In the present case, fortunately, none of these complications occurred at this stage.

4. Conclusions

Type V tibial tubercle avulsion fractures are extremely rare. To the best of our knowledge, this is the first report to describe a case of tubercle avulsion fractures with detailed evaluation using MRI and arthroscopy. Based on our report, if intra-articular injury is suspected, an MRI evaluation should be performed without hesitation.

5. Clinical Message

MRI should be performed to evaluate the presence of concomitant injuries, such as periprosthetic ligament and intra-articular injuries.

Author Contributions: Conceptualization, H.I.; software, S.F.; writing—original draft preparation, H.O.; writing—review and editing, T.O.; visualization, K.I.; supervision, Y.K.; project administration, K.N. All authors have read and agreed to the published version of the manuscript.

Funding: This research received no external funding.

Institutional Review Board Statement: Not applicable.

Informed Consent Statement: Informed consent regarding the use of patient information in this study was obtained.

Data Availability Statement: The data presented in this study are available on request from the corresponding author. The data are not publicly available due to them containing information that could compromise the privacy of research participants.

Conflicts of Interest: The authors declare no conflict of interest.

References

1. Bolesta, M.J.; Fitch, R.D. Tibial tubercle avulsions. *J. Pediatr. Orthop.* **1986**, *6*, 186–192. [CrossRef] [PubMed]
2. Shelton, W.R.; Canale, S.T. Fractures of the tibia through the proximal tibial epiphyseal cartilage. *J. Bone Joint Surg. Am.* **1979**, *61*, 167–173. [CrossRef] [PubMed]
3. Ryu, R.K.; Debenham, J.O. An unusual avulsion fracture of the proximal tibial epiphysis. Case report and proposed addition to the Watson-Jones classification. *Clin. Orthop. Relat. Res.* **1985**, *194*, 181–184.
4. McKoy, B.E.; Stanitski, C.L. Acute tibial tubercle avulsion fractures. *Orthop. Clin. N. Am.* **2003**, *34*, 397–403. [CrossRef] [PubMed]
5. Ogden, J.A.; Tross, R.B.; Murphy, M.J. Fractures of the tibial tuberosity in adolescents. *J. Bone Joint Surg. Am.* **1980**, *62*, 205–215. [CrossRef] [PubMed]
6. Curtis, J.F. Type IV tibial tubercle fracture revisited: A case report. *Clin. Orthop. Relat. Res.* **2001**, *389*, 191–195. [CrossRef] [PubMed]
7. Pace, J.L.; McCulloch, P.C.; Momoh, E.O.; Nasreddine, A.Y.; Kocher, M.S. Operatively treated type IV tibial tubercle apophyseal fractures. *J. Pediatr. Orthop.* **2013**, *33*, 791–796. [CrossRef] [PubMed]
8. Cole, W.W., 3rd; Brown, S.M.; Vopat, B.; Heard, W.M.R.; Mulcahey, M.K. Epidemiology, diagnosis, and management of tibial tubercle avulsion fractures in adolescents. *JBJS Rev.* **2020**, *8*, e0186. [CrossRef] [PubMed]
9. Ehrenborg, G.; Engfeldt, B. The insertion of the ligamentum patellae on the tibial tuberosity. Some views in connection with the Osgood-Schlatter lesion. *Acta Chir. Scand.* **1961**, *121*, 491–499. [PubMed]
10. Pandya, N.K.; Edmonds, E.W.; Roocroft, J.H.; Mubarak, S.J. Tibial tubercle fractures: Complications, classification, and the need for intra-articular assessment. *J. Pediatr. Orthop.* **2012**, *32*, 749–759. [CrossRef] [PubMed]
11. Schiller, J.; DeFroda, S.; Blood, T. Lower extremity avulsion fractures in the pediatric and adolescent athlete. *J. Am. Acad. Orthop. Surg.* **2017**, *25*, 251–259. [CrossRef] [PubMed]
12. Nicolini, A.P.; Carvalho, R.T.; Ferretti, M.; Cohen, M. Simultaneous bilateral tibial tubercle avulsion fracture in a male teenager: Case report and literature review. *J. Pediatr. Orthop. B* **2018**, *27*, 40–46. [CrossRef] [PubMed]
13. Checa Betegón, P.; Arvinius, C.; Cabadas González, M.I.; Martínez García, A.; Del Pozo Martín, R.; Marco Martínez, F. Management of pediatric tibial tubercle fractures: Is surgical treatment really necessary? *Eur. J. Orthop. Surg. Traumatol.* **2019**, *29*, 1073–1079. [CrossRef] [PubMed]
14. Ishibashi, Y.; Tsuda, E.; Sasaki, T.; Toh, S. Magnetic resonance imaging AIDS in detecting concomitant injuries in patients with tibial spine fractures. *Clin. Orthop. Relat. Res.* **2005**, *434*, 207–212. [CrossRef] [PubMed]
15. Yamauchi, S.; Sasaki, S.; Kimura, Y.; Yamamoto, Y.; Tsuda, E.; Ishibashi, Y. Tibial eminence fracture with midsubstance anterior cruciate ligament tear in a 10-year-old boy: A case report. *Int. J. Surg. Case Rep.* **2020**, *67*, 13–17. [CrossRef] [PubMed]
16. Rodriguez, I.; Sepúlveda, M.; Birrer, E.; Tuca, M.J. Fracture of the anterior tibial tuberosity in children. *EFORT Open. Rev.* **2020**, *5*, 260–267. [CrossRef] [PubMed]
17. Burkhart, S.S.; Peterson, H.A. Fractures of the proximal tibial epiphysis. *J. Bone Joint Surg. Am.* **1979**, *61*, 996–1002. [CrossRef] [PubMed]
18. Gautier, E.; Ziran, B.H.; Egger, B.; Slongo, T.; Jakob, R.P. Growth disturbances after injuries of the proximal tibial epiphysis. *Arch. Orthop. Trauma. Surg.* **1998**, *118*, 37–41. [CrossRef] [PubMed]
19. Frey, S.; Hosalkar, H.; Cameron, D.B.; Heath, A.; David Horn, B.; Ganley, T.J. Tibial tuberosity fractures in adolescents. *J. Childs Orthop.* **2008**, *2*, 469–474. [CrossRef] [PubMed]
20. Pretell-Mazzini, J.; Kelly, D.M.; Sawyer, J.R.; Esteban, E.M.; Spence, D.D.; Warner, W.C., Jr.; Beaty, J.H. Outcomes and complications of tibial tubercle fractures in pediatric patients: A systematic review of the literature. *J. Pediatr. Orthop.* **2016**, *36*, 440–446. [CrossRef]

Disclaimer/Publisher's Note: The statements, opinions and data contained in all publications are solely those of the individual author(s) and contributor(s) and not of MDPI and/or the editor(s). MDPI and/or the editor(s) disclaim responsibility for any injury to people or property resulting from any ideas, methods, instructions or products referred to in the content.

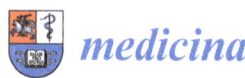

Systematic Review

Does Surgical Approach Influence Complication Rate of Hip Hemiarthroplasty for Femoral Neck Fractures? A Literature Review and Meta-Analysis

Matteo Filippini [1,2], Marta Bortoli [1], Andrea Montanari [1], Andrea Pace [1], Lorenzo Di Prinzio [1], Gianluca Lonardo [2], Stefania Claudia Parisi [1], Valentina Persiani [2], Roberto De Cristofaro [2], Andrea Sambri [2], Massimiliano De Paolis [2,*] and Michele Fiore [1,2]

[1] Alma Mater Studiorum, University of Bologna, 40126 Bologna, Italy; matteo.filippini@ior.it (M.F.); marta.bortoli@ior.it (M.B.); andrea.montanari36@studio.unibo.it (A.M.); andrea.pace@ior.it (A.P.); lorenzo.diprinzio@ior.it (L.D.P.); stefaniaclaudiaparisi@hotmail.it (S.C.P.); michele.fiore@ior.it (M.F.)

[2] Orthopedics and Traumatology Department, IRCCS Azienda Ospedaliero-Universitaria di Bologna, 40138 Bologna, Italy; gianluca.lonardo@gmail.com (G.L.); valentina.persiani@aosp.bo.it (V.P.); roberto.decristofaro@aosp.bo.it (R.D.C.); andrea.sambri2@unibo.it (A.S.)

* Correspondence: massimiliano.depaolis@aosp.bo.it

Abstract: *Background:* Femoral neck fractures are an epidemiologically significant issue with major effects on patients and health care systems, as they account for a large percentage of bone injuries in the elderly. Hip hemiarthroplasty is a common surgical procedure in the treatment of displaced femoral neck fractures. Several surgical approaches may be used to access the hip joint in case of femoral neck fractures, each with its own benefits and potential drawbacks, but none of them has consistently been found to be superior to the others. This article aims to systematically review and compare the different approaches in terms of the complication rate at the last follow-up. *Methods:* an in-depth search on PubMed/Scopus/Web of Science databases and a cross-referencing search was carried out concerning the articles comparing different approaches in hemiarthroplasty and reporting detailed data. *Results:* A total of 97,576 hips were included: 1030 treated with a direct anterior approach, 4131 with an anterolateral approach, 59,110 with a direct lateral approach, and 33,007 with a posterolateral approach. Comparing the different approaches, significant differences were found in both the overall complication rate and the rate of revision surgery performed ($p < 0.05$). In particular, the posterolateral approach showed a significantly higher complication rate than the lateral approach (8.4% vs. 3.2%, $p < 0.001$). Furthermore, the dislocation rate in the posterolateral group was significantly higher than in the other three groups considered ($p < 0.026$). However, the posterolateral group showed less blood loss than the anterolateral group ($p < 0.001$), a lower intraoperative fractures rate than the direct anterior group ($p < 0.035$), and shorter mean operative time than the direct lateral group ($p < 0.018$). *Conclusions:* The posterolateral approach showed a higher complication rate than direct lateral approach and a higher prosthetic dislocation rate than the other three types of surgical approaches. On the other hand, patients treated with posterolateral approach showed better outcomes in other parameters considered, such as mean operative time, mean blood loss and intraoperative fractures rate. The knowledge of the limitations of each approach and the most common associated complications can lead to choosing a surgical technique based on the patient's individual risk.

Keywords: hip hemiarthroplasty; femoral neck fracture; postero-lateral approach; lateral approach; antero-lateral approach; anterior approach

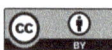

1. Introduction

Fractures of the femoral neck are one of the most common bone injuries among the elderly, often caused by accidental trauma or bone fragility due to osteoporosis. This injury can cause intense pain and significantly limit a patient's mobility, affecting their quality of life.

Hip hemiarthroplasty (HHA), also known as partial hip replacement is a common surgical procedure in the treatment of displaced femoral neck fractures. In this type of surgery, only the femoral head is replaced; the acetabulum is left intact and the joint is realigned to provide a smooth and stable surface for movement. HHA is considered a less invasive surgical technique than total hip arthroplasty and may be indicated especially for elderly patients or those with poor health conditions [1–3].

There are several surgical approaches that may be used to access the hip joint, each with its own benefits and potential drawbacks. The most appropriate approach for each patient depends on many factors, including general health status, the specific pathology, and the preference of the surgeon [3]. The direct lateral approach (DL) and posterolateral approach (PL) are the most commonly used according to the literature [4,5], but the antero-lateral approach (AL) and the direct anterior approach (DA) have also been extensively described [6–9].

The complication rate of these approaches has been compared in several studies but none of them has consistently been found to be superior to the others. However, to our knowledge, there is no study in which all approaches have been analyzed simultaneously.

The aim of this systematic review of the literature is to offer an up-to-date overview of the evidence regarding hemiarthroplasty by comparing all the most used different approaches in terms of complication rate at last follow-up.

2. Materials and Methods

This systematic review was conducted in accordance with the 2020 PRISMA guidelines (Preferred reporting items of systematic reviews) (Figure 1).

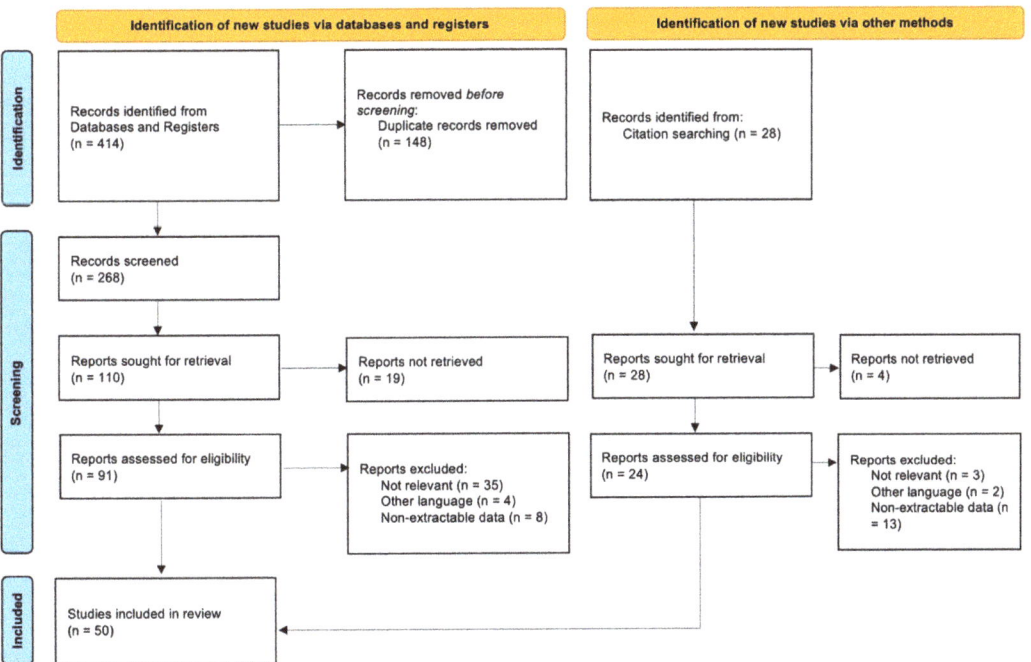

Figure 1. PRISMA flow diagram and the selection of studies.

All studies (randomized controlled trials-RCT, prospective and retrospective comparative studies and case series) reporting on 'hemiarthroplasty' as treatment of femoral neck fractures were included. The diagnosis has been made based on clinical features and radiograph by the individual authors.

Studies reporting the results of femoral neck fractures treatment other than HHA (including THA and internal fixation techniques) were excluded. Studies reporting the results of HHA were included only if the results obtained in patients undergoing different surgical approaches were clearly distinguishable.

Only studies comparing two different surgical approaches were included. Only studies with a minimum follow-up of 6 months and a minimum of 5 patients treated with hemiarthroplasty available for analysis were considered for inclusion. Only studies in English were included. Case series reporting on a single technique were excluded. Biomechanical studies, cadaveric studies, in vitro studies, and animal model studies were also excluded.

Studies eligible for this systematic review have been identified, through an electronic systematic search with no restriction on date of publication, up to the end of February 2023, performed on PubMed (https://pubmed.ncbi.nlm.nih.gov/ (accessed on 28 February 2023)), Scopus (https://www.scopus.com (accessed on 28 February 2023)), and Web of Science (www.webofscience.com (accessed on 28 February 2023)) databases. Articles that were considered relevant by electronic search were retrieved in full-text, and a cross-referencing search of their bibliography was performed, to find further related articles. Reviews and meta-analyses were also analyzed, in order to broaden the search for studies that might have been missed through the electronic search. All duplicates were removed, and all the articles retrieved were analyzed.

After the first screening, records without eligibility criteria were excluded.

Remnant studies were categorized by type, according to the Oxford Centre for Evidence-Based Medicine (OCEBM). To assess the quality of the articles, Cochrane risk-of-bias tool for randomized trials (RoB 2) (Figure 2) and Cochrane's risk of bias tool for non-randomized studies (ROBINS-I) (Figure 3) were used. These tools assign a categorical value based on the risk of bias of each single aspect of each study and allow to obtain a summary value that quantifies its overall quality.

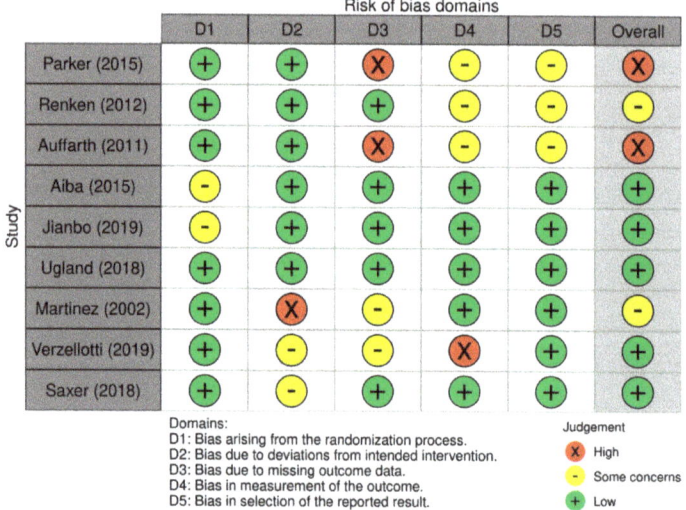

Figure 2. Cochrane risk-of-bias tool for randomized trials (RoB 2) [10–18].

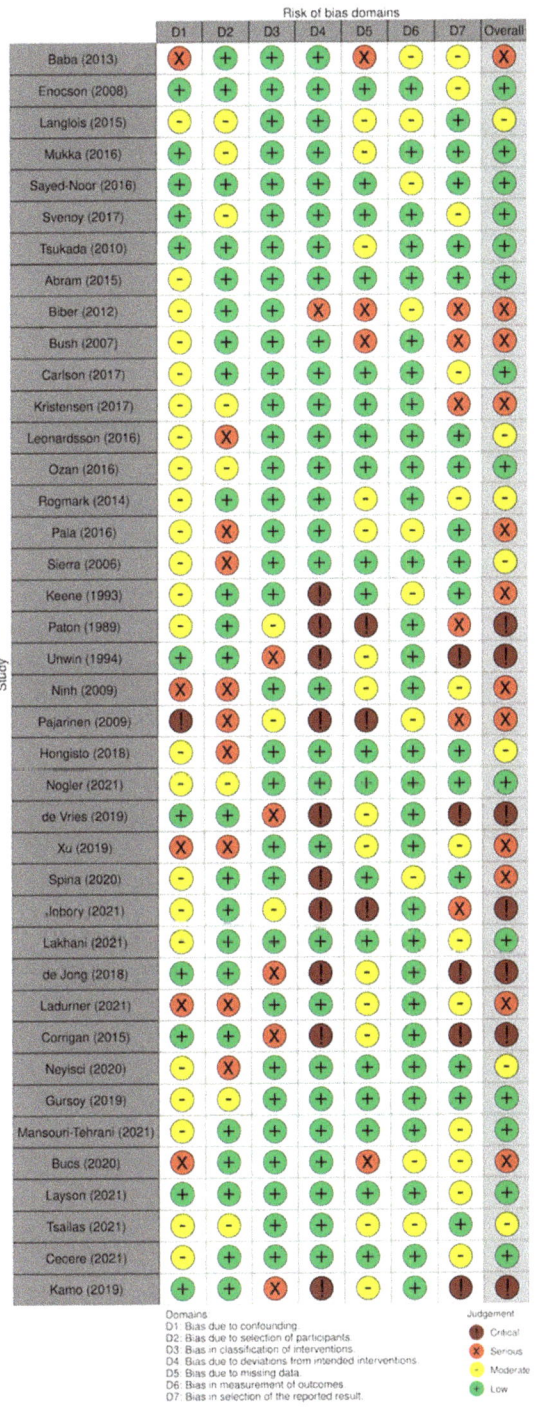

Figure 3. Cochrane risk-of-bias tool for non-randomized studies (ROBINS-I) [5,19–58].

All the included studies were analyzed. The data extracted included mean age, mean follow-up, number of hips, mean operative time, mean estimated blood loss, number and type of peri-operative complications, number of revision surgeries, mean length of stay. Based on the type of surgical approach, four groups were formed: (1) direct lateral approach, (2) anterolateral approach, (3) direct anterior approach, (4) posterolateral approach. Functional outcomes were not reported in this review, due to the lack of these data in the vast majority of the included studies.

Studies with reported quantitative data were used for statistical analysis. Weighted means and standard deviations were calculated to summarize the values reported in the individual studies and to compare them. For quantitative variables, Shapiro–Wilk test was used to verify normal distribution. Levene test was used to assess the equality of variances. Chi-square statistics (Pearson's chi-square, Yates' chi-square, Fisher's exact test, Fisher–Freeman–Halton test), ANOVA, or Kruskal–Wallis tests were used to assess associations and homogeneity among the groups, depending on the type of variables considered. The meta-analysis was conducted when at least 4 studies were available for comparison. Quantification of the extent of statistical heterogeneity across studies included in the meta-analysis employed the inconsistency statistic ($I^2 > 75\%$ was considered as highly heterogeneity). Potential sources of heterogeneity by study-level and clinically relevant characteristics were explored using stratified analysis and meta-regression. Publication bias was assessed using Egger's regression symmetry test. p-value < 0.05 was considered to be significant. All statistical analyses were performed with IBM SPSS v26.0 for MacOS (SPSS Inc., Chicago, IL, USA) and ProMeta 3 (Internovi, Cesena, Italy) softwares.

3. Results

A total of 268 studies were found through the electronic search and 3 studies were added follwing cross-referenced research on the bibliography of the examined full-text articles. After a preliminary analysis, a total of 50 studies were included in this systematic review [5,10–58] (Table 1).

The DL approach was compared to the AL approach in 3 studies [40,41,57], to the DA approach in 8 studies [10,18,39,41,44,46,57,58], and to the PL approach in 18 studies [5,11,20,23,25–28,34,36,37,40–42,45,51,52,57]. The AL approach was compared to the DA approach in five studies [13,41,48,49,57], and to the PL approach in nine studies [19,22,24,38,40,41,49,55,57]. The DA and the PL approach were compared in 10 studies [12,15,30–33,41,49,50,57].

Nine studies were randomized control trials [10–18], six were prospective comparative cohort studies [19,30–32,35,37], thirty-two were retrospective comparative cohort studies [20–24,26–29,33,34,36,38–44,46–58] and three were registry studies [5,25,45].

The overall quality of the series assessed (with Rob 2; Robins-I) was classified as high [12,14–16,18,22,24,33,35–37,39,41,46,51,52,54,56] or moderate [5,13,26,34,40,50,55] in most of the cases (Figures 2 and 3). No significant differences were found between the different groups analyzed regarding the mean age and the mean follow-up time (Table 2).

Table 1. Data from the studies included in this review.

Study	Design	Approach	Total n. of Patients	N. of Patients for Group	Mean Age (Years)	Mean FU (Months)	Mean OT (min)	Mean EBL (mL)	Dislocation n.	Dislocation %	Stem Loosening n.	Stem Loosening %	Periprosthetic Fracture n.	Periprosthetic Fracture %	Deep Infection n.	Deep Infection %	Wound Dehiscence/Superficial Infection n.	Wound Dehiscence/Superficial Infection %	Intraoperative Fracture n.	Intraoperative Fracture %	Others * n.	Others * %	TOTAL n.	TOTAL %	Revision Surgeries n.	Revision Surgeries %	Mean LOS (Days)
Kersee (1993) [19]	PCCS	AL / PL	531	302 / 229	81 / 81	12	56 / 48	251 / 197	5 / 10	1.7 / 4.3	0 / 0	0 / 0	0 / 8	0 / 3.5	6 / 2	2 / 0.9	18 / 6	6 / 2.6	6 / 4	2 / 1.7	4 / 22	1.3 / 9.6	39 / 52	12.9% / 22.7%	0 / 0	0 / 0	N/A
Paton (1989) [20]	RCCS	DL / PL	171	78 / 93	79.3 / 79.3	N/A	N/A / N/A	N/A / N/A	2 / 8	2.6 / 8.6	N/A / N/A	N/A / N/A	N/A / N/A	N/A / N/A	N/A / N/A	N/A / N/A	N/A / N/A	N/A / N/A	N/A / N/A	N/A / N/A	N/A / N/A	N/A / N/A	2 / 8	2.6% / 8.6%	N/A / N/A	N/A / N/A	34 / 33
Unwin (1994) [21]	RCCS	DL / PL	2906	1250 / 1656	N/A	N/A	N/A / N/A	N/A / N/A	41 / 149	3.3 / 9	N/A / N/A	N/A / N/A	N/A / N/A	N/A / N/A	N/A / N/A	N/A / N/A	N/A / N/A	N/A / N/A	N/A / N/A	N/A / N/A	N/A / N/A	N/A / N/A	41 / 149	3.3% / 9.0%	N/A / N/A	N/A / N/A	N/A / N/A
Abram (2014) [22]	RCCS	AL / PL	807	753 / 54	N/A / N/A	12	N/A / N/A	N/A / N/A	16 / 7	2.1 / 13	0 / 0	0 / 0	0 / 0	0 / 0	33	4.1	0 / 0	0 / 0	15	1.9	N/A	N/A	64 / 7	8.5% / 13.0%	33	4.1	26
Biber (2012) [23]	RCCS	PL / DL	704	487 / 217	80.4 / 80.3	N/A / N/A	N/A / N/A	N/A / N/A	19 / 1	3.9 / 0.5	0 / 0	0 / 0	0 / 0	0 / 0	12 / 7	2.5 / 3.2	0 / 0	0 / 0	3 / 1	0.6 / 0.5	15 / 14	3 / 6.4	49 / 23	10.1% / 10.6%	N/A / N/A	N/A / N/A	N/A / N/A
Enocson (2008) [24]	RCCS	AL / PL	739	431 / 308	84 / 85	2.3	N/A / N/A	N/A / N/A	13 / 32	3 / 10.4	0 / 0	0 / 0	0 / 0	0 / 0	0 / 0	0 / 0	0 / 0	0 / 0	0 / 0	0 / 0	0 / 0	0 / 0	13 / 32	3.0% / 10.4%	13	1.8	N/A / N/A
Kristensen (2016) [25]	RS	DL / PL	20,908	18,918 / 1990	83 / 83	36	76 / 67	N/A / N/A	N/A / N/A	N/A / N/A	N/A / N/A	N/A / N/A	N/A / N/A	N/A / N/A	N/A / N/A	N/A / N/A	N/A / N/A	N/A / N/A	N/A / N/A	N/A / N/A	N/A / N/A	N/A / N/A	0 / 0	0.0% / 0.0%	757 / 139	4 / 7	N/A / N/A
Leonardsson (2016) [26]	RCCS	DL / PL	2118	1140 / 978	85 / 85	N/A / N/A	N/A / N/A	N/A / N/A	10 / 20	0.9 / 2	0 / 0	0 / 0	6 / 4	0.5 / 0.4	12 / 13	1.1 / 1.3	0 / 0	0 / 0	0 / 0	0 / 0	8 / 3	0.7 / 0.3	36 / 40	3.2% / 4.1%	36 / 40	3 / 4	N/A / N/A
Ninh (2009) [27]	RCCS	PL / DL	144	115 / 29	77.3 / 77.3	12	N/A / N/A	N/A / N/A	9 / 2	7.8 / 6.9	N/A / N/A	N/A / N/A	N/A / N/A	N/A / N/A	N/A / N/A	N/A / N/A	N/A / N/A	N/A / N/A	N/A / N/A	N/A / N/A	N/A / N/A	N/A / N/A	9 / 2	7.8% / 6.9%	N/A / N/A	N/A / N/A	N/A / N/A
Pajarinen (2009) [28]	RCCS	PL / DL	338	86 / 252	83.2 / 83.2	6	N/A / N/A	N/A / N/A	14 / 8	16.3 / 3.2	N/A / N/A	N/A / N/A	N/A / N/A	N/A / N/A	N/A / N/A	N/A / N/A	N/A / N/A	N/A / N/A	N/A / N/A	N/A / N/A	N/A / N/A	N/A / N/A	14 / 8	16.3% / 3.2%	N/A / N/A	N/A / N/A	N/A / N/A
Parker (2015) [11]	RCT	DL / PL	216	108 / 108	84.3 / 83.6	12	53.6 / 54	N/A / N/A	2 / 1	1.9 / 0.9	0 / 0	0 / 0	1 / 4	0.9 / 3.8	0 / 2	0 / 1.9	3 / 2	2.9 / 1.9	6 / 2	5.6 / 1.9	1 / 2	0.9 / 1.9	13 / 13	12.0% / 12.0%	2 / 1	1.9 / 0.9	20.3 / 18.5
Rogmark (2014) [15]	RS	PL / DL	33,205	11,999 / 21,206	84 / 84	32	N/A / N/A	N/A / N/A	443	1.3	13	0.04	154	0.5	424	1.3	N/A / N/A	N/A / N/A	N/A / N/A	N/A / N/A	130	0.4	1164 / 0	9.7% / 0.0%	477 / 687	4 / 3.2	N/A / N/A
Svenoy (2017) [29]	RCCS	PL / DL	583	186 / 397	83.2 / 82.6	12	69.2 / 66.7	N/A / N/A	15 / 4	8.1 / 1	N/A / N/A	N/A / N/A	N/A / N/A	N/A / N/A	N/A / N/A	N/A / N/A	12 / 20	6.5 / 5	3 / 8	1.6 / 2			30 / 32	16.1% / 8.1%	8 / 2	4.3 / 0.5	N/A / N/A
Alba (2015) [12]	RCT	DA / PA	29	13 / 16	81.5 / 78.6	N/A	85.6 / 61.8	198.3 / 146.7	0 / 0	0 / 0	0 / 0	0 / 0	0 / 0	0 / 0	0 / 0	0 / 0	0 / 0	0 / 0	2 / 1	15 / 0	4 / 3	13.8 / 10.3	6 / 3	46.2% / 18.8%	0 / 0	0 / 0	N/A / N/A
Auffarth (2011) [10]	RCT	DA / DL	48	24 / 24	82.6 / 83.7	6	N/A / N/A	N/A / N/A	0 / 0	0 / 0	0 / 0	0 / 0	0 / 0	0 / 0	0 / 1	0 / 4.2	0 / 0	0 / 0	0 / 1	0 / 4.2	6 / 2	25 / 8.3	6 / 4	25.0% / 16.7%	1 / 1	4.2 / 4.2	N/A / N/A
Renken (2012) [13]	RCT	DA / AL	57	30 / 27	84 / 87.5	1.3	73.6 / 64.8	N/A / N/A	0 / 0	0 / 0	0 / 0	0 / 0	0 / 0	0 / 0	0 / 1	0 / 3.7	0 / 1	0 / 3.3	0 / 0	0 / 0	1 / 2	3.3 / 7.4	2 / 3	6.7% / 11.1%	0 / 0	0 / 0	29.9 / 29.3
Baba (2013) [30]	PCCS	DA / PL	79	40 / 39	76.7 / 74.9	36	65.3 / 76.7	121 / 146	0 / 1	0 / 2.6	0 / 0	0 / 0	0 / 0	0 / 0	0 / 0	0 / 0	0 / 0	0 / 0	1 / 1	2.5 / 2.6	0 / 0	0 / 0	1 / 2	2.5% / 5.1%	0 / 0	0 / 0	N/A / N/A
Langlois (2015) [31]	PCCS	DA / PL	82	38 / 44	86 / 75	22	65 / 54	N/A / N/A	1 / 9	2.6 / 20.5	0 / 0	0 / 0	0 / 0	0 / 0	0 / 1	0 / 2.3	0 / 0	0 / 0	0 / 1	0 / 2.3	2 / 1	5.3 / 2.3	3 / 12	7.9% / 27.3%	1 / 1	2.6 / 2.3	N/A / N/A
Pala (2016) [32]	PCCS	DA / PL	109	55 / 54	89 / 87.6	24	47 / 57	289 / 213	1 / 4	1.8 / 7.4	0 / 0	0 / 0	0 / 1	0 / 1.8	0 / 0	0 / 0	0 / 0	0 / 0	1 / 0	1.8 / 0	3 / 1	5.5 / 1.8	5 / 6	9.1% / 11.1%	N/A / N/A	N/A / N/A	12 / 14
Tsukada (2010) [33]	RCCS	DA / PL	83	44 / 39	80.4 / 81.9	12	75.1 / 79.3	370.1 / 230	0 / 1	0 / 2.6	0 / 0	0 / 0	0 / 0	0 / 0	0 / 0	0 / 0	0 / 0	0 / 0	2 / 0	4.5 / 0	1 / 0	2.3 / 0	3 / 1	6.8% / 2.6%	0 / 0	0 / 0	35.4 / 36.1

Table 1. Cont.

Study	Design	Approach	Total n. of Patients	N. of Patients for Group	Mean Age (Years)	Mean FU (Months)	Mean OT (min)	Mean EBL (mL)	Dislocation		Stem Loosening		Periprosthetic Fracture		Local Peri-Operative Complications Deep Infection		Wound Dehiscence/Superficial Infection		Intraoperative Fracture		Others *		TOTAL		Revision Surgeries		Mean LOS (Days)
									n.	%	n.	%	n.	%	n.	%	n.	%	n.	%	n.	%	n.	%	n.	%	
Hongisto (2018) [34]	RCCS	DL PL	269	151 118	82.9 82.5	12	N/A N/A	N/A N/A	0 4	0 3.4	N/A N/A	N/A N/A	N/A N/A	N/A N/A	N/A N/A	N/A N/A	N/A N/A	N/A N/A	N/A N/A	N/A N/A	N/A N/A	N/A N/A	0 4	0.0% 3.4%	N/A N/A	N/A N/A	N/A N/A
Sayed-Noor (2016) [35]	PCCS	DL PL	48	24 24	83.4 82.7	12	N/A N/A	N/A N/A	N/A N/A	N/A N/A	N/A N/A	N/A N/A	N/A N/A	N/A N/A	N/A N/A	N/A N/A	N/A N/A	N/A N/A	N/A N/A	N/A N/A	N/A N/A	N/A N/A	0 0	0.0% 0.0%	N/A N/A	N/A N/A	N/A N/A
Ozan (2016) [36]	RCCS	DL PL	233	86 147	78.3 78.7	17.1	90 66	254 239	4 17	4.6 11.5	0 0	0 0	0 0	0 0	3 11	3.4 7.4	N/A N/A	N/A N/A	0 0	0 0	N/A N/A	N/A N/A	7 28	8.1% 19.0%	N/A N/A	N/A N/A	N/A N/A
Muaka (2016) [37]	PCCS	DL PL	185	76 58	83.5 85.5	12	N/A N/A	N/A N/A	3 9	3.9 15.5	0 0	0 0	1 0	1.3 0	5 5	6.6 8.6	0 2	0 3.4	0 0	0 0	0 1	0 1.7	9 17	11.8% 29.3%	15 9	19.7 15.5	N/A N/A
Bush (2007) [38]	RCCS	AL PL	385	186 199	80.5 79.2	6	N/A N/A	N/A N/A	0 9	0 4.5	0 1	0 0.5	0 0	0 0	0 0	0 0	0 0	0 0	0 0	0 0	0 1	0 0.5	0 11	0.0% 5.5%	N/A N/A	N/A N/A	7.3 6.4
Carlson (2017) [39]	RCCS	DA DL	160	85 75	82.7 82.9	6	42.9 N/A	N/A N/A	2 0	2.4 0	0 0	0 0	3 4	3.5 4	1 2	1.2 2.7	0 0	0 0	0 0	0 0	2 3	2.4 4	8 8	9.4% 10.7%	4 5	4.7 6.7	6.2 8.9
Sierra (2006) [40]	RCCS	AL PL DL	1802	1432 245 125	N/A N/A N/A	N/A N/A N/A	N/A N/A N/A	N/A N/A N/A	22 5 5	1.5 2 4	N/A N/A N/A	N/A N/A N/A	3 1 0	0.2 0.4 0	N/A N/A N/A	N/A N/A N/A	N/A N/A N/A	N/A N/A N/A	N/A N/A N/A	N/A N/A N/A	N/A N/A N/A	N/A N/A N/A	25 6 5	1.7% 2.4% 4.0%	15 2 4	1 0.8 3.2	N/A N/A N/A
Nogler (2021) [41]	RCCS	PL DL DA AL	1158	656 312 116 74	89.1 86.7 85 84.7	N/A N/A N/A N/A	N/A N/A N/A N/A	N/A N/A N/A N/A	8 3 1 1	1.2 0.96 0.86 1.35	N/A N/A N/A N/A	N/A N/A N/A N/A	15 8 1 1	2.28 2.56 0.86 1.35	N/A N/A N/A N/A	N/A N/A N/A N/A	N/A N/A N/A N/A	N/A N/A N/A N/A	6 4 2 2	0.9 1.28 1.7 2.7	N/A N/A N/A N/A	N/A N/A N/A N/A	29 15 4 4	4.4% 4.8% 3.4% 5.4%	N/A N/A N/A N/A	N/A N/A N/A N/A	4.2 4.8 2.3 2.8
de Vries (2019) [42]	RCCS	DL PL	1009	493 516	87 86	N/A N/A	N/A N/A	N/A N/A	7 15	1.4 2.9	N/A N/A	N/A N/A	14 12	2.8 2.3	23 23	4.5 4.7	11 16	2.2 3.1	N/A N/A	N/A N/A	N/A N/A	N/A N/A	55 66	11.2% 12.8%	N/A N/A	N/A N/A	7 7
Spina (2020) [44]	RCCS	DA DL	75	37 38	87.6 87	12	87.7 82	N/A N/A	1 2	2.7 5.3	0 0	0 0	0 0	0 0	0 1	0 2.6	0 0	0 0	0 0	0 0	N/A N/A	N/A N/A	1 3	2.7% 7.9%	N/A N/A	N/A N/A	N/A N/A
Joborry (2021) [45]	RS	DL PL	25,603	13,769 11,834	N/A N/A	12	N/A N/A	N/A N/A	366 850	2.7 7.2	N/A N/A	N/A N/A	N/A N/A	N/A N/A	N/A N/A	N/A N/A	N/A N/A	N/A N/A	N/A N/A	N/A N/A	N/A N/A	N/A N/A	366 850	2.7% 7.2%	162 241	1.2 2	N/A N/A
Lakhani (2021) [46]	RCCS	DA DL	94	40 54	85.4 85.8	19.2	90 90	N/A N/A	1 2	2.5 3.7	0 0	0 0	0 0	0 0	2 4	5 7.4	0 0	0 0	0 2	0 3.7	2 2	5 3.7	5 10	12.5% 18.5%	2 5	5 9.26	8 9
Verzellotti (2021) [15]	RCT	DA PL	100	50 50	85.3 85	6	72.6 64.1	N/A N/A	0 0	0 0	0 0	0 0	0 0	0 0	0 0	0 0	0 0	0 0	0 0	0 0	5 6	10 12	5 6	10.0% 12.0%	0 0	0 0	N/A N/A
Ugland (2018) [16]	RCT	AL DL	150	75 75	81.4 81.3	12	N/A N/A	N/A N/A	N/A N/A	N/A N/A	N/A N/A	N/A N/A	N/A N/A	N/A N/A	N/A N/A	N/A N/A	N/A N/A	N/A N/A	N/A N/A	N/A N/A	N/A N/A	N/A N/A	0 0	0.0% 0.0%	N/A N/A	N/A N/A	N/A N/A
Ladurner (2021) [48]	RCCS	DA AL	237	79 158	85.5 86	N/A	72.5 89.5	285.5 287	0 1	0 0.6	0 0	0 0	0 0	0 0	1 2	1.3 1.3	0 0	0 0	0 0	0 0	2 8	2.5 5.1	3 11	3.8% 7.0%	2 5	2.5 3.2	8.3 8.4

Table 1. Cont.

Study	Design	Approach	Total n. of Patients	N. of Patients for Group	Mean Age (Years)	Mean FU (Months)	Mean OT (min)	Mean EBL (mL)	Dislocation n.	Dislocation %	Stem Loosening n.	Stem Loosening %	Periprosthetic Fracture n.	Periprosthetic Fracture %	Deep Infection n.	Deep Infection %	Wound Dehiscence/Superficial Infection n.	Wound Dehiscence/Superficial Infection %	Intraoperative Fracture n.	Intraoperative Fracture %	Others * n.	Others * %	TOTAL n.	TOTAL %	Revision Surgeries n.	Revision Surgeries %	Mean LOS (Days)
Corrigan (2015) [49]	RCCS	DA AL PL	82	26 32 24	78.5 77.3 81.7	N/A	N/A N/A N/A	N/A N/A N/A	N/A N/A N/A	N/A N/A N/A	N/A N/A N/A	N/A N/A N/A	N/A N/A N/A	N/A N/A N/A	N/A N/A N/A	N/A N/A N/A	N/A N/A N/A	N/A N/A N/A	N/A N/A N/A	N/A N/A N/A	5 11 6	19 34 25	5 11 6	19.2% 34.4% 25.0%	N/A N/A N/A	N/A N/A N/A	N/A N/A N/A
Neyisci (2020) [50]	RCCS	PL DA	110	54 56	83 82	15.5	110 90	N/A N/A	0 0	0 0	0 0	0 0	0 0	0 0	0 0	0 0	0 0	0 0	0 1	0 1.8	0 3	0 5.4	0 4	0.0% 7.1%	0 0	0 0	11.3 8.2
Gursoy (2019) [51]	RCCS	PL DL	112	48 64	86.5 87.1	42	66.6 60	N/A N/A	8 3	16.7 4.7	0 0	0 0	0 0	0 0	2 2	4.2 3.1	0 0	0 0	0 0	0 0	N/A N/A	N/A N/A	10 5	20.8% 7.8%	N/A N/A	N/A N/A	N/A N/A
Mansouri-Tehrani (2021) [52]	RCCS	DL PL	154	99 55	78 75.4	36.5	N/A N/A	N/A N/A	6 1	6.1 1.81	0 0	0 0	0 0	0 0	4 2	4.04 3.63	0 0	0 0	0 0	0 0	29 15	29.3 27.3	39 18	39.4% 32.7%	3 1	3.03 1.81	N/A N/A
Bucs (2020) [53]	RCCS	DA AL	94	51 43	79.4 79.3	4	52.3 53.7	738.23 810.47	N/A N/A	N/A N/A	N/A N/A	N/A N/A	N/A N/A	N/A N/A	N/A N/A	N/A N/A	N/A N/A	N/A N/A	N/A N/A	N/A N/A	N/A N/A	N/A N/A	0 0	0.0% 0.0%	N/A N/A	N/A N/A	1.4 3.1
Layson (2021) [54]	RCCS	DA AL	173	93 80	81.6 79.1	N/A	95.1 74.8	N/A N/A	N/A N/A	N/A N/A	N/A N/A	N/A N/A	N/A N/A	N/A N/A	N/A N/A	N/A N/A	N/A N/A	N/A N/A	N/A N/A	N/A N/A	N/A N/A	N/A N/A	0 0	0.0% 0.0%	N/A N/A	N/A N/A	N/A N/A
Saxer (2018) [18]	RCT	DL DA	181	99 82	84 84.4	12	100.1 96.3	N/A N/A	0 0	0 0	0 0	0 0	0 0	0 0	0 7	0 8.5	5 0	5.1 0	0 0	0 0	46 0	46.5 0	51 7	51.5% 8.5%	N/A N/A	N/A N/A	N/A N/A
Tsailas (2021) [55]	RCCS	AL PL	100	50 50	80.9 82.3	47	75 67.5	N/A N/A	1 2	2 4	0 0	0 0	0 0	0 0	0 0	0 0	0 0	0 0	2 2	4 4	2 5	4 10	5 9	10.0% 18.0%	N/A N/A	N/A N/A	N/A N/A
Kamo (2019) [57]	RCCS	AL DA DL PL	194	25 21 9 50	82.2 83 87.1 83.6	10	80 63 82 72	N/A N/A N/A N/A	2 0 0 1	8 0 0 2	0 0 0 0	0 0 0 0	0 0 0 6	0 0 0 3.1	0 0 0 0	0 0 0 0	0 0 0 0	0 0 0 0	4 4 0 2	16 19 0 4	6	3.1	18 4 0 3	72.0% 19.0% 0.0% 6.0%	N/A N/A N/A N/A	N/A N/A N/A N/A	N/A N/A N/A N/A
Orth (2022) [58]	RCCS	DA DL	100	50 50	82.5 79.9	12	86.9 90.7	72.5 155.4	1 1	0 2	0 0	0 0	0 0	0 0	1 2	2 2	0 0	0 0	0 3	0 6	N/A N/A	N/A N/A	1 4	2.0% 8.0%	N/A N/A	N/A N/A	13.3 13.1

* Deep vein thrombosis, pulmonary embolism, hematoma, seroma, sepsis, cardiovascular accident, acetabular erosion, nerve palsy, heterotopic ossification. Abbreviations: FU, follow-up; OT, operative time; EBL, estimated blood loss; LOS, length of stay; PCCS, prospective comparative cohort study; RCCS, retrospective comparative cohort study; RS, registry study; RCT, randomized controlled trial; DA, direct anterior approach; AL, anterolateral approach; DL, direct lateral approach; PL, posterolateral approach; N/A, not available.

Table 2. Summarized data from the included studies of this review.

	DA	AL	DL	PL	Total
Studies (n.)	20	16	27	41	50
N. of patients	1030	4131	59,110	33,007	97,576
Mean age (yrs)	83.5	82.2	83.6	83.8	83.4
Mean follow-up (months)	13.1	9.8	28.0	22.7	25.5
Complications (%)	79 (7.7)	258 (6.2)	1901 (3.2)	2762 (8.4)	3773 (3.9)
Revision surgery (%)	10 (2.0)	70 (2.9)	1677 (3.0)	965 (3.4)	2678 (3.0)

Abbreviations: DA, direct anterior approach; AL, anterolateral approach; DL, direct lateral approach; PL, posterolateral approach.

A total of 97,278 hips were included: 1030 treated with the DA approach, 4131 treated with the AL approach, 59,110 treated with the DL approach, and 33,007 treated with the PL approach (Table 1). Mean age was comparable between the four groups (83.5 ± 3.0 in DA group; 82.2 ± 2.8 in AL group; 83.6 ± 3.0 in DL group; 83.8 ± 3.4 in PL group). The mean follow-up was 25.5 ± 11.3 months, comparable between the four groups.

Regarding the overall complication rate, significant differences were found between the different surgical approaches ($p < 0.001$). In particular, the PL approach showed a significantly higher complication rate than the DL approach (8.4% vs. 3.2%, $p < 0.001$, $I^2 = 86.13\%$) (Figure 4).

The revision surgery rate also differed significantly between the individual surgical approaches ($p < 0.001$). In particular, compared to the DL approach, the PL group showed a significantly higher revision surgery rate (3.41% vs. 3.00%; $p < 0.007$, $I^2 = 71.52\%$), while the AL group showed a significantly lower revision surgery rate than the DL group (1.96% vs. 3.00%; $p < 0.046$; $I^2 \approx 0\%$) (Figure 5).

In this study, we compared the rate of each complication in the groups analyzed. It was found that the PL approach showed a significantly higher dislocation rate than the DA approach (5.10% vs. 0.68%; $p < 0.035$; $I^2 \approx 0\%$), the AL group (5.10% vs. 1.62%; $p < 0.001$; $I^2 = 46.78\%$), and the DL group (5.10% vs. 1.54%; $p < 0.018$; $I^2 = 37.42\%$). No significant differences were found in dislocation rate when comparing the other three groups (DA, AL, DL) to each other (Figure 6). On the other hand, the PL group showed less mean blood loss than the AL group (359.63 mL vs. 449.5 mL; $p < 0.001$; $I^2 \approx 0\%$), a lower intraoperative fractures rate than the DA group (0.13% vs. 1.26%; $p < 0.035$; $I^2 \approx 0\%$) (Figure 7), and a shorter mean operative time than the DL group (69.38 min. vs. 78.04 min.; $p < 0.018$; $I^2 = 92.72\%$) (Figure 8a).

Furthermore, a significant difference was found concerning the mean length of stay between the AL and the DL group, with the AL group showing a greater length of stay (11.95 days vs. 8.56 days; $p < 0.001$; $I^2 \approx 0\%$).

Other differences were observed between the DA group and the DL group, showing a lower mean operative time (74.23 min. vs. 78.04 min.; $p < 0.046$; $I^2 = 82.11\%$) (Figure 8b), but a higher mean blood loss (296.38 mL vs. 204.70 mL; $p < 0.001$; $I^2 \approx 0\%$) in the DA group.

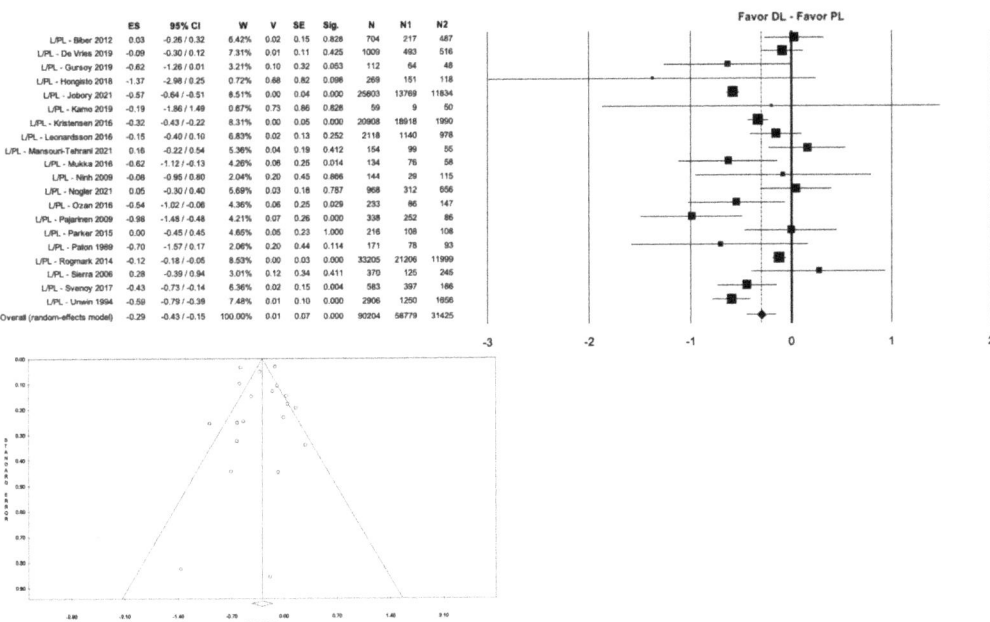

Figure 4. Forest plot and funnel plot of overall meta-analysis evaluating studies with data on overall complications in patients treated with direct lateral approach vs. posterolateral approach. The figure shows the highest estimated risk of complications in the posterolateral group. Abbreviations: ES, effect size; 95% CI, 95% confidence interval; W, weight; N, sample size [5,11,20,21,23,25–29,34,36,37,40–42,45,51,52,57].

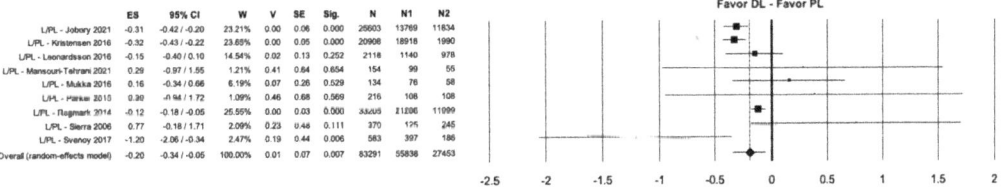

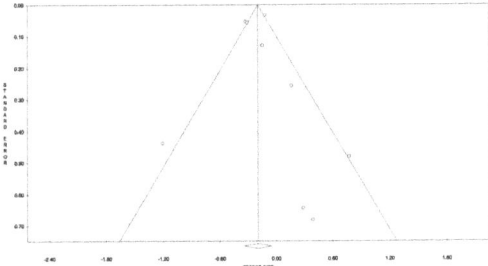

Figure 5. Forest plot and funnel plot of overall meta-analysis evaluating studies with data about revision surgeries in patients treated with direct lateral approach vs. posterolateral approach. The figure shows the highest estimated risk of revision surgeries in the posterolateral group. Abbreviations: ES, effect size; 95% CI, 95% confidence interval; W, weight; N, sample size [5,11,25,26,29,37,40,45,52].

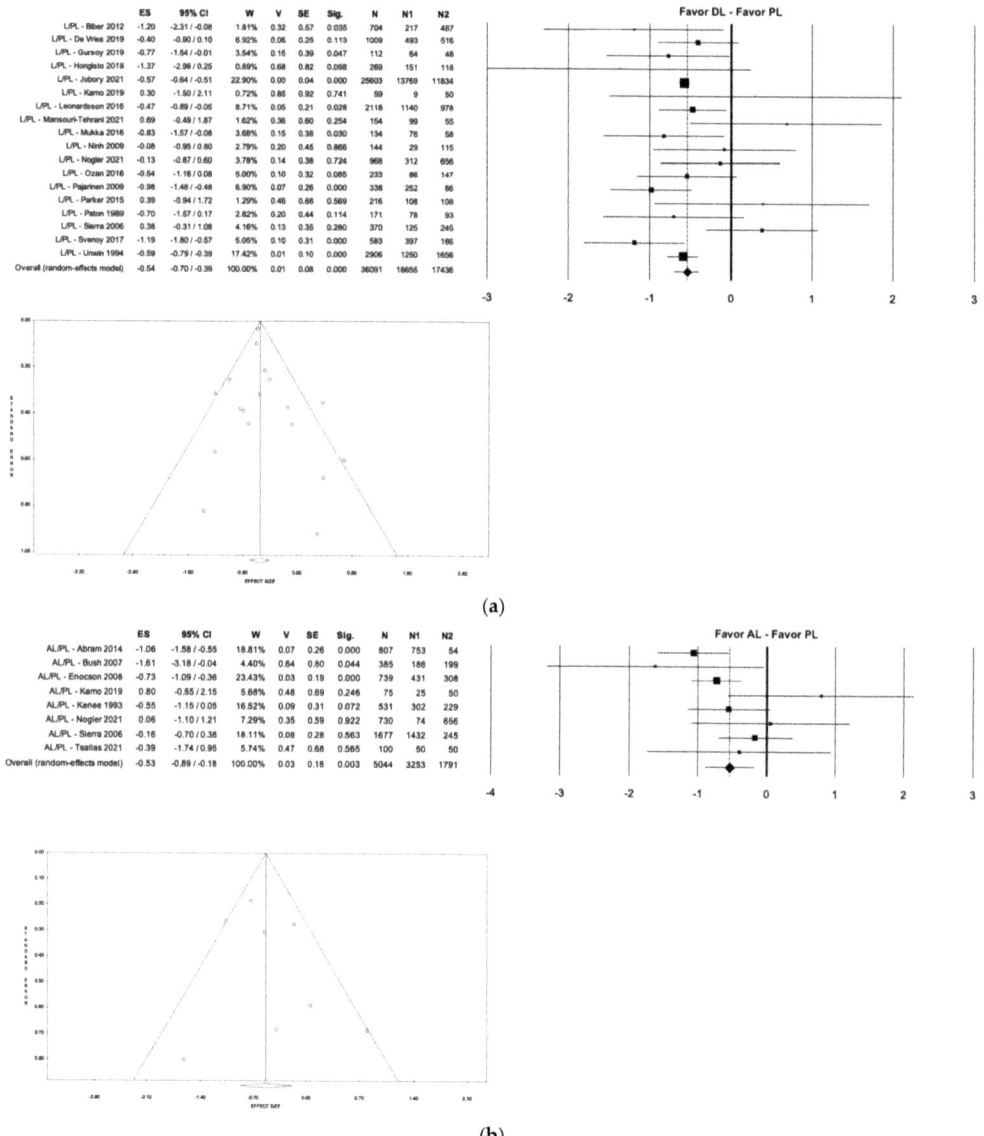

Figure 6. Cont.

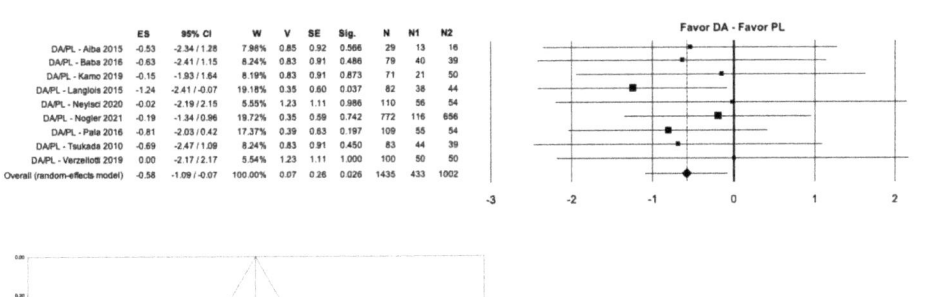

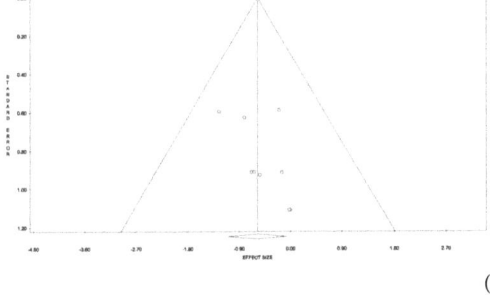

(c)

Figure 6. Forest plot and funnel plot of overall meta-analysis evaluating studies with data about dislocations in patients treated with direct lateral approach vs. posterolateral approach. (**a**) the figure shows the highest estimated risk of dislocations in the posterolateral group; anterolateral approach vs. posterolateral approach; (**b**) the figure shows the highest estimated risk of dislocations in the posterolateral group; direct anterior approach vs. posterolateral approach; (**c**) the figure shows the highest estimated risk of dislocations in the posterolateral group. Abbreviations: ES, effect size; 95% CI, 95% confidence interval; W, weight; N, sample size [11,12,15,19–24,26–34,36–38,40–42,45,50–52,55,57].

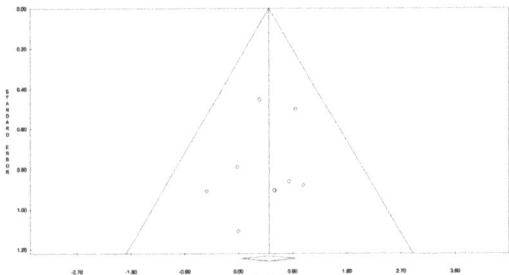

Figure 7. Forest plot and funnel plot of overall meta-analysis evaluating studies with data about intraoperative fractures in patients treated with direct anterior approach vs. posterolateral approach. The figure shows the highest estimated risk of dislocations in the direct anterior group. Abbreviations: ES, effect size; 95% CI, 95% confidence interval; W, weight; N, sample size [12,15,30–33,41,50,57].

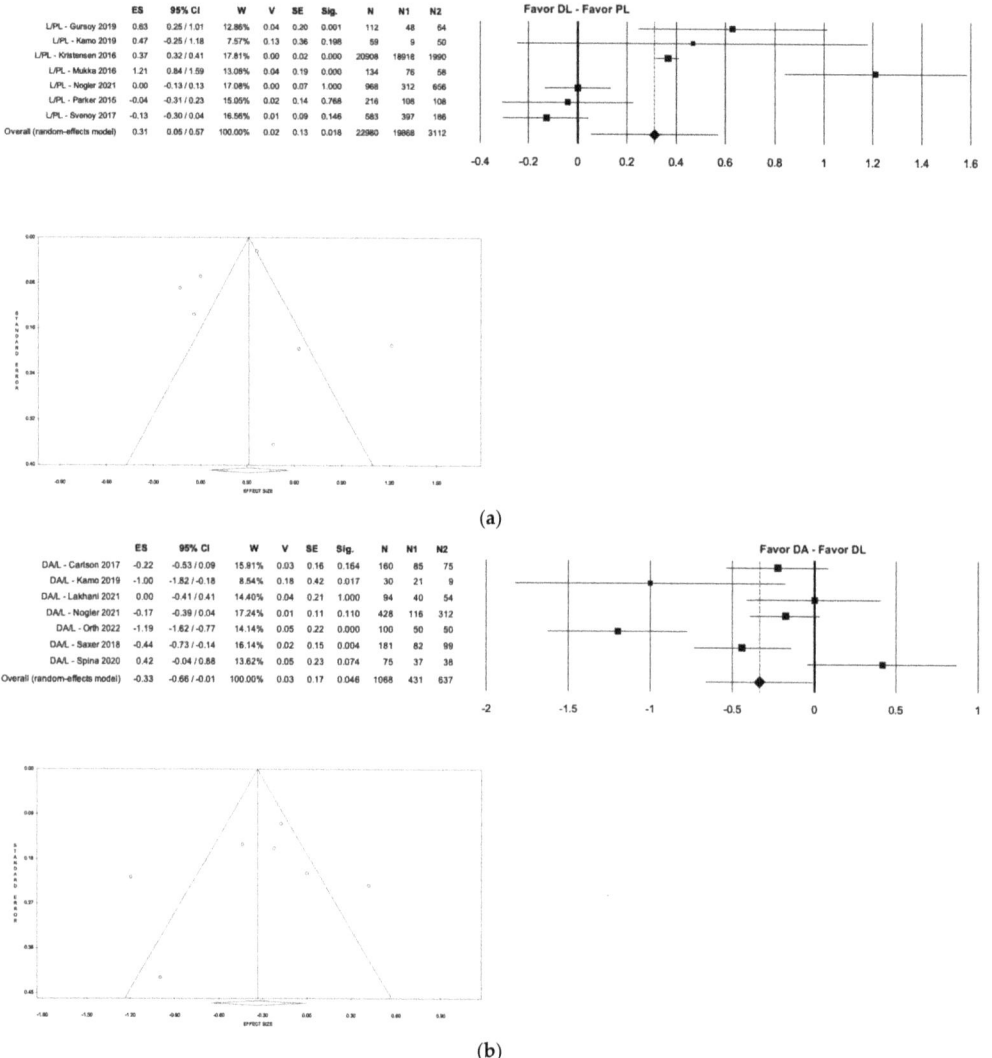

Figure 8. Forest plot and funnel plot of overall meta-analysis evaluating studies with data about mean operative time in patients treated with: direct lateral approach vs. posterolateral approach (**a**): the figure shows the shortest mean operative time in the posterolateral group; direct anterior approach vs. direct lateral approach (**b**): the figure shows the shortest mean operative time in the direct anterior group. Abbreviations: ES, effect size; 95% CI, 95% confidence interval; W, weight; N, sample size [11,18,25,29,37,39,41,44,46,51,57,58].

4. Discussion

This review was conducted with the aim of evaluating the evidence available in the literature regarding the differences between the four most common surgical approaches used for hemiarthroplasty surgery for femoral neck fractures. We found a large amount of data in the literature, but we decided to utilize only comparative studies, in order to conduct an "approach vs. approach" meta-analysis of good quality studies.

The distribution of patients according to the approach was not homogeneous, with a prevalence of cases treated with a PL and a DL approach. This is not to be understood as representative data of surgical practice, but is probably the consequence of the inclusion of registry studies, in which the included patients had been mainly treated with the PL or DL approach.

This study showed that none of the approaches analyzed was significantly worse overall in terms of total complications, in line with the findings of the study by Fullam et al. in 2018 [59]. The only cases in which significant differences were found has been when single "approach vs. approach" comparisons were conducted, also in line with the literature [11,23,31,32,37].

Significant differences in the overall complication rate were found only when comparing the DL approach with the PL approach, with the highest rate in the PL group. This finding contrasts with what was found by Tol et al. in 2021, with their systematic review, which showed no significant difference between the two groups [60]. This might be explained by the higher number of patients considered in the present review and the different quality of the studies included.

With regard to the rate of revision surgeries, this study appears to be in line with the literature. The re-operation rate in patients treated with the PL approach was significantly higher than in the DL group, similar to what emerged in the review by Van der Sijp et al. [61]. It deserves attention that the revision surgery rate in this review was found to be higher in the DL approach than in the AL approach. The reason might be related to the fact that the AL approach involves less muscle than the DL approach, despite the other similarities between these two approaches.

As far as single complications are concerned, significant differences emerged in the various comparisons with regard to the dislocation rate, intraoperative fractures, average blood loss, and mean operative time.

Data from this study suggest that the PL approach exposes the patient to an increased risk of dislocation than the other three surgical approaches analyzed. Tol et al. stated that the PL approach, compared with the DL approach, is associated with more dislocations, but patients have less walking problems and a lower risk of abductor insufficiency [60]. In addition, lateral patient positioning has the advantage of needing fewer operators for the procedure [61]. Similar results were found by Leonardsson et al., whose data showed that patients treated with the PL approach were affected by an increased risk of needing revision surgery due to dislocation, but had a better functional score at follow-up in terms of quality of life [26]. The review of the literature conducted by Van der Sijp et al. showed a higher risk of dislocation and reoperation in patients treated with the PL approach when compared with those treated with the DL and the DA approach [62]. It is interesting to note that the results of both this study and previous reviews regarding the higher dislocation rate of HHA performed with the PL approach differ from the results of total hip replacement (THA), according to the literature. In fact, with regard to THA, the dislocation rate appears to be comparable between the PL approach and the other ones. This is probably due both to the greater retention of the cup and to the possibility of positioning the acetabular components with different orientations, according to the chosen approach [63].

Another interesting finding from this review is the risk of intraoperative fractures, which was significantly lower in the PL approach than the DA approach, in agreement with the studies by Pala et al. and Langlois et al., who have previously compared complications related to these surgical approaches [31,32]. The higher rate of intraoperative fractures in the DA approach is probably due to the greater difficulty in correctly exposing the femur for its preparation, a maneuver which requires the application of greater force than in other approaches. These observations should be coupled with reporting the method of stem fixation used (cemented or uncemented), as this could be an important factor influencing fracture risk, regardless of the approach employed. However, as emphasized below in the section on study limitations, it was not possible to stratify data from many studies according to cementation. Nevertheless, considering the homogeneity of the mean age of patients for each approach (Table 2), always above 80 years, it might be reasonable to assume that the use of cemented stems was prominent in most studies, thus making it a non-determinant variable in influencing the results of this review on intraoperative fractures. This finding differs from what was found in the literature for THA surgery, for which, despite the absolute number of intraoperative fractures for the DA approach being higher, the difference does not appear to be significant when compared to the PL approach, as was found in the systematic review by Wang et al. [64]. This could be explained by advanced age and the greater number of comorbidities that can affect bone quality in patients treated with HA.

Few studies in the literature have compared the surgical time for the different approaches. The recent review by Kunkel et al. showed that there were no significant differences between the DA approach's surgical time compared to the other approaches [65]. In this review, it was found that the PL approach has a significantly shorter surgical time than the DL approach. However, one aspect that should be considered is the time needed for patient positioning on the surgical bed, which is usually longer in the PL approach, as the patient lies on their side, compared to DL and DA approaches, in which the patient lies supine.

There are major limitations to this systematic review and meta-analysis. The studies included in this review have allowed a deep analysis for some comparisons between surgical approaches, but, on the other hand, have not allowed all possible comparisons, due to a lack of extensive data in the literature. Moreover, the limited number of randomized control studies available necessitated the inclusion of many non-randomized studies. Nevertheless, the rigorous methodological quality analysis performed has allowed us to identify several types of potential bias in the included studies. The analysis of functional outcomes was severely limited by cross-study variability, in the type of metrics used and patient follow-up duration. For these reasons, functional aspect was not included in this review. Moreover, analyzing the outcomes for every surgical approach by stratifying the cohorts according to the type of cup (unipolar versus bipolar) and the use of cement would have led to an excessive dispersion of data. In fact, these aspects were not able to be discriminated in most of the included studies. Therefore, a multivariate analysis that would allow the type of approach to be identified as an independent risk factor for specific outcomes was not performed.

5. Conclusions

In conclusion, there is no approach which appears worse overall, in terms of complications. This systematic literature review has showed that each approach has strengths and weaknesses. The posterolateral approach has the disadvantage of being characterized by a higher dislocation rate and a higher rate of complications than the DL approach. However, it has the advantage of having a shorter operative time, less blood loss, and the need for fewer operators. On the other hand, the DA approach carries the advantage of less blood loss, a shorter operating time, and a lower rate of dislocations compared to the PL approach. The disadvantage is the higher rate of intraoperative femoral fractures, which is why it would be less suitable for patients with greater risk of fracture due to poor bone quality. The DL approach shows a lower rate of complications and revisions than the PL, but has a longer operative time and greater blood loss. Knowledge of the limitations of each approach and the most common associated complications can lead to choosing a surgical technique based on the patient's individual risk.

Author Contributions: Conceptualization, M.F. (Michele Fiore), A.S. and R.D.C.; methodology, M.F. (Matteo Filippini) and A.M.; software, M.B., A.M and L.D.P.; investigation, M.F. (Matteo Filippini), A.P. and S.C.P.; data curation, A.P., L.D.P. and V.P.; writing—original draft preparation, M.F. (Matteo Filippini) and G.L.; writing—review and editing, M.F. (Michele Fiore), G.L. and A.S.; supervision, R.D.C. and M.D.P. All authors have read and agreed to the published version of the manuscript.

Funding: This research received no external funding.

Institutional Review Board Statement: Not applicable.

Informed Consent Statement: Not applicable.

Data Availability Statement: Data are available on current Literature.

Conflicts of Interest: The authors declare no conflict of interest.

References

1. Butler, M.; Forte, M.; Kane, R.L.; Joglekar, S.; Duval, S.J.; Swiontkowski, M.; Wilt, T. Treatment of Common Hip Fractures. *Evid. Rep. Technol. Assess* **2009**, *184*, 1–85.
2. Butler, M.; Forte, M.L.; Joglekar, S.B.; Swiontkowski, M.F.; Kane, R.L. Evidence Summary: Systematic Review of Surgical Treatments for Geriatric Hip Fractures. *J. Bone Jt. Surg.* **2011**, *93*, 1104–1115. [CrossRef] [PubMed]
3. Gjertsen, J.-E.; Vinje, T.; Lie, S.A.; Engesæter, L.B.; Havelin, L.I.; Furnes, O.; Fevang, J.M. Patient Satisfaction, Pain, and Quality of Life 4 Months after Displaced Femoral Neck Fractures: A Comparison of 663 Fractures Treated with Internal Fixation and 906 with Bipolar Hemiarthroplasty Reported to the Norwegian Hip Fracture Register. *Acta Orthop.* **2008**, *79*, 594–601. [CrossRef]
4. Norwegian National Advisory Unit on Arthroplasty and Hip Fractures. Available online: https://helse-bergen.no/nasjonal-kompetansetjeneste-for-leddproteser-og-hoftebrudd/norwegian-national-advisory-unit-on-arthroplasty-and-hip-fractures (accessed on 10 April 2023).
5. Rogmark, C.; Fenstad, A.M.; Leonardsson, O.; Engesæter, L.B.; Kärrholm, J.; Furnes, O.; Garellick, G.; Gjertsen, J.-E. Posterior Approach and Uncemented Stems Increases the Risk of Reoperation after Hemiarthroplasties in Elderly Hip Fracture Patients: An Analysis of 33,205 Procedures in the Norwegian and Swedish National Registries. *Acta Orthop.* **2014**, *85*, 18–25. [CrossRef] [PubMed]
6. Bauer, R.; Kerschbaumer, F.; Poisel, S.; Oberthaler, W. The Transgluteal Approach to the Hip Joint. *Arch. Orthop. Traumat. Surg.* **1979**, *95*, 47–49. [CrossRef]
7. Gibson, A. Posterior Exposure of the Hip Joint. *J. Bone Jt. Surg. Br. Vol.* **1950**, *32*, 183–186. [CrossRef]
8. Weber, M.; Ganz, R. The Anterior Approach to Hip and Pelvis. *Orthop. Traumatol.* **2002**, *10*, 245–257. [CrossRef]
9. Light, T.R.; Keggi, K.J. Anterior Approach to Hip Arthroplasty. *Clin. Orthop. Relat. Res.* **1980**, *152*, 255–260. [CrossRef]
10. Auffarth, A.; Resch, H.; Lederer, S.; Karpik, S.; Hitzl, W.; Bogner, R.; Mayer, M.; Matis, N. Does the Choice of Approach for Hip Hemiarthroplasty in Geriatric Patients Significantly Influence Early Postoperative Outcomes? A Randomized-Controlled Trial Comparing the Modified Smith-Petersen and Hardinge Approaches. *J. Trauma Inj. Infect. Crit. Care* **2011**, *70*, 1257–1262. [CrossRef]
11. Parker, M.J. Lateral versus Posterior Approach for Insertion of Hemiarthroplasties for Hip Fractures: A Randomised Trial of 216 Patients. *Injury* **2015**, *46*, 1023–1027. [CrossRef]
12. Watanabe, N.; Aiba, H.; Sagara, G. Prospective Randomised Study of Direct Anterior Approach Versus Posterior Approach for Bipolar Hemiarthroplasty of the Hip. *Orthop. Procs.* **2016**, *98*, 123. [CrossRef]
13. Renken, F.; Renken, S.; Paech, A.; Wenzl, M.; Unger, A.; Schulz, A.P. Early Functional Results after Hemiarthroplasty for Femoral Neck Fracture: A Randomized Comparison between a Minimal Invasive and a Conventional Approach. *BMC Musculoskelet. Disord.* **2012**, *13*, 141. [CrossRef] [PubMed]
14. Jianbo, J.; Ying, J.; Xinxin, L.; Lianghao, W.; Baoqing, Y.; Rongguang, A. Hip Hemiarthroplasty for Senile Femoral Neck Fractures: Minimally Invasive SuperPath Approach versus Traditional Posterior Approach. *Injury* **2019**, *50*, 1452–1459. [CrossRef] [PubMed]
15. Verzellotti, S.; Candrian, C.; Molina, M.; Filardo, G.; Alberio, R.; Grassi, F.A. Direct Anterior versus Posterolateral Approach for Bipolar Hip Hemiarthroplasty in Femoral Neck Fractures: A Prospective Randomised Study. *HIP Int.* **2020**, *30*, 810–817. [CrossRef]
16. Ugland, T.O.; Haugeberg, G.; Svenningsen, S.; Ugland, S.H.; Berg, Ø.H.; Pripp, A.H.; Nordsletten, L. Biomarkers of Muscle Damage Increased in Anterolateral Compared to Direct Lateral Approach to the Hip in Hemiarthroplasty: No Correlation with Clinical Outcome: Short-Term Analysis of Secondary Outcomes from a Randomized Clinical Trial in Patients with a Displaced Femoral Neck Fracture. *Osteoporos. Int.* **2018**, *29*, 1853–1860. [CrossRef]
17. Martínez, Á.; Herrera, A.; Cuenca, J.; Panisello, J.; Tabuenca, A. Comparison of Two Different Posterior Approaches for Hemiarthroplasty of the Hip. *Arch. Orthop. Trauma Surg.* **2002**, *122*, 51–52. [CrossRef]
18. Saxer, F.; Studer, P.; Jakob, M.; Suhm, N.; Rosenthal, R.; Dell-Kuster, S.; Vach, W.; Bless, N. Minimally Invasive Anterior Muscle-Sparing versus a Transgluteal Approach for Hemiarthroplasty in Femoral Neck Fractures-a Prospective Randomised Controlled Trial Including 190 Elderly Patients. *BMC Geriatr.* **2018**, *18*, 222. [CrossRef]
19. Keene, G.S.; Parker, M.J. Hemiarthroplasty of the Hip—The Anterior or Posterior Approach? A Comparison of Surgical Approaches. *Injury* **1993**, *24*, 611–613. [CrossRef]
20. Paton, R.W.; Hirst, P. Hemiarthroplasty of the Hip and Dislocation. *Injury* **1989**, *20*, 167–169. [CrossRef]
21. Unwin, A.J.; Thomas, M. Dislocation after Hemiarthroplasty of the Hip: A Comparison of the Dislocation Rate after Posterior and Lateral Approaches to the Hip. *Ann. R. Coll. Surg. Engl.* **1994**, *76*, 327–329.
22. Abram, S.G.F.; Murray, J.B. Outcomes of 807 Thompson Hip Hemiarthroplasty Procedures and the Effect of Surgical Approach on Dislocation Rates. *Injury* **2015**, *46*, 1013–1017. [CrossRef] [PubMed]

23. Biber, R.; Brem, M.; Singler, K.; Moellers, M.; Sieber, C.; Bail, H.J. Dorsal versus Transgluteal Approach for Hip Hemiarthroplasty: An Analysis of Early Complications in Seven Hundred and Four Consecutive Cases. *Int. Orthop.* **2012**, *36*, 2219–2223. [CrossRef] [PubMed]
24. Enocson, A.; Tidermark, J.; Törnkvist, H.; Lapidus, L.J. Dislocation of Hemiarthroplasty after Femoral Neck Fracture: Better Outcome after the Anterolateral Approach in a Prospective Cohort Study on 739 Consecutive Hips. *Acta Orthop.* **2008**, *79*, 211–217. [CrossRef] [PubMed]
25. Kristensen, T.B.; Vinje, T.; Havelin, L.I.; Engesæter, L.B.; Gjertsen, J.-E. Posterior Approach Compared to Direct Lateral Approach Resulted in Better Patient-Reported Outcome after Hemiarthroplasty for Femoral Neck Fracture: 20,908 Patients from the Norwegian Hip Fracture Register. *Acta Orthop.* **2017**, *88*, 29–34. [CrossRef]
26. Leonardsson, O.; Rolfson, O.; Rogmark, C. The Surgical Approach for Hemiarthroplasty Does Not Influence Patient-Reported Outcome: A National Survey of 2118 Patients with One-Year Follow-Up. *Bone Jt. J.* **2016**, *98*, 542–547. [CrossRef]
27. Ninh, C.C.; Sethi, A.; Hatahet, M.; Les, C.; Morandi, M.; Vaidya, R. Hip Dislocation After Modular Unipolar Hemiarthroplasty. *J. Arthroplast.* **2009**, *24*, 768–774. [CrossRef]
28. Pajarinen, J.; Savolainen, V.; Lindahl, J.; Hirvensalo, E. Factors Predisposing to Dislocation of the Thompson Hemiarthroplasty: 22 Dislocations in 338 Patients. *Acta Orthop. Scand.* **2003**, *74*, 45–48. [CrossRef]
29. Svenøy, S.; Westberg, M.; Figved, W.; Valland, H.; Brun, O.C.; Wangen, H.; Madsen, J.E.; Frihagen, F. Posterior versus Lateral Approach for Hemiarthroplasty after Femoral Neck Fracture: Early Complications in a Prospective Cohort of 583 Patients. *Injury* **2017**, *48*, 1565–1569. [CrossRef]
30. Baba, T. Bipolar Hemiarthroplasty for Femoral Neck Fracture Using the Direct Anterior Approach. *WJO* **2013**, *4*, 85. [CrossRef]
31. Langlois, J.; Delambre, J.; Klouche, S.; Faivre, B.; Hardy, P. Direct Anterior Hueter Approach Is a Safe and Effective Approach to Perform a Bipolar Hemiarthroplasty for Femoral Neck Fracture: Outcome in 82 Patients. *Acta Orthop.* **2015**, *86*, 358–362. [CrossRef]
32. Pala, E.; Trono, M.; Bitonti, A.; Lucidi, G. Hip Hemiarthroplasty for Femur Neck Fractures: Minimally Invasive Direct Anterior Approach versus Postero-Lateral Approach. *Eur. J. Orthop. Surg. Traumatol.* **2016**, *26*, 423–427. [CrossRef] [PubMed]
33. Tsukada, S.; Wakui, M. Minimally Invasive Intermuscular Approach Does Not Improve Outcomes in Bipolar Hemiarthroplasty for Femoral Neck Fracture. *J. Orthop. Sci.* **2010**, *15*, 753–757. [CrossRef] [PubMed]
34. Hongisto, M.T.; Nuotio, M.S.; Luukkaala, T.; Väistö, O.; Pihlajamäki, H.K. Lateral and Posterior Approaches in Hemiarthroplasty. *Scand. J. Surg.* **2018**, *107*, 260–268. [CrossRef] [PubMed]
35. Sayed-Noor, A.S.; Hanas, A.; Sköldenberg, O.G.; Mukka, S.S. Abductor Muscle Function and Trochanteric Tenderness after Hemiarthroplasty for Femoral Neck Fracture. *J. Orthop. Trauma* **2016**, *30*, e194–e200. [CrossRef] [PubMed]
36. Ozan, F.; Öncel, E.S.; Koyuncu, S.; Gürbüz, K.; Doğar, F.; Vatansever, F.; Duygulu, F. Effects of Hardinge versus Moore approach on postoperative outcomes in elderly patients with hip fracture. *Int. J. Clin. Exp. Med.* **2016**, *9*, 4425–4431.
37. Mukka, S.; Mahmood, S.; Kadum, B.; Sköldenberg, O.; Sayed-Noor, A. Direct Lateral vs. Posterolateral Approach to Hemiarthroplasty for Femoral Neck Fractures. *Orthop. Traumatol. Surg. Res.* **2016**, *102*, 1049–1054. [CrossRef]
38. Bush, J.B.; Wilson, M.R. Dislocation after Hip Hemiarthroplasty: Anterior Versus Posterior Capsular Approach. *Orthopedics* **2007**, *30*, 138–144. [CrossRef]
39. Carlson, V.R.; Ong, A.C.; Orozco, F.R.; Lutz, R.W.; Duque, A.F.; Post, Z.D. The Direct Anterior Approach Does Not Increase Return to Function following Hemiarthroplasty for Femoral Neck Fracture. *Orthopedics* **2017**, *40*, e1055–e1061. [CrossRef]
40. Sierra, R.J.; Schleck, C.D.; Cabanela, M.E. Dislocation of Bipolar Hemiarthroplasty: Rate, Contributing Factors, and Outcome. *Clin. Orthop. Relat. Res.* **2006**, *442*, 230–238. [CrossRef]
41. Nogler, M.; Randelli, F.; Macheras, G.A.; Thaler, M. Hemiarthroplasty of the Hip Using the Direct Anterior Approach. *Oper. Orthop. Traumatol.* **2021**, *33*, 304–317. [CrossRef]
42. de Vries, E.N.; Gardenbroek, T.J.; Ammerlaan, H.; Steenstra, F.; Vervest, A.M.J.S.; Hogervorst, M.; van Velde, R. The Optimal Approach in Hip Hemiarthroplasty: A Cohort of 1009 Patients. *Eur. J. Orthop. Surg. Traumatol.* **2020**, *30*, 569–573. [CrossRef] [PubMed]
43. Xu, K.; Anwaier, D.; He, R.; Zhang, X.; Qin, S.; Wang, G.; Duan, X.; Tong, D.; Ji, F. Hidden Blood Loss after Hip Hemiarthroplasty Using the SuperPATH Approach: A Retrospective Study. *Injury* **2019**, *50*, 2282–2286. [CrossRef] [PubMed]
44. Spina, M.; Luppi, V.; Chiappi, J.; Bagnis, F.; Balsano, M. Direct Anterior Approach versus Direct Lateral Approach in Total Hip Arthroplasty and Bipolar Hemiarthroplasty for Femoral Neck Fractures: A Retrospective Comparative Study. *Aging Clin. Exp. Res.* **2021**, *33*, 1635–1644. [CrossRef] [PubMed]
45. Jobory, A.; Rolfson, O.; Åkesson, K.E.; Arvidsson, C.; Nilsson, I.; Rogmark, C. Hip Precautions Not Meaningful after Hemiarthroplasty Due to Hip Fracture. Cluster-Randomized Study of 394 Patients Operated with Direct Anterolateral Approach. *Injury* **2019**, *50*, 1318–1323. [CrossRef] [PubMed]
46. Lakhani, K.; Mimendia, I.; Porcel, J.A.; Martín-Domínguez, L.A.; Guerra-Farfán, E.; Barro, V. Direct Anterior Approach Provides Better Functional Outcomes When Compared to Direct Lateral Approach in Hip Hemiarthroplasty following Femoral Neck Fracture. *Eur. J. Orthop. Surg. Traumatol.* **2022**, *32*, 137–143. [CrossRef] [PubMed]
47. de Jong, L.; Klem, T.M.A.L.; Kuijper, T.M.; Roukema, G.R. The Minimally Invasive Anterolateral Approach versus the Traditional Anterolateral Approach (Watson-Jones) for Hip Hemiarthroplasty after a Femoral Neck Fracture: An Analysis of Clinical Outcomes. *Int. Orthop.* **2018**, *42*, 1943–1948. [CrossRef]

48. Ladurner, A.; Schöfl, T.; Calek, A.K.; Zdravkovic, V.; Giesinger, K. Direct Anterior Approach Improves In-Hospital Mobility Following Hemiarthroplasty for Femoral Neck Fracture Treatment. *Arch. Orthop. Trauma Surg.* **2021**, *142*, 3183–3192. [CrossRef]
49. Corrigan, C.M.; Greenberg, S.E.; Sathiyakumar, V.; Mitchell, P.M.; Francis, A.; Omar, A.; Thakore, R.V.; Obremskey, W.T.; Sethi, M.K. Heterotopic Ossification after Hemiarthroplasty of the Hip—A Comparison of Three Common Approaches. *J. Clin. Orthop. Trauma* **2015**, *6*, 1–5. [CrossRef]
50. Neyisci, C.; Erdem, Y.; Bilekli, A.B.; Bek, D. Direct Anterior Approach Versus Posterolateral Approach for Hemiarthroplasty in the Treatment of Displaced Femoral Neck Fractures in Geriatric Patients. *Med. Sci. Monit.* **2020**, *26*, e919993. [CrossRef]
51. Gursoy, S.; Simsek, M.E.; Akkaya, M.; Dogan, M.; Bozkurt, M. Transtrochanteric Approach Can Provide Better Postoperative Care and Lower Complication Rate in the Treatment of Hip Fractures. *CIA* **2019**, *14*, 137–143. [CrossRef]
52. Mansouri-Tehrani, M.M.; Yavari, P.; Pakdaman, M.; Eslami, S.; Nourian, S.M.A. Comparison of Surgical Complications Following Hip Hemiarthroplasty between the Posterolateral and Lateral Approaches. *Int. J. Burns Trauma* **2021**, *11*, 406–411. [PubMed]
53. Bűcs, G.; Dandé, Á.; Patczai, B.; Sebestyén, A.; Almási, R.; Nöt, L.G.; Wiegand, N. Bipolar Hemiarthroplasty for the Treatment of Femoral Neck Fractures with Minimally Invasive Anterior Approach in Elderly. *Injury* **2021**, *52*, S37–S43. [CrossRef] [PubMed]
54. Layson, J.T.; Coon, M.S.; Sharma, R.; Diedring, B.; Afsari, A.; Best, B. Comparing Postoperative Leg Length Discrepancy and Femoral Offset Using Two Different Surgical Approaches for Hemiarthroplasty of the Hip. *Spartan Med. Res. J.* **2021**, *6*, 25096. [CrossRef]
55. Tsailas, P.G.; Argyrou, C.; Valavanis, A. Management of Femoral Neck Fractures with the ALMIS Approach in Elderly Patients: Outcomes Compared to Posterior Approach. *Injury* **2021**, *52*, 3666–3672. [CrossRef] [PubMed]
56. Cecere, A.B.; De Cicco, A.; Bruno, G.; Toro, G.; Errico, G.; Braile, A.; Schiavone Panni, A. SuperPath Approach Is a Recommendable Option in Frail Patients with Femoral Neck Fractures: A Case–Control Study. *Arch. Orthop. Trauma Surg.* **2021**, *142*, 3265–3270. [CrossRef] [PubMed]
57. Kamo, K.; Kido, H.; Kido, S. Comparison of the Incidence of Intra-Operative Fractures in Hip Hemi-Arthroplasty Performed in Supine and Lateral Positions. *Hip Pelvis* **2019**, *31*, 33. [CrossRef] [PubMed]
58. Orth, M.; Osche, D.; Mörsdorf, P.; Holstein, J.H.; Rollmann, M.F.; Fritz, T.; Pohlemann, T.; Pizanis, A. Minimal-Invasive Anterior Approach to the Hip Provides a Better Surgery-Related and Early Postoperative Functional Outcome than Conventional Lateral Approach after Hip Hemiarthroplasty following Femoral Neck Fractures. *Arch. Orthop. Trauma Surg.* **2022**, *143*, 3173–3181. [CrossRef]
59. Fullam, J.; Theodosi, P.G.; Charity, J.; Goodwin, V.A. A Scoping Review Comparing Two Common Surgical Approaches to the Hip for Hemiarthroplasty. *BMC Surg.* **2019**, *19*, 32. [CrossRef]
60. Tol, M.C.J.M.; Willigenburg, N.W.; Willems, H.C.; Gosens, T.; Rasker, A.; Heetveld, M.J.; Schotanus, M.G.M.; Van Dongen, J.M.; Eggen, B.; Kormos, M.; et al. Posterolateral or Direct Lateral Approach for Cemented Hemiarthroplasty after Femoral Neck Fracture (APOLLO): Protocol for a Multicenter Randomized Controlled Trial with Economic Evaluation and Natural Experiment Alongside. *Acta Orthop.* **2022**, *93*, 732–738. [CrossRef]
61. Aofoundation.org. Available online: https://surgeryreference.aofoundation.org/orthopedic-trauma/adult-trauma/proximal-femur/femoral-neck-fracture-subcapital-displaced/hemiarthroplasty#general-considerations (accessed on 1 May 2023).
62. van der Sijp, M.P.L.; van Delft, D.; Krijnen, P.; Niggebrugge, A.H.P.; Schipper, I.B. Surgical Approaches and Hemiarthroplasty Outcomes of Femoral Neck Fractures: A Meta-Analysis. *J. Arthroplast.* **2018**, *33*, 1617–1627.e9. [CrossRef]
63. Graves, S.C.; Dropkin, B.M.; Keeney, B.J.; Lurie, J.D.; Tomek, I.M. Does Surgical Approach Affect Patient-Reported Function After Primary THA? *Clin. Orthop. Relat. Res.* **2016**, *474*, 971–981. [CrossRef] [PubMed]
64. Wang, Z.; Hou, J.; Wu, C.; Zhou, Y.; Gu, X.; Wang, H.; Feng, W.; Cheng, Y.; Sheng, X.; Bao, H. A Systematic Review and Meta-Analysis of Direct Anterior Approach versus Posterior Approach in Total Hip Arthroplasty. *J. Orthop. Surg. Res.* **2018**, *13*, 229. [CrossRef] [PubMed]
65. Kunkel, S.T.; Sabatino, M.J.; Kang, R.; Jevsevar, D.S.; Moschetti, W.E. A Systematic Review and Meta-Analysis of the Direct Anterior Approach for Hemiarthroplasty for Femoral Neck Fracture. *Eur. J. Orthop. Surg. Traumatol.* **2018**, *28*, 217–232. [CrossRef] [PubMed]

Disclaimer/Publisher's Note: The statements, opinions and data contained in all publications are solely those of the individual author(s) and contributor(s) and not of MDPI and/or the editor(s). MDPI and/or the editor(s) disclaim responsibility for any injury to people or property resulting from any ideas, methods, instructions or products referred to in the content.

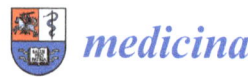

Systematic Review

Updated Meta-Analysis of Randomized Controlled Trials Comparing External Fixation to Intramedullary Nailing in the Treatment of Open Tibial Fractures

Danilo Jeremić [1,2,*], Nina Rajovic [3], Boris Gluscevic [1,2], Branislav Krivokapic [1,2], Stanislav Rajkovic [1,2], Nikola Bogosavljevic [1,2], Kristina Davidovic [2,4] and Slavko Tomic [1,2]

[1] Institute for Orthopedic Surgery "Banjica", 11000 Belgrade, Serbia; glborismmm@gmail.com (B.G.); branislav.krivokapic@iohbb.edu.rs (B.K.); stanbgd@hotmail.com (S.R.); boga19@gmail.com (N.B.); tomicslavko1956@gmail.com (S.T.)
[2] Faculty of Medicine, University of Belgrade, 11000 Belgrade, Serbia; dr.kristina.davidovic@gmail.com
[3] Institute for Medical Statistics and Informatics, Faculty of Medicine, University of Belgrade, 11000 Belgrade, Serbia; nina.rajovic@med.bg.ac.rs
[4] Department of Radiology, Clinical Center of Serbia, 11000 Belgrade, Serbia
* Correspondence: danilo.jeremic@iohbb.edu.rs

Abstract: *Background:* The purpose of this study was to collect all available randomized controlled trials (RCT) on the treatment of open tibial fractures with an external fixator (EF) and intramedullary nailing (IMN) for meta-analysis to provide reliable evidence-based data for clinical decision-making. *Material and methods:* The systematic review was undertaken in accordance with Preferred Reporting Items for Systematic Reviews and Meta-Analyses (PRISMA) and AMSTAR (Assessing the Methodological Quality of Systematic Review). An electronic search of PubMed, Cochrane Library, and Web of Science was performed until 1 March 2023 to identify RCTs which compared either IMN or EF to fix the open tibial fracture. Outcome measures were: postoperative superficial and deep infection, time to union, delayed union, malunion, nonunion and hardware failure. In addition, pain and health-related quality of life were evaluated after 3 and 12 months of follow-up. *Results:* Sixteen publications comprising 1011 patients were included in the meta-analysis. The pooled results suggested that the IMN technique had a lower postoperative superficial infection and malunion rate (RR = 3.56, 95%CI = 2.56–4.95 and RR = 1.96, 95%CI = 1.12–3.44, respectively), but higher hardware failure occurrence in contrast to EF (RR = 0.30; 95%CI = 0.13–0.69). No significant differences were found in the union time, delayed union or nonunion rate, and postoperative deep infection rate between the treatments. Lower levels of pain were found in the EF group (RR = 0.05, 95%CI = 0.02–0.17, $p < 0.001$). A difference in quality of life favoring IMN after 3 months was found (RR = −0.04, 95%CI = −0.05–−0.03, $p < 0.001$), however, no statistical difference was found after 12 months (RR = 0.03, 95%CI = −0.05–0.11, $p = 0.44$). *Conclusions:* Meta-analysis presented reduced incidence rates of superficial infection, malunion, and health-related quality of life 3 months after treatment in IMN. However, EF led to a significant reduction in pain and incidence rate of hardware failure. Postoperative deep infection, delayed union, nonunion and health-related quality of life 12 months following therapy were similar between groups. More high-quality RCTs should be conducted to provide reliable evidence-based data for clinical decision-making.

Keywords: meta-analysis; open tibial fractures; external fixator; intramedullary nailing

Citation: Jeremić, D.; Rajovic, N.; Gluscevic, B.; Krivokapic, B.; Rajkovic, S.; Bogosavljevic, N.; Davidovic, K.; Tomic, S. Updated Meta-Analysis of Randomized Controlled Trials Comparing External Fixation to Intramedullary Nailing in the Treatment of Open Tibial Fractures. *Medicina* **2023**, *59*, 1301. https://doi.org/10.3390/medicina59071301

Academic Editor: Woo Jong Kim

Received: 19 June 2023
Revised: 6 July 2023
Accepted: 10 July 2023
Published: 14 July 2023

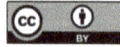

Copyright: © 2023 by the authors. Licensee MDPI, Basel, Switzerland. This article is an open access article distributed under the terms and conditions of the Creative Commons Attribution (CC BY) license (https://creativecommons.org/licenses/by/4.0/).

1. Introduction

The most common type of open fracture of the long bones in the extremities is the open tibial fracture, which is frequently observed in traffic accidents [1,2]. For patients suffering from this type of fracture, emergency wound debridement, exploration of vascular and nerve damage, early soft tissue coverage, and fracture stabilization are agreed-upon treatments [3–5]. Two common surgical methods used to treat this fracture are external fixators (EF) and intramedullary nailing (IMN). However, both methods have their own advantages and disadvantages, making it controversial which one is better [6].

In the past, EF was widely used due to its rapid operation, lack of surgical incision, and no negative effect on blood supply to the fracture site [7]. However, postoperative patients with EF often suffer from complications such as pin-track infections, fracture malunion, reduction loss, and joint contracture [8,9]. Additionally, the long-term use of EF can be inconvenient for nurses and patients. Nowadays, IMN is widely used because of its advantages of central fixation, early weight-bearing, minimal invasiveness, and convenient postoperative care [10,11]. However, there are still risks of hardware failure and infection diffusion through the medullary cavity [12].

Several meta-analyses on the treatment of open tibial fractures with IMN and EF were conducted, but there have been limitations. Some did not compare fracture healing time [13], others did not conduct heterogeneity analysis [14], and some included retrospective studies and case reports [15], which impacted the level of evidence. Aiming to collect the best available evidence, Liu et al. published meta-analysis based on randomized clinical trials (RCTs) comparing the treatment of open tibial fractures with EF and IMN, and recommended IMN as a preferred method of fracture fixation for patients with open tibial fractures [16]. However, none of these meta-analyses assessed the level of pain and quality of life of patients undergoing EF or IMN, which may influence decisions about treatment modalities. In addition, a new RCT on functional and radiological outcomes of primary ring fixator versus antibiotic nails in open tibial diaphyseal fractures has been reported recently [17]. Therefore, the purpose of this study was to collect all available RCTs on the treatment of open tibial fractures with EF and IMN for meta-analysis to provide reliable evidence-based data for clinical decision-making.

2. Materials and Methods

The systematic review was undertaken in accordance with Preferred Reporting Items for Systematic Reviews and Meta-Analyses (PRISMA) [18,19] and AMSTAR (A Measurement Tool to Assess Systematic Reviews) [20] (Supplementary Material Tables S1 and S2). Review methods were established prior to the conduct of the review and there were no significant deviations from the protocol.

2.1. Study Selection

Screening for inclusion of publications in the systematic review was performed in two phases, with the discussion or consensus of two reviewers at each stage and with the inclusion of a third reviewer to resolve all possible discrepancies. Eligible studies were published RCT trials which compared the use of either IMN or EF to fix the tibial fracture. Studies were excluded if: (1) did not make a comparison between IMN and EF; (2) had other populations (animal, femur etc.); (3) assessed other techniques in fixing tibial fracture; (4) did not have the outcomes of interest; (5) were abstracts; (6) were not original articles; (7) were not confined to the English language.

2.2. Search Strategy

The search strategy was developed by two reviewers, one with a background in orthopedics and one with experience in developing search strategy. An electronic search of databases such as PubMed, Cochrane Library, and Web of Science until 1 March 2023 was conducted to identify published studies containing the following keywords: "fracture external fixation" and "tibial intramedullary nailing".

2.3. Data Abstraction and Quality Assessment

The following data were abstracted independently by two reviewers: title of the study, author(s), year of publication, country where research was performed, sample size, gender and age of patients included, duration of follow-up, intervention type, and types of fracture.

Data of the following outcomes of interest were abstracted: presence of superficial and deep infections, union time, delayed union, malunion, nonunion, and hardware failure. Health-related quality of life data measured using the EQ-5D and data on the presence of pain were additionally obtained from the related articles. If data were unclear or missing, the authors of relevant articles were contacted.

2.4. Risk of Bias

The risk of bias within each study and the overall quality of the gathered evidence was assessed independently by two reviewers using a quality assessment The Risk of Bias 2 (RoB 2) tool of "Cochrane Collaboration's tool to assess the risk of bias in randomized trials". The domains included in RoB 2: bias arising from the randomization process, bias due to deviations from intended interventions, bias due to missing outcome data, bias in the measurement of the outcome, and bias in the selection of the reported result covered all types of bias that are currently understood to affect the results of RCTs [21]. Publication bias was assessed by funnel plots (Supplementary Material Figure S1). The sources of funding for individual studies included in the review were not reported by the study authors.

2.5. Data Analysis

Analyses of the included studies were performed using Review Manager Version 5.4 (Cochrane, 2021). Continuous outcomes, such as time to union and health-related quality of life were expressed with mean difference (MD) and 95% confidence interval (CI). The mean difference for time to union was calculated as MD = μIMN − μEF, whereas the mean difference for health-related quality of life was calculated as MD = μEF − μIMN. If continuous data were presented with mean and ranges, standard deviations were estimated as (max-min)/6. Dichotomous variables, such as postoperative superficial and deep infection, delayed union, malunion, nonunion, hardware failure, and pain were expressed by risk ratio (RR) and 95% CI. The risk ratio was calculated as the ratio of the risk of postoperative superficial and deep infection, delayed union, malunion, and nonunion in the EF group in contrast to the IMN group. The risk ratio was calculated as the ratio of the risk of hardware failure and pain in the IMN group in contrast to the EF group. Chi-square Q and I^2 statistics were used to assess heterogeneity. Based on the Cochrane Handbook [22], I2 categorization of heterogeneity states that $I^2 < 30\%$ corresponds to low, $I^2 = 30$–60% corresponds to moderate, and $I^2 > 60$ corresponds to high heterogeneity of the included studies. Fixed-effect analysis and random-effect analysis were used for data with low and high heterogeneity, respectively. For each analysis, a separate forest plot was constructed, showing the RR (box), 95% CI (lines), and weight (size of box) for each study. The overall effect size was represented by a diamond. A p-value of <0.05 was considered to be statistically significant for all analyses.

3. Results

3.1. Search Results

A total of 1157 potentially eligible articles were extracted from three electronic databases. After duplicates were removed, 896 titles and abstracts were screened for relevance. Eventually, 856 studies did not meet the eligibility criteria and a total of 40 articles were sought for retrieval. Due to one article not being retrieved, 39 articles were assessed for eligibility. After screening the full text, two studies were excluded because they had a wrong population, four had the wrong study design, two had the wrong outcome, three were the wrong publication type, nine represented follow-up studies, two were ongoing clinical trials, and one clinical trial failed. The study selection process using the PRISMA flow diagram is shown in Figure 1.

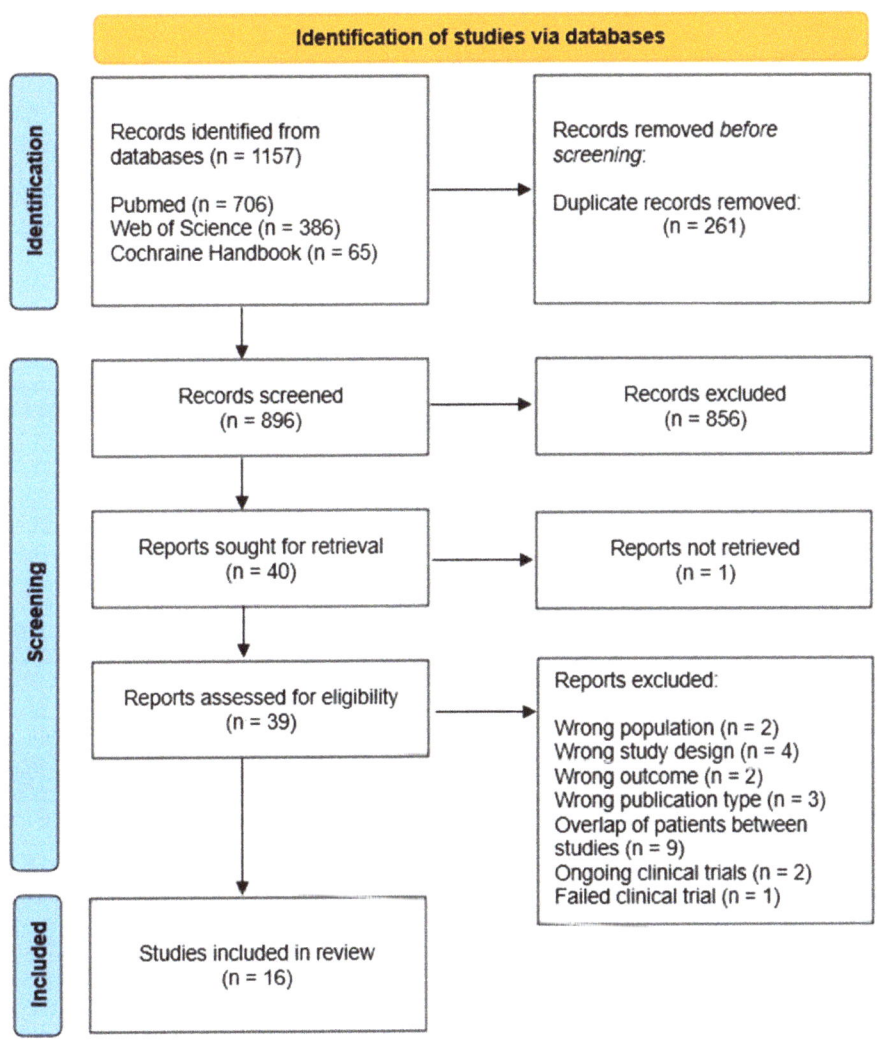

Figure 1. Flowchart of the study selection process.

3.2. Characteristics of Eligible Studies

Characteristics of all 16 publications included in the meta-analysis are presented in detail in Table 1. The studies were published between 1994 and 2022, with a minimum sample size of 29 [23] and a maximum of 221 [24]. Five eligible studies were conducted from Asian countries, three from African countries, four from European countries, three from the USA, and one eligible study was conducted from South America (Figure 2). The average age varied from 25 years to 46 years, and studies comprised a total of 1011 patients (811 male and 200 female). The average duration of follow-up ranged from 4.5 to 46.5 months, and in eligible studies fracture types ranged from I to IIIb according to the Gustilo–Anderson classification.

Table 1. Characteristics of studies included in the meta-analysis.

Study	Year	Country	No. of Patients IMN	No. of Patients EF	Gender (Male/Female) IMN	Gender (Male/Female) EF	Age (Yrs), Mean ± Sd IMN	Age (Yrs), Mean ± Sd EF	Follow Up (Month), Mean ± Sd IMN	Follow Up (Month), Mean ± Sd EF	GA	Type IMN	Type EF
Holbrook et al. [25]	1989	USA	29	28	NA	NA	28 (15–66) †	25 (7–65) †	16.8 (14–21) †	18.5 (12–24) †	I, II, III	Ender	Half-pin
Rohilla et al. [26]	2022	India	16	16	13/3	13/3	33.1 ± 11.2	31.1 ± 9.7	24.1	23.3	II, III	Antibiotic, interlocking	Standard ring frame
Kisitu et al. [27]	2022	Uganda	31	24	21/10	16/8	39 ± 11	39 ± 13	12	4.5	II, IIIa	Unreamed	NA
Haonga et al. [24]	2020	Tanzania	111	110	98/13	91/19	33.3 ± 11.8	31.8 ± 9.5	12	12	I, II, IIIa	Hand-reamed, interlocking (SIGN)	AO uniplanar DISPOFIX
Ramos et al. [28]	2014	Sweden	27	31	19/8	22/9	38 (19–70) †	46 (18–71) †	12	12	I, II;	Reamed, locked, cannulated (Syntes)	Original Ilizarov design
Inan et al. [8]	2007	Turkey	29	32	24/5	28/4	31.7 (17–54) †	32.3 (15–64) †	43.3 (30–61) †	46.5 (33–67) †	IIIa	Unreamed	Hybrid Ilizarov
Li Y et al. [29]	2014	China	46	45	41/5	37/8	44 (18–78) †	43 (20–82) †	14.6 (13–17) †	14.6 (12–17) †	I, II	Reamed and static locking	Combined with limited open reduction and absorbable internal fixation
Garg et al. [30]	2019	India	25	25	18/7	19/6	Mean: 40.4	Mean: 38.8	36 weeks *		IIIa, IIIb	Unreamed	Half-pin
Mohseni et al. [31]	2011	Iran	25	25	20/5	22/3	30.8 ± 5.2	28.9 ± 8.9	12	12	IIIa, IIIb	Unreamed	AO tubular external fixation
Braten et al. [32]	2005	Norway	36	39	NA	NA	43 (16–90) †	41 (16–83) †			I, II	Grosse-Kempf reamed	Ex-fi-re device
Henley et al. [33]	1998	USA	104	70	79/21	53/15	33 (14–81) †	33 (16–77) †	472 days	529 days	II, IIIa, IIIb	Unreamed interlocking	Half-pin
Tu et al. [34]	1995	Taiwan	18	18	30/6 *		38.5 (16–65) *†		20.5 (18–24) *		IIIa, IIIb	Unreamed interlocking	Hoffmann skeletal fixation
Tornetta et al. [23]	1994	USA	15	14	11/4	9/5	41 (21–73) †	37 (19–86) †	21 (19–36) *†		IIIb	Non reamed, statically locked (Gross-Kempf, Alta, AO)	Hoffmann anterior and ACE multiplane
Rodrigues et al. [35]	2014	Brazil	26	31	24/2	28/3	30.5 ± 2	30.3 ± 2.2	12	12	I, II, IIIa	Reamed	Biplanar
Frihagen et al. [36]	2020	Norway	32	31	22/10	20/11	41.8 ± 14.7	43.4 ± 13.5	24	24	42 A-B ‡	Reamed, locked	TSF ring
Esan et al. [37]	2014	Nigeria	20	20	17/3	16/4	38.1 ± 16.3	40.7 ± 17.1	24	24	II, IIIa	Interlocking (SIGN)	AO/ASIF and Orthofix

NA, Not available; GA—Gustilo-Anderson classification; SIGN—The Surgical Implant Generation Network; AO/ASIF—Association for Osteosynthesis/Association for the Study of Internal Fixation; TSF—Taylor Spatial Fixator. * information for all patients included in study, not according to treatment. † median (range) ‡ AO/OTA classification.

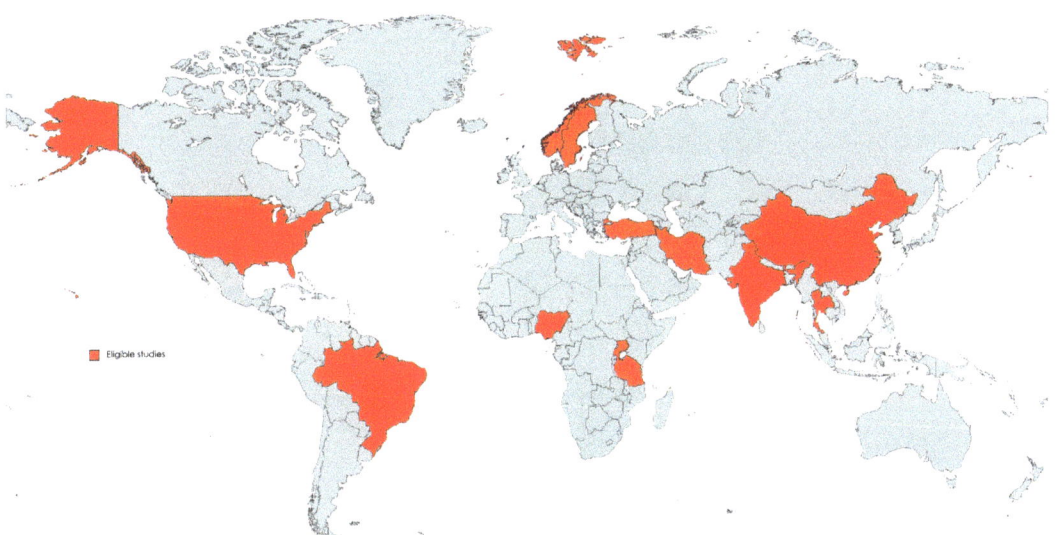

Figure 2. Geographical overview of the eligible studies included in the meta-analyses.

3.3. Quality Assessment of the Eligible Studies

Sixteen studies which reported the randomization method [8,23–37] were assessed for the risk of bias according to the Cochrane Handbook. Six studies reported that the method of randomization in their study was based on even or odd medical record number [8,23,25,31,33,34]. In studies conducted by Kisitu et al. [27], Ramos et al. [28], Li [29], Braten et al. [32], and Rodrigues [35], sealed opaque envelopes were used for randomization; Li et al. [29] stated that the randomization was performed by computer allocation and that sequentially numbered opaque envelopes were assigned to included patients prospectively. However, Kisitu et al. [27] reported in their study that computer randomization was not logistically viable, therefore opaque envelopes were sorted in random sequence. A centralized web-based electronic randomization tool was the randomization method used in the study by Rohilla et al. [26], Haonga et al. [24], and Frihagen et al. [36]. Garg et al. [30] reported that the randomization chit box was used, whereas Esan et al. [37] randomized patients with simple random sampling using a balloting process. In the study conducted by Kisitu et al. [27], it was stated that patients and the treating staff were not blinded to their study group allocation. All studies showed a low risk of bias due to missing outcome data and the measurement of the outcome. Detailed information about the quality assessment of the eligible studies is shown in Figure 3a,b.

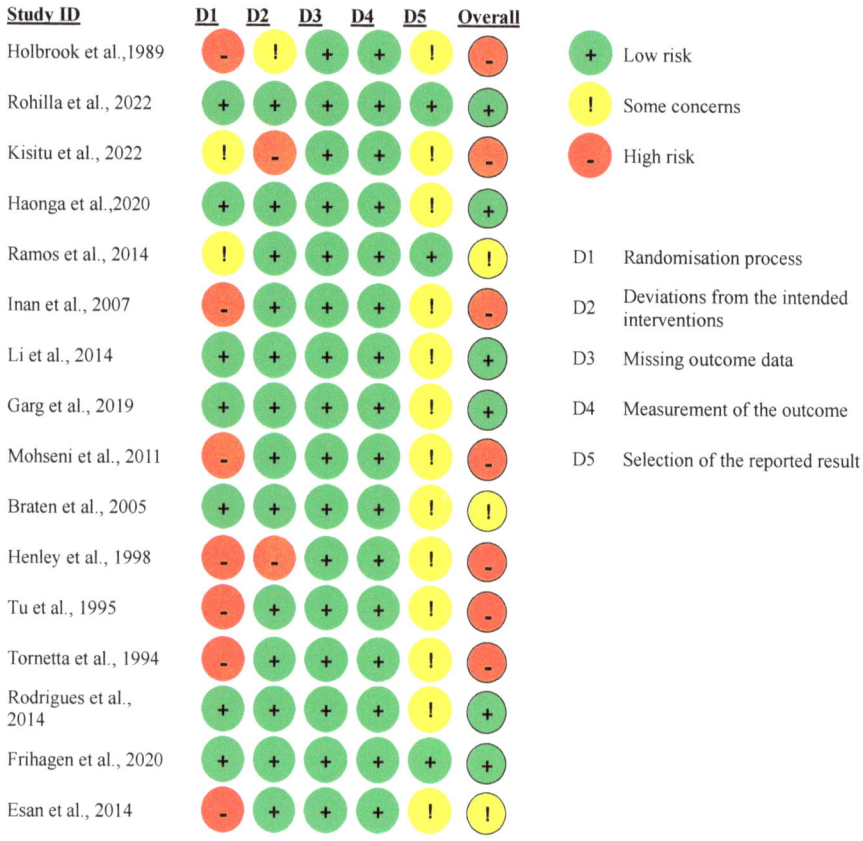

(a)

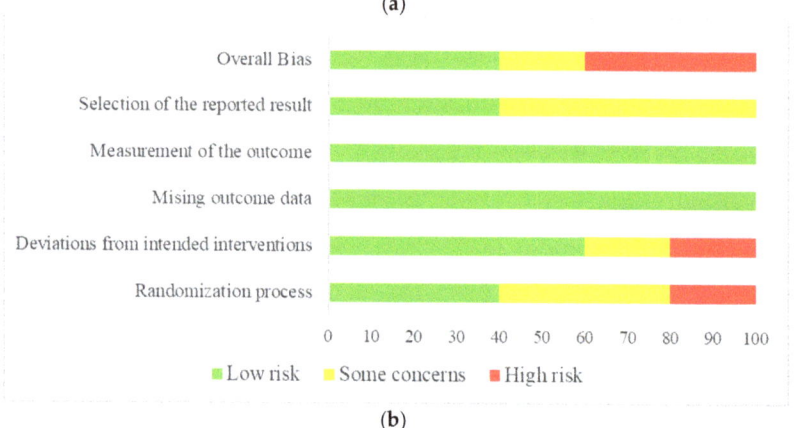

(b)

Figure 3. (a) Risk of bias according to domains [8,23–37]. (b) Overall risk of bias.

4. Results of Meta-Analysis

4.1. Postoperative Superficial Infection

Twelve studies [8,23–30,32,33,36] with a total of 966 cases (EF = 465, IMN = 501) reported the presence of postoperative superficial infection. The fixed-effects model was used due to low heterogeneity among studies ($I^2 = 35\%$). The presence of postoperative superficial infection was significantly higher in the EF group compared to the IMN group (RR = 3.56, 95%CI = 2.56–4.95, $p < 0.001$) (Figure 4).

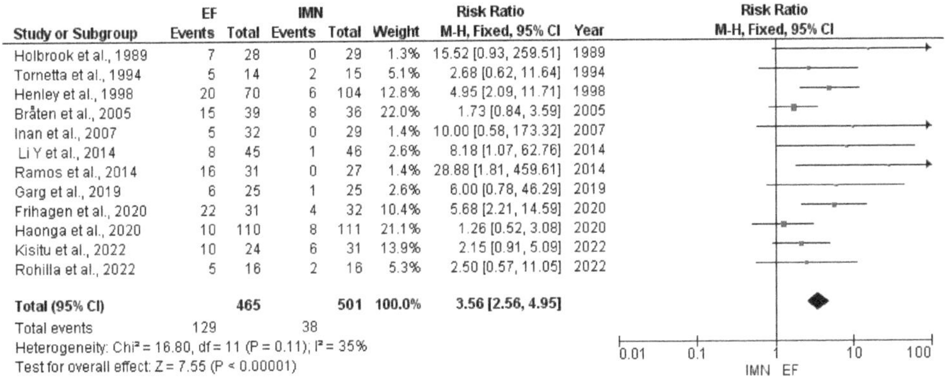

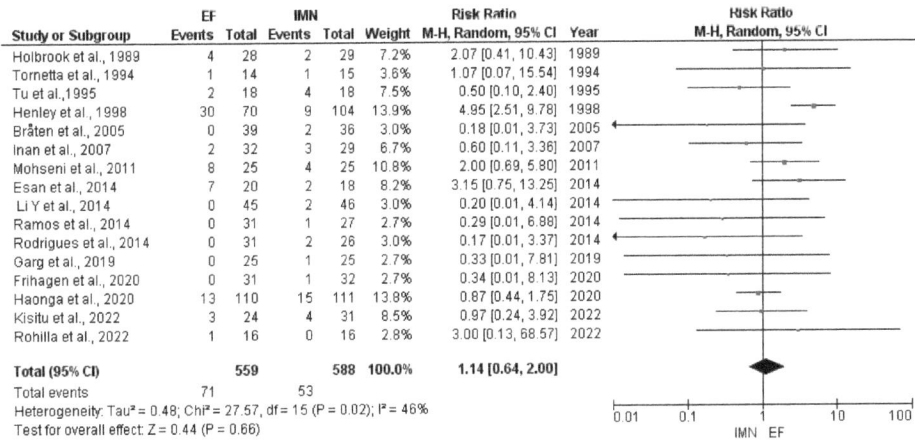

Figure 4. Forest plot presenting the comparison of postoperative superficial infections occurrence between EF and IMN; Blue squares—the individual study effect; Diamond—pooled effect [8,23–29,31,32,34,36].

4.2. Postoperative Deep Infection

Data on postoperative deep infection were provided by all sixteen studies [8,23–37] included in the meta-analysis. Due to moderate heterogeneity ($I^2 = 46\%$) among included studies, random-effect analysis was performed, and the results showed that no statistical difference was found in the presence of postoperative deep infections between EF and IMN groups (RR = 1.14, 95%CI = 0.64–2.00, $p = 0.66$) (Figure 5).

Figure 5. Forest plot presenting the comparison of postoperative deep infections occurrence between EF and IMN; Blue squares—the individual study effect; Diamond—pooled effect [8,23–37].

4.3. Time to Union

Eight studies [8,23,25,28–30,32,37] comprising a total of 459 cases (EF = 234, IMN = 225) provided data about union time. The random-effects model was adopted due to high heterogeneity among studies ($I^2 = 81\%$). The results of meta-analysis showed no statistical difference in time to union between IMN and EF groups (MD = -0.87, 95%CI = -2.42–0.68), $p = 0.27$) (Figure 6).

	IMN			EF				Mean Difference		Mean Difference
Study or Subgroup	Mean	SD	Total	Mean	SD	Total	Weight	IV, Random, 95% CI	Year	IV, Random, 95% CI
Holbrook et al., 1989	5.9	2	29	6.6	2.3	28	17.3%	-0.70 [-1.82, 0.42]	1989	
Tornetta et al., 1994	23	2	15	28.3	4	14	13.3%	-5.30 [-7.63, -2.97]	1994	
Bråten et al., 2005	16	5.8	36	17	6.4	39	11.9%	-1.00 [-3.76, 1.76]	2005	
Inan et al., 2007	21	3.3	29	19	1.5	32	16.8%	2.00 [0.69, 3.31]	2007	
Ramos et al., 2014	13	17.3	27	12.5	39.5	31	1.0%	0.50 [-14.86, 15.86]	2014	
Esan et al., 2014	14.4	5.8	18	14.8	9.9	20	6.2%	-0.40 [-5.50, 4.70]	2014	
Li Y et al., 2014	15.6	3.2	46	15.2	3.5	45	16.5%	0.40 [-0.98, 1.78]	2014	
Garg et al., 2019	32.6	1.8	25	34.4	2.6	25	17.0%	-1.80 [-3.04, -0.56]	2019	
Total (95% CI)			225			234	100.0%	-0.87 [-2.42, 0.68]		

Heterogeneity: Tau² = 3.30; Chi² = 36.49, df = 7 (P < 0.00001); I² = 81%
Test for overall effect: Z = 1.10 (P = 0.27)

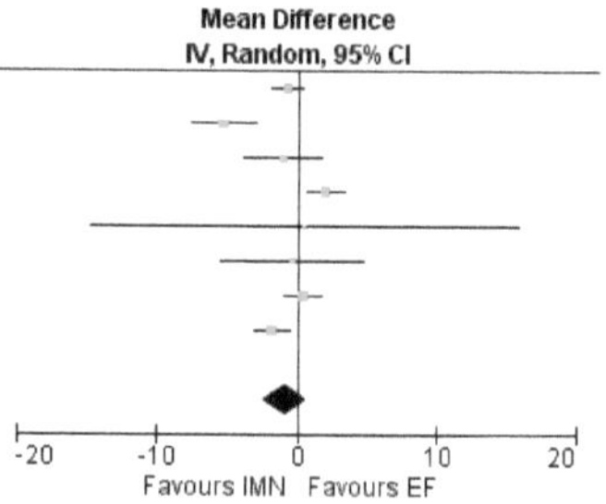

Favours IMN   Favours EF

Figure 6. Forest plot presenting the mean difference in time to union between EF and IMN; Green squares—the individual study effect; Diamond—pooled effect [8,23,27–29,31,34,37].

4.4. Delayed union

Data on delayed union were provided by nine studies [8,23,25,28,29,32,33,36,37] included in the meta-analysis. Due to no heterogeneity ($I^2 = 0\%$) among included studies, fixed-effect analysis was performed, and the results showed that no statistical difference was found in the presence of delayed union between EF and IMN groups (RR = 1.30, 95%CI = 0.84–2.02, $p = 0.23$) (Figure 7).

	EF		IMN			Risk Ratio		Risk Ratio
Study or Subgroup	Events	Total	Events	Total	Weight	M-H, Fixed, 95% CI	Year	M-H, Fixed, 95% CI
Holbrook et al., 1989	6	28	4	29	12.8%	1.55 [0.49, 4.92]	1989	
Tornetta et al., 1994	2	14	2	15	6.3%	1.07 [0.17, 6.61]	1994	
Henley et al., 1998	12	70	13	104	34.1%	1.37 [0.67, 2.83]	1998	
Bråten et al., 2005	1	39	0	36	1.7%	2.77 [0.12, 66.02]	2005	
Inan et al., 2007	4	32	3	29	10.3%	1.21 [0.29, 4.95]	2007	
Esan et al., 2014	6	20	3	18	10.3%	1.80 [0.53, 6.16]	2014	
Li Y et al., 2014	3	45	5	46	16.1%	0.61 [0.16, 2.42]	2014	
Ramos et al., 2014	0	31	1	27	5.2%	0.29 [0.01, 6.88]	2014	
Frihagen et al., 2020	3	31	1	32	3.2%	3.10 [0.34, 28.19]	2020	
Total (95% CI)		310		336	100.0%	1.30 [0.84, 2.02]		
Total events	37		32					

Heterogeneity: Chi² = 3.26, df = 8 (P = 0.92); I² = 0%
Test for overall effect: Z = 1.19 (P = 0.23)

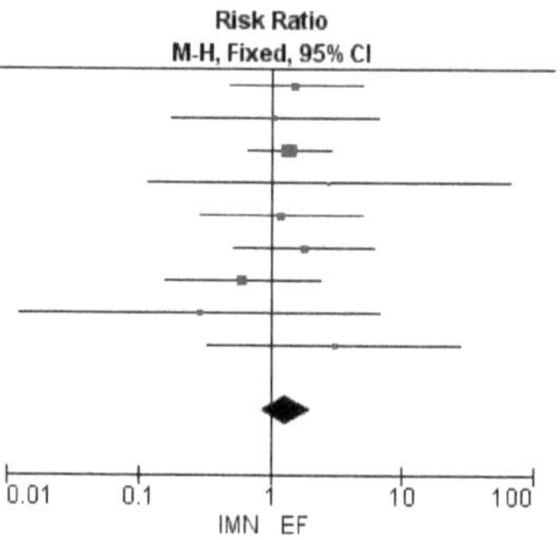

IMN   EF

Figure 7. Forest plot presenting the comparison of delayed union occurrence between EF and IMN; Blue squares—the individual study effect; Diamond—pooled effect [8,23,27,28,31,32,34,36,37].

4.5. Malunion

Fourteen studies [8,23–25,27–36] with a total of 1077 cases (EF = 523, IMN = 554) reported the presence of malunion. The random-effects model was used due to high heterogeneity among studies ($I^2 = 57\%$). The results of the meta-analysis showed significant difference in malunion occurrence between EF and IMN group, favoring IMN (RR = 1.96, 95%CI = 1.12–3.44, $p = 0.02$) (Figure 8).

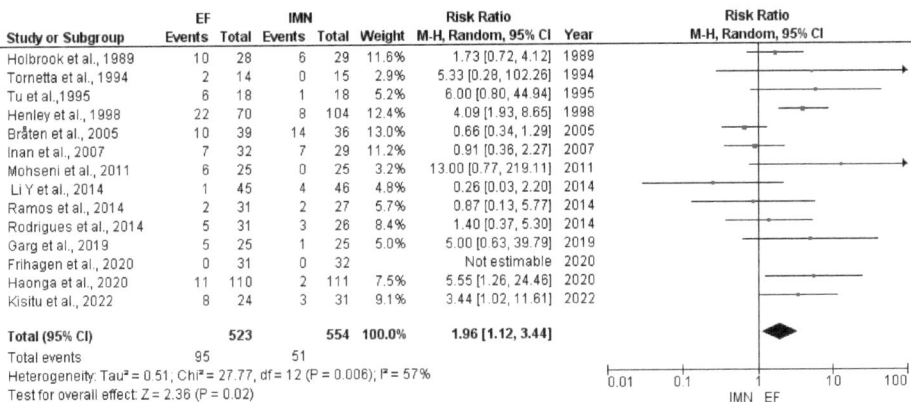

Figure 8. Forest plot presenting the comparison of malunion occurrence between EF and IMN; Blue squares—the individual study effect; Diamond—pooled effect [8,23,25–36].

4.6. Nonunion

Data on nonunion were provided by fourteen studies [8,23–27,29–31,33–37] included in the meta-analysis. Due to no heterogeneity ($I^2 = 0\%$) among included studies, fixed-effect analysis was performed, and the results showed that no statistical difference was found in the presence of nonunion between EF and IMN groups (RR = 1.31, 95%CI = 0.86—2.00, $p = 0.21$) (Figure 9).

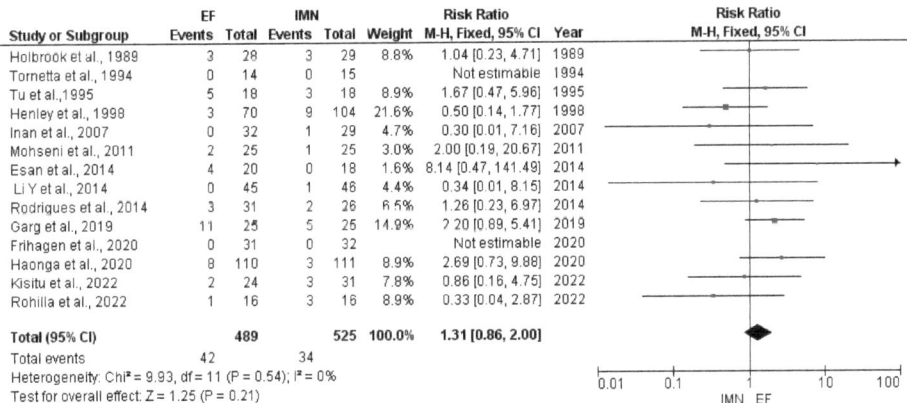

Figure 9. Forest plot presenting the comparison of nonunion occurrence between EF and IMN; Blue squares—the individual study effect; Diamond—pooled effect [8,23–26,28–30,32–37].

4.7. Hardware Failure

Six studies [8,25,28,30,33,34] with a total of 436 cases (EF = 204, IMN = 232) reported the presence of hardware failure. The fixed-effects model was adopted due to no heterogeneity among studies ($I^2 = 0\%$). The results of the meta-analysis showed significant difference in hardware failure between EF and IMN group, favoring EF (RR = 0.30, 95%CI = 0.13–0.69, $p = 0.004$) (Figure 10).

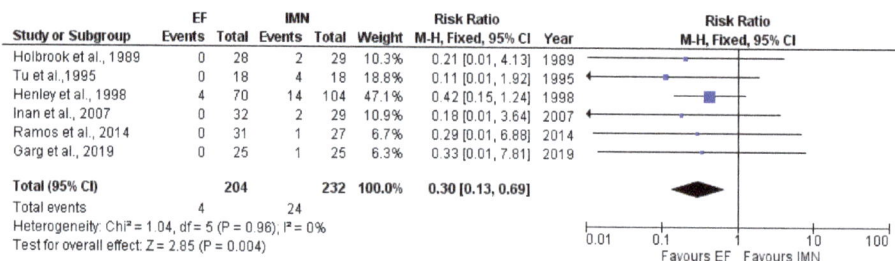

Figure 10. Forest plot presenting the comparison of hardware failure occurrence between EF and IMN; Blue squares—the individual study effect; Diamond—pooled effect [8,23,27,29,32,33].

4.8. Pain

Data on pain were provided by four studies [25,26,28,32] included in the meta-analysis. Due to low heterogeneity ($I^2 = 28\%$) among included studies, fixed-effect analysis was performed, and the results showed that statistical difference was found in the presence of pain between EF and IMN groups, favoring EF (RR = 0.05, 95%CI = 0.02–0.17, $p < 0.001$) (Figure 11).

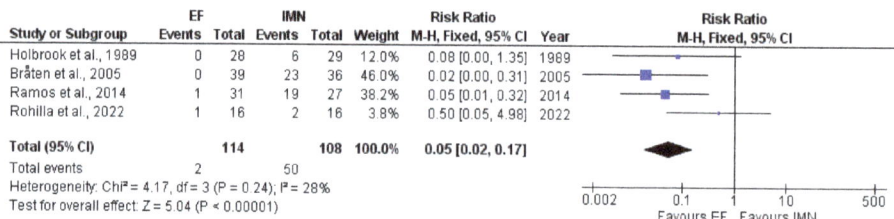

Figure 11. Forest plot presenting the comparison of pain occurrence between EF and IMN; Blue squares—the individual study effect; Diamond—pooled effect [23,24,27,31].

4.9. Health-Related Quality of Life Measured after 3 Months

Three studies [24,27,28] with a total of 334 cases (EF = 165, IMN = 169) provided data about the quality of life related to health. The fixed-effects model was adopted due to no heterogeneity among studies ($I^2 = 0\%$). The results of the meta-analysis showed a significant difference in quality of life between EF and IMN groups after 3 months of procedure, favoring IMN (RR = −0.04, 95%CI = −0.05–0.03, $p < 0.001$) (Figure 12).

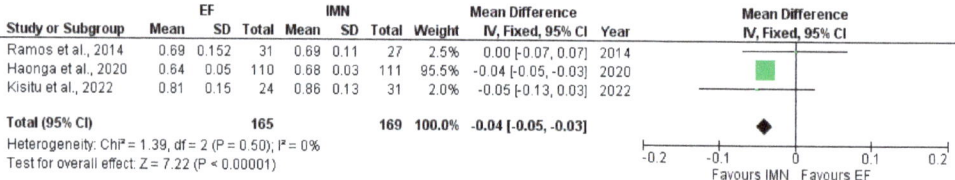

Figure 12. Forest plot presenting the comparison of Health-related quality of life measured after 3 months between EF and IMN; Green squares—the individual study effect; Diamond—pooled effect [25–27].

4.10. Health-Related Quality of Life Measured after 12 Months

Data on health-related quality of life measured after 12 months were provided by three studies [24,27,28] included in the meta-analysis. Due to high heterogeneity ($I^2 = 89\%$) among included studies, random-effect analysis was performed, and the results showed that no statistical difference was found in the presence of quality of life measured after 12 months between EF and IMN groups (RR = 0.03, 95%CI = −0.05–0.11, $p = 0.44$) (Figure 13).

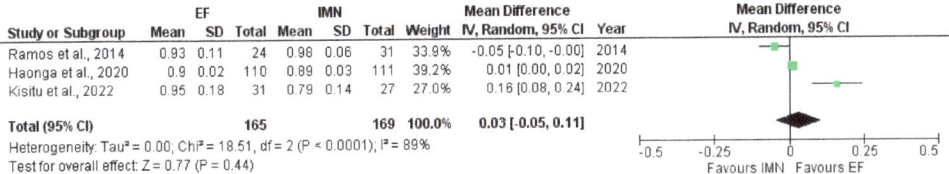

Figure 13. Forest plot presenting the comparison of health-related quality of life measured after 12 months between EF and IMN; Green squares—the individual study effect; Diamond—pooled effect [25–27].

5. Discussion

The findings of this meta-analysis showed that EF was superior in the treatment of open tibia fractures as it was associated with lower rates of hardware failure and pain, but it was inferior in terms of higher rates of superficial infection and malunion, as well as lower health-related quality of life 3 months after treatment. Furthermore, our findings demonstrated no significant difference in deep infection, delayed union and nonunion rates, time to union, and health-related quality of life 12 months following therapy between EF and IMN groups.

The debate over the best surgical treatment technique for open tibia fractures has still been challenging and a subject of discussion for a long time. In 2015. Foote et al. [6] published a network meta-analysis with the objective to compare the relative effects of various treatment options on the risk of requiring unscheduled revision surgery after open fractures of the tibial diaphysis. Independent of the Gustilo classification of the fracture, Foote et al. [6] discovered that the unreamed nail fixation was associated with a lower risk of reoperation in contrast to EF. Results of the meta-analysis conducted by Foote et al. [6] further validated current knowledge that EF of open fractures was associated with increased infection rates [38], many of which may require reoperation. As secondary study endpoints were to quantify differences in malunion, deep infection, and superficial infection in unreamed nail fixation and EF, Foote et al. [6] were unable to identify any significant differences between treatment options due to the small number of reported events. Not long after, in 2016. a research paper reflecting the current status of both IMN and EF for treating Gustilo grade IIIB open tibial fractures was published [15]. This study's meta-analyses demonstrated similar results to Foote et al. [6], moreover that unreamed IMN was superior in the treatment of Gustilo IIIB tibial fractures, with shorter time to union and decreased incidence of superficial infection and malunion, while without increasing the risk of delayed union, non-union, deep infection, and fixation failure compared to EF.

As meta-analyses of RCTs are regarded to provide the strongest evidence for clinical interventions, as compared to observational studies and solitary randomized trials, it is of immense importance to mention Fu et al.'s [13] 2018. meta-analysis of RCT, aimed to compare EF with tibial nailing treatment modality of open tibial fractures. Six RCTs with a total of 407 cases were included in the Fu et al.'s [13] meta-analysis and their results suggest that nailing treatment is superior to EF in preventing post-fixation complications, such as superficial infection and malunion. Consistent with previously published research, their meta-analysis revealed a higher incidence of superficial infections among EF patients, however, Fu et al. [13] pointed out that with effective debridement, stringent wound management, and prudent antibiotic use the risk of superficial infections among these patients can be reduced to a manageable level. In contrast to superficial infection, deep infections and osteomyelitis are more concerning complications of open tibia fractures treatment. Due to exposure of the marrow cavity, the risk of its further contamination and even amputation is increased in patients treated by IMN. However, in EF patients, osteomyelitis is more often presented after early infection and massive soft-tissue defects and is rarely developed from the pin tract infection. Antibiotic-coated nails have recently been introduced to address this issue since they deliver a high concentration of local antibiotic elution in addition to providing stability at the fracture site. A recent study carried out by Rohilla and colleagues [26] found that both the antibiotic-coated tibial interlocking nail and ring fixator obtained equivalent rates of union and similar complications. The findings of this study showed that, although ring fixation is a well-established alternative for treating open tibial fractures, an antibiotic-coated intramedullary nail may also be a viable choice.

EF patients, on the other hand, had a much lower incidence of hardware failure compared to patients in whom nailing was the treatment modality. With a frequency of up to 3–16%, hardware failure remains the most often reported nailing complication across studies, due to the breakage of locking screws [13]. A total of 22 cases of nailing hardware failure were reported in the study by Fu et al. [13], compared to the six EF cases. Additionally, results of the meta-analysis conducted by Fu et al. [13] showed similar treatment effects for postoperative deep infection, delayed union, and nonunion between groups. The pooled results of the most recent meta-analysis including 9 RCTs with 733 cases [16], suggested that the IMN technique had a lower postoperative superficial infection and malunion rate ($RR = 2.84$, 95%CI = 1.83–4.39 and $RR = 3.05$, 95%CI = 2.06–4.52, respectively), but higher hardware failure occurrence in contrast to EF ($RR = 0.38$; 95%CI = 0.17–0.83). No significant differences were found in the union time, delayed union or nonunion rate, and postoperative deep infection rate between the treatments. These findings are in accordance with the results of our meta-analyses based on 16 RCTs and 1011 cases, where patients treated with IMN had higher rates of hardware failure, however lower rates of complications such as superficial infection and malunion. It is worth mentioning that although several RCTs compared health-related quality of life and pain between EF and IMN patients, no meta-analysis has been performed in this regard. In 2014, a randomized prospective study comparing the Ilizarov circular fixator and locked IMN methods in patients with tibia shaft fractures was published [28]. Results of Ramos et al. [28] demonstrated that despite the fact that the Ilizarov group had more open fractures, the absolute number of severe complications was greater in the IMN group. With respect to assessing major complications between groups, such as compartment syndrome, deep infection, hardware failure, delayed union, pseudarthrosis, and malunion, several self-report measures of pain and functionality were included in this study additionally. There was a statistically significant difference between the Ilizarov and IMN groups of patients on both pain and satisfaction at 1 year, showing that patients in the Ilizarov group scored better than patients in the IMN group. Ramos et al. [28] concluded that diaphyseal tibial fractures may be effectively treated utilizing the Ilizarov method, a minimally invasive procedure that allows for immediate weight-bearing, tend to decrease anterior knee discomfort and benefit patients with leaving no implant behind.

In addition to assessing the composite primary event of reoperation or mortality for deep infection, nonunion, or malalignment at 1 year, Haonga et al. [24] assessed the quality of life between uniplanar EF and IMN patients. The results of this RCT conducted at a tertiary orthopedic center in Tanzania showed significant early differences in quality of life in favor of IMN, however, these differences did not persist at 12 months. Haonga et al. [24] stated that given the inconveniences of an external fixator, the improved early quality of life following intramedullary nailing is not unexpected. Despite variations in radiographic healing and ultimate alignment, quality of life in the treatment groups equilibrated between 6 and 12 weeks, the time during which external fixators were removed. Our meta-analysis, to our knowledge, is the first to evaluate both pain and health-related quality of life, as important outcome measures after open tibia fracture treatment. Pooled results of our meta-analysis revealed a significant difference in quality of life 3 months after the procedure between the EF and IMN groups, favoring IMN. However, the assessment of quality of life evaluated 12 months following interventions presented findings comparable to Haonga et al. [24]. Given that only four studies assessing pain and three studies assessing health-related quality of life were eligible for meta-analysis, more high-quality RCTs should be conducted to provide reliable evidence-based data for clinical decision-making.

There are several limitations of this meta-analysis. The first limitation of this study was that out of the 16 studies included, 7 studies showed a high overall risk of bias. Next, six studies had the method of randomization based on even or odd medical record numbers, not meeting the strict randomization criteria. Furthermore, only 3 studies provided data of pain and health-related quality of life, therefore more RCTs are needed to generate more convincing evidence.

6. Conclusions

This meta-analysis presented reduced incidence rates of superficial infection, malunion, and health-related quality of life 3 months after treatment in IMN. However, EF led to a significant reduction in pain and incidence rate of hardware failure. Postoperative deep infection, delayed union, nonunion and health-related quality of life 12 months following therapy were similar between groups. More high-quality RCTs should be conducted to provide reliable evidence-based data for clinical decision-making.

Supplementary Materials: The following supporting information can be downloaded at: https://www.mdpi.com/article/10.3390/medicina59071301/s1, Table S1: Prisma Checklist [39,40]; Table S2: AMSTAR 2 Checklist; Figure S1: Funnel plots of: (**a**) Superficial infection; (**b**) Deep infection; (**c**) Delayed union; (**d**) Malunion; (**e**) Nonunion; (**f**) Hardware failure; (**g**) Pain.

Author Contributions: Conceptualization, D.J., N.R. and S.T.; methodology, D.J., N.R., B.G., B.K., S.R., N.B., K.D. and S.T; software, D.J., N.R. and S.T.; validation, D.J., N.R., B.G., B.K., S.R., N.B., K.D. and S.T.; formal analysis, D.J., N.R. and S.T.; investigation, D.J., N.R., B.G., B.K., S.R., N.B., K.D. and S.T.; resources, D.J., N.R., B.G., B.K., S.R., N.B., K.D. and S.T.; data curation, D.J., N.R., B.G., B.K., S.R., N.B., K.D. and S.T.; writing—original draft preparation, D.J., N.R., B.G., B.K., S.R., N.B., K.D. and S.T.; writing—review and editing, D.J., N.R., B.G., B.K., S.R., N.B., K.D. and S.T.; visualization, D.J. and S.T.; supervision, D.J. and S.T.; project administration, D.J. and S.T.; funding acquisition, D.J. and S.T. All authors have read and agreed to the published version of the manuscript.

Funding: This research received no external funding.

Institutional Review Board Statement: Not applicable.

Informed Consent Statement: Not applicable.

Data Availability Statement: The data that support the findings of this study are available on request from the corresponding author.

Conflicts of Interest: The authors declare no conflict of interest.

References

1. Court-Brown, C.M.; Rimmer, S.; Prakash, U.; McQueen, M.M. The epidemiology of open long bone fractures. *Injury* **1998**, *29*, 529–534. [CrossRef]
2. Weiss, R.J.; Montgomery, S.M.; Ehlin, A.; Al Dabbagh, Z.; Stark, A.; Jansson, K.A. Decreasing incidence of tibial shaft fractures between 1998 and 2004, information based on 10,627 Swedish inpatients. *Acta Orthop.* **2008**, *79*, 526–533. [CrossRef]
3. Okike, K. Current concepts review: Trends in the management of open fractures. *J. Bone Jt. Surg. A* **2006**, *88*, 2739–2747. [CrossRef]
4. Elniel, A.R.; Giannoudis, P.V. Open fractures of the lower extremity: Current management and clinical outcomes. *EFORT Open Rev.* **2018**, *3*, 316–325. [CrossRef] [PubMed]
5. Zalavras, C.G.; Patzakis, M.J. Open fractures: Evaluation and management. *JAAOSJ Am. Acad. Orthopaed. Surg.* **2003**, *11*, 212–219. [CrossRef] [PubMed]

6. Foote, C.J.; Guyatt, G.H.; Vignesh, K.N.; Mundi, R.; Chaudhry, H.; Heels-Ansdell, D.; Thabane, L.; Tornetta, P., 3rd; Bhandari, M. Which Surgical Treatment for Open Tibial Shaft Fractures Results in the Fewest Reoperations? A Network Meta-analysis. *Clin. Orthop. Relat. Res.* **2015**, *473*, 2179–2192. [CrossRef] [PubMed]
7. Hosny, G.; Fadel, M. Ilizarov external fixator for open fractures of the tibial shaft. *Int. Orthop.* **2003**, *27*, 303–306. [CrossRef] [PubMed]
8. Inan, M.; Halici, M.; Ayan, I.; Tuncel, M.; Karaoglu, S. Treatment of type IIIA open fractures of tibial shaft with Ilizarov external fixator versus unreamed tibial nailing. *Arch. Orthop. Trauma Surg.* **2007**, *127*, 617–623. [CrossRef]
9. Court-Brown, C.M.; Wheelwrigh, E.F.; Christie, J.; McQueen, M.M. External fixation for type III open tibial fractures. *J. Bone Jt. Surg. Br.* **1990**, *72*, 801–804. [CrossRef]
10. Whitelaw, G.P.; Cimino, W.G.; Segal, D. The treatment of open tibial fractures using nonreamed fexible intramedullary fixation. *Orthop. Rev.* **1990**, *19*, 244–256.
11. Greco, T.; Vitiello, R.; Cazzato, G.; Cianni, L.; Malerba, G.; Maccauro, G.; Perisano, C. Intramedullary antibiotic coated nail in tibial fracture: A systematic review. *J. Biol. Regul. Homeost. Agents* **2020**, *34*, 63–69. [PubMed]
12. Rohde, C.; Greives, M.R.; Cetrulo, C.; Lerman, O.Z.; Levine, J.P.; Hazen, A. Gustilo grade IIIB tibial fractures requiring microvascular free faps: External fxation versus intramedullary rod fixation. *Ann. Plast. Surg.* **2007**, *59*, 14–17. [CrossRef] [PubMed]
13. Fu, Q.; Zhu, L.; Lu, J.; Ma, J.; Chen, A. External fixation versus unreamed tibial intramedullary nailing for open tibial fractures: A meta-analysis of randomized controlled trials. *Sci. Rep.* **2018**, *8*, 12753. [CrossRef]
14. Xu, X.; Li, X.; Liu, L.; Wu, W. A meta-analysis of external fixator versus intramedullary nails for open tibial fracture fixation. *J. Orthop. Surg. Res.* **2014**, *9*, 75. [CrossRef] [PubMed]
15. Zhang, F.; Zhu, Y.; Li, W.; Chen, W.; Tian, Y.; Zhang, Y. Unreamed Intramedullary Nailing is a better alternative than External Fixator for Gustilo grade IIIB Tibial Fractures based on a meta-analysis. *Scand. J. Surg.* **2016**, *105*, 117–124. [CrossRef] [PubMed]
16. Liu, J.; Xie, L.; Liu, L.; Gao, G.; Zhou, P.; Chu, D.; Qiu, D.; Tao, J. Comparing external fixators and intramedullary nailing for treating open tibia fractures: A meta-analysis of randomized controlled trials. *J. Orthop. Surg. Res.* **2023**, *18*, 13. [CrossRef]
17. Fang, X.; Jiang, L.; Wang, Y.; Zhao, L. Treatment of Gustilo grade III tibial fractures with unreamed intramedullary nailing versus external fxator: A meta-analysis. *Med. Sci. Monit.* **2012**, *18*, RA49–RA56. [CrossRef]
18. Stroup, D.F.; Berlin, J.A.; Morton, S.C.; Olkin, I.; Williamson, G.D.; Rennie, D.; Moher, D.; Becker, B.J.; Sipe, T.A.; Thacker, S.B. Meta-analysis of observational studies in epidemiology: A proposal for reporting. Meta-analysis Of Observational Studies in Epidemiology (MOOSE) group. *JAMA* **2000**, *283*, 2008–2012. [CrossRef]
19. Liberati, A.; Altman, D.G.; Tetzlaff, J.; Mulrow, C.; Gøtzsche, P.C.; Ioannidis, J.P.; Clarke, M.; Devereaux, P.J.; Kleijnen, J.; Moher, D. The PRISMA statement for reporting systematic reviews and meta-analyses of studies that evaluate health care interventions: Explanation and elaboration. *PLoS Med.* **2009**, *6*, e1000100. [CrossRef]
20. Shea, B.J.; Reeves, B.C.; Wells, G.; Thuku, M.; Hamel, C.; Moran, J.; Moher, D.; Tugwell, P.; Welch, V.; Kristjansson, E.; et al. AMSTAR 2, a critical appraisal tool for systematic reviews that include randomised or non-randomised studies of healthcare interventions, or both. *BMJ* **2017**, *358*, j4008. [CrossRef]
21. Higgins, J.P.T.; Savović, J.; Page, M.J.; Elbers, R.G.; Sterne, J.A.C. Chapter 8, Assessing risk of bias in a randomized trial. In *Handbook for Systematic Reviews of Interventions Version 6.3*, updated February 2022, 2nd ed.; Higgins, J.P.T., Thomas, J., Chandler, J., Cumpston, M., Li, T., Page, M.J., Welch, V.A., Eds.; John Wiley & Sons: Chichester, UK, 2019. Available online: www.training.cochrane.org/handbook (accessed on 5 January 2023).
22. Higgins, J.P.; Thomas, J.; Chandler, J.; Cumpston, M.; Li, T.; Page, M.J.; Welch, V. *Cochrane Handbook for Systematic Reviews of Interventions*; John Wiley & Sons: Hoboken, NJ, USA, 2019.
23. Tornetta, P., 3rd; Bergman, M.; Watnik, N.; Berkowitz, G.; Steuer, J. Treatment of grade-IIIb open tibial fractures: A prospective randomised comparison of external fixation and non-reamed locked nailing. *J. Bone Jt. Surg. Br.* **1994**, *76*, 13–19. [CrossRef]
24. Haonga, B.T.; Liu, M.; Albright, P.; Challa, S.T.; Ali, S.H.; Lazar, A.A.; Eliezer, E.N.; Shearer, D.W.; Morshed, S. Intramedullary Nailing Versus External Fixation in the Treatment of Open Tibial Fractures in Tanzania: Results of a Randomized Clinical Trial. *J. Bone Jt. Surg. Am.* **2020**, *102*, 896–905. [CrossRef] [PubMed]
25. Holbrook, J.L.; Swiontkowski, M.F.; Sanders, R. Treatment of open fractures of the tibial shaft: Ender nailing versus external fixation: A randomized, prospective comparison. *J. Bone Jt. Surg. Am.* **1989**, *71*, 1231–1238. [CrossRef]
26. Rohilla, R.; Arora, S.; Kundu, A.; Singh, R.; Govil, V.; Khokhar, A. Functional and radiological outcomes of primary ring fixator versus antibiotic nail in open tibial diaphyseal fractures: A prospective study. *Injury* **2022**, *53*, 3464–3470. [CrossRef] [PubMed]
27. Kisitu, D.K.; O'Hara, N.N.; Slobogean, G.P.; Howe, A.L.; Blachut, P.A.; O'Brien, P.J.; Stockton, D.J. Unreamed Intramedullary Nailing Versus External Fixation for the Treatment of Open Tibial Shaft Fractures in Uganda: A Randomized Clinical Trial. *J. Orthop. Trauma* **2022**, *36*, 349–357. [CrossRef]
28. Ramos, T.; Eriksson, B.I.; Karlsson, J.; Nistor, L. Ilizarov external fixation or locked intramedullary nailing in diaphyseal tibial fractures: A randomized, prospective study of 58 consecutive patients. *Arch. Orthop. Trauma Surg.* **2014**, *134*, 793–802. [CrossRef]
29. Li, Y.; Jiang, X.; Guo, Q.; Zhu, L.; Ye, T.; Chen, A. Treatment of distal tibial shaft fractures by three different surgical methods: A randomized, prospective study. *Int. Orthop.* **2014**, *38*, 1261–1267. [CrossRef]
30. Garg, S.; Khanna, V.; Goyal, M.P.; Joshi, N. Unreamed Intra-Medullary Nail Versus Half Pin External Fixator in Grade III [A & B] Open tibia fractures. *J. Clin. Orthop. Trauma* **2019**, *10*, 941–948.

31. Mohseni, M.A.; Soleimanpour, J.; Mohammadpour, H.; Shahsavari, A. AO tubular external fixation vs. unreamed intramedullary nailing in open grade IIIA-IIIB tibial shaft fractures: A single-center randomized clinical trial. *Pak. J. Biol. Sci.* **2011**, *14*, 490–495. [CrossRef]
32. Bråten, M.; Helland, P.; Grøntvedt, T.; Aamodt, A.; Benum, P.; Mølster, A. External fixation versus locked intramedullary nailing in tibial shaft fractures: A prospective, randomised study of 78 patients. *Arch. Orthop. Trauma Surg.* **2005**, *125*, 21–26. [CrossRef]
33. Henley, M.B.; Chapman, J.R.; Agel, J.; Harvey, E.J.; Whorton, A.M.; Swiontkowski, M.F. Treatment of type II, IIIA, and IIIB open fractures of the tibial shaft: A prospective comparison of unreamed interlocking intramedullary nails and half-pin external fixators. *J. Orthop. Trauma* **1998**, *12*, 1–7. [CrossRef]
34. Tu, Y.K.; Lin, C.H.; Su, J.I.; Hsu, D.T.; Chen, R.J. Unreamed interlocking nail versus external fixator for open type III tibia fractures. *J. Trauma* **1995**, *39*, 361–367. [CrossRef] [PubMed]
35. Rodrigues, F.L.; de Abreu, L.C.; Valenti, V.E.; Valente, A.L.; da Costa Pereira Cestari, R.; Pohl, P.H.; Rodrigues, L.M. Bone tissue repair in patients with open diaphyseal tibial fracture treated with biplanar external fixation or reamed locked intramedullary nailing. *Injury* **2014**, *45* (Suppl. S5), S32–S35. [CrossRef] [PubMed]
36. Frihagen, F.; Madsen, J.E.; Sundfeldt, M.; Flugsrud, G.B.; Andreassen, J.S.; Andersen, M.R.; Andreassen, G.S. Taylor Spatial Frame or Reamed Intramedullary Nailing for Closed Fractures of the Tibial Shaft: A Randomized Controlled Trial. *J. Orthop. Trauma* **2020**, *34*, 612–619. [CrossRef] [PubMed]
37. Esan, O.; Ikem, I.C.; Oginni, L.M.; Esan, O.T. Comparison of unreamed interlocking nail and external fixation in open tibia shaft fracture management. *West Afr. J. Med.* **2014**, *33*, 16–20.
38. Melvin, J.S.; Dombroski, D.G.; Torbert, J.T.; Kovach, S.J.; Esterhai, J.L.; Mehta, S. Open tibial shaft fractures: II. Definitive management and limb salvage. *J. Am. Acad. Orthop. Surg.* **2010**, *18*, 108–117. [CrossRef]
39. Page, M.J.; McKenzie, J.E.; Bossuyt, P.M.; Boutron, I.; Hoffmann, T.C.; Mulrow, C.D.; Shamseer, L.; Tetzlaff, J.M.; Akl, E.A.; Brennan, S.E.; et al. The PRISMA 2020 statement: An updated guideline for reporting systematic reviews. *BMJ* **2021**, *372*, n71. [CrossRef]
40. Available online: http://www.prisma-statement.org/ (accessed on 6 July 2023).

Disclaimer/Publisher's Note: The statements, opinions and data contained in all publications are solely those of the individual author(s) and contributor(s) and not of MDPI and/or the editor(s). MDPI and/or the editor(s) disclaim responsibility for any injury to people or property resulting from any ideas, methods, instructions or products referred to in the content.

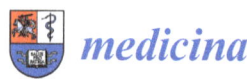

Article

A Comparative Analysis of Pain Control Methods after Ankle Fracture Surgery with a Peripheral Nerve Block: A Single-Center Randomized Controlled Prospective Study

Jeong-Kil Lee [1], Gi-Soo Lee [1,*], Sang-Bum Kim [1], Chan Kang [1], Kyong-Sik Kim [2] and Jae-Hwang Song [3]

1. Department of Orthopedic Surgery, Chungnam National University School of Medicine, Daejeon 34134, Republic of Korea
2. Department of Anaesthesia, Chungnam National University Sejong Hospital, Sejong 30099, Republic of Korea
3. Department of Orthopedic Surgery, Konyang University College of Medicine, Daejeon 35365, Republic of Korea
* Correspondence: gslee1899@gmail.com; Tel.: +82-44-995-4730

Abstract: *Background and Objectives*: Patients experience severe pain after surgical correction of ankle fractures. Although their exact mechanism is unknown, dexamethasone and epinephrine increase the analgesic effect of anesthetics in peripheral nerve blocks. This study aimed to compare the postoperative pain control efficacy of peripheral nerve blocks with ropivacaine combined with dexamethasone/epinephrine and peripheral nerve blocks with only ropivacaine and added patient-controlled analgesia in patients with ankle fractures. *Materials and Methods*: This randomized, controlled prospective study included patients aged 18–70 years surgically treated for ankle fractures between December 2021 and September 2022. The patients were divided into group A (n = 30), wherein pain was controlled using patient-controlled analgesia after lower extremity peripheral nerve block, and group B (n = 30), wherein dexamethasone/epinephrine was combined with the anesthetic solution during peripheral nerve block. In both groups, ropivacaine was used as the anesthetic solution for peripheral nerve block, and this peripheral nerve block was performed just before ankle surgery for the purpose of anesthesia for surgery. Pain (visual analog scale), patient satisfaction, and side effects were assessed and compared between the two groups. *Results*: The patients' demographic data were similar between groups. Pain scores were significantly lower in group B than in group A postoperatively. Satisfaction scores were significantly higher in group B (p = 0.003). There were no anesthesia-related complications in either group. *Conclusions*: Dexamethasone and epinephrine as adjuvant anesthetic solutions can effectively control pain when performing surgery using peripheral nerve blocks for patients with ankle fractures.

Keywords: ankle fracture; anesthetic; nerve block; pain management; postoperative pain control

Citation: Lee, J.-K.; Lee, G.-S.; Kim, S.-B.; Kang, C.; Kim, K.-S.; Song, J.-H. A Comparative Analysis of Pain Control Methods after Ankle Fracture Surgery with a Peripheral Nerve Block: A Single-Center Randomized Controlled Prospective Study. *Medicina* **2023**, *59*, 1302. https://doi.org/10.3390/medicina59071302

Academic Editor: Woo Jong Kim

Received: 24 June 2023
Revised: 11 July 2023
Accepted: 13 July 2023
Published: 14 July 2023

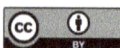

Copyright: © 2023 by the authors. Licensee MDPI, Basel, Switzerland. This article is an open access article distributed under the terms and conditions of the Creative Commons Attribution (CC BY) license (https://creativecommons.org/licenses/by/4.0/).

1. Introduction

Severe pain after orthopedic surgery contributes to fear of surgery and post-traumatic stress disorder [1]. Postoperative pain control in patients with lower extremity fractures is an ongoing research topic. The peripheral nerve block (PNB) has recently gained popularity as an anesthetic technique for lower extremity surgery.

Ropivacaine is usually used as an anesthetic solution for PNB. The analgesic effect of PNBs with ropivacaine is brief, generally lasting <24 h postoperatively [2]. Dexamethasone and epinephrine increase anesthetic effects and may also be effective in PNBs [3]. However, few studies have investigated the usefulness of combining dexamethasone and epinephrine for PNBs [4–7]. To our knowledge, no comparative studies on pain control using conventional PNB for ankle fractures are available.

We hypothesized that PNB with dexamethasone and epinephrine is more effective than other pain control methods after conventional PNB. Therefore, this study aimed to prospectively compare PNB combined with dexamethasone/epinephrine and patient-controlled analgesia (PCA) using ketorolac after PNB anesthesia in patients with ankle fractures.

2. Materials and Methods

2.1. Patients

This single-center randomized, controlled prospective study enrolled patients aged 18–70 years surgically treated for ankle fractures between December 2021 and September 2022. Unilateral open reduction and internal fixation for ankle fractures were performed on the patients by a single surgeon who has been operating in this field for >10 years. Fracture types included fractures involving the articular surface of the distal tibia and fibula, including simple fibula fractures, bimalleolar fractures, trimalleolar fractures, and pilon fractures. Patients were blinded to their group assignment and hospitalized for at least three days for postoperative pain control.

The exclusion criteria were contraindication for PNBs; uncontrolled diabetes mellitus, peripheral vascular disease, renal or hepatic disease, or any neurologic disease; and contraindication for regional anesthesia (coagulopathy or injection site infection). Patients with body mass index <18.5 kg/m^2, which is considered underweight according to the World Health Organization standard [8], were excluded for anesthesia safety. Patients with suspected nerve injuries or nerve injuries requiring careful postoperative observation and those at risk of compartment syndrome were also excluded (Figure 1).

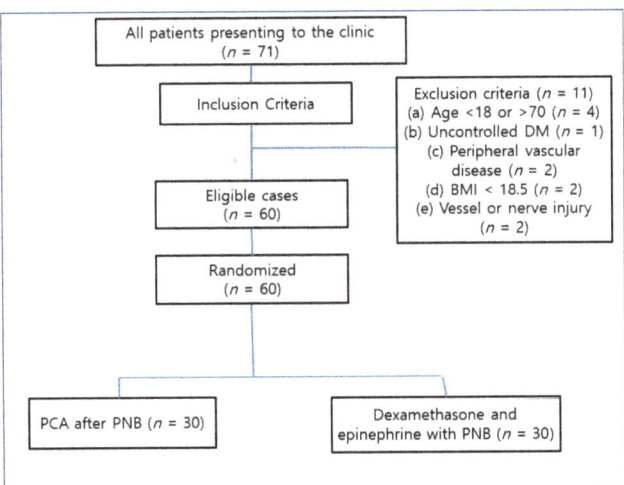

Figure 1. CONSORT (Consolidated Standards of Reporting Trials) flow diagram. Abbreviations: DM; diabetes mellitus, BMI; body mass index, PCA; patient-controlled analgesia, PNB; peripheral nerve block.

This study was approved by the institutional review board (CNUSH 2021-11-003) and was conducted in accordance with the Declaration of Helsinki. This study was registered with the ISRCTN registry (ISRCTN17431025). Written informed consent was obtained from all patients. A single researcher explained and conducted the study. Patients understood, and agreed to be hospitalized for more than three days according to their will, which is common in this research institution for hospitalization of more than three days after ankle fracture surgery, and is related to the medical system. All authors approved the final version of this manuscript.

2.2. Study Design

All patients were anesthetized using ultrasound-guided PNB with ropivacaine. We randomly allocated 60 participants (1:1) into two groups using blinded randomization blocks. Group A received PCA with ketorolac for postoperative pain management after PNB. Group B received PCA with normal saline; instead, dexamethasone and epinephrine were added to ropivacaine during PNB. The allocation sequence was concealed from the researchers and participants in sequentially numbered, opaque sealed envelopes. The envelopes were opened only for the researchers after the enrolled participants had completed all baseline assessments, when it was time to perform the intervention in the operating room. A sample size of 59 patients was determined based on the following parameters: significance level (5%), statistical power (90%), sample ratio (1:1), variance (2.5), and difference between the two groups (1.5). To obtain a 1:1 ratio between groups, we included 60 cases (30 in each group).

In group A, PCA was initiated approximately 10 h after PNB induction [2,9]. The treatment comprised 4 mL ketorolac (120 mg) and 100 mL normal saline. An initial bolus of 8 mL was injected, followed by an additional 96 mL slowly administered with a PCA instrument (Auto Selector; Tecnica Scientifica Service, Torino, Italy) over 48 h. A maintenance dose of 2 mL/h was administered, with each additional PCA bolus containing 1 mL and a lockout interval of 15 min.

In group B, PNB was performed using an anesthetic solution of ropivacaine (Naropin®, AstraZeneca AB, Sodertalje, Sweden) combined with dexamethasone disodium phosphate 5 mg (5 mg/mL, Daewon Pharm. Co., Ltd., Seoul, Republic of Korea) and epinephrine 0.1 mg (1 mg/mL, Daihan Pharm. Co., Ltd., Seoul, Republic of Korea); epinephrine was added in a ratio of 1:200,000. The same PCA instrument was also used for all patients in group B. However, only normal saline was administered in the same way as in group A. We kept all patients unaware of which group they belonged to until the end of the study. To do so, the same PCA instrument was applied to all patients included in this study. In both groups, patients with visual analog scale (VAS) scores ≥ 5 received intravenous acetaminophen (Kabi paracetamol 100 mL, 1 mg/mL, Fresenius Kabi, Friedberg, Germany) for rescue analgesia. VAS scores obtained within 8 h of intravenous acetaminophen injection were excluded from the analysis. No other pain control medications or methods were used in either group.

Pain intensity (VAS score: 0, no pain; 10, worst pain imaginable) was compared between the two groups at 6, 12, 18, 24, 32, 40, 48, and 60 h after PNB. The time at which the sensation began (analgesia time) and the time at which motor function was restored were recorded. After three days of administering pain control, a questionnaire was completed to assess patients' satisfaction with the pain control method (Likert scale). The clinical researcher collected the questionnaires and confirmed that the patients had filled them correctly (Figure 2). The clinical researcher, blinded to group allocation and not involved in the block procedure, investigated the other surgical and anesthetic data. The number of additional analgesic doses required during the same 60 h period and complications were measured by a surgeon.

2.3. Anesthetic and Operative Procedures

The surgeon administered the anesthetic solution (30 mL 0.75% ropivacaine) via a 50-mL syringe connected to a venous catheter with a 100-mm, 23-gauge spinal needle. A registered nurse prepared the anesthetic solution by adding dexamethasone and epinephrine to the ropivacaine (Figure 3).

A standard noninvasive monitor was used in the operating room, and an intravenous line was secured. A 3–12 MHz linear transducer with an ultrasonic device (LOGIQ S7; GE Healthcare, Seoul, Republic of Korea) was used. All patients received an ultrasound-guided single-injection sciatic nerve block at the mid-thigh level on the lateral side, and a femoral nerve block in the inguinal area. The femoral and sciatic nerves were each injected with 15 mL of the solution under aseptic conditions.

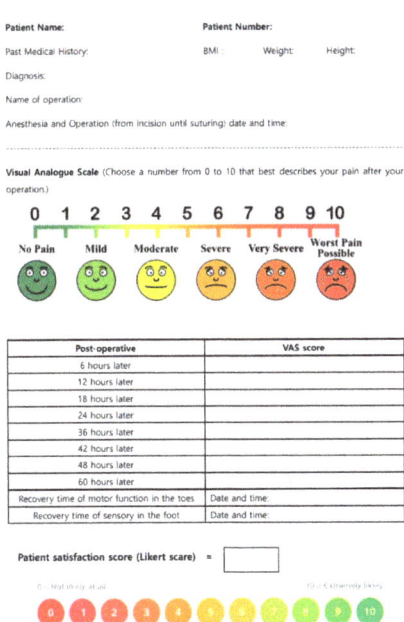

Figure 2. The questionnaires. Abbreviation: BMI; body mass index.

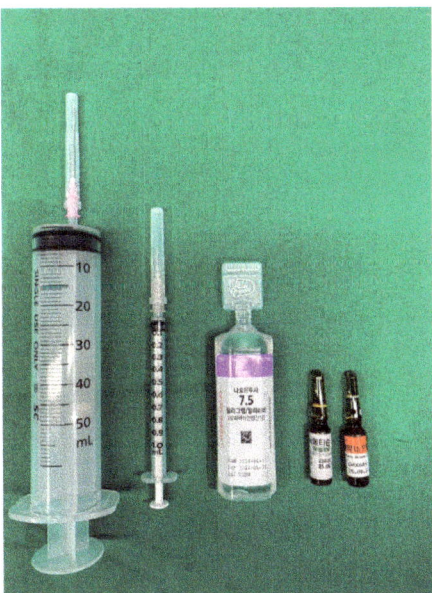

Figure 3. Preparations for peripheral nerve block: anesthetic drugs (ropivacaine) with dexamethasone, epinephrine, tools for mixing, and tools prepared for injection.

The patients were placed in a supine position, and a femoral nerve block was performed. A spinal needle was inserted via an in-plane approach while ultrasonographically visualizing the short axis of the femoral nerve at the inguinal level. Ultrasound visualization helped confirm the correct needle position. Following this, a negative aspiration was performed and 15 mL of local anesthesia was injected in fractionated doses over a minute. A sciatic nerve block was performed in the proximal 15 cm of the popliteal fossa before separating the tibial and peroneal nerves, while the patient was in a supine position with their knee flexed at 60 degrees. Local anesthesia injection around the sciatic nerve was performed with the same technique employed for the femoral nerve block (Figure 4).

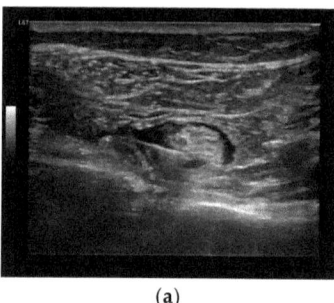 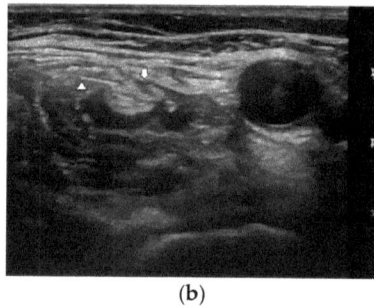

(a) (b)

Figure 4. Ultrasound images. (a) Anesthetic fluid is injected around the sciatic nerve epineurium, and the needle tip position is confirmed via ultrasound. (b) The appearance following injection around the femoral nerve. An image showing the injection of anesthetics near the femoral nerve (arrow) and the needle tip (arrowhead) position is confirmed via ultrasound.

After confirming the loss of a cold sensation in the ankle and lower leg, surgery was started. The same orthopedic team conducted all surgeries. At surgery commencement, patients complaining of mild pain in the medial malleolar area received 5 mL local injections of 1% lidocaine hydrochloride (20 mg/mL, Daihan Pharm. Co., Ltd., Seoul, Republic of Korea) for analgesia. A tourniquet was applied to the distal thigh in all patients. In some patients, thigh pain during the surgery was relieved by removing the tourniquet after a rubber bandage was wrapped around the proximal tibia. A scrub nurse recorded the operation start and end times.

2.4. Statistical Analyses

All statistical analyses were performed using SPSS software (v.24.0; IBM Corp., Armonk, NY, USA). VAS and satisfaction scores were compared between pain control methods using a Mann–Whitney U test. Sex and diagnoses were compared using a chi-square or Fisher's exact test. Operation time and motor and sensory function recovery times were compared between the groups using an independent t-test. Results are considered statistically significant at $p \leq 0.05$.

3. Results

All 60 enrolled patients completed the study. Patient characteristics were similar between the two groups. Group A included 20 men, and Group B comprised 19 men. The fracture types in both groups are shown in Table 1.

The anesthesia procedure and operation times were similar between the groups. It took an average of 14.4 and 13.4 min to perform the skin incision in groups A and B, respectively. The incision was delayed by approximately 5 min if there was insufficient anesthesia. In three group A and two group B patients, 1% lidocaine (5 mL) was locally injected into the surgical site at the start of the operation due to medial malleolar pain. The average time between the groups from anesthesia initiation to surgery completion was similar. After surgery, the surgeon confirmed that all patients' ankles and lower extremities were completely paralyzed. Analgesia duration and the time of recovery of motor function after surgery differed significantly between the groups. In group A, the analgesia time was an average of 11.6 h (8–14), and motor function recovery began at an average of 12.0 h (8–15.5). In group B, sensation was restored at 35.8 h (20–42), and movement at 35.6 h

(21–41) ($p < 0.001$). There were no complaints of pain in both groups at 6 h. In group A, sensation began to return before PCA was applied in some cases, at approximately 10 h, but no cases of severe pain were reported until the beginning of PCA. If additional pain control was required postoperatively, intravenous acetaminophen was administered. In group A, five patients received intravenous acetaminophen between 12 and 18 h, and one had an additional same dose injection. In group B, three patients received intravenous acetaminophen, two between 24 and 32 h and one between 32 and 40 h. Satisfaction scores (Likert scale) differed significantly between the groups (group A: 7.3; group B: 8.5; $p = 0.003$). Complications related to anesthesia or surgery were not reported in any group (Table 2).

Table 1. Patient demographic data ($n = 60$).

	Group A ($n = 30$)	Group B ($n = 30$)	p-Value
Age at surgery, years	35.5 ± 15.2 (19–70)	48 ± 14.9 (20–70)	0.002 *
Sex, male	20	19	0.787
BMI (kg/m^2)	24.2 ± 2.3	24.9 ± 2.4	0.234
Affected ankle, right	16	17	1.000
Fracture type			0.808
Unimalleolar	9	9	
Bimalleolar	12	9	
Trimalleolar	7	9	
Pilon	2	3	

Abbreviation: BMI, body mass index. * Significant difference ($p < 0.05$). The statistical analysis method is as follows. Age was analyzed using a Mann–Whitney test, sex with a chi-square test, BMI with an independent t-test, and fracture type Fisher's exact test.

Table 2. Anesthesia and surgical outcomes in both groups.

Case	Group A ($n = 30$)	Group B ($n = 30$)	p-Value
Operation time (min)	54.8 ± 16.7	51.4 ± 17.8	0.448
Time from anesthesia to start of surgery (min)	14.37 ± 4.20	13.40 ± 4.04	0.458
Additional injections (n)	5	3	0.704
Analgesia time (h)	11.6 ± 2.3	35.8 ± 8.3	<0.001 *
Motor block time (h)	12 ± 2.5	35.6 ± 7.0	<0.001 *
Likert scale	7.3 ± 1.8	8.5 ± 1.2	0.003 *

* Significant difference ($p < 0.05$). An independent t-test and Mann–Whitney test were used for analysis.

At 12, 18, 24, 40, 48, and 60 h after surgery, group B had significantly lower VAS pain scores ($p < 0.001$, <0.001, <0.001, 0.007, 0.001, 0.001, respectively); no significant difference was noted at 6 and 32 h ($p = 1.000$ and 0.082, respectively) (Figure 5, Table 3).

Table 3. Postoperative VAS pain score in both groups, stratified by treatment.

Postoperative Hour	VAS Pain Score		
	Group A	Group B	p-Value
6	0 ± 0	0 ± 0	1.000
12	3.2 ± 1.1	0 ± 0	<0.001 *
18	3.3 ± 0.9	0 ± 0	<0.001 *
24	4.4 ± 1	0.3 ± 1.0	<0.001 *

Table 3. Cont.

Postoperative Hour	VAS Pain Score		p-Value
	Group A	Group B	
32	3.4 ± 0.9	2.8 ± 1.6	0.082
40	3.5 ± 0.9	2.7 ± 1.5	0.007 *
48	3.2 ± 0.8	2.3 ± 1.2	0.001 *
60	2.6 ± 1.0	1.7 ± 0.8	0.001 *

Abbreviation: VAS, visual analog scale. * Significant difference ($p < 0.05$). A Mann–Whitney test was used for analysis.

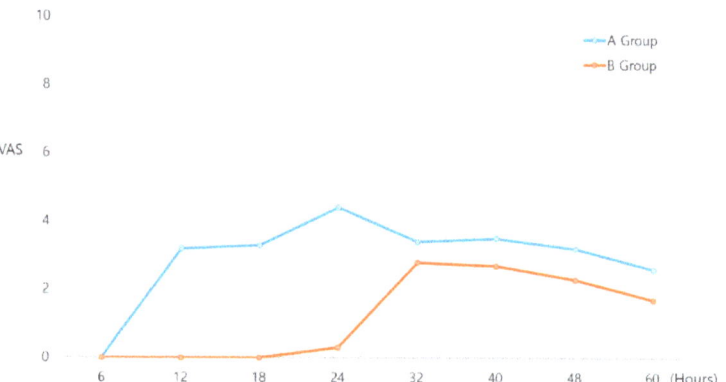

Figure 5. Postoperative visual analog scale (VAS) pain scores for both groups. VAS scores are significantly different between the two groups most of the time. After 32 h, similar patterns are observed between the two groups. Group A: patient-controlled analgesia after lower extremity peripheral nerve block; group B: dexamethasone/epinephrine combined with an anesthetic solution during peripheral nerve block.

4. Discussion

The combined use of ropivacaine with dexamethasone and epinephrine for PNB provided significantly prolonged and better analgesic effects than PCA after PNB anesthesia with ropivacaine alone. Moreover, patients who received dexamethasone and epinephrine experienced significantly less pain than the controls, even after the anesthetic effect had worn off. This finding may be related to the drug effect of dexamethasone or epinephrine, or a psychological effect related to delayed pain onset after anesthesia. Two patients in the dexamethasone and epinephrine group reported VAS pain scores of 0 throughout the investigation, even after recovering motor and sensory nerve function.

However, no significant difference was noted in VAS scores between the two groups at 32 h after surgery. In group A, patients complained of peak pain about 24 h after surgery, which gradually decreased. However, patients in group B complained of peak pain at around 32 h, when the effect of PNB disappeared; then, the pain level decreased further over time. Therefore, the pain difference between the two groups was considered to be the smallest at around 32 h. This finding is thought to be associated with some rebound pain, with complaints of high repulsive pain in some cases at the point at which the effects of PNB disappear [7].

In orthopedics, morphine, non-steroidal anti-inflammatory drugs (NSAIDs), and acetaminophen are common postoperative pain control medications, but they all have limitations. Patients may experience severe pain after surgery, but morphine often has side effects and can be fatal when overused [10]. NSAIDs and acetaminophen are safer than morphine, but oral administration is not ideal, given the possibility of hepatotoxicity and nephrotoxicity [11].

Ropivacaine is a long-acting amide local anesthetic. The major concern when using high doses of local anesthetic is systemic toxicity, which develops when the free serum concentration of ropivacaine exceeds the toxic threshold [12]. Ropivacaine is relatively long-acting and safe compared to other anesthetics, and is often used for PNBs.

There are conflicting reports on whether adding epinephrine to ropivacaine is effective. Most studies showing its effectiveness found that it reduced the risk of toxicity by slowing systemic absorption. However, the studies did not identify a significant effect on analgesic duration. Several researchers advocate the addition of epinephrine to large doses of local anesthetics to reduce the maximum plasma concentration [13]. Adding epinephrine to reduce the maximum plasma concentration induces local vasoconstriction at the injection site [14], thereby slowing absorption. Several studies have reported decreased Cmax and increased Tmax when adding epinephrine to ropivacaine for epidural [7], caudal [15], or regional [16] (thoracic paravertebral block) anesthesia. Conversely, for the perivascular subclavian block, Hickey et al. [17] found no effect on pharmacokinetics (Cmax, Tmax, or area under the curve) after adding epinephrine to ropivacaine.

The glucocorticoid, dexamethasone, appeared to be effective in one preclinical [18] and several clinical [4,19,20] studies. The mechanism by which dexamethasone prolongs regional anesthesia is debatable. As steroids induce vasoconstriction, one theory holds that the drug acts by reducing local anesthetic absorption [21]. A more plausible theory states that dexamethasone increases inhibitory potassium channel activity on nociceptive C-fibers (via glucocorticoid receptors), thereby decreasing their activity [22]. Most studies have reported that dexamethasone enhances the analgesic effect [4,6,23]; however, accurate dosage information is unavailable.

Given the conflicting reports of the pharmacokinetic effects of the addition of dexamethasone or epinephrine to PNBs [7,24–26], we investigated the results of adding a small amount of both drugs when performing PNBs with ropivacaine, with promising results.

During our study, we considered the possibility of anesthetic drug toxicity [13,27]. First, individuals with a low body mass index (<18.5 kg/m^2) and those with systemic diseases were excluded. Second, we were careful not to cause toxicity reactions while administering the drugs to the patients. The authors restricted the use of additional drugs other than those approved in this study for patients. Additionally, 1% lidocaine administered during the surgery was minimized to 5 mL because of the aforementioned problems.

As expected, pain scores remained significantly different, with a block duration at most time points. The total number of additional analgesic injections administered over the first 60 h differed significantly between the groups. No significant complications occurred in either group; no neurological symptoms were reported.

In cases in which sensation remained on the medial side after anesthesia induction, a part of the posterior division of the femoral nerve was not completely anesthetized [28]. Additionally, since only ropivacaine was used, the anesthesia onset time was longer than in cases wherein lidocaine was used [2,9]. In such cases, additional anesthesia with 1% lidocaine was required for the superficial layer. Considering the duration of the action of lidocaine, it did not contribute to the postoperative VAS scores in our study.

In our study, both sensation and movement returned gradually. In group A, sensation returned first, whereas in group B, movement returned first. The sensation was determined based on when patients reported starting to feel pain. However, because the pain increased gradually, patients had difficulty specifying the point at which sensation was restored, and recovery of movement was often only identified after the patient had started moving their foot to some extent, which can be difficult to measure and can produce inaccuracies. In addition, accurate measurements were difficult when sensation and movement were recovered late at night or while the patient was sleeping. In some cases, the exact time point could not be identified. Therefore, investigating the exact time of motor and sensory function recovery was difficult in this study.

Most patients with ankle fractures can be discharged immediately after surgery. Administration of dexamethasone and epinephrine with PNB may be useful in cases wherein patients with fractures require or want hospitalization. Moreover, when managing an ankle fracture, we thought this method could be beneficial for pain control at home after hospital discharge, even in non-hospitalized patients. However, delayed motor and sensory function recovery caused discomfort in some patients. The transfer process at discharge, motor and sensory function recovery progress after discharge, and related precautions should be sufficiently explained. Alternatively, a saphenous nerve block in the adductor canal, rather than a femoral block, can also reduce the above problems. An ankle block can be convenient and require little concern for patient safety in some cases.

In addition, postoperative sensory loss can cause problems in terms of detecting if or when compartment syndrome occurs. We must be aware of the possibility of postoperative compartment syndrome and prepare diagnostic methods, because the period without motor and sensory functions lasts very long after PNB.

Normal pressure within a compartment is less than 10 mmHg. An intra-compartmental pressure greater than 30 mmHg indicates acute compartment syndrome and the need for fasciotomy. However, a single normal intra-compartmental pressure reading does not exclude acute compartment syndrome. Intra-compartmental pressure should be monitored serially or continuously. Several methods can be used for monitoring. Before the 1960s, most measurements of intra-compartmental pressure used needles to inject saline. When intra-compartmental pressure increases to within 10 mmHg to 30 mmHg of the patient's diastolic blood pressure, it indicates inadequate perfusion and relative ischemia of the involved extremity. A Stryker Intra-Compartmental Pressure Monitor System (Stryker Orthopaedics, Mahwah, NJ, USA) has been used recently to evaluate compartment pressure. It is a portable monitor that uses a side port needle, a disposable syringe of saline flush, and a digital read-out manometer to allow for simple measurement of compartment pressure [29].

If there is even a slight suspicion of compartment syndrome after PNB, one should be ready to apply these methods. This may reduce the risk to some extent. However, according to research, even this can often be inaccurate and insufficient [30]. In conclusion, when compartment syndrome occurs after surgery with PNBs, it may be more difficult to diagnose than when surgery is performed with a usual anesthetic method. Therefore, anesthesia and pain control using a PNB should be applied to patients with a low risk of developing compartment syndrome, such as low-energy single and bimalleolar fractures. In patients with severe soft tissue damage or preoperative swelling, a PNB method should preferably be avoided.

It is important to note that complications may occur when applying PNB to patients and using anesthetic drugs. When high-dose local anesthetics are used, the main problem is systemic toxicity when the free ropivacaine serum concentration exceeds the threshold. However, when anesthetics are mixed with dexamethasone and epinephrine, they cause local vasoconstriction near the injection site, which slows the drug absorption, thus lowering the maximum plasma concentration of the free ropivacaine [14,21]. Thus, the combination of dexamethasone and epinephrine is considered to have a less adverse effect on systemic drug toxicity when using ropivacaine. However, one should always pay attention and be careful of the complications of drug interactions. In our study, no systemic toxicity or complications occurred. However, after using anesthetics mixed with dexamethasone during PNB in another clinical study [6], complaints of numbness and tingling sensations in the innervation area for two weeks were reported, although without statistical significance. Therefore, caution is required when using the drug, and anesthetics should be used after a detailed investigation of the patient's medical and drug history and systemic condition.

This study is considered a well-compared study, with no dropouts of patients and measurement errors. However, this study had limitations. First, our study only included a few patients. Second, we did not perform mid- to long-term observations; thus, longer-term complications and sequelae should be studied in larger study populations after using the combination of medicines. Further research is needed to determine whether this medication combination will be effective for other types of surgery, or if this combination can be applied to nerves in other body parts. In our study, we used ropivacaine with dexamethasone and epinephrine; hence, it was unknown which of the two drugs played a major role in sustaining the anesthetic effect. In addition, it was impossible to provide the dose of the drug combination appropriate for a single use of epinephrine or dexamethasone. Moreover, future comparative studies should determine the effect of adding only dexamethasone or epinephrine to ropivacaine, and the optimal concentration of these drugs for achieving the maximum effect while reducing side effects.

5. Conclusions

PNB is a useful anesthetic method for patients with an ankle fracture. The adjuvant use of dexamethasone and epinephrine as anesthetic agents had an excellent effect on pain control by extending the duration of the anesthetic effect. The anesthesia method described herein could be useful if surgery is selected after carefully considering the exclusion criteria.

Author Contributions: Conceptualization, C.K., J.-K.L. and G.-S.L.; methodology, K.-S.K., J.-K.L. and G.-S.L.; software, G.-S.L. and J.-H.S.; validation, C.K., G.-S.L. and S.-B.K.; formal analysis, G.-S.L. and S.-B.K.; investigation, G.-S.L.; resources, C.K., G.-S.L. and J.-K.L.; data curation, J.-H.S.; writing—original draft preparation, G.-S.L.; writing—review and editing, G.-S.L. and J.-K.L.; visualization, G.-S.L.; supervision, C.K. and S.-B.K. All authors have read and agreed to the published version of the manuscript.

Funding: This research received no external funding.

Institutional Review Board Statement: The study was conducted in accordance with the Declaration of Helsinki and approved by the Chungnam National University Sejong Hospital institutional review board (protocol code: CNUSH 2021-11-003, approved on 21 December 2021).

Informed Consent Statement: Informed consent was obtained from all subjects involved in the study.

Data Availability Statement: The data presented in this study are available on request from the corresponding author.

Acknowledgments: This work was supported by Chungnam National University.

Conflicts of Interest: The authors declare no conflict of interest.

References

1. Cremeans-Smith, J.K.; Contrera, K.; Speering, L.; Miller, E.T.; Pfefferle, K.; Greene, K.; Delahanty, D.L. Using established predictors of post-traumatic stress to explain variations in recovery outcomes among orthopedic patients. *J. Health Psychol.* **2015**, *20*, 1296–1304. [CrossRef] [PubMed]
2. Kang, C.; Lee, G.S.; Kim, S.B.; Won, Y.G.; Lee, J.K.; Jung, Y.S.; Cho, H.J. Comparison of postoperative pain control methods after bony surgery in the foot and ankle. *Foot Ankle Surg.* **2018**, *24*, 521–524. [CrossRef] [PubMed]
3. Mikjunovikj-Derebanova, L.; Kartalov, A.; Kuzmanovska, B.; Donev, L.; Lleshi, A.; Toleska, M.; Dimitrovski, A.; Demjanski, V. Epinephrine and dexamethasone as adjuvants in upper extremity peripheral nerve blocks in pediatric patients. *Prilozi* **2021**, *42*, 79–88. [CrossRef] [PubMed]
4. Aoyama, Y.; Sakura, S.; Abe, S.; Uchimura, E.; Saito, Y. Effects of the addition of dexamethasone on postoperative analgesia after anterior cruciate ligament reconstruction surgery under quadruple nerve blocks. *BMC Anesthesiol.* **2021**, *21*, 218. [CrossRef]
5. Weber, A.; Fournier, R.; Van Gessel, E.; Riand, N.; Gamulin, Z. Epinephrine does not prolong the analgesia of 20 mL ropivacaine 0.5% or 0.2% in a femoral three-in-one block. *Anesth. Analg.* **2001**, *93*, 1327–1331. [CrossRef]
6. De Oliveira, G.S.; Castro Alves, L.J.; Nader, A.; Kendall, M.C.; Rahangdale, R.; McCarthy, R.J. Perineural dexamethasone to improve postoperative analgesia with peripheral nerve blocks: A meta-analysis of randomized controlled trials. *Pain Res. Treat.* **2014**, *2014*, 179029. [CrossRef]
7. Lee, B.B.; Kee, W.D.N.; Plummer, J.L.; Karmakar, M.K.; Wong, A.S. The effect of the addition of epinephrine on early systemic absorption of epidural ropivacaine in humans. *Anesth. Analg.* **2002**, *95*, 1402–1407. [CrossRef]
8. World Health Organization; Interagency Oncology Task Force Fellowship/International Association for the Study of Obesity. *The Asia-Pacific Perspective: Redefining Obesity and Its Treatment*; World Health Organization: Geneva, Switzerland, 2000.

9. Lee, J.K.; Kang, C.; Hwang, D.S.; Lee, G.S.; Hwang, J.M.; Park, E.J.; Ga, I.H. An innovative pain control method using peripheral nerve block and patient-controlled analgesia with ketorolac after bone surgery in the ankle area: A prospective study. *J. Foot Ankle Surg.* **2020**, *59*, 698–703. [CrossRef]
10. Van, A.H.; Thys, L.; Veekman, L.; Buerkle, H. Assessing analgesia in single and repeated administrations of propacetamol for postoperative pain: Comparison with morphine after dental surgery. *Anesth. Analg.* **2004**, *98*, 159–165.
11. Gago, M.A.; Escontrela, R.B.; Planas, R.A.; Martínez, R.A. Intravenous ibuprofen for treatment of post-operative pain: A multicenter, double blind, placebo-controlled, randomized clinical trial. *PLoS ONE* **2016**, *11*, e0154004.
12. Bleckner, L.L.; Bina, S.; Kwon, K.H.; McKnight, G.; Dragovich, A.; Buckenmaier, C.C., III. Serum ropivacaine concentrations and systemic local anesthetic toxicity in trauma patients receiving long-term continuous peripheral nerve block catheters. *Anesth. Analg.* **2010**, *110*, 630–634. [CrossRef] [PubMed]
13. Rosenberg, P.H.; Veering, B.T.; Urmey, W.F. Maximum recommended doses of local anesthetics: A multifactorial concept. *Reg. Anesth. Pain Med.* **2004**, *29*, 564–575. [CrossRef]
14. Bernards, C.M.; Kopacz, D.J. Effect of epinephrine on lidocaine clearance in vivo: A microdialysis study in humans. *Anesthesiology* **1999**, *91*, 962–968. [CrossRef]
15. Van Obbergh, L.J.; Roelants, F.A.; Veyckemans, F.; Verbeeck, R.K. In children, the addition of epinephrine modifies the pharmacokinetics of ropivacaine injected caudally. *Can. J. Anaesth.* **2003**, *50*, 593–598. [CrossRef]
16. Karmakar, M.K.; Ho, A.M.; Law, B.K.; Wong, A.S.; Shafer, S.L.; Gin, T. Arterial and venous pharmacokinetics of ropivacaine with and without epinephrine after thoracic paravertebral block. *Anesthesiology* **2005**, *103*, 704–711. [CrossRef] [PubMed]
17. Hickey, R.; Blanchard, J.; Hoffman, J.; Sjovall, J.; Ramamurthy, S. Plasma concentrations of ropivacaine given with or without epinephrine for brachial plexus block. *Can. J. Anaesth.* **1990**, *37*, 878–882. [CrossRef] [PubMed]
18. Colombo, G.; Padera, R.; Langer, R.; Kohane, D.S. Prolonged duration local anesthesia with lipid–protein–sugar particles containing bupivacaine and dexamethasone. *J. Biomed. Mater. Res. A* **2005**, *75*, 458–464. [CrossRef]
19. Movafegh, A.; Razazian, M.; Hajimaohamadi, F.; Meysamie, A. Dexamethasone added to lidocaine prolongs axillary brachial plexus blockade. *Anesth. Analg.* **2006**, *102*, 263–267. [CrossRef]
20. Vieira, P.A.; Pulai, I.; Tsao, G.C.; Manikantan, P.; Keller, B.; Connelly, N.R. Dexamethasone with bupivacaine increases duration of analgesia in ultrasound-guided interscalene brachial plexus blockade. *Eur. J. Anaesthesiol.* **2010**, *27*, 285–288. [CrossRef]
21. Marks, R.; Barlow, J.; Funder, J. Steroid-induced vasoconstriction: Glucocorticoid antagonist studies. *J. Clin. Endocrinol. Metab.* **1982**, *54*, 1075–1077. [CrossRef]
22. Kopacz, D.J.; Lacouture, P.G.; Wu, D.; Nandy, P.; Swanton, R.; Landau, C. The dose response and effects of dexamethasone on bupivacaine microcapsules for intercostal blockade (T9 to T11) in healthy volunteers. *Anesth. Analg.* **2003**, *96*, 576–582. [CrossRef]
23. Cummings, K.C., III; Napierkowski, D.; Parra-Sanchez, I.; Kurz, A.; Dalton, J.E.; Brems, J.J.; Sessler, D.I. Effect of dexamethasone on the duration of interscalene nerve blocks with ropivacaine or bupivacaine. *Br. J. Anaesth.* **2011**, *107*, 446–453. [CrossRef]
24. Albrecht, E.; Reynvoet, M.; Fournier, N.; Desmet, M. Dose–response relationship of perineural dexamethasone for interscalene brachial plexus block: A randomised, controlled, triple-blind trial. *Anaesthesia* **2019**, *74*, 1001–1008. [CrossRef]
25. Parrington, S.J.; O'Donnell, D.; Chan, V.W.; Brown-Shreves, D.; Subramanyam, R.; Qu, M.; Brull, R. Dexamethasone added to mepivacaine prolongs the duration of analgesia after supraclavicular brachial plexus blockade. *Reg. Anesth. Pain Med.* **2010**, *35*, 422–426. [CrossRef]
26. Schoenmakers, K.P.; Vree, T.B.; Jack, N.T.; van den Bemt, B.; van Limbeek, J.; Stienstra, R. Pharmacokinetics of 450 mg ropivacaine with and without epinephrine for combined femoral and sciatic nerve block in lower extremity surgery. A pilot study. *Br. J. Clin. Phamacol.* **2013**, *75*, 1321–1327. [CrossRef] [PubMed]
27. Kuthiala, G.; Chaudhary, G. Ropivacaine: A review of its pharmacology and clinical use. *Indian J. Anaesth.* **2011**, *55*, 104. [CrossRef]
28. Short, A.J.; Barnett, J.J.G.; Gofeld, M.; Baig, E.; Lam, K.; Agur, A.M.R.; Peng, P.W.H. Anatomic study of innervation of the anterior hip capsule: Implication for image-guided intervention. *Reg. Anesth. Pain Med.* **2018**, *43*, 186–192. [CrossRef] [PubMed]
29. Torlincasi, A.M.; Lopez, R.A.; Waseem, M. Acute Compartment Syndrome. In *StatPearls*; StatPearls Publishing: Treasure Island, FL, USA, 2022.
30. Morris, M.R.; Harper, B.L.; Hetzel, S.; Shaheen, M.; Davis, A.; Nemeth, B.; Halanski, M.A. The effect of focused instruction on orthopaedic surgery residents' ability to objectively measure intracompartmental pressures in a compartment syndrome model. *J. Bone Joint Surg. Am.* **2014**, *96*, e171. [CrossRef] [PubMed]

Disclaimer/Publisher's Note: The statements, opinions and data contained in all publications are solely those of the individual author(s) and contributor(s) and not of MDPI and/or the editor(s). MDPI and/or the editor(s) disclaim responsibility for any injury to people or property resulting from any ideas, methods, instructions or products referred to in the content.

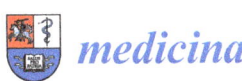

Case Report

Isolated Avulsion Fracture of the Tibial Tuberosity in an Adult Treated with Suture-Bridge Fixation: A Rare Case and Literature Review

Dong Hwan Lee [1], Hwa Sung Lee [1], Chae-Gwan Kong [2] and Se-Won Lee [1,*]

[1] Department of Orthopedic Surgery, Yeouido St. Mary's Hospital, College of Medicine, The Catholic University of Korea, 10, 63-Ro, Seoul 07345, Republic of Korea; ldh850606@naver.com (D.H.L.)
[2] Department of Orthopaedic Surgery, Uijeongbu St. Mary's Hospital, College of Medicine, The Catholic University of Korea, 271, Cheonbo-Ro, Uijeongbu-si 11765, Republic of Korea
* Correspondence: ssewon@naver.com or ssewon@gmail.com; Tel.: +82-2-3779-1068; Fax: +82-2-783-0252

Abstract: *Background and objectives*: Isolated tibial tuberosity avulsion fractures are exceptionally uncommon among adults, with limited instances documented in published literature. Here, we describe a case of an isolated tibial tuberosity avulsion fracture in an adult that was treated successfully with the suture bridge repair technique. *Patient concerns*: A 65-year-old female visited the outpatient department with left knee pain after a slip and fall. Lateral radiographs and sagittal MR images of the left knee revealed the tibial tuberosity avulsion fracture, but the fracture line did not extend into the knee joint space. Surgical intervention was performed on the patient's knee using an anterior midline approach, involving open reduction and internal fixation. The avulsed tendon was grasped and pulled, and an appropriate suture location was identified. Using a suture hook, the suture was guided through the patellar tendon as near to its uppermost point of the fragment as achievable, and tied over tendon. A single suture limb from each anchor was fastened over the tibial tuberosity to the distally positioned foot print anchor, effectively anchoring the tibial tuberosity using the suture bridge technique. The patient started walking on crutches after one week and was able to walk independently with a brace after two weeks from the operation day. After three months, the patient had regained her mobility to the level prior to the injury and exhibited painless active range of motion from 0 to 130 degrees. Hardware positioning and bony union were maintained at the one-year follow-up. *Conclusions*: In our case, the open suture bridge fixation method for tibial tuberosity avulsion fractures produced satisfactory results. Open suture bridge fixation may be considered for isolated tibial tuberosity avulsion fractures in adults, especially when the avulsion tip is too small for screw fixation.

Keywords: tibial tuberosity; avulsion fracture; suture bridge fixation; surgical technique

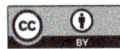

1. Introduction

Though they comprise less than 3% of all physical injuries in children, tibial tuberosity avulsion fractures are exceptionally uncommon among adults, with limited instances documented in published literature [1–7]. Tibial tuberosity fractures are mainly treated by two methods: using lag screws to secure the main fragment from anterior to posterior direction and tension band wiring with cerclage wires at the patella tendon insertion site on the tibial tuberosity [8]. The suture bridge fixation technique was first introduced as an effective method for repairing rotator cuff tears. By promoting a broad contact surface, healing is improved and results in stronger fixation. Its application has subsequently expanded to the greater tuberosity avulsion fractures of the humerus [9]. Moreover, the employment of the suture bridge repair technique for surgical intervention in Achilles insertional tendinopathy is widely recognized [10,11], and a suture bridge fixation approach has also been introduced for Achilles tendon avulsion fractures of the calcaneus [12].

Additionally, a similar approach has been employed in cases involving the triceps insertion at the elbow [13]. Thus, the suture bridge repair technique for avulsions at large tendon insertion sites across the body appears to be considered an effective therapeutic approach.

However, to the best of our knowledge, this technique has yet to be adopted for treatment of tibial tuberosity avulsion fractures in adults. Here, we describe a case report in which the suture bridge technique was adopted to repair an isolated tibial tuberosity avulsion fracture in an adult. Additionally, a literature review of previously reported cases of tibial tuberosity avulsion fracture was conducted to emphasize the advantages of fixation using the suture bridge technique. Furthermore, the rehabilitation protocols outlined in the existing reports were reviewed and compared to our approach.

2. Case Presentation

A 65-year-old female visited the outpatient department with left knee pain after a slip and fall. The patient had a past history of surgery with tension band wiring for a left (ipsilateral side) displaced patellar fracture one year prior. The hardware had been removed six months before the present injury. The patient's plain radiography of the left knee exhibited osteoporotic bone quality in the patella, distal femur, and proximal tibia, which is presumed to be a result of previous trauma and two prior surgeries. She had difficulty in performing active knee extension and complete leg straightening. Lateral radiographs and sagittal MR images of the left knee revealed the tibial tuberosity avulsion fracture, but the fracture line did not extend into the knee joint space (Figure 1).

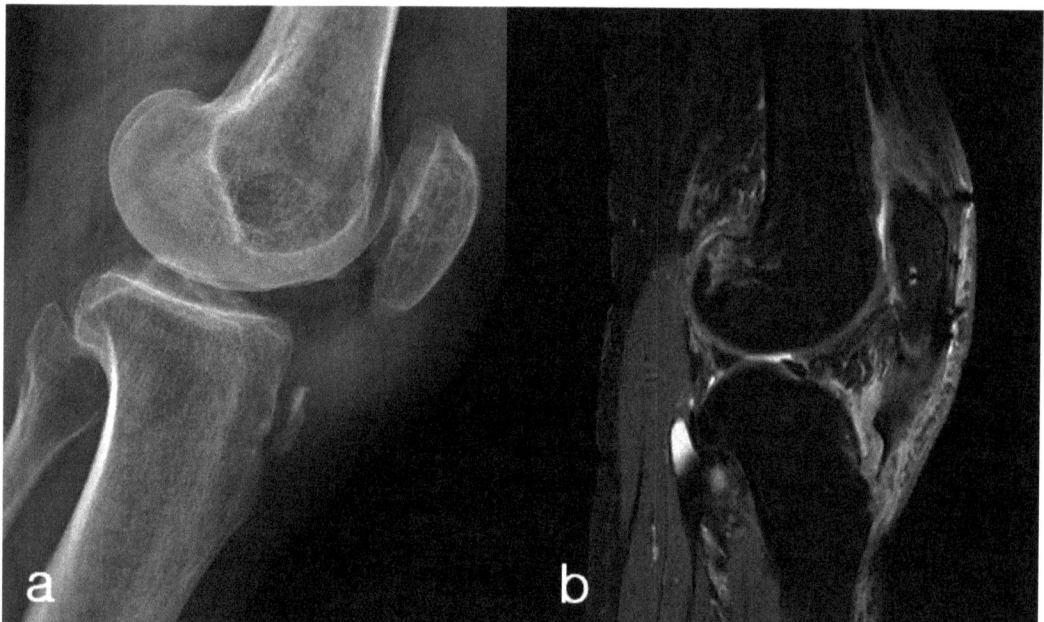

Figure 1. Lateral radiograph (**a**) and sagittal MR image (**b**) of the left knee, revealing the tibial tuberosity avulsion fracture, but the fracture line does not extend into the knee joint space. Plain radiography exhibited osteoporotic bone quality in the patella, distal femur, and proximal tibia, which is presumed to be a result of previous trauma and two prior surgeries.

Surgical intervention was performed on the patient's knee using an anterior midline approach, involving open reduction and internal fixation. The avulsed tendon was grasped and pulled, and an appropriate suture location was identified. In the knee-full-extension state, No. 2 Ethibond sutures were applied for temporary traction while two metal suture anchors (5.5 mm TwinFix; Smith & Nephew, Andover, MA, USA) were inserted 15 mm from each other. A temporary K-wire was inserted under the image intensifier for fixation of the fragment in its anatomical position. Using a suture hook, the suture was guided through the patellar tendon as near to its uppermost point of the fragment as achievable and tied over tendon. After that, a single suture limb from each anchor was fastened over the tibial tuberosity to the distally positioned 5.5-mm Footprint anchors (Smith and Nephew, Andover, MA, USA), effectively anchoring the tibial tuberosity using the suture bridge technique (Figures 2 and 3). To achieve firm fixation, maintaining proper tension during the crossing of suture limbs and fixation is crucial, along with the placement of the anchors. The temporary K-wire and traction sutures were subsequently removed. Postoperatively, the patient was placed in a functional brace that limited up to 90 degree flexion for four weeks.

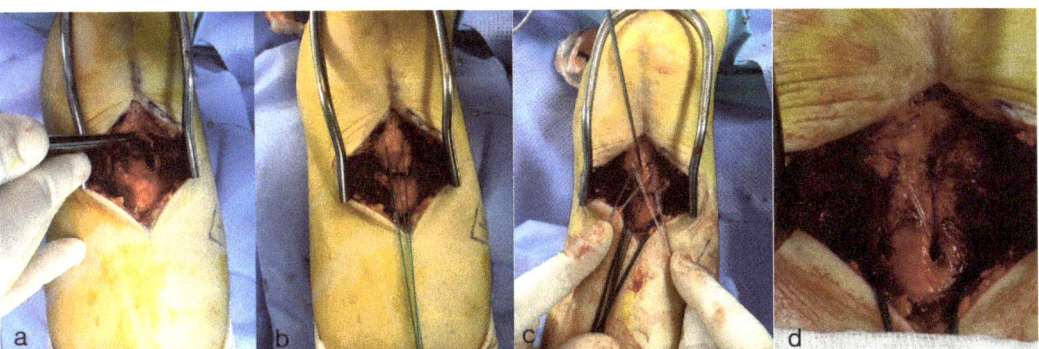

Figure 2. Intra-operative images. (**a**) Image depicts a tibial tuberosity avulsion fracture, as indicated by the forceps holding the avulsed fragment. (**b**) The avulsed tendon was grasped and pulled using No. 2 Ethibond suture, and an appropriate suture anchor location was identified. (**c**) Image shows the fixation method using the suture bridge technique. A single suture limb from each anchor was secured over the tibial tuberosity and fastened to the distally positioned footprint anchors. (**d**) A well-reduced state was observed with the suture bridge repair technique.

The patient initiated passive range of motion (ROM) exercises one day after surgery. The range of motion was gradually increased, with a restriction of up to 90 degrees for the first 4 weeks. The patient was permitted to bear weight according to their comfort level. She started walking on crutches after one week from the operation day and was able to walk independently with a brace after two weeks. Until the sixth week, only ambulation on level ground was allowed, and, after 6 weeks, the patient started ambulation with active stretching, including stair climbing. After three months, the patient had regained her mobility to the level prior to the injury and exhibited painless active range of motion from 0 to 130 degrees (Figure 4). On the 12-month postoperative X-ray, the position of the metal anchor remained unchanged, and the fracture fragment was well-maintained without any displacement and had successfully achieved union (Figure 5).

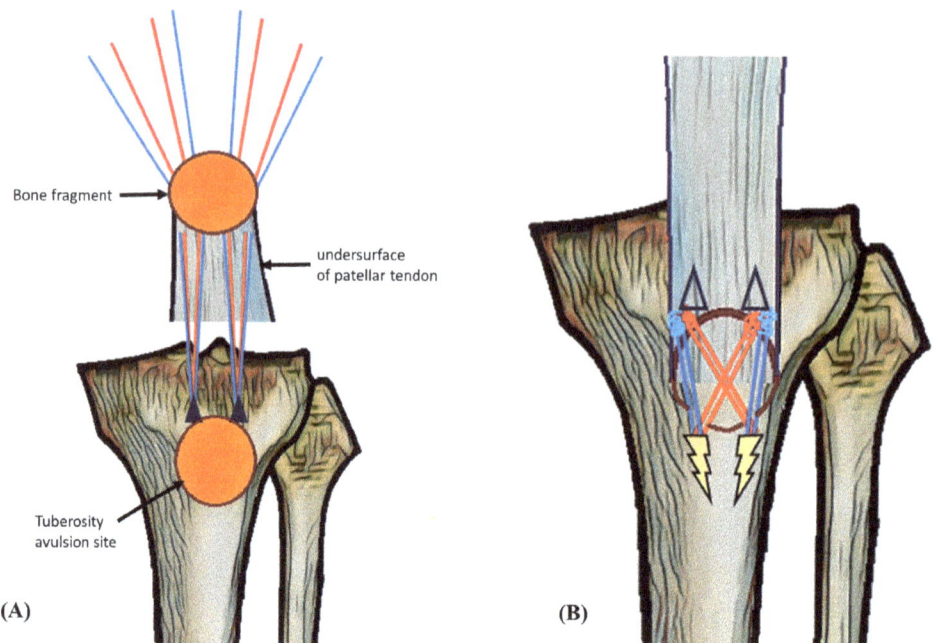

Figure 3. Schematic image of surgical techniques. (**A**) An image viewed from the undersurface of the patellar tendon showing the passage of the suture. Two orange circles indicate the fracture surfaces. Two navy blue triangles indicate the position of the 5.5 mm metal anchors. The red and blue lines indicate the sutures that are attached to the anchors. (**B**) An image depicting the appearance after suture bridge fixation. Two yellow markers indicate the positions of the 5.5 mm footprint anchors. The image shows the crossing of suture limbs from each anchor to secure the avulsed tibial tuberosity fragment using the distally positioned footprint anchor. To achieve firm fixation, maintaining proper tension during the crossing of suture limbs and fixation is crucial, along with the placement of the anchors.

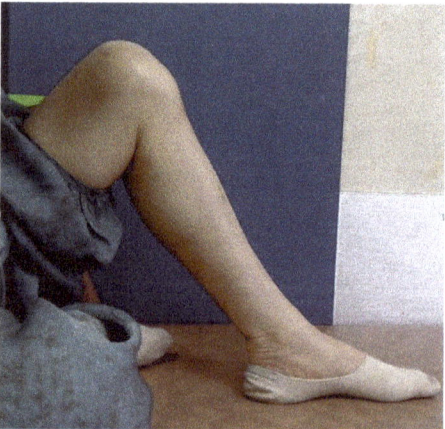

Figure 4. Clinical image of the patient's lower extremity with recovery of range of motion at three months after the operation.

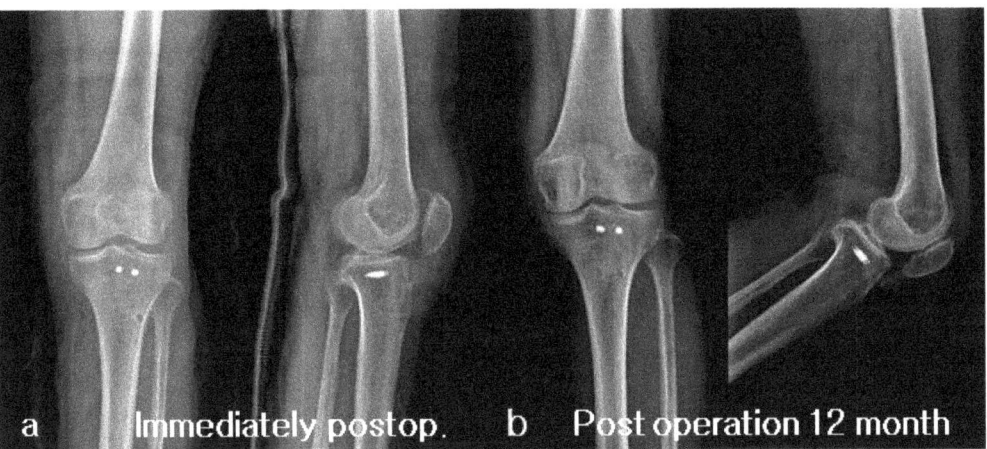

Figure 5. Post-operative X-rays. (**a**) Immediate postoperative X-rays show that the avulsed tibial tuberosity fragment has been successfully reduced to its anatomical position. (**b**) 12-month postoperative X-rays show that the fracture fragment is well-maintained without any displacement and has successfully achieved union.

3. Discussion

Isolated tibial tuberosity avulsion fractures are exceptionally uncommon among adults. Only six previous case were documented in the published literature [1–3,5–7]. In adolescents, they are a kind of growth plate injury and make up less than 3% of all such injuries [14–17]. They are believed to occur due to sudden quadriceps contraction against knees that are partially flexed, like during the landing after a fall or jump [4,18,19].

The closing growth plate during adolescence is vulnerable to pulling forces and can be easily avulsed [20]. In adults, the exact cause is not clear. In general cases, sudden contraction of the quadriceps muscle may result in injury to weaker structures such as the quadriceps or patellar tendons. However, in patients with osteoporotic bone quality, it appears that the bone in the tibial tuberosity becomes weak, leading to fractures in that area [3]. Moreover, even in cases of good bone quality, tibial tuberosity fractures can occur with high energy traumas, such as falling from a height. Another possibility is to consider that avulsion fractures can occur due to direct trauma towards the tibial tuberosity. In the previous six documented cases in adults, one fell from a ladder, and two suffered direct injuries to the tibial tuberosity. The other three cases involved relatively low-energy traumas, specifically fall and twisting injuries. Among them, two cases were observed in super-elderly patients, while the remaining case was associated with Paget's disease, indicating that all cases occurred in osteoporotic bone (Table 1). In our case, avulsion of the tibial tuberosity is theorized to have occurred due to forceful full flexion of the knee, prompted by patellar baja caused by the previously healed patellar fracture. We believe that this is a rare complication that can occur at the end stage of full flexion in patellar fractures in adults and was not previously reported.

Various techniques for surgically treating avulsion fractures of the tibial tuberosity have been reported for individuals across all age groups. The AO Foundation suggests two techniques for fixation of tibial tuberosity fractures [8]. One technique uses lag screws to secure the main fragment from anterior to posterior direction [20]. The other method utilizes tension band wiring with cerclage wires inserted through the Sharpey's fibers at the patellar tendon insertion site on the tibial tuberosity [3]. In our case, the main fragment was too small for either screw fixation or tension band wiring. Therefore, we considered the use of suture anchors for fixation and decided to perform the suture bridge technique, which we deemed more suitable for fixation of an avulsed fragment.

Table 1. Review of reported isolated tibial tuberosity avulsion fractures.

	Age (Years)	Injury Mechanism	Fixation Method	Remarks
Mounasamy et al. [5]	49	Fall from ladder	Plate and screws	Immobilized in a knee brace for three weeks
Pires et al [6].	62	Direct injury	Lag screw	Immobilized with a long brace for six weeks
Choi et al. [2]	67	Direct injury	Two suture anchor and fiber-tape	Functional brace for four weeks; 0 to 30° at first week, 0 to 120° at four weeks
Brown et al. [1]	86	Fall with twist	Screw and spike	Second fall caused implant loosening.
			Tendon repair using suture anchor at the second surgery.	Immobilized with a cylindrical cast for four weeks and changed to a genu brace.
K AJ et al. [3]	88	Fall with twist	Lag screw and tension band wiring	Immobilized with an extension splint for six weeks and tolerable weight bearing.
Raad et al. [7]	54	Fall with twist	Lag screw and tension band wiring	Underlying Paget's disease. Immobilized with a cast for six weeks and non-weight bearing. Changed to functional brace with progressive weight-bearing until 12 weeks.

In the majority of previously reported cases, patients were advised to restrict weight-bearing for an extended period after the surgery. Furthermore, in the majority of cases, the initiation of knee range-of-motion exercises was delayed, and the duration of immobilization was extended. Among the six reported cases, in four of them, immobilization was maintained using a cast or brace for approximately 4–6 weeks. In older patients, like ours, this could lead to decreased physical fitness and atrophy of the quadriceps muscles. Furthermore, these older patients often have a weaker motivation for rehabilitation and may find it challenging to endure a painful rehabilitation process. Therefore, if immobilization is prolonged, there is a higher risk of developing knee stiffness. The potential advantages of using suture bridge fixation are early rehabilitation and weight-bearing. It took one week for our patient to start walking on crutches and two weeks to walk by herself with a brace applied on the affected knee. She regained her mobility to the level prior to the injury and exhibited painless active range of motion from 0 to 130 degrees at 12 months after surgery. Among the previously reported cases, Choi et al. utilized suture anchors and employed a different fixation approach from ours for treatment [2].

They reported applying a functional brace immediately after surgery, allowing 0–30° of motion in the first week, and gradually increasing the range of motion through rehabilitation. By the fourth week, they were able to achieve a knee motion of 0–120°. Considering our case alongside theirs, the use of suture anchors for fixation appears to provide sufficient fixation power to enable early ambulation and range-of-motion exercises without problems. However, even when utilizing alternative methods, such as screws, plates, or tension band wiring, if a sufficiently secure fixation can be achieved, early ambulation and range-of-motion exercises can be performed without any difficulties or issues. Regarding ambulation, we believe that weight bearing itself does not pose a problem for the fracture recovery, as long as early activities involving active stretching, such as climbing stairs or steep inclines, are avoided. Therefore, in cases where the fracture fragment is large, using plates, screws, or tension band wiring for surgery, it is recommended to ensure firm fixation during the surgery and initiate early rehabilitation after the procedure.

Another advantage of using the suture bridge technique for repair is its usefulness in stabilizing small bone fragments. In addition, the advantage of our proposed procedure is that there is no need for additional surgery to remove any inserted instrument. Although the removal of instruments is not a major surgery, it can provide a great advantage in terms of relieving patients from the burden of surgery. Given these advantages, the suture bridge technique could become a valuable option for surgical management of tibial tuberosity avulsion fractures in adults, especially when the avulsion tip is too small for screw fixation.

4. Conclusions

In our case, the open suture bridge fixation method for tibial tuberosity avulsion fractures produced satisfactory results. Open suture bridge fixation may be considered for isolated tibial tuberosity avulsion fractures in adults, especially when the avulsion tip is too small for screw fixation. After surgery, early ambulation and early range-of-motion exercises are possible and recommended. Through early rehabilitation exercise, optimal therapeutic outcomes can be achieved.

Author Contributions: D.H.L., H.S.L. and C.-G.K. prepared the figures and collected the data. S.-W.L. performed the surgery. D.H.L. and S.-W.L. wrote the manuscript. All authors have read and agreed to the published version of the manuscript.

Funding: Authors received research funding from IL-YANG Pharm. Co., Ltd. for the conduct of the present work.

Institutional Review Board Statement: All of the consent procedures and details were approved by the Institutional Review Board of our hospital.

Informed Consent Statement: Informed consent was obtained from all subjects involved in the study.

Data Availability Statement: All data concerning the case are presented in the manuscript.

Conflicts of Interest: The authors declare no conflict of interest.

Abbreviations

MR   magnetic resonance

References

1. Liu, Y.-P.; Hao, Q.-H.; Lin, F.; Wang, M.-M.; Hao, Y.-D. Tibial Tuberosity Avulsion Fracture and Open Proximal Tibial Fracture in an Adult: A Case Report and Literature Review. *Medicine* **2015**, *94*, e1684. [CrossRef] [PubMed]
2. Pires e Albuquerque, R.; Campos, A.S.; de Araújo, G.C.; Gameiro, V.S. Fracture of tibial tuberosity in an adult. *BMJ Case Rep.* **2013**, *2013*, bcr2013202411. [CrossRef] [PubMed]
3. Colton, C.; Krikler, S.; Schatzker, J.; Trafton, P. *AO Surgery Reference*; AO Foundation: Graubünden, Switzerland, 2012.
4. Greenhagen, R.M.; Shinabarger, A.B.; Pearson, K.T.; Burns, P.R. Intermediate and long-term outcomes of the suture bridge technique for the management of insertional Achilles tendinopathy. *Foot Ankle Spec.* **2013**, *6*, 185–190. [CrossRef] [PubMed]
5. Furuhata, R.; Kamata, Y.; Kono, A.; Nishimura, T.; Otani, S.; Morioka, H. Surgical Repair Using Suture Bridge Technique for Triceps Tendon Avulsion. *Case Rep. Orthop.* **2021**, *2021*, 5572126. [CrossRef] [PubMed]
6. Mirbey, J.; Besancenot, J.; Chambers, R.T.; Durey, A.; Vichard, P. Avulsion fractures of the tibial tuberosity in the adolescent athlete. Risk factors, mechanism of injury, and treatment. *Am. J. Sports Med.* **1988**, *16*, 336–340. [CrossRef] [PubMed]
7. Ogden, J.A.; Tross, R.B.; Murphy, M.J. Fractures of the tibial tuberosity in adolescents. *J. Bone Jt. Surg. Am.* **1980**, *62*, 205–215. [CrossRef]
8. Choi, Y.H.; Park, D. A novel technique of tibial tuberosity fracture fixation with two knotless suture anchors in an adult: A case report and literature review. *Acta Orthop. Traumatol. Turc.* **2022**, *56*, 416–420. [CrossRef] [PubMed]
9. Kim, K.-C.; Rhee, K.-J.; Shin, H.-D.; Kim, Y.-M. Arthroscopic fixation for displaced greater tuberosity fracture using the suture-bridge technique. *Arthrosc. J. Arthrosc. Relat. Surg.* **2008**, *24*, 120.e121–120.e123. [CrossRef] [PubMed]
10. Raad, M.; Ndlovu, S.; Høgsand, T.; Ahmed, S.; Norris, M. Fracture of tibial tuberosity in an adult with Paget's disease of the bone—An interesting case and review of literature. *Trauma Case Rep.* **2021**, *32*, 100440. [CrossRef] [PubMed]
11. Levi, J.H.; Coleman, C.R. Fracture of the tibial tubercle. *Am. J. Sports Med.* **1976**, *4*, 254–263. [CrossRef] [PubMed]
12. Mounasamy, V.; Brown, T.E. Avulsion fracture of the tibial tuberosity with articular extension in an adult: A novel method of fixation. *Eur. J. Orthop. Surg. Traumatol.* **2008**, *18*, 157–159. [CrossRef]
13. Brown, E.; Sohail, M.T.; West, J.; Davies, B.; Mamarelis, G.; Sohail, M.Z. Tibial Tuberosity Fracture in an Elderly Gentleman: An Unusual Injury Pattern. *Case Rep. Orthop.* **2020**, *2020*, 8650927. [CrossRef] [PubMed]
14. K AJ, L.P. Avulsion Fracture of the Tibial Tubercle in an Adult Treated with Tension-Band Wiring: A Case Report. *Internet J. Orthop. Surg.* **2009**, *18*, 2–5.
15. Cho, B.-K.; Park, J.-K.; Choi, S.-M. Reattachment using the suture bridge augmentation for Achilles tendon avulsion fracture with osteoporotic bony fragment. *Foot* **2017**, *31*, 35–39. [CrossRef] [PubMed]

16. Georgiou, G.; Dimitrakopoulou, A.; Siapkara, A.; Kazakos, K.; Provelengios, S.; Dounis, E. Simultaneous bilateral tibial tubercle avulsion fracture in an adolescent: A case report and review of the literature. *Knee Surg. Sports Traumatol. Arthrosc. Off. J. ESSKA* **2007**, *15*, 147–149. [CrossRef]
17. Nimityongskul, P.; Montague, W.L.; Anderson, L.D. Avulsion fracture of the tibial tuberosity in late adolescence. *J. Trauma* **1988**, *28*, 505–509. [CrossRef] [PubMed]
18. Rigby, R.B.; Cottom, J.M.; Vora, A. Early weightbearing using Achilles suture bridge technique for insertional Achilles tendinosis: A review of 43 patients. *J. Foot Ankle Surg.* **2013**, *52*, 575–579. [CrossRef] [PubMed]
19. Silva Júnior, A.T.D.; Silva, L.J.D.; Silva Filho, U.C.D.; Teixeira, E.M.; Araújo, H.R.S.; Moraes, F.B.d. Anterior avulsion fracture of the tibial tuberosity in adolescents—Two case reports. *Rev. Bras. Ortop.* **2016**, *51*, 610–613. [CrossRef] [PubMed]
20. Slobogean, G.P.; Mulpuri, K.; Alvarez, C.M.; Reilly, C.W. Comminuted simultaneous bilateral tibial tubercle avulsion fractures: A case report. *J. Orthop. Surg.* **2006**, *14*, 319–321. [CrossRef] [PubMed]

Disclaimer/Publisher's Note: The statements, opinions and data contained in all publications are solely those of the individual author(s) and contributor(s) and not of MDPI and/or the editor(s). MDPI and/or the editor(s) disclaim responsibility for any injury to people or property resulting from any ideas, methods, instructions or products referred to in the content.

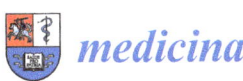

Article

COVID-19 Infection Was Associated with the Functional Outcomes of Hip Fracture among Older Adults during the COVID-19 Pandemic Apex

Hua-Yong Tay [1,2], Wen-Tien Wu [1,3], Cheng-Huan Peng [1], Kuan-Lin Liu [1,3], Tzai-Chiu Yu [1], Ing-Ho Chen [1,3], Ting-Kuo Yao [1], Chia-Ming Chang [1], Jian-Yuan Chua [1], Jen-Hung Wang [4] and Kuang-Ting Yeh [1,2,3,5,*]

1. Department of Orthopedics, Hualien Tzu Chi Hospital, Buddhist Tzu Chi Medical Foundation, Hualien 97002, Taiwan; nonametay@gmail.com (H.-Y.T.); timwu@tzuchi.com.tw (W.-T.W.); peng0913@tzuchi.com.tw (C.-H.P.); knlnliu@tzuchi.com.tw (K.-L.L.); feyu@tzuchi.com.tw (T.-C.Y.); ihchen@tzuchi.com.tw (I.-H.C.); tkyao0318@me.com (T.-K.Y.); newfresheric@gmail.com (C.-M.C.); chua.jian.yuan@hotmail.com (J.-Y.C.)
2. Department of Medical Education, Hualien Tzu Chi Hospital, Buddhist Tzu Chi Medical Foundation, Hualien 97002, Taiwan
3. School of Medicine, Tzu Chi University, Hualien 970374, Taiwan
4. Department of Medical Research, Hualien Tzu Chi Hospital, Buddhist Tzu Chi Medical Foundation, Hualien 97002, Taiwan; paulwang@tzuchi.com.tw
5. Graduate Institute of Clinical Pharmacy, Tzu Chi University, Hualien 970374, Taiwan
* Correspondence: micrograft@tzuchi.com.tw

Abstract: *Background and Objectives*: Hip fractures are associated with mortality and poor functional outcomes. The COVID-19 pandemic has affected patterns of care and health outcomes among fracture patients. This study aimed to determine the influence of COVID-19 infection on hip fracture recovery. *Materials and Methods*: We prospectively collected data on patients with hip fractures who presented at Hualien Tzu Chi Hospital between 9 March 2022 and 9 September 2022. The data included demographic information and functional scores taken before, during, and after surgery. The patients were divided into two groups: COVID-19 (+) and COVID-19 (−). *Results*: This study recruited 85 patients, 12 of whom (14.12%) were COVID-19 (+). No significant differences in preoperative or perioperative parameters between the two groups were observed. The postoperative Barthel index score was significantly impacted by COVID-19 infection ($p = 0.001$). The incidence of postoperative complications was significantly correlated with general anesthesia ($p = 0.026$) and the length of stay ($p = 0.004$) in hospital. Poor postoperative functional scores were associated with lower preoperative Barthel index scores ($p < 0.001$). Male sex ($p = 0.049$), old age ($p = 0.012$), a high American Society of Anesthesiologists grade ($p = 0.029$), and a high Charlson comorbidity index score ($p = 0.028$) were associated with mortality. *Conclusions*: Hip fracture surgeries were not unduly delayed in our hospital during the COVID-19 pandemic, but the patients' postoperative Barthel index scores were significantly influenced by COVID-19 (+). The preoperative Barthel index score may be a good predictive tool for the postoperative functional recovery of these patients.

Keywords: COVID-19; hip fracture; postoperative complications; activities of daily living; mortality

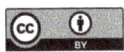

1. Introduction

Hip fracture is a medical condition associated with mortality and poor functional outcomes. According to the International Osteoporosis Foundation, 1.6 million hip fractures were recorded worldwide in 2000, and this number is expected to increase to 4.5–6.3 million by 2050 because of the ageing of the population [1,2]. The mortality risk from a hip fracture persists beyond 5 years, and the 1-year mortality rate is estimated to be 20–24% [3,4]. Among patients who experience hip fractures, 40% cannot walk independently, 60% require assistance, and 33% are completely dependent or living in a nursing home 1 year after they experience the hip fracture [3,5,6].

COVID-19 is an infectious disease transmitted through air droplets and small airborne particles. The first known COVID-19 infection occurred on 31 December 2019 in China [7]. The COVID-19 pandemic was a burden on healthcare systems worldwide. Orthopedic clinics performed fewer elective and nonelective surgeries during the COVID-19 pandemic. However, orthopedic surgeries for trauma cases were still performed. The number of older adult patients presenting to hospitals with hip fractures was the same during the COVID-19 pandemic as it was before the pandemic, even in regions that experienced severe outbreaks of the virus [8]. Moldovan et al. conducted a multicenter study in Romania in 2023 and found that the COVID-19 pandemic has had a severe impact on the volume of elective arthroplasty cases in Romania's 120 hospitals, with a dramatic decrease in the volume of primary interventions for hip and knee patients of up to 69.14% and a corresponding decline in the quality of patient care [9]. The COVID-19 pandemic has influenced patterns of care and health outcomes among patients with hip fractures [10].

In Taiwan, the COVID-19 pandemic reached a critical stage in March 2022. To prevent the spread of the virus, the government implemented strict hospital care and visitation policies. These policies influenced the quality of care, including daily living care and bedside rehabilitation, received by patients with hip fractures. An inferior quality of care has been associated with increased mortality, adverse outcomes, and poor functional improvement.

We hypothesized that the COVID-19 pandemic has led to the launch of policies that could affect hip fracture postoperative care. This includes nursing care and family care, where a decrease in the number of early bedside rehabilitation programs may further increase mortality and poor functional outcomes. Our study aimed to compare mortality and functional outcomes between patients with and without COVID-19 after surgery for hip fractures in our medical center during the COVID-19 pandemic apex in Taiwan.

2. Materials and Methods

2.1. Study Design and Population

We conducted this prospective cohort study in a single medical center in eastern Taiwan, enrolling patients aged 60 and above who were diagnosed with hip fractures between 9 March 2022 and 9 September 2022. The patients with pertrochanteric fractures received open reduction and internal fixation with a cephalomedullary nail, while the patients with displaced femoral neck fractures received hemiarthroplasty. Patients with high-energy trauma, periprosthetic or peri-implant fractures, as well as those who did not undergo surgery or underwent revision surgery for a prior hip fracture, were excluded from the study. The patients' data were included, collected, and classified, as shown in Figure 1.

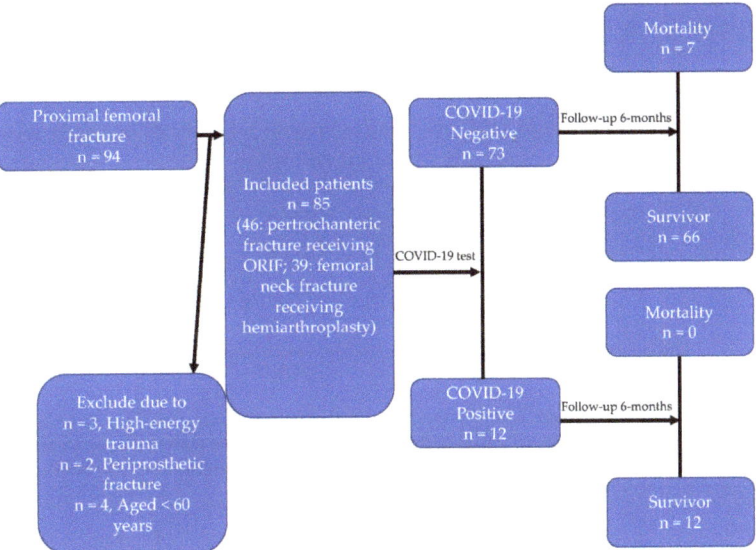

Figure 1. Flowchart of this study.

2.2. Data Collection

Demographic and clinical data were meticulously extracted from electronic medical records. Preoperative functional scores were assessed upon patient admission through validated tools. Follow-up postoperative functional scores were obtained during scheduled outpatient consultations or structured telephone interviews conducted by trained medical staff. The parameters were as listed as below: (1) preoperative data: age, gender, body mass index, fracture type, American Society of Anesthesiologists grade, blood chemistry, Charlson comorbidity index, Barthel index score (activities of daily living), Eastern Cooperative Oncology Group (ECOG) score, and COVID-19 status, as confirmed using polymerase chain reaction tests; (2) operative data: surgical approach, anesthesia type, use of a nerve block, preoperative NPO time, time from admission to operation, the duration of the operation, anesthesia time, estimated blood loss, and immediate postoperative hemoglobin levels; (3) postoperative data: the length of hospital stay, complication incidence (e.g., pneumonia, sepsis, acute urinary retention, ileus, electrolyte imbalance, urinary tract infection, anemia, moderate to severe hip pain), mortality, and postoperative functional scores (ECOG, Barthel index, and modified Harris hip score).

2.3. Statistical Analysis

All statistical analyses were performed using SPSS version 23.0 (IBM, Armonk, NY, USA). The descriptive statistics included continuous variables presented as means ± standard deviations and categorical variables shown as numbers and percentages. The univariate analysis included Student's *t*-test, employed for comparing continuous variables between groups, and chi-square tests, used for categorical variables. The multivariable analysis included a multiple linear regression analysis conducted to assess the impact of the covariates and postoperative comorbidities on changes in the ECOG, Barthel index, and Harris hip scores, with adjustments made for potential confounders. The variable selection was based on a stepwise backward elimination process. The outcome analysis included logistic regression models used to identify factors independently associated with mortality, adjusted for confounding variables. Odds ratios and 95% confidence intervals were reported for all the logistic regression analyses. Statistical significance was defined as a p-value of <0.05, and all tests were two-tailed.

3. Results

This study comprised 85 patients, 12 of whom (14.12%) were COVID-19-positive. There were 29 (34.1%) males and 56 (65.9%) females with a mean age of 79.42 years and mean body mass index of 22.58 ± 3.72 kg/m² (Table 1). In total, 39 (45.9%) of them had femoral pertrochanteric fractures and 46 (54.1%) had femoral neck fractures (Table 1). No statistically significant differences in age, body mass index, gender, ASA grade, fracture type, Charlson comorbidity index score, comorbidity status, preoperative blood chemistry data, or preoperative Barthel index score were observed between the COVID-19-positive and -negative groups (Table 1).

Table 1. Preoperative demographics of patients with proximal femoral fractures receiving ORIF (n = 85).

Variable	COVID-19 Infection Negative	COVID-19 Infection Positive	Total	p
N	73	12	85	
Age	79.18 ± 9.43	80.92 ± 10.44	79.42 ± 9.53	0.561
Body mass index (kg/m²)	22.42 ± 3.76	23.54 ± 3.48	22.58 ± 3.72	0.339
Gender	-	-	-	0.051
Male	28 (38.4%)	1 (8.3%)	29 (34.1%)	
Female	45 (61.6%)	11 (91.7%)	56 (65.9%)	
ASA physical status classification	-	-	-	0.755
1	7 (9.6%)	0 (0.0%)	7 (8.2%)	
2	25 (34.2%)	4 (33.3%)	29 (34.1%)	
3	31 (42.5%)	7 (58.3%)	38 (44.7%)	
4	10 (13.7%)	1 (8.3%)	11 (12.9%)	
Fracture type	-	-	-	0.119
Pertrochanteric	31 (42.5%)	8 (66.7%)	39 (45.9%)	
Femoral neck fracture	42 (57.5%)	4 (33.3%)	46 (54.1%)	
Preoperative blood test				
Hemoglobin (g/dL)	11.34 ± 2.12	10.86 ± 2.50	11.27 ± 2.17	0.478
Platelet (×10³/uL)	205.21 ± 64.4	218.83 ± 88.46	207.13 ± 67.85	0.522
PT (s)	11.10 ± 2.22	10.96 ± 0.63	11.08 ± 2.07	0.822
aPTT (s)	26.65 ± 4.26	28.97 ± 3.99	26.98 ± 4.27	0.082
INR	1.07 ± 0.22	1.07 ± 0.06	1.07 ± 0.21	0.949
ALT (U/L)	22.01 ± 18.43	28.83 ± 36.49	22.98 ± 21.71	0.316
BUN (mg/dL)	27.86 ± 21.61	16.67 ± 6.97	26.28 ± 20.55	0.080
Creatinine (mg/dL)	1.32 ± 1.39	0.75 ± 0.19	1.24 ± 1.30	0.164
Na (mmol/L)	137.16 ± 4.37	135.92 ± 6.73	136.71 ± 4.86	0.055
K (mmol/L)	5.76 ± 15.70	3.92 ± 0.63	5.50 ± 14.55	0.687
Charlson comorbidity index	5.26 ± 2.04	4.92 ± 1.93	5.21 ± 2.02	0.588
Comorbidity number	1.81 ± 1.25	2.25 ± 0.97	1.87 ± 1.22	0.248
Preoperative Barthel index	93.01 ± 14.71	93.75 ± 11.31	93.12 ± 14.23	0.869

Data are presented as n or mean ± standard deviation. aPTT: activated partial thromboplastin time; ASA: American Society of Anesthesiologists; PT: prothrombin time; INR: international normalized ratio.

The COVID-19-negative group had a shorter anesthesia time than the positive group (137.73 ± 32.30 vs. 158.25 ± 40.24 min, p = 0.046; Table 2). No statistically significant differences in the surgical method, anesthesia method, use of perioperative nerve block, preoperative NPO time, time to operation, operation time, blood loss, or hemoglobin level were observed between the COVID-19-positive and -negative groups (Table 2). The postoperative Barthel index scores were significantly lower in the COVID-19-positive group (74.58 ± 17.64) than in the negative group (88.03 ± 16.82) (p = 0.014; Table 3). No significant differences in the length of hospital stay, incidence of complications, ECOG status, Harris hip score, or mortality rate were observed between the groups (Table 3).

Table 2. Perioperative demographics of patients with proximal femoral fractures receiving ORIF (n = 85).

Variable	COVID-19 Infection Negative	COVID-19 Infection Positive	Total	p
Surgical method	-	-	-	0.119
Hemiarthroplasty	42 (57.5%)	4 (33.3%)	46 (54.1%)	
ORIF	31 (42.5%)	8 (66.7%)	39 (45.9%)	
Anesthesia method	-	-	-	1.000
General	45 (61.6%)	8 (66.7%)	53 (62.4%)	
Neuroaxial	28 (38.4%)	4 (33.3%)	32 (37.6%)	
Perioperative nerve block	57 (78.1%)	11 (91.7%)	68 (80.0%)	0.445
Preoperative NPO time (h)	12.18 ± 3.34	13.00 ± 3.81	12.29 ± 3.40	0.441
Time to operation (day)	1.38 ± 0.49	1.58 ± 0.51	1.41 ± 0.50	0.197
Operation time (min)	67.34 ± 20.92	73.83 ± 22.76	68.26 ± 21.17	0.328
Anesthesia time (min)	137.73 ± 32.30	158.25 ± 40.24	140.62 ± 34.03	0.046
Blood loss (mL)	190.41 ± 135.61	245.83 ± 178.96	198.24 ± 142.60	0.214
Postoperative hemoglobin level (g/dL)	10.07 ± 1.81	9.85 ± 2.03	10.04 ± 1.83	0.696

Data are presented as n or mean ± standard deviation ORIF = open reduction and internal fixation.

Table 3. Postoperative demographics of patients with proximal femoral fractures receiving ORIF (n = 85).

Variable	COVID-19 Infection Negative	COVID-19 Infection Positive	Total	p
Length of stay (day)	11.00 ± 9.85	11.08 ± 5.16	11.01 ± 9.31	0.977
Postoperative complication numbers	1.00 ± 0.91	0.92 ± 1.24	0.99 ± 0.96	0.782
Postoperative ECOG performance status	1.79 ± 0.83	2.00 ± 0.74	1.82 ± 0.82	0.412
Postoperative Barthel index	88.03 ± 16.82	74.58 ± 17.64	85.96 ± 17.53	0.014 *
Postoperative modified Harrison hip score	73.42 ± 14.01	66.00 ± 11.79	72.28 ± 13.89	0.089
Mortality	7 (9.6%)	0 (0.0%)	7 (8.2%)	0.586

Data are presented as n or mean ± standard deviation. * $p < 0.05$ was considered statistically significant after the test.

Subgroup analyses were performed to investigate the relationships between postoperative complications and functional outcomes after 6 months in terms of the ECOG, Barthel index, and Harris hip score. A higher incidence of complications was associated with general anesthesia (β: 0.50, 95% confidence interval (CI): 0.06–0.94, $p = 0.026$) and a longer length of hospital stay (β: 0.04, 95% CI: 0.01–0.06, $p = 0.004$) (Table 4). Poor ECOG status was associated with a lower preoperative Barthel index score (β: −0.03, 95% CI: −0.04 to −0.02, $p < 0.001$) (Table 4). A lower postoperative Barthel index score was correlated with COVID-19 infection (β: −15.59, 95% CI: −24.29 to −6.89, $p = 0.001$), a higher Charlson comorbidity index score (β: −3.30, 95% CI: −5.18 to −1.42, $p = 0.001$), and a lower preoperative Barthel index score (β: 0.65, 95% CI: 0.43–0.87, $p < 0.001$) (Table 4). A lower postoperative Harris hip score was correlated with COVID-19 infection (β: −8.20, 95% CI: −16.75 to −0.35, $p = 0.048$), a higher Charlson comorbidity index score (β: −1.78, 95% CI: −3.62 to −0.07, $p = 0.049$), and a lower preoperative Barthel index (β: 0.36, 95% CI: 0.15–0.58, $p = 0.001$) (Table 4). We investigated the factors which were associated with postoperative mortality. After adjustment for various factors, age (adjusted odd ratio (aOR): 1.25, 95% CI: 1.001–1.55, $p = 0.049$), gender (aOR: 342.45, 95% CI: 3.56–32910.44, $p = 0.012$), ASA grade (aOR: 28.96, 95% CI: 1.42–590.37, $p = 0.029$), and Charlson comorbidity index score (aOR: 0.22, 95% CI: 0.06–0.85, $p = 0.028$) were closely associated with postoperative mortality (Table 5).

Table 4. Factors associated with postoperative complications, ECOG performance status, barthel index and modified Harrison hip score at postoperative 6 months (n = 85).

Variable	Incidence of Complications		ECOG Status		Bathal Index		HHS	
	β (95% CI)	p	β (95% CI)	p	β (95% CI)	p	β (95% CI)	p
Age	0.004 (−0.021, 0.029)	0.762	0.004 (−0.016, 0.023)	0.699	0.02 (−0.36, 0.40)	0.906	−0.09 (−0.46, 0.28)	0.637
Gender (Male vs. Female)	−0.09 (−0.53, 0.35)	0.689	0.06 (−0.30, 0.42)	0.732	−0.16 (−7.19, 6.86)	0.963	−3.71 (−10.62, 3.20)	0.287
COVID-19 infection (Positive vs. Negative)	−0.19 (−0.78, 0.40)	0.523	0.37 (−0.07, 0.82)	0.098	−15.59 (−24.29, −6.89)	0.001 *	−8.20 (−16.75, −0.35)	0.048 *
ASA physical status classification	0.13 (−0.18, 0.43)	0.408	−0.07 (−0.31, 0.17)	0.567	4.62 (−0.10, 9.34)	0.055	1.77 (−2.87, 6.41)	0.449
Fracture type (Pertrochanteric vs. Femoral neck)	0.08 (−0.35, 0.51)	0.725	0.04 (−0.30, 0.37)	0.829	−3.22 (−9.73, 3.28)	0.326	−1.98 (−8.38, 4.41)	0.538
Anesthesia (General vs. Neuraxial)	0.50 (0.06, 0.94)	0.026 *	0.14 (−0.20, 0.48)	0.416	−1.74 (−8.47, 5.00)	0.608	−3.95 (−10.57, 2.67)	0.238
Peripheral Nerve block (Yes vs. No)	0.11 (−0.40, 0.63)	0.660	0.03 (−0.38, 0.44)	0.882	−2.25 (−10.23, 5.72)	0.575	−3.06 (−10.89, 4.78)	0.439
Charlson Comorbidity Index	0.08 (−0.05, 0.20)	0.238	0.08 (−0.02, 0.18)	0.099	−3.30 (−5.18, −1.42)	0.001 *	−1.78 (−3.62, −0.07)	0.049 *
Preoperative Barthel Index	0.01 (−0.01, 0.02)	0.194	−0.03 (−0.04, −0.02)	<0.001*	0.65 (0.43, 0.87)	<0.001 *	0.36 (0.15, 0.58)	0.001 *
Time to operation	−0.02 (−0.46, 0.42)	0.943	−0.31 (−0.65, 0.03)	0.073	1.18 (−5.51, 7.87)	0.726	2.29 (−4.29, 8.86)	0.489
Operation time	−0.004 (−0.014, 0.006)	0.473	−0.004 (−0.012, 0.003)	0.266	−0.04 (−0.19, 0.12)	0.651	−0.03 (−0.18, 0.12)	0.674
Blood loss	0.001 (−0.001, 0.002)	0.411	−0.001 (−0.002, 0.001)	0.439	0.01 (−0.01, 0.04)	0.325	−0.004 (−0.029, 0.021)	0.726
Length of Stay	0.04 (0.01, 0.06)	0.004 *	0.01 (−0.01, 0.03)	0.195	0.01 (−0.37, 0.39)	0.958	0.00 (−0.37, 0.37)	0.998

Data are presented as β (95% CI). * p value < 0.05 was considered statistically significant after test. ASA = American Society of Anaesthesiologists, ECOG = Eastern Cooperative Oncology Group, HHS = modified Harrison hip score.

Table 5. Factors associated with mortality at 6 postoperative months (n = 85).

Variable	Crude		Adjusted	
	OR (95% CI)	p	OR (95% CI)	p
Age	1.03 (0.94, 1.12)	0.533	1.25 (1.001, 1.55)	0.049 *
Gender (Male vs. Female)	14.35 (1.63, 125.94)	0.016 *	342.45 (3.56, 32,910.44)	0.012 *
COVID-19 infection (Positive vs. Negative)	0.00 (NA)	0.999		
ASA physical status classification	2.60 (0.87, 7.74)	0.086	28.96 (1.42, 590.37)	0.029 *
Fracture type (Pertrochanteric vs. Femoral neck)	0.88 (0.18, 4.17)	0.867	3.48 (0.13, 95.13)	0.460
Anesthesia (General vs. Neuraxial)	2.46 × 10^8 (NA)	0.998		
Peripheral nerve block (Yes vs. No)	0.60 (0.11, 3.37)	0.558	8.88 (0.16, 505.33)	0.289
Charlson comorbidity index	0.98 (0.66, 1.45)	0.924	0.22 (0.06, 0.85)	0.028 *
Preoperative Barthel index	0.99 (0.94, 1.04)	0.742	1.03 (0.91, 1.16)	0.663
Time to operation	2.02 (0.42, 9.66)	0.378	0.23 (0.01, 6.44)	0.390
Operation time	0.98 (0.94, 1.02)	0.355	0.97 (0.90, 1.05)	0.486
Blood loss	1.001 (0.996, 1.006)	0.672	1.01 (0.998, 1.02)	0.101
Length of stay	1.04 (0.98, 1.10)	0.170	1.06 (0.93, 1.20)	0.390

Data are presented as odds ratio (95% CI). * p value < 0.05 was considered statistically significant after the test. ASA: American Society of Anaesthesiologists. NA: not applicable.

4. Discussion

In our study, we noticed that time to operation did not significantly differ between the positive and negative groups (1.58 ± 0.51 vs. 1.38 ± 0.39 days, respectively). No significant differences were observed in the length of hospital stay or postoperative complications between the groups. Kim discovered that during the COVID-19 pandemic, hip fracture surgeries were postponed for 24 to 36 h, and the rate of postoperative complications did not increase [11]. Wang observed no change in the 30-day mortality rate, time to surgery, or length of hospital stay in a level-1 trauma center in the United States before, during, and after the COVID-19 pandemic [8]. However, a systematic review of 11 cohort studies and a total of 336 patients discovered that the in-hospital mortality rate of hip fracture patients was 29.8% (95% CI: 26.6–35.6%), the 30-day postoperative mortality rate was 35% (95% CI: 29.9–40.5%), and the average hospital stay was 11.29 days [12]. Another systematic review and meta-analysis discovered that patients with hip fractures who had concomitant COVID-19 infection had a 34% short-term mortality rate [13]. Mastan et al. found that COVID-19 status was associated with a 4-fold increase in mortality among patients with hip fractures [14]. In a study conducted by Raheman, patients with hip fractures who had COVID-19 had a 4-fold risk of mortality (risk ratio: 4.59, $p < 0.0001$), and the 30-day mortality rate was 38% (hazard ratio: 4.73, $p < 0.0001$). Raheman et al. discovered that male sex, diabetes, dementia, and extracapsular fractures were risk factors for mortality in patients with COVID-19 [15]. However, in our study, the mortality rate did not significantly differ between patients who had COVID-19 and those who did not have COVID-19. None of the seven patients who died had COVID-19.

The postoperative Barthel index score was significantly lower in the COVID-19-positive group (74.58 ± 17.64) than in the COVID-19-negative group. The postoperative Barthel index score and Harris hip score were associated with COVID-19 status (Table 4). Two factors may have contributed to this result. First, COVID-19 may have made the patients more vulnerable to health problems or caused their existing health problems to worsen. Second, the delayed initiation of rehabilitation may have had a significant impact on the surgical results because of the isolation policy for COVID-19 infection. Early mobilization is essential for the optimal postoperative management of patients with hip fractures, including activities such as getting in and out of bed, performing sit-to-stand exercises, rising from chairs with assistance, and walking with the aid of a walker [16–19]. Patients with hip fractures experience an average loss of muscle strength in their affected limbs of more than 50% in the first postoperative week [20–23].

The COVID-19 pandemic clearly impacted surgical treatment for patients with a hip pathology. Moldovan et al. quantified the effects of COVID-19 on elective arthroplasty interventions in Romania. He found that the COVID-19 pandemic had a severe impact on the volume of elective arthroplasty cases in Romania's 120 hospitals [9], and this impact had significant financial ramifications for the hospitals. The author proposed the development of new clinical procedures and personalized home recovery programs for future outbreaks. Telemedicine through virtual consultations may also be integrated into emergency orthopedics in the future to maintain the care quality of patients during infectious disease pandemics [24,25]. The COVID-19 pandemic has placed unprecedented strain on healthcare systems worldwide, affecting various medical specialties, including orthopedics [26]. The pandemic apex has led to specific challenges in managing hip fractures among older adults in Taiwan in terms of both surgical quality and postoperative care. In terms of the impact of hip fractures on surgical quality, it can be divided into four parts: (1) Resource Allocation and Triage: The pandemic has forced many hospitals to reprioritize surgeries, with centers often postponing elective surgeries to focus on emergency cases [27]. In Taiwan, this has impacted the availability of resources like surgical suites, specialized orthopedic teams, and even equipment, which could potentially affect the surgical outcomes for hip fractures. (2) Surgical Delays: With hospitals at or near capacity due to COVID-19 patients, surgical delays have become common. A study in the *Journal of Bone and Joint Surgery* indicated that even a delay of just over 48 h could lead to a significant increase in 30-day mortality rates for hip fractures [28]. Delays may be exacerbated if the patient is COVID-19-positive, given the need for special protocols and isolation measures. (3) Surgical Technique and Team Experience: Due to the need for staff redeployment to care for COVID-19 patients, less experienced teams may sometimes handle surgeries, possibly affecting the surgical outcomes. Additionally, some studies suggest that less invasive surgical techniques might be preferred during pandemic conditions to reduce the operation time and hospital stay, although this could affect long-term outcomes [29]. (4) Perioperative Care: Special precautions have to be taken if the patient is COVID-19-positive. These include changes in anesthesia protocols and more intensive monitoring, which could affect the overall surgical experience and potentially lead to complications [30]. In terms of the impact on postoperative care quality for hip fractures, it can be divided into six parts: (1) Hospital Stay: During the pandemic's apex, the focus was on reducing the length of hospital stays to free up beds. Quick discharge protocols may not always align with the optimal recovery paths for hip fracture patients, especially older adults, who often have comorbid conditions requiring complex care [9]. (2) Physical Rehabilitation: Given the social distancing norms and limitations on in-person interactions, physical rehabilitation schedules may be disrupted. A meta-analysis study in *Medicine* indicates that reduced postoperative mobility can lead to complications such as joint stiffness and an increased fall risk [31]. (3) Psychological Impact: Isolation due to COVID-19 protocols, coupled with the natural apprehension arising from being in a hospital during a pandemic, can lead to mental health issues like depression or anxiety [32]. These psychological factors can adversely affect postoperative recovery. (4) Follow-Up and Long-Term Care: Telehealth has often replaced in-person consultations for follow-up care, but not all aspects of postoperative care can be adequately managed remotely [24]. Moreover, older adults may face challenges in accessing or using digital platforms. (5) Economic Impact: In Taiwan, as elsewhere, the economic repercussions of the pandemic have led to funding cuts and resource allocation changes that could affect the quality of postoperative care. (6) Complications: According to an article in the *World Journal of Orthopedics*, the incidence of postoperative complications like pneumonia, urinary tract infections, or deep vein thrombosis may rise due to the strains and changes in standard care protocols during a pandemic [33]. As Taiwan navigates the challenges of COVID-19, innovative strategies like tele-rehabilitation, personalized home-based recovery plans, and the integration of artificial intelligence into the monitoring of postoperative care are becoming more relevant. Research and healthcare policies must adapt to ensure that the surgical and postoperative care quality of hip fracture patients is not compromised, irrespective of pandemic conditions. The apex of the COVID-19 pandemic has had a multifaceted impact on the quality of surgical and postoperative care for hip fractures in Taiwan. With shifting resources and strained healthcare systems, the implications are vast and warrant urgent attention to mitigate adverse outcomes.

The COVID-19 pandemic has significantly disrupted healthcare systems, and its impact extends beyond immediate medical care to longer-term functional outcomes in various patient groups. Patients recovering from surgeries often require extensive postoperative care, including physical therapy [31]. The pandemic has led to limitations in access to physical rehabilitation services due to social distancing measures and the diversion of healthcare resources. A study in *Clinical Rehabilitation* has indicated that this reduction in physical therapy access can have negative implications for long-term functional recovery, especially in the first 6 months post-surgery, which is a critical period for regaining function [34]. For patients with chronic conditions like COPD, diabetes, or heart disease, routine care and regular exercise are vital for maintaining functional ability. A study in *Experimental Gerontology* found that the interruption of regular healthcare visits and reduced physical activity due to lockdown measures can result in deteriorated functional quality over a 6-month period [35]. For instance, decreased exercise can exacerbate issues with glycemic control in diabetics, and reduced pulmonary rehabilitation can affect respiratory function in COPD patients. Regarding COVID-19 survivors, a number of studies have examined the "long COVID" phenomenon, where symptoms persist for months after the initial infection has resolved [36]. These symptoms can range from fatigue and muscle weakness to difficulties with concentration and memory, all affecting functional quality. A study in *The Lancet Global Health* found that even mild cases of COVID-19 can have lingering functional impacts up to 6 months after recovery, affecting the ability to return to work and carry out daily activities [37]. Elderly patients are at high risk of functional decline due to both age and an increased susceptibility to COVID-19. Social isolation measures, although necessary, have contributed to reduced physical activity, and studies in *The Journal of Frailty*

& *Aging* have highlighted how this inactivity can lead to rapid functional decline in elderly populations [38]. The pandemic also had a widespread psychological impact, exacerbating conditions like depression and anxiety, which can have a direct effect on physical health and functional ability [39]. Psychological stress can influence pain perception, sleep quality, and overall well-being, factors that are critical in functional recovery from any illness or surgical intervention [32]. The above conditions may explain why the apex of the COVID-19 pandemic had a profound impact on the 6-month functional quality of patients with hip fractures in our study. Reduced access to healthcare services, interruptions in routine care, and the lingering effects of COVID-19 itself pose challenges that need urgent attention. Telemedicine and home-based care models are emerging as potential alternatives, but there is a dire need for more research in order to understand how to effectively mitigate these functional impairments.

This study has several limitations. First, this was a single-center study with a small sample ($n = 85$). The unexpected phenomenon whereby all the patients who died were in the COVID-19-negative group is due to the small sample size. Second, this study compared patients with and without COVID-19 during the pandemic and did not evaluate patients before the pandemic. Third, we did not include other parameters such as bone density, sarcopenia, and nutrition status that may have also impacted the patients' postoperative function scores. In the future, we could design a matching study to reduce the bias from other interfering causes. The strength of our study is that it is based on real-world data obtained during patient admission and during follow-up in the outpatient clinic department or using telephone interviews. Few studies have investigated functional outcomes in patients with hip fractures who have COVID-19. Our study provides information on the association between functional outcomes and COVID-19 in patients with hip fractures.

5. Conclusions

At our hospital, orthopedic surgeries were not unduly delayed during the COVID-19 pandemic. No significant differences in the length of hospital stay, postoperative complications, or mortality were observed between patients with and without COVID-19. The key finding of this study is that among patients with hip fractures, those with COVID-19 may have worse functional outcomes in terms of the Barthel index and Harris hip score than those without COVID-19.

Author Contributions: Conceptualization, W.-T.W. and K.-T.Y.; methodology, T.-K.Y.; software, J.-Y.C.; validation, I.-H.C.; formal analysis, J.-H.W.; investigation, C.-M.C. and C.-I.P.; data curation, K.-L.L. and T.-C.Y.; writing—original draft preparation, H.-Y.T.; writing—review and editing, K.-T.Y.; supervision, W.-T.W. and K.-T.Y. All authors have read and agreed to the published version of the manuscript.

Funding: This research received no external funding.

Institutional Review Board Statement: This study was conducted in accordance with the Declaration of Helsinki and approved by the Research Ethics Committee of Hualien Tzu Chi Hospital (Approval Code: IRB112-035-B Approval Date: 23 February 2023), Buddhist Tzu Chi Medical Foundation. Informed consent was obtained from all individuals. All patients provided written informed consent prior to participation.

Informed Consent Statement: Informed consent was obtained from all subjects involved in the study.

Data Availability Statement: The data are contained within the article.

Conflicts of Interest: The authors declare no conflict of interest.

References

1. Cooper, C.; Campion, G.; Melton, L.J., 3rd. Hip fractures in the elderly: A world-wide projection. *Osteoporos. Int.* **1992**, *2*, 285–289. [CrossRef] [PubMed]
2. Gullberg, B.; Johnell, O.; Kanis, J.A. World-wide projections for hip fracture. *Osteoporos. Int.* **1997**, *7*, 407–413. [CrossRef] [PubMed]

3. Leibson, C.L.; Tosteson, A.N.; Gabriel, S.E.; Ransom, J.E.; Melton, L.J. Mortality, disability, and nursing home use for persons with and without hip fracture: A population-based study. *J. Am. Geriatr. Soc.* **2002**, *50*, 1644–1650. [CrossRef] [PubMed]
4. Magaziner, J.; Lydick, E.; Hawkes, W.; Fox, K.M.; Zimmerman, S.I.; Epstein, R.S.; Hebel, J.R. Excess mortality attributable to hip fracture in white women aged 70 years and older. *Am. J. Public Health* **1997**, *87*, 1630–1636. [CrossRef] [PubMed]
5. Riggs, B.L.; Melton, L.J., 3rd. The worldwide problem of osteoporosis: Insights afforded by epidemiology. *Bone* **1995**, *17* (Suppl. S5), 505S–511S. [CrossRef]
6. Magaziner, J.; Simonsick, E.M.; Kashner, T.M.; Hebel, J.R.; Kenzora, J.E. Predictors of functional recovery one year following hospital discharge for hip fracture: A prospective study. *J. Gerontol.* **1990**, *45*, M101–M107. [CrossRef]
7. Cheng, S.C.; Chang, Y.C.; Fan Chiang, Y.L.; Chien, Y.C.; Cheng, M.; Yang, C.H.; Huang, C.H.; Hsu, Y.N. First case of Coronavirus Disease 2019 (COVID-19) pneumonia in Taiwan. *J. Formos. Med. Assoc.* **2020**, *119*, 747–751. [CrossRef]
8. Wang, K.C.; Xiao, R.; Cheung, Z.B.; Barbera, J.P.; Forsh, D.A. Early mortality after hip fracture surgery in COVID-19 patients: A systematic review and meta-analysis. *J. Orthop.* **2020**, *22*, 584–591. [CrossRef]
9. Moldovan, F.; Gligor, A.; Moldovan, L.; Bataga, T. An Investigation for Future Practice of Elective Hip and Knee Arthroplasties during COVID-19 in Romania. *Medicina* **2023**, *59*, 314. [CrossRef]
10. Zhong, H.; Poeran, J.; Liu, J.; Wilson, L.A.; Memtsoudis, S.G. Hip fracture characteristics and outcomes during COVID-19: A large retrospective national database review. *Br. J. Anaesth.* **2021**, *127*, 15–22. [CrossRef]
11. Kim, K.K.; Lee, S.W.; Choi, J.K.; Won, Y.Y. Epidemiology and postoperative complications of hip fracture during COVID-19 pandemic. *Osteoporos. Sarcopenia* **2022**, *8*, 17–23. [CrossRef] [PubMed]
12. Tayyebi, H.; Hasanikhah, M.; Heidarikhoo, M.; Fakoor, S.; Aminian, A. Length of hospital stay and mortality of hip fracture surgery in patients with Coronavirus disease 2019 (COVID-19) infection: A systematic review and meta-analysis. *Curr. Orthop. Pract.* **2022**, *33*, 172–177. [CrossRef] [PubMed]
13. Isla, A.; Landy, D.; Teasdall, R.; Mittwede, P.; Albano, A.; Tornetta, P., 3rd; Bhandari, M.; Aneja, A. Postoperative mortality in the COVID-positive hip fracture patient, a systematic review and meta-analysis. *Eur. J. Orthop. Surg. Traumatol.* **2023**, *33*, 927–935. [CrossRef]
14. Mastan, S.; Hodhody, G.; Sajid, M.; Malik, R.; Charalambous, C.P. COVID-19 Is Associated With a 4-Fold Increase in 30-day Mortality Risk in Hip Fracture Patients in the United Kingdom: A Systematic Review and Meta-Analysis. *Geriatr. Orthop. Surg. Rehabil.* **2022**, *13*, 21514593221099375. [CrossRef] [PubMed]
15. Raheman, F.J.; Rojoa, D.M.; Nayan Parekh, J.; Berber, R.; Ashford, R. Meta-analysis and metaregression of risk factors associated with mortality in hip fracture patients during the COVID-19 pandemic. *Sci. Rep.* **2021**, *11*, 10157. [CrossRef]
16. Parker, M.; Johansen, A. Hip fracture. *BMJ* **2006**, *333*, 27–30. [CrossRef]
17. Mak, J.C.; Cameron, I.D.; March, L.M.; National Health and Medical Research Council. Evidence-based guidelines for the management of hip fractures in older persons: An update. *Med. J. Aust.* **2010**, *192*, 37–41. [CrossRef]
18. Ftouh, S.; Morga, A.; Swift, C.; Guideline Development Group. Management of hip fracture in adults: Summary of NICE guidance. *BMJ* **2011**, *342*, d3304. [CrossRef]
19. Swierstra, B.A.; Vervest, A.M.; Walenkamp, G.H.; Schreurs, B.W.; Spierings, P.T.; Heyligers, I.C.; van Susante, J.L.; Ettema, H.B.; Jansen, M.J.; Hennis, P.J.; et al. Dutch guideline on total hip prosthesis. *Acta. Orthop.* **2011**, *82*, 567–576. [CrossRef]
20. Kristensen, M.T.; Bandholm, T.; Bencke, J.; Ekdahl, C.; Kehlet, H. Knee-extension strength, postural control and function are related to fracture type and thigh edema in patients with hip fracture. *Clin. Biomech.* **2009**, *24*, 218–224. [CrossRef]
21. Lamb, S.E.; Morse, R.E.; Evans, J.G. Mobility after proximal femoral fracture: The relevance of leg extensor power, postural sway and other factors. *Age Ageing.* **1995**, *24*, 308–314. [CrossRef] [PubMed]
22. Sherrington, C.; Lord, S.R.; Herbert, R.D. A randomised trial of weight-bearing versus non-weight-bearing exercise for improving physical ability in inpatients after hip fracture. *Aust. J. Physiother.* **2003**, *49*, 15–22. [CrossRef] [PubMed]
23. Kronborg, L.; Bandholm, T.; Palm, H.; Kehlet, H.; Kristensen, M.T. Feasibility of progressive strength training implemented in the acute ward after hip fracture surgery. *PLoS ONE* **2014**, *9*, e93332. [CrossRef] [PubMed]
24. Rizkalla, J.M.; Gladnick, B.P.; Bhimani, A.A.; Wood, D.S.; Kitziger, K.J.; Peters, P.C., Jr. Triaging Total Hip Arthroplasty during the COVID-19 Pandemic. *Curr. Rev. Musculoskelet. Med.* **2020**, *13*, 416–424. [CrossRef]
25. Teo, S.H.; Abd Rahim, M.R.; Nizlan, N.M. The impact of COVID-19 pandemic on orthopaedic specialty in Malaysia: A cross-sectional survey. *J. Orthop. Surg.* **2020**, *28*, 2309499020938877. [CrossRef] [PubMed]
26. Moldovan, F.; Gligor, A.; Moldovan, L.; Bataga, T. The Impact of the COVID-19 Pandemic on the Orthopedic Residents: A Pan-Romanian Survey. *Int. J. Environ. Res. Public Health.* **2022**, *19*, 9176. [CrossRef] [PubMed]
27. Shih, C.L.; Huang, P.J.; Huang, H.T.; Chen, C.H.; Lee, T.C.; Hsu, C.H. Impact of the COVID-19 pandemic and its related psychological effect on orthopedic surgeries conducted in different types of hospitals in Taiwan. *J. Orthop. Surg.* **2021**, *29*, 2309499021996072. [CrossRef]
28. Siegmeth, A.W.; Gurusamy, K.; Parker, M.J. Delay to surgery prolongs hospital stay in patients with fractures of the proximal femur. *J. Bone Jt. Surg. Br.* **2005**, *87*, 1123–1126. [CrossRef]
29. Qin, H.C.; He, Z.; Luo, Z.W.; Zhu, Y.L. Management of hip fracture in COVID-19 infected patients. *World J. Orthop.* **2022**, *13*, 544–554. [CrossRef]
30. Shin, S.; Kim, S.H.; Park, K.K.; Kim, S.J.; Bae, J.C.; Choi, Y.S. Effects of Anesthesia Techniques on Outcomes after Hip Fracture Surgery in Elderly Patients: A Prospective, Randomized, Controlled Trial. *J. Clin. Med.* **2020**, *9*, 1605. [CrossRef]

31. Liu, Y.; Yang, Y.; Liu, H.; Wu, W.; Wu, X.; Wang, T. A systematic review and meta-analysis of fall incidence and risk factors in elderly patients after total joint arthroplasty. *Medicine* **2020**, *99*, e23664. [CrossRef] [PubMed]
32. Hwang, T.J.; Rabheru, K.; Peisah, C.; Reichman, W.; Ikeda, M. Loneliness and social isolation during the COVID-19 pandemic. *Int. Psychogeriatr.* **2020**, *32*, 1217–1220. [CrossRef] [PubMed]
33. Obamiro, E.; Trivedi, R.; Ahmed, N. Changes in trends of orthopedic services due to the COVID-19 pandemic: A review. *World J. Orthop.* **2022**, *13*, 955–968. [CrossRef] [PubMed]
34. Berggren, M.; Karlsson, Å.; Lindelöf, N.; Englund, U.; Olofsson, B.; Nordström, P.; Gustafson, Y.; Stenvall, M. Effects of geriatric interdisciplinary home rehabilitation on complications and readmissions after hip fracture: A randomized controlled trial. *Clin. Rehabil.* **2019**, *33*, 64–73. [CrossRef]
35. Markotegi, M.; Irazusta, J.; Sanz, B.; Rodriguez-Larrad, A. Effect of the COVID-19 pandemic on the physical and psychoaffective health of older adults in a physical exercise program. *Exp. Gerontol.* **2021**, *155*, 111580. [CrossRef]
36. Sykes, D.L.; Holdsworth, L.; Jawad, N.; Gunasekera, P.; Morice, A.H.; Crooks, M.G. Post-COVID-19 Symptom Burden: What Is Long-COVID and How Should We Manage It? *Lung* **2021**, *199*, 113–119. [CrossRef]
37. Dryden, M.; Mudara, C.; Vika, C.; Blumberg, L.; Mayet, N.; Cohen, C.; Tempia, S.; Parker, A.; Nel, J.; Perumal, R.; et al. Post-COVID-19 condition 3 months after hospitalisation with SARS-CoV-2 in South Africa: A prospective cohort study. *Lancet Glob. Health* **2022**, *10*, e1247–e1256. [CrossRef]
38. Risbridger, S.; Walker, R.; Gray, W.K.; Kamaruzzaman, S.B.; Ai-Vyrn, C.; Hairi, N.N.; Khoo, P.L.; Pin, T.M. Social Participation's Association with Falls and Frailty in Malaysia: A Cross-Sectional Study. *J. Frailty Aging* **2022**, *11*, 199–205. [CrossRef]
39. Clemente-Suárez, V.J.; Martínez-González, M.B.; Benitez-Agudelo, J.C.; Navarro-Jiménez, E.; Beltran-Velasco, A.I.; Ruisoto, P.; Diaz Arroyo, E.; Laborde-Cárdenas, C.C.; Tornero-Aguilera, J.F. The Impact of the COVID-19 Pandemic on Mental Disorders. A Critical Review. *Int. J. Environ. Res. Public Health* **2021**, *18*, 10041. [CrossRef]

Disclaimer/Publisher's Note: The statements, opinions and data contained in all publications are solely those of the individual author(s) and contributor(s) and not of MDPI and/or the editor(s). MDPI and/or the editor(s) disclaim responsibility for any injury to people or property resulting from any ideas, methods, instructions or products referred to in the content.

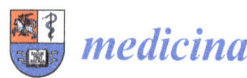

Article

Treatment of Soft Tissue Defects after Minimally Invasive Plate Osteosynthesis in Fractures of the Distal Tibia: Clinical Results after Reverse Sural Artery Flap

Jun Young Lee [1,†], Hyo Jun Lee [1,†], Sung Hoon Yang [1], Je Hong Ryu [1], Hyoung Tae Kim [1], Byung Ho Lee [2], Sung Hwan Kim [3], Ho Sung Kim [3] and Young Koo Lee [3,*]

1. Department of Orthopaedic Surgery, College of Medicine, Chosun University, 365 Pilmundae-ro, Dong-gu, Gwangju 61453, Republic of Korea; leejy88@chosun.ac.kr (J.Y.L.); whogus12@kakao.com (H.J.L.); shyang1234@naver.com (S.H.Y.); ryujh9950@naver.com (J.H.R.); kht2769@naver.com (H.T.K.)
2. Department of Orthopaedic Surgery, Daejung Hospital, 180 Daein-ro, Dong-gu, Gwangju 61473, Republic of Korea; hand8150@naver.com
3. Department of Orthopaedic Surgery, Soonchunhyang University Hospital Bucheon, 170 Jomaru-ro, Wonmi-gu, Bucheon-si 14584, Republic of Korea; shk9528@naver.com (S.H.K.); nine4141@naver.com (H.S.K.)
* Correspondence: brain0808@hanmail.net
† These authors contributed equally to this work and are co-first authors.

Abstract: *Introduction*: Distal tibial fractures make up approximately 3% to 10% of all tibial fractures or about 1% of lower extremity fractures. MIPO is an appropriate procedure and method to achieve stable metal plate fixation and osseointegration by minimizing soft tissue damage and vascular integrity at the fracture site. MIPO to the medial tibia during distal tibial fractures induces skin irritation due to the thickness of the metal plate, which causes discomfort and pain on the medial side of the distal leg, and if severe, complications such as infection and skin defect may occur. The reverse sural flap is a well-researched approach for covering defects in the lower third of the leg, ankle, and foot. *Materials and Methods*: Among 151 patients with distal tibia fractures who underwent minimally invasive metal plate fixation, soft tissue was injured due to postoperative complications. We treated 13 cases with necrosis and exposed metal plates by retrograde nasogastric artery flap surgery. For these patients, we collected obligatory patient records, radiological data, and wound photographs of the treatment results and complications of reconstructive surgery. *Results*: In all the cases, flap survival was confirmed at the final outpatient follow-up. The exposed area of the metal plate was well coated, and there was no plate failure due to complete necrosis. Three out of four women complained of aesthetic dissatisfaction because the volume of the tunnel through which the skin mirror passed and the skin plate itself were thick. In two cases, defatting was performed to reduce the thickness of the plate while removing the metal plate. *Conclusions*: Metal plate exposure after distal tibial fractures have been treated with minimally invasive metal plate fusion and can be successfully treated with retrograde nasogastric artery flaps, and several surgical techniques are used during flap surgery.

Keywords: distal tibia fracture; MIPO; reverse sural artery flap

Citation: Lee, J.Y.; Lee, H.J.; Yang, S.H.; Ryu, J.H.; Kim, H.T.; Lee, B.H.; Kim, S.H.; Kim, H.S.; Lee, Y.K. Treatment of Soft Tissue Defects after Minimally Invasive Plate Osteosynthesis in Fractures of the Distal Tibia: Clinical Results after Reverse Sural Artery Flap. *Medicina* 2023, 59, 1751. https://doi.org/10.3390/medicina59101751

Academic Editor: Johannes Mayr

Received: 8 August 2023
Revised: 27 September 2023
Accepted: 28 September 2023
Published: 30 September 2023

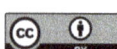

Copyright: © 2023 by the authors. Licensee MDPI, Basel, Switzerland. This article is an open access article distributed under the terms and conditions of the Creative Commons Attribution (CC BY) license (https://creativecommons.org/licenses/by/4.0/).

1. Introduction

Distal tibial fractures make up approximately 3% to 10% of all tibial fractures or about 1% of lower extremity fractures. In 70% to 85% of cases, there is also a concomitant fibular fracture, indicating more complex injuries [1]. It is a break in the lower part of the shinbone that includes the metaphyseal region and can potentially extend to the weight-bearing joint surface. It is also referred to as a tibial pilon fracture or tibial plafond fracture when the joint surface is involved [2]. Intra-articular fractures occurring at the distal end of the tibia, which involve a substantial portion of the weight-bearing articular surface, present formidable complexities and difficulties in their therapeutic management [3]. Distal tibial fractures are caused by high-energy shear and rotational forces [4] and have a high probability of complications such as delayed union, nonunion, joint stiffness, and soft tissue necrosis due to the small amount of surrounding soft tissue, poor blood flow, and thin periosteum. Fractures located at the distal tibia typically necessitate surgical intervention, as non-operative approaches involving lengthy application of long leg casts, extended immobilization, and the inherent risk of malunion are less favored. Non-operative treatment is predominantly reserved for individuals with significant comorbidities that might hinder their ability to undergo anesthesia, as well as for patients with minimally displaced fractures [5].

The most appropriate treatment for distal tibial fractures is a subject of controversy [6]. Surgical treatment methods include open reduction, internal fixation using a metal plate, intramedullary nailing, minimally invasive plate osteosynthesis (MIPO), and external fixation [7,8]. Over the past six decades, there has been remarkable and rapid growth in the field of surgical techniques and understanding of fracture treatment. This progress can be highlighted by comparing Robert Danis' original principles of osteosynthesis to the current principles advocated by the AO (Arbeitsgemeinschaft für Osteosynthesefragen). While Danis emphasized the precise anatomic restoration of bones and achieving absolute stability, the contemporary theory has evolved to allow for the restoration of anatomic relationships (such as length, alignment, and rotation), even if not directly at the articular surfaces. Current approaches also accept the concept of relative stability, promoting callus formation and giving importance to cautious soft tissue handling. These differences clearly distinguish traditional and minimally invasive plating techniques, signifying the advancements that have taken place in fracture management over the years [9]. The primary goal of surgical intervention is to rectify the anatomical positioning of the lowermost tibia and furnish adequate stability, thereby fostering the mending of fractures and reducing delayed complications [10].

Extensive scholarly material exists concerning the management of fractures situated along the tibial diaphysis, and intramedullary nailing (IMN) is commonly characterized as the foremost therapeutic option for the vast majority of cases [11]. Intramedullary nailing (IMN) offers the advantage of being minimally invasive, leading to smaller skin incisions, reduced soft-tissue trauma, and preservation of blood supply around the bone. The fixation achieved through IMN is stable, allowing for early mobilization. However, there is a possibility of experiencing anterior knee pain, and malunions have been reported in cases of distal tibial fractures treated with this method [5]. Inserting the nail tip within the uppermost third between the tibial plateau and tibial tuberosity, and exhibiting nail prominence of over 5 mm beyond the front surface of the tibial cortex, emerged as variables correlated with post-intramedullary nailing (IMN) knee discomfort following tibial diaphyseal fractures [11]. While intramedullary fixation offers benefits such as better preservation of soft tissue and blood supply, the management of fracture fragments becomes increasingly difficult as the fracture approaches the articular surface, transitioning from the diaphysis to the metaphysis. As the gap between the intramedullary nail and the cortex widens, the likelihood of malreduction and malunion also increases [9]. Within the central region of the tibial shaft, IMN may enable adequate alignment, yet this length remains abbreviated. The upper or lower portion of the shaft presents variability, precluding IMNs from interacting with the tibial cortex in these regions. In such cases, sustaining the alignment relies exclusively on anchoring the locking nails at the proximal or distal area. As a result, the IMN fixation manifests relative fragility, leading to limited torsional resilience [12].

On the other hand, open reduction and internal fixation (ORIF) carry a lower risk of malunion but require a longer time before weight-bearing is allowed and pose an increased risk of wound complications [5]. ORIFs were utilized to restore the anatomical integrity of the joint surface. Spiral oblique and spiral wedge fractures arise from different mechanisms than transverse fractures. These fractures materialize due to rotational forces, and such rotational dynamics can engender extensive fracture patterns extending toward metaphyseal regions. Plates exhibit superior resistance against torsional forces in comparison to intramedullary nails (IMNs), rendering them a potentially more fitting selection for managing spiral oblique and spiral wedge fractures [12]. Nevertheless, the extensive dissection of soft tissue resulted in elevated infection rates and complications related to the soft tissue. Furthermore, it has been observed that open reduction and plate fixation can modify the blood supply to the tibia, potentially leading to delayed union or nonunion [3]. Using external fixators in the management of high-energy distal tibia fractures provides the benefit of significantly reducing soft tissue dissection and minimizing disruption of the blood supply. This proves advantageous in cases where there is extensive soft tissue damage and traumatized skin. Moreover, high-energy distal tibia fractures are frequently associated with other bodily trauma. Therefore, the temporary application of an external fixation device allows for additional time to attain hemodynamic stability and address other life-threatening injuries [13].

MIPO is a procedure that accounts for the biomechanics of fractures and is an appropriate method for achieving stable metal plate fixation and osseointegration by minimizing soft tissue damage and vascular integrity at the fracture site using an indirect reduction technique [14]. The MIPO technique offers clear advantages, such as reduced soft tissue damage and improved osteointegration; when compared to conventional surgical methods, it still faces several significant issues that remain unresolved. In research conducted by Hasenboehler et al., 32 patients with distal tibial fractures were subjected to minimally invasive plate osteosynthesis (MIPO). The study revealed a tendency for delayed union in cases of simple fracture patterns. Despite the advantage of preserving the blood supply, MIPO does not facilitate optimal fracture reduction. In simple fractures, the fragments may not be anatomically aligned, and interfragmentary compression might be inadequate, leading to delayed union. Furthermore, there have been reports of other intraoperative complications, including damage to the saphenous nerve and vein [7]. In addition, MIPO to the medial tibia during distal tibial fractures induces skin irritation due to the thickness of the metal plate, which causes discomfort and pain on the medial side of the distal leg, and if severe, complications such as infection and skin defect may occur. According to T.W. Lau et al., of a total of 48 patients who underwent MIPO after distal tibia fracture, infection occurred in 7 patients (15%) and skin irritation due to exposed metal plates was reported in 25 patients (52%) [15]. Treating postoperative soft-tissue defects on the lower legs presents significant challenges due to arterial and venous insufficiency, compromised skin quality characterized by epidermal and dermal atrophy, limited tissue laxity, and an elevated risk of infection [16]. Due to this anatomical characteristic and frequent bone exposure, most surgeons have come to regard free flaps as the primary treatment option [17]. Microvascular flaps are outstanding alternatives, but their surgical procedure is challenging and demands a skilled team, advanced equipment, and specialized hospital centers. Cutaneous and fasciocutaneous flaps with a distal pedicle are another viable option to be taken into consideration. The reverse sural flap is a well-researched approach for covering defects in the lower third of the leg, ankle, and foot. It relies on the communicating and perforating branches of the fibular artery, originating approximately 5 to 6 cm cranially to the lateral malleolus [18].

Therefore, the present authors performed retrograde superficial sural artery flap surgery for the distal metal plate exposure, which occurred as a complication after MIPO for distal tibial fracture. The aim of this study is to suggest some surgical tips with a small cohort to improve the outcome and success rate after MIPO for distal tibia fracture.

2. Materials and Methods

From June 2010 to December 2020, among 151 patients with distal tibia fractures who underwent MIPO at our hospital, 13 patients (9%) had soft tissue injury due to postoperative necrosis. We treated 13 cases with necrosis and exposed metal plates by retrograde superficial sural artery flap surgery, and for these patients, we collected patients' hospital records, radiological data, and wound photographs of the treatment results and complications of reconstructive surgery. A retrospective analysis was originally performed, and patients who could be followed up for at least 12 months after surgery were included (Table 1). The female-to-male ratio was 44.4%.

Table 1. Patients Demographics.

	Age/Sex	Injury Mechanism	MIPO Op. interval (Days)	MIPO to RSSA Op. interval (mo.)	Wound Culture
1	49/F	IncarTA	7	0.5	No growth
2	28/M	Sports	8	1.5	No growth
3	59/M	IncarTA	4	1.3	No growth
4	64/M	Fall down	21	0.6	GNR
5	81/M	IncarTA	9	1.1	GPC
6	63/F	Fall down	11	0.8	No growth
7	52/M	Sports	13	1.4	GPC
8	79/M	Fall down	2	1.0	No growth
9	37/F	IncarTA	6	0.4	No growth
10	22/M	IncarTA	14	0.9	No growth
11	77/F	Fall down	10	1.1	No growth
12	56/M	Sports	8	1.5	No growth
13	23/M	Fall down	6	1.6	No growth

TA: traffic accident. GNR: Gram-negative bacillus. GPC: Gram-positive coccus.

Surgical Technique

Initially, the patient was placed in a prone position under spinal or general anesthesia, and the pneumatic tourniquet was at 300 mmHg. Then, debridement on the metal plate exposed area was performed. A circular or oval shape was drawn with a marking pen along the area of the skin, which is considered normal around the visible metal plate exposed area, and then excised with a scalpel. In order to suture the sural artery flap, a relatively thick pedicle flap containing subcutaneous fat and fascia, skin-to-skin without tension at the defect, even if the exposed area is small during excision, the defect is at least 4 × 3 cm^2 in size, which was enlarged and excised.

The axis of the flap draws an imaginary line connecting the center of the back of the lower leg from the point approximately 3–5 cm proximal to the lateral malleolus of the ankle joint to the popliteal fossa, considering the travel of the small saphenous vein and the peroneal artery. A donor flap was drawn on this line.

The pivot point of the arc of rotation is set at a point approximately 8–10 cm proximal in the lateral malleolus of ankle joint surgery to maximize preservation of the perforator from the peroneal artery, maintain arterial blood flow, and make it possible to rotate the flap without twisting to the defect in the ankle joint area.

Next, the length of the skin mirror was measured with a tape along the movement path of the skin mirror from the reference point of the rotation arc to the metal plate exposed area, and about 1 cm was added to this to determine the length of the skin mirror. The shape of the flap was circular or oval, depending on the shape of the defect, and the distal portion of the flap was shaped like a teardrop with a length of about 2 cm. When the skin was sutured in the defect, the inlet of the skin mirror was cut in a straight line of the same size and sutured with the distal flap to reduce the pressure on the skin mirror. The size of the flap was set to be about 0.5 cm larger than the defect in men and about 1 cm larger in diameter than the defect in women with relatively large amounts of subcutaneous fat.

The elevation of the flap proceeded from the proximal part to the distal part, and the dissection between the fascial layer and the muscular layer was bluntly dissected with a Hemostat, etc., and the distal part was elevated. In this process, the peroneal nerve was preserved as much as possible if possible, and when the peroneal nerve entered the upper fascial layer, it was cut. In this study, the peroneal nerve was preserved without cutting in 5 cases. After lifting the flap to the center of rotation, the flap was moved to the defect, and when it was determined that the flap could be moved without tension, the dissection of the fascia and muscular layer was stopped.

Afterwards, the pressure tourniquet was released to ensure the flap had good blood circulation, and the suture aligned the transferred flap skin-to-skin with the skin of the defect. The donor site, considering the size and condition of the site, was sutured, and the procedure was completed after placing a drainage tube to prevent complications such as venous congestion. The operation site was covered with a transparent cover to check for complications, such as postoperative necrosis around the flap suture, and the flap was protected with splint fixation to strictly limit the range of motion of the ankle joint and bearing of weight.

3. Results

In all cases, flap survival was confirmed at the final outpatient follow-up. The exposed area of the metal plate was well coated, and there was no plate failure due to complete necrosis. In one case (8%), there were color changes and slight blister formation due to venous congestion, but they survived without partial necrosis. Venous congestion and marginal skin necrosis were found in the other case; however, it was healed by secondary healing after antibiotics and daily dressing of the flap wound site, and no additional surgical treatment was required. Additionally, patients with sural nerve damage immediately after surgery had side effects such as hypoesthesia and numbness of the lateral leg in one case (8%); however, they gradually adapted over time, and there was no occurrence of a neuroma.

Three out of four women complained of aesthetic dissatisfaction because the volume of the tunnel through which the skin mirror passed and the skin plate itself were thick. In two cases, defatting was performed to reduce the thickness of the plate while removing the metal plate.

Case 1.

A 22-year-old man visited our emergency center with a pilon fracture caused by a 2 m fall down accident. Radiological examination revealed severe shortening of the tibial joint surface, and emergency surgical treatment using external fixation was performed. Two weeks later, conversion using the MIPO technique for tibia and plate fixation in the fibula was performed (Figure 1A–C). One month after internal fixation, soft tissue defects and metal plate exposure were observed on the medial side of the left ankle (Figure 1D,E).; therefore, a reverse sural artery flap was performed (Figure 2A–D). The size of the flap was 2×3 cm^2, and the length of the flap pedicle was 7 cm. The donor site was sutured, and the donor site and flap survived without complications at the final outpatient follow-up.

Case 2.

A 64-year-old man visited our emergency center with a closed distal tibial fracture caused by a pedestrian TA. At the time of the injury, the swelling around the ankle joint was severe, and there were many bulla in the soft tissue and abrasions. Therefore, internal fixation was performed using the MIPO technique 3 weeks after the injury. In the subsequent wound management process, signs of infection, accompanied by redness, heat, and pain on the medial side of the shin and soft tissue defects, were observed (Figure 3A). Bacterial identification tests on the wound area confirmed the presence of GNR. Under antibiotic maintenance, the wound was in good condition, and a reverse sural artery flap was performed (Figure 3B,C). The size of the flap was 4×4 cm^2, and the length of the flap pedicle was 9 cm. Postoperatively, venous congestion around the flap and marginal skin necrosis were observed (Figure 3D,E). Additional surgical treatment was considered; however, the flap site recovered through secondary healing using antibiotics and daily dressing (Figure 3F).

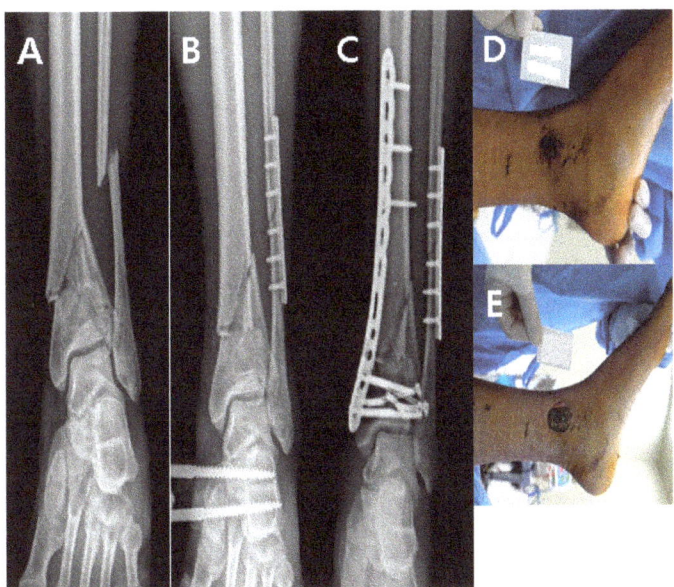

Figure 1. (**A**) Pilon fracture by 2 m F/D. (**B**) For the two-stage operation, EF was done. (**C**) Conversion operation was performed using the MIPO technique. (**D,E**) One month after MIPO, skin defect and plate exposure occurred.

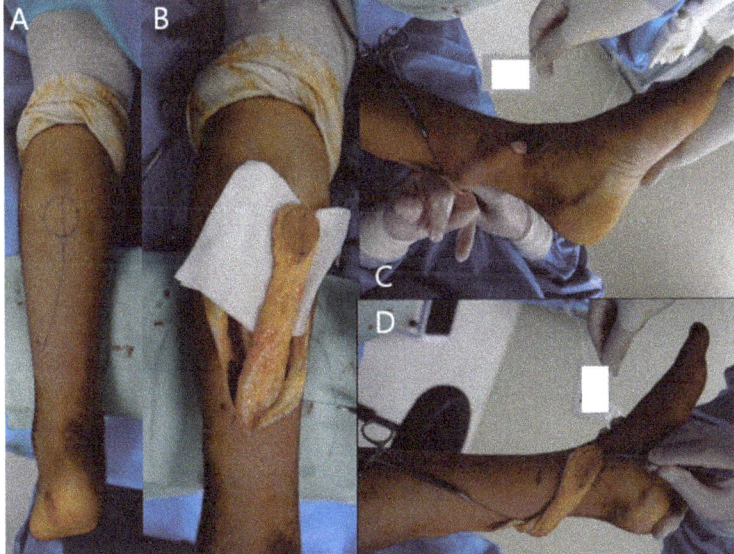

Figure 2. (**A**) A flap on the donor site was designed. (**B**) Drawing the line from the popliteal fossa to the lateral malleolus; the pivot point was set to 10 cm proximal to approximate the vascular axis of the flap. (**C,D**) The flap was passed through the subcutaneous tunnel to the defect site.

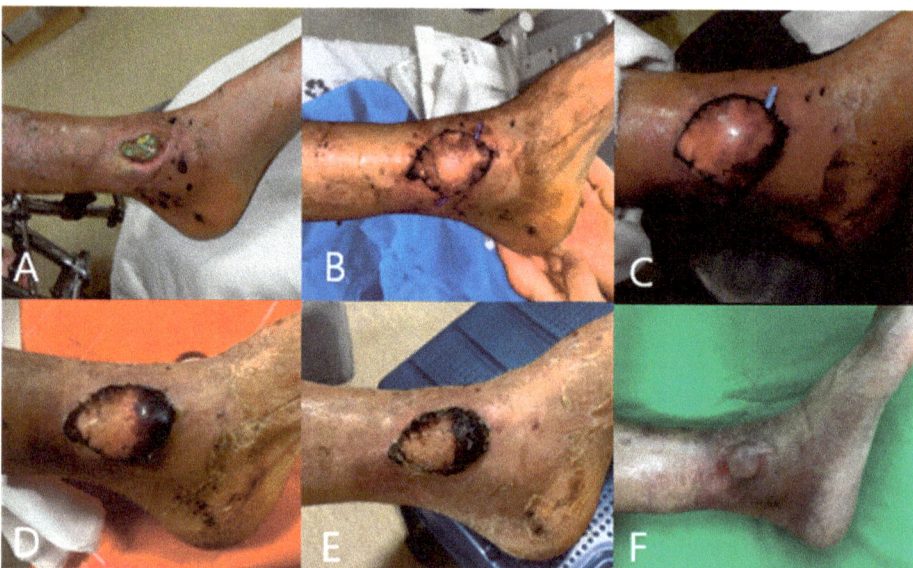

Figure 3. A 64-year-old man with a distal tibia extra-articular fracture by a car accident. (**A**) The wound before doing reverse sural artery flap. (**B–D**) After reversing the sural artery flap, venous congestion and marginal skin necrosis occurred. (**E,F**) Using antibiotics and dressing daily, the flap site wound healed by secondary healing.

4. Discussion

Distal tibial fractures have a high risk of complications such as infection and soft tissue defects due to their complex fracture pattern and the small amount of soft tissue around the ankle joint [19], making it challenging for surgeons to select an appropriate treatment method. Owing to its biomechanical advantage of minimizing damage to the injured soft tissue and maintaining the vascular integrity of the periosteum, MIPO is one of the preferred procedures for treating distal tibial fractures [20–22]. However, when a metal plate is inserted into the inside of the ankle joint, the metal plate and the bone often float without being in close contact with each other, which can cause discomfort and pain (Figure 4). Due to this, skin irritation of the ankle causes soft tissue defects, resulting in complications such as metal plate exposure. The present authors also experienced such soft tissue defects. When a soft tissue defect occurs in which the metal plate is exposed in the distal tibia, the operator has no choice but to suffer embarrassing complications. When the metal plate is exposed at the distal tibia, primary suturing is almost impossible, no matter how small the defect is. It is also not easy to cover the defect by using regional flap or muscle flap transposition.

In this study, a reverse sural artery flap was used, which has been proven to be clinically effective in treating defects in the distal lower extremities, such as the tibia ankle and heel defects [23,24]. Similar to the results of this study, several studies have shown good results with the procedure in the lower limbs [25–27]. This procedure is a myofascial skin flap based on the sural artery network; therefore, unlike the free flap, it does not require microsurgery using a microscope, making the procedure simple. Moreover, it provides stable blood flow to the flap without damaging major arteries of the lower leg, and this whole procedure can be performed by a single operator [28–30]. The authors attempted to suggest some surgical methods to consider during surgical treatment, along with the results of the patient treatment outcomes.

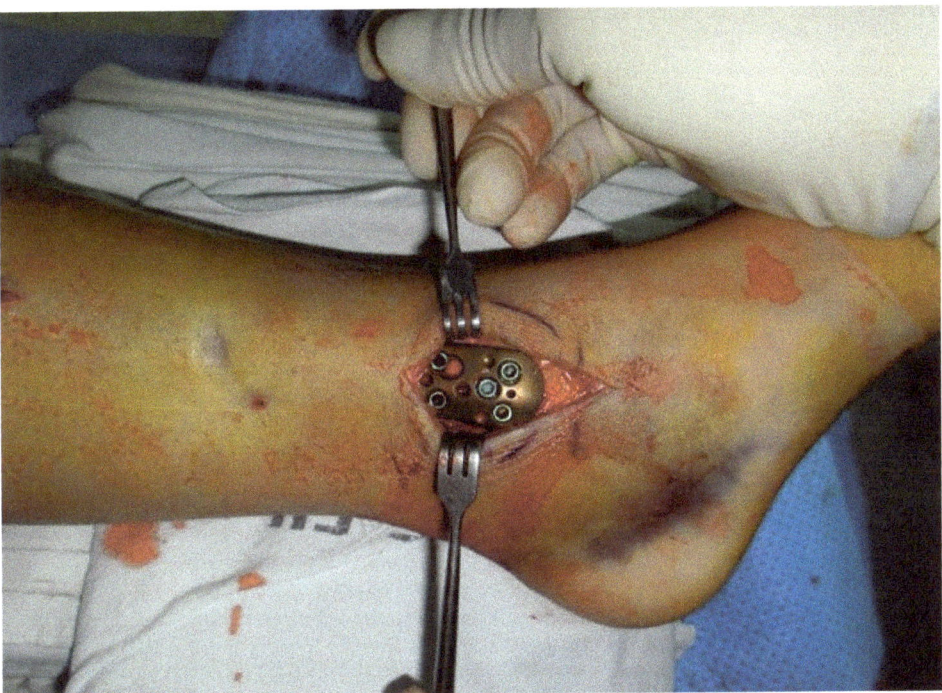

Figure 4. Minimally Invasive Plate Osteosynthesis (MIPO) procedures.

First, the skin plate size must be determined by performing a marginectomy on the exposed metal plate. The size of the defect after the procedure was larger than before the marginectomy. We kept the defect size to be at least 4×3 cm^2 after marginectomy. It was for the sural artery flap (comparatively thick pedicle flap containing subcutaneous fat and fascia), which is being sutured skin-to-skin without tension. The width of the flap diameter is a minimum of 4 cm; it was thought that if it was smaller than this, it would be difficult to place the flap on the defect without tension.

The superficial sural artery originates from the proximal popliteal artery anastomoses with the venous and neuroskin perforators of the peroneal artery approximately 3–5 cm proximal to the lateral malleolus. Through this anastomosis, retrograde blood flows back into the sural artery. These venous skin perforators play a critical role in the blood circulation of the flap [24,31,32]. Considering this, when performing reverse sural artery flap, we set a pivot point approximately 3–5 cm proximal to the last venous and neuroskin perforators. However, the authors set 8–10 cm points for saving the perforated area that is as close to the plate as possible, and the plate can be applied to the more proximal part, near the center of the back of the inferior part, and the donor part can be completed through primary suturing without partial or full-thickness skin grafting. This was to allow the plate to move to the defect without twisting the plate-receiving mirror. The peroneal artery runs along the fascia, and therefore, fascia must be included to facilitate the supply of the retrograde reverse sural artery flap. The suprafascial network plays an especially important role, and venous drainage is accomplished by a connection between the subcutaneous lesser saphenous vein and the deep-lying Venae comitantes of the sural nerve.

In contrast, the reverse sural artery flap is known to have some disadvantages, such as venous congestion, necrosis of the soft tissue around the flap suture, and neuroma from sural nerve damage. According to Hasegawa et al., venous congestion is a common complication of the reverse sural artery flap, which is caused by the presence of valves in the deep venous system that obstructs retrograde venous blood flow. If the flap is not elevated with the fascia during the operation, soft tissue necrosis around the flap suture site may occur [31]. To prevent such complications, several studies have reported that pedicle width plays an important role in flap survival. Sugg et al. recommended a pedicle width of a minimum of 4 cm to preserve the venous drainage and Colossus at the Adipofascial skin plate containing subcutaneous tissue on the skin mirror and improve flap survival rate during reverse sural artery flap [33]. Considering that the thin, soft tissue and flap of the distal tibial defect must pass through the subcutaneous tunnel to the defect, the authors used a 3 cm width of the subcutaneous tissue for the flap pedicle and an inferior width of the fascia of the skin is 5 cm. This method reduces the volume of the flap diameter, facilitates passage of the flap through the tunnel and, at the same time, secures the stability of blood circulation. The fascia part of the plate was also 1 cm wider than the skin and made a colossus.

When making a subcutaneous tunnel through which the flap pedicle passes, it is expanded wide enough to pass two fingers so that the flap pedicle is not pushed. The distal part of the flap was set in a teardrop shape, and a 2 cm incision was made at the proximal part of the connection line so that the flap can be sutured without pressure and tension when the flap and the skin of the defect are sutured.

The authors found that the flap survived in the previous case, partial necrosis along the skin suture boundary occurred in one case, which healed with the use of prophylactic antibiotics and dressings alone, and venous congestion occurred in one case from the day after surgery. Discoloration occurred but healed well with Colossus alone without the use of medical leeches. In the authors' case, the better results compared to other studies were flap coverage performed in the same setting of plate exposure occurring after minimally invasive metal plate fixation, and the size of the flap was relatively small. In addition to the fact that it was in the site, it is thought that the fact that the authors designed and colossalized the flaps and provided technical modifications also helped.

This is thought to be caused by insufficient dissection of the flap, which left out some fascia during flap elevation. Each operator performs reverse sural artery flap surgery in a slightly different manner, depending on the patient's clinical experience. If the sural nerve is cut during surgery, the patient complains of muscle weakness in the ankle, paresthesia, or pain in the distal lower extremities. According to Touam et al., there are sometimes cases that require additional surgical treatment due to the development of neuroma [34]. The authors sought to preserve possible affected peroneal nerves during flap coverage. However, in the remaining cases, the peroneal nerve migrated to the upper fascia relatively early during flap colossus, necessitating fasciotomy for nerve preservation, and nerve preservation was abandoned due to concerns about flap blood circulation and disconnected. A nerve amputation patient had numbness and cramping in the lateral foot, but this patient appeared to improve over time and did not develop a nerve amputation neuroma.

The limitations of this study are as follows: First, given that the number of cases was small and this was a retrospective study based on medical records and radiological data, more studies based on a larger number of cases are needed to confirm that the reverse sural artery flap is indeed an effective treatment for patients who underwent internal fixation through the MIPO procedure. The fact that this study did not mention a correlation with the patient's underlying disease, such as the presence of vascular diseases that may affect the survival rate of the flap, should also be supplemented in future studies.

However, for the treatment of metal plate exposures that occur after MIPO procedures for peripheral tibial fractures, retrograde superficial sural artery flaps may be an effective treatment. This study is meaningful in that it suggested a surgical technique which could improve outcomes and success rates.

5. Conclusions

Metal plate exposure treatments that occur after distal tibial fractures that have been treated with the MIPO procedure can be successfully treated with a retrograde superficial sural artery flap, and it is believed that more successful flap survival can be achieved by applying several surgical techniques during the flap.

Author Contributions: Conceptualization, J.Y.L.; methodology, H.J.L.; software, S.h.Y.; validation, J.H.R.; formal analysis, H.T.K.; investigation, B.H.L.; resources, H.S.K.; data curation, S.H.Y.; writing—original draft preparation, S.H.K.; writing—review and editing, Y.K.L.; visualization, H.J.L.; supervision, J.Y.L.; project administration, S.H.K.; funding acquisition, J.Y.L. All authors have read and agreed to the published version of the manuscript.

Funding: This study was supported by research fund from Chosun University, 2022.

Institutional Review Board Statement: The study was conducted in accordance with the Declaration of Helsinki and approved by the Institutional Review Board and Human Research Ethics Committee of Chosun University Hospital (IRB No. 2022-02-005-001).

Informed Consent Statement: Informed consent was obtained from all subjects involved in the study.

Data Availability Statement: Data sharing is not applicable to this article because there were no datasets made or analyzed during this study.

Conflicts of Interest: The authors declare no conflict of interest.

References

1. Sitnik, A.; Beletsky, A.; Schelkun, S. Intra-articular fractures of the distal tibia: Current concepts of management. *EFORT Open Rev.* **2017**, *2*, 352–361. [CrossRef]
2. Rushdi, I.; Che-Ahmad, A.; Abdul-Ghani, K.; Mohd-Rus, R. Surgical management of distal tibia fracture: Towards an outcome-based treatment algorithm. *Malays. Orthop. J.* **2020**, *14*, 57.
3. Barış, A.; Çirci, E.; Demirci, Z.; Öztürkmen, Y. Minimally invasive medial plate osteosynthesis in tibial pilon fractures: Longterm functional and radiological outcomes. *Acta Orthop. Traumatol. Turc.* **2020**, *54*, 20. [CrossRef] [PubMed]
4. Im, G.-I.; Tae, S.-K. Distal metaphyseal fractures of tibia: A prospective randomized trial of closed reduction and intramedullary nail versus open reduction and plate and screws fixation. *J. Trauma Acute Care Surg.* **2005**, *59*, 1219–1223. [CrossRef]
5. Ekman, E.; Lehtimäki, K.; Syvänen, J.; Saltychev, M. Comparison between nailing and plating in the treatment of distal tibial fractures: A meta-analysis. *Scand. J. Surg.* **2021**, *110*, 115–122. [CrossRef]
6. Kuo, L.T.; Chi, C.C.; Chuang, C.H. Surgical interventions for treating distal tibial metaphyseal fractures in adults. *Cochrane Database Syst. Rev.* **2015**, *2015*, CD010261. [CrossRef] [PubMed]
7. Vidović, D.; Matejčić, A.; Ivica, M.; Jurišić, D.; Elabjer, E.; Bakota, B. Minimally-invasive plate osteosynthesis in distal tibial fractures: Results and complications. *Injury* **2015**, *46*, S96–S99. [CrossRef] [PubMed]
8. Biz, C.; Angelini, A.; Zamperetti, M.; Marzotto, F.; Sperotto, S.P.; Carniel, D.; Iacobellis, C.; Ruggieri, P. Medium-long-term radiographic and clinical outcomes after surgical treatment of intra articular tibial pilon fractures by three different techniques. *BioMed Res. Int.* **2018**, *2018*, 6054021. [CrossRef] [PubMed]
9. Toogood, P.; Huang, A.; Siebuhr, K.; Miclau, T. Minimally invasive plate osteosynthesis versus conventional open insertion techniques for osteosynthesis. *Injury* **2018**, *49*, S19–S23. [CrossRef]
10. Wang, C.; Huang, Q.; Lu, D.; Wang, Q.; Ma, T.; Zhang, K.; Li, Z. A clinical comparative study of intramedullary nailing and minimally invasive plate osteosynthesis for extra-articular distal tibia fractures. *Am. J. Transl. Res.* **2023**, *15*, 1996.
11. Kang, H.; Song, J.-K.; Rho, J.Y.; Lee, J.; Choi, J.; Choi, S. Minimally invasive plate osteosynthesis (MIPO) for mid-shaft fracture of the tibia (AO/OTA classification 42): A retrospective study. *Ann. Med. Surg.* **2020**, *60*, 408–412. [CrossRef]
12. Katı, Y.A.; Öken, Ö.F.; Yıldırım, A.Ö.; Köse, Ö.; Ünal, M. May minimally invasive plate osteosynthesis be an alternative to intramedullary nailing in selected spiral oblique and spiral wedge tibial shaft fractures? *Jt. Dis. Relat. Surg.* **2020**, *31*, 494. [CrossRef] [PubMed]
13. Kwan, Y.H.; Decruz, J.; Premchand, A.X.; Khan, S.A. Complex distal tibia fractures treated with multi-planar external fixation-a single center experience. *Int. J. Burn. Trauma* **2022**, *12*, 98.
14. Jha, A.K.; Bhattacharyya, A.; Kumar, S.; Ghosh, T.K. Evaluation of results of minimally invasive plate osteosynthesis (MIPO) of distal tibial fractures in adults. *J. Indian Med. Assoc.* **2012**, *110*, 823–824. [PubMed]
15. Lau, T.; Leung, F.; Chan, C.; Chow, S. Wound complication of minimally invasive plate osteosynthesis in distal tibia fractures. *Int. Orthop.* **2008**, *32*, 697–703. [CrossRef] [PubMed]
16. Rich, M.D.; Mazloom, S.E.; Sorenson, T.J.; Phillips, M.A. Management of surgical soft tissue defects of the lower extremities. *Dermatol. Online J.* **2021**, *27*. [CrossRef] [PubMed]
17. Chaput, B.; Meresse, T.; Bekara, F.; Grolleau, J.; Gangloff, D.; Gandolfi, S.; Herlin, C. Lower limb perforator flaps: Current concept. *Ann. Chir. Plast. Esthet.* **2020**, *65*, 496–516. [CrossRef] [PubMed]
18. Clivatti, G.M.; Nascimento, B.B.; Ribeiro, R.D.A.; Milcheski, D.A.; Ayres, A.M.; Gemperli, R. Reverse sural flap for lower limb reconstruction. *Acta Ortop. Bras.* **2022**, *30*, e248774. [CrossRef]

19. McFerran, M.A.; Smith, S.W.; Boulas, H.J.; Schwartz, H.S. Complications encountered in the treatment of pilon fractures. *J. Orthop. Trauma* **1992**, *6*, 195–200. [CrossRef]
20. Khoury, A.; Liebergall, M.; London, E.; Mosheiff, R. Percutaneous plating of distal tibial fractures. *Foot Ankle Int.* **2002**, *23*, 818–824. [CrossRef]
21. Krackhardt, T.; Dilger, J.; Flesch, I.; Höntzsch, D.; Eingartner, C.; Weise, K. Fractures of the distal tibia treated with closed reduction and minimally invasive plating. *Arch. Orthop. Trauma Surg.* **2005**, *125*, 87–94. [CrossRef]
22. Moldovan, F.; Gligor, A.; Bataga, T. Dimensional optimization in screw fixation for personalized treatment of the tibial plateau fracture. In *International Conference Interdisciplinarity in Engineering*; Springer: Cham, Switzerland, 2021; pp. 772–783.
23. Donski, P.K.; Fogdestam, I. Distally based fasciocutaneous flap from the sural region. *Scand. J. Plast. Reconstr. Surg.* **1983**, *17*, 191–196. [CrossRef] [PubMed]
24. Masquelet, A.; Romana, M.; Wolf, G. Skin island flaps supplied by the vascular axis of the sensitive superficial nerves: Anatomic study and clinical experience in the leg. *Plast. Reconstr. Surg.* **1992**, *89*, 1115–1121. [CrossRef]
25. Han, S.-H.; Hong, I.-T.; Choi, S.; Kim, M. Reverse Superficial Sural Artery Flap for the Reconstruction of Soft Tissue Defect Accompanied by Fracture of the Lower Extremity. *J. Korean Orthop. Assoc.* **2020**, 253–260. [CrossRef]
26. Muppireddy, S.; Srikanth, R. Distally based reverse sural artery flap as an interpolation flap. *Int. J. Res. Orthop.* **2017**, *3*, 61–65. [CrossRef]
27. Choi, Y.R.; Lee, S.Y.; Lee, S.C.; Lee, H.J.; Han, S.H. Reverse Superficial Sural artery flap for the Reconstruction of Soft Tissue Defect on Posterior side of heel exposing Achilles tendon. *J. Korean Soc. Surg. Hand* **2012**, *21*, 159–164.
28. Costa-Ferreira, A.; Reis, J.; Pinho, C.; Martins, A.; Amarante, J. The distally based island superficial sural artery flap: Clinical experience with 36 flaps. *Ann. Plast. Surg.* **2001**, *46*, 308–313. [CrossRef] [PubMed]
29. Follmar, K.E.; Baccarani, A.; Baumeister, S.P.; Levin, L.S.; Erdmann, D. The distally based sural flap. *Plast. Reconstr. Surg.* **2007**, *119*, 138e–148e. [CrossRef]
30. Yilmaz, M.; Karatas, O.; Barutcu, A. The distally based superficial sural artery island flap: Clinical experiences and modifications. *Plast. Reconstr. Surg.* **1998**, *102*, 2358–2367. [CrossRef]
31. Hasegawa, M.; Torii, S.; Katoh, H.; Esaki, S. The distally based superficial sural artery flap. *Plast. Reconstr. Surg.* **1994**, *93*, 1012–1020. [CrossRef]
32. Singh, S.; Naasan, A. Use of distally based superficial sural island artery flaps in acute open fractures of the lower leg. *Ann. Plast. Surg.* **2001**, *47*, 505–510. [CrossRef] [PubMed]
33. Sugg, K.B.; Schaub, T.A.; Concannon, M.J.; Cederna, P.S.; Brown, D.L. The reverse superficial sural artery flap revisited for complex lower extremity and foot reconstruction. *Plast. Reconstr. Surg. Glob. Open* **2015**, *3*, e519. [CrossRef] [PubMed]
34. Touam, C.; Rostoucher, P.; Bhatia, A.; Oberlin, C. Comparative study of two series of distally based fasciocutaneous flaps for coverage of the lower one-fourth of the leg, the ankle, and the foot. *Plast. Reconstr. Surg.* **2001**, *107*, 383–392. [CrossRef] [PubMed]

Disclaimer/Publisher's Note: The statements, opinions and data contained in all publications are solely those of the individual author(s) and contributor(s) and not of MDPI and/or the editor(s). MDPI and/or the editor(s) disclaim responsibility for any injury to people or property resulting from any ideas, methods, instructions or products referred to in the content.

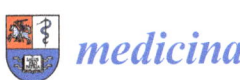

Article

A Comparative Analysis of Fasciotomy Results in Children and Adults Affected by Crush-Induced Acute Kidney Injury following the Kahramanmaraş Earthquakes

Mustafa Yalın * and Fatih Gölgelioğlu

Department of Orthopaedics and Traumatology, Elazığ Fethi Sekin City Hospital, Elazığ 23050, Turkey; fatihgolgelioglu@gmail.com
* Correspondence: mustiyalin1988@gmail.com

Abstract: *Background and Objectives*: The current study aims to determine the impact of fasciotomy on mortality and morbidity in children and adults with crush-related AKI following the 2023 Kahramanmaraş earthquakes. *Materials and Methods*: The study included individuals who had suffered crush injuries after the 2023 Kahramanmaraş earthquakes and were identified as having an acute kidney injury (AKI). Patients with an AKI were divided into two groups based on age: those under 18 years and those over 18 years. A comparative analysis was conducted between the mortality and morbidity rates of patients who underwent fasciotomy and those who did not. Disseminated intravascular coagulopathy (DIC), sepsis, and adult respiratory distress syndrome (ARDS) have all been identified as contributors to morbidity. *Results*: The study was conducted with a total of 40 patients (21 males and 19 females) aged between 4 and 83 years. A total of 21 patients underwent fasciotomy, and the patients underwent varying numbers of fasciotomy, ranging from 0 to 11. The mortality rate was 12.5%, corresponding to five adult patients. No instances of mortality were reported in the paediatric cohort. The application of fasciotomy in instances of crush-induced AKI did not result in elevated levels of mortality in either the paediatric or adult demographic. Within the adult population, a substantial difference in the duration of dialysis was observed between individuals who underwent fasciotomy and those who did not. A statistically significant increase in the number of fasciotomy incisions was observed in patients diagnosed with sepsis compared with those without sepsis. The study found a significant positive correlation between the number of fasciotomy incisions and dialysis days. *Conclusions*: Neither adult nor paediatric patients with crush-induced AKI showed an increased risk of death after fasciotomy. The number of fasciotomy incisions significantly correlated with the development of sepsis. Despite experiencing delays in hospital admission for paediatric patients, the incidence of both crush syndrome and mortality rates among children remained relatively low.

Keywords: crush-related acute kidney injury; fasciotomy; morbidity; earthquake

Citation: Yalın, M.; Gölgelioğlu, F. A Comparative Analysis of Fasciotomy Results in Children and Adults Affected by Crush-Induced Acute Kidney Injury following the Kahramanmaraş Earthquakes. *Medicina* **2023**, *59*, 1593. https://doi.org/10.3390/medicina59091593

Academic Editor: Woo Jong Kim

Received: 9 August 2023
Revised: 29 August 2023
Accepted: 1 September 2023
Published: 3 September 2023

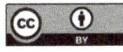

Copyright: © 2023 by the authors. Licensee MDPI, Basel, Switzerland. This article is an open access article distributed under the terms and conditions of the Creative Commons Attribution (CC BY) license (https://creativecommons.org/licenses/by/4.0/).

1. Introduction

On 6 February 2023, Kahramanmaraş, southeastern Turkey, experienced two devastating earthquakes. The first earthquake had a magnitude of 7.7 on the Richter scale, followed by a second earthquake nine hours later, with a magnitude of 7.6. These back-to-back earthquakes were accompanied by over 1000 aftershocks, some of which exceeded a magnitude of 6. The impact of these consecutive earthquakes has been unprecedented in recent Turkish history, causing widespread destruction and resulting in a current estimate of 35,000 reported fatalities and 105,000 injured individuals within one week of the earthquakes [1]. In the aftermath of the earthquake, the widespread destruction of medical facilities posed a significant challenge to delivering immediate healthcare to the affected population. Consequently, a considerable number of patients must be transferred to hospitals located on the periphery of the affected area. Notably, the emergency department (ED) of our institution has emerged as a vital hub for receiving a substantial influx of patients from neighbouring provinces. This strategic measure played a pivotal role in mitigating the burden on the strained local health system, thereby enabling the hospital to allocate approximately 1000 beds exclusively to address the urgent needs of earthquake victims.

Earthquake catastrophes not only lead to a significant number of instantaneous fatalities due to injury to essential organs, but also bring with them a cluster of severely injured victims, in whom crush incidents and prolonged entrapment of extremities are prevalent types of trauma. When a limb is trapped under debris, muscle cells experience mechanical strain, leading to the release of their cellular contents [2]. Increased intracompartmental pressure may result from an increase in both interstitial and intracellular fluid volumes. When the pressure surpasses the capillary perfusion pressure, which is approximately 30 mmHg, muscular veins collapse. Furthermore, tissue oxygenation is disrupted if the pressure exceeds the diastolic blood pressure threshold. Consequently, the resulting ischemic damage causes necrosis in the muscles, known as rhabdomyolysis, as well as in nerves [3]. According to estimates, acute compartment syndrome may lead to muscle necrosis in up to 35% of patients within 2 h following the injury [4]. The consensus in the medical community is that prompt initiation of early fasciotomy is crucial to achieve the best outcomes in cases of compartment syndrome [5–10]. Disruption of renal blood flow due to hypovolemia and the accumulation of nephrotoxic deposits increase the likelihood of acute kidney injury (AKI) in patients with crush injury [11]. In this already problematic scenario, fasciotomy's open incision might worsen preexisting coagulopathy and increase the risk of death from sepsis. Dialysis for patients with an AKI will be more difficult, and the risk of an AKI will increase as a result of these factors. The current study aimed to determine the impact of fasciotomy on mortality and morbidity in children and adults with crush-related AKIs following the Kahramanmaraş earthquakes in Turkey.

2. Materials and Methods

Injuries from the 2023 Kahramanmaraş earthquakes were the focus of the current retrospective investigation conducted at a single centre. The present study was approved by the local ethics committee (Approval Number: 2023/07-12). In accordance with established ethical guidelines, written informed consent was obtained from all participants, thereby ensuring voluntary participation and authorisation for the utilisation of their anonymised data in the current study. The study strictly adhered to the principles outlined in the Declaration of Helsinki governing the ethical conduct of clinical research. Stringent measures were implemented throughout the study to maintain patient confidentiality and to safeguard the privacy of their personal information. The study included individuals who had suffered crush injuries subsequent to an earthquake and were identified by experts as having an AKI based on the analysis of biochemical markers. The information for this research was gathered through a comprehensive review of existing medical files. X34 (earthquake victim) identification was issued to individuals who self-reported injuries sustained during the earthquake or were transported via ambulance from a nearby province. Disseminated intravascular coagulopathy (DIC), sepsis, and adult respiratory distress syndrome (ARDS) have all been identified as contributors to morbidity. Patients with a prior medical condition of chronic renal failure or an AKI resulting from unrelated factors were excluded from the study. Additionally, individuals with injuries or circumstances that could not be directly attributed to earthquakes were excluded. Patients diagnosed with an AKI were stratified into two distinct age cohorts: those below and those above the age of 18. A comparative analysis was conducted within each age group and between the two age groups. The objective of the current study was to conduct a comparative analysis of the demographic characteristics, biochemistry profiles, and clinical outcomes of patients who were diagnosed with an AKI, with a specific focus on whether they underwent fasciotomy. A comparative analysis was conducted on the mortality and morbidity rates of patients who underwent fasciotomies and those who did not. The decision of whether or not to proceed with a fasciotomy operation was made by in-clinic evaluations conducted by physicians with a minimum of five years of expertise in trauma medicine.

These assessments included both the viability of the affected limb and the cost–benefit analysis associated with performing the fasciotomy. Patients who received emergency fasciotomy upon initial presentation, as well as those who were eligible for fasciotomy but needed careful monitoring, were admitted to the intensive care unit. The patients were closely monitored by nephrology and intensive care physicians, with regular visits from orthopaedic doctors to assess their circulation and wound healing. The fasciotomy procedures involved the performing of two wide incisions, one on the medial side and the other on the lateral side, for the cruris and thigh. Additionally, two incisions were made in the dorsal region of the foot, specifically in the second and fourth web intervals. A wide volar incision was performed on the forearm, while three incisions were made in the dorsal region of the hand, specifically in the second and fourth web intervals and the tenar region. In the current study, all individuals who had fasciotomy were subjected to vacuum-assisted debridement and irrigation at regular 3-day intervals. Additionally, the wound lip approximation method, aimed at facilitating quicker closure of the wound lips, was performed during each debridement process. In cases where primary delayed closure was not achievable due to skin retraction, full-thickness skin grafting was scheduled for all patients. Support for this procedure was sought from the plastic surgery department. Wound culture samples were routinely taken from patients during the debridement process to investigate suspected infections at the wound site or any deterioration observed during clinical follow-up. The results of these samples were then referred to the infectious diseases department for consultation. In individuals diagnosed with foot drop or radial nerve palsy, the use of splints and orthoses was promptly initiated in order to maintain joint neutrality and stability. Based on the outcomes of in-clinic assessments, the decision was made to proceed with amputation of the limb that experienced a loss of viability.

2.1. Acute Kidney Injury Definition

Owing to the retrospective nature of the study, conventional AKI criteria were not used [12]. In the case of crush-related acute kidney injury, the victim must have had a crush injury and have shown at least one of the following symptoms: serum potassium > 6 mEq/L, phosphorus > 8 mg/dL, or calcium < 8 mg/dL; oliguria (urine production < 400 mL/day); blood urea nitrogen > 40 mg/dL; serum creatinine > 2 mg/dL; and serum uric acid > 8 mg/dL [13].

2.2. Definitions of Disseminated Intravascular Coagulation (DIC), Acute Respiratory Distress Syndrome (ARDS), and Sepsis

The diagnosis of DIC was determined by integrating clinical observations with laboratory measurements [14]. The definitive diagnosis of DIC can only be established when there is a recognised primary ailment that has been determined to be linked with DIC and when the clinical manifestations and symptoms align with this underlying medical condition. Common results in routine laboratory tests include thrombocytopenia as well as a rapid decline in the number of platelets; unusual monitoring assessments such as prothrombin time (PT) or activated partial thromboplastin time (aPTT); and a significant increase in markers of the formation of fibrin and subsequent collapse, such as D-dimer or other forms of fibrin products of degradation [14]. Thromboembolism affecting larger blood vessels will manifest with symptoms consistent with the blockage of blood flow. Another common observation is the occurrence of extensive bleeding from mucosal tissue, such as the gingiva, nose, or digestive tract, as well as from the insertion sites of indwelling catheters [15]. Patients suspected of having DIC were referred for haematology consultations as part of their intensive care unit (ICU) follow-up. The final diagnoses were established in collaboration with the haematology department.

ARDS is characterised by sudden hypoxemia and bilateral pulmonary oedema caused by increased permeability of the alveolocapillary membrane. ARDS was defined clinically by the Berlin description (panel 1) and included stages that assess mortality risk. However, there is no singular test available to definitively diagnose or rule out ARDS [16]. The pulmonology department diagnosed and monitored ARDS during the ICU follow-up.

Sepsis is characterised as a severe condition in which the body's response to infection becomes uncontrolled, leading to life-threatening dysfunction of organs. The clinical criteria for sepsis consisted of suspected or confirmed infection and an unexpected rise of a minimum of two Sequential Organ Failure Assessment (SOFA) points, which served as an indicator of failure of the organs [17]. The diagnosis of sepsis was established by the analysis of culture samples obtained during vacuum-assisted debridements, in conjunction with an assessment of the patients' clinical condition, in collaboration with the infectious diseases department.

2.3. Statistics

Statistical analyses of the study's findings were conducted using IBM SPSS Statistics 22 software (Version 22.0. Armonk, NY, USA: IBM Corp; 2013; IBM SPSS, Elazığ, Turkey). The normality of the parameters was assessed using the Shapiro–Wilk test. The study employed both descriptive statistical techniques, such as means, standard deviations, and frequencies, as well as inferential statistical methods. Specifically, the Student t test was used to compare quantitative data between two groups with normally distributed parameters, while the Mann–Whitney U test was employed to compare non-normally distributed parameters between the two groups. Fisher's exact test was used to compare the qualitative datasets. Spearman's rho correlation analysis was employed to examine the associations among variables that did not adhere to a normal distribution. Statistical significance was set at a significance level of $p < 0.05$.

3. Results

The current study was conducted with a total of 40 patients: 21 (52.5%) males and 19 (47.5%) females, aged between four and 83 years, with a mean age of 32.63 ± 18.99 years. The study included a total of 40 participants, with 10 being paediatric patients and 30 being adult patients. The children's ages ranged from 4 to 17 years, with a mean age of 10.6 ± 4.48 years. The age range of the adult participants in the study was 19 to 83 years, with a mean age of 39.97 ± 15.98. Table 1 represents the descriptive characteristics of the participants. A total of 21 patients (15 adults and 6 children) underwent fasciotomy, and the patients underwent varying numbers of fasciotomy, ranging from 0 to 11, with a mean of 2.43 ± 3.16. All paediatric patients who underwent a fasciotomy procedure were diagnosed with compartment syndrome upon arrival at the ED, prompting the immediate initiation of an emergency fasciotomy procedure. All fasciotomy operations conducted on paediatric patients included cruris and thigh fasciotomy procedures for the lower extremities. Fasciotomy procedures were performed on three adult patients during their ICU follow-up, after discussions held within the clinic. Emergency fasciotomy was performed in 12 adult patients who presented to the ED. Additional fasciotomies were subsequently performed in 5 patients due to the development of compartment syndrome in other extremities during follow-up. We admitted one patient for further treatment with below-knee amputation. Additionally, we performed pinky toe amputation in two patients due to the development of necrosis during follow-up. The mortality rate was 12.5%, corresponding to five adult patients. All deaths occurred within the initial week of ICU follow-up. The causes of death were cardiac arrest in three patients, cardiac arrest and DIC in one patient, and sepsis and DIC in one patient.

Table 1. The distribution of general characteristics of the patients. DIC: Disseminated intravascular coagulation. ARDS: Acute respiratory distress syndrome.

		Min–Max	Mean ± SD (Median)
Age		4–83	32.63 ± 18.99
		N	%
Gender	Male	21	52.5
	Female	19	47.5
Time-to-admission from the earthquake (TAE) (hours)		14–144	44.5 ± 25.87 (36)
Time under the debris (TUD) (hours)		2–40	11.68 ± 8.29 (9.5)
The number of fasciotomy		0–11	2.43 ± 3.16 (1)
Fasciotomy	Absent	19	47.5
	Present	21	52.5
Death	Absent	35	87.5
	Present	5	12.5
The reason for death (n = 5)	Cardiac arrest	3	60
	DIC and Cardiac Arrest	1	20
	Sepsis and DIC	1	20
Nerve Injury	Peroneal nerve injury	23	57.5
	Ulnar nerve injury	8	20
	Radial nerve injury	8	20
	Medain nerve injury	7	17.5
Dialysis day		0–30	5.15 ± 6.72 (3)
DIC	Absent	33	82.5
	Present	7	17.5
ARDS	Absent	32	80
	Present	8	20
Sepsis	Absent	32	80
	Present	8	20
Amputation	Absent	38	95
	Present	2	5

The study was conducted in two groups: 10 (25%) children and 30 (75%) adults. In the paediatric population, hospital admission time varied from 18 to 144 h, with a mean of 65.1 ± 36.18 and a median of 60. The hospital admission time for adults varied from 14 to 70 h, with a mean of 37.63 ± 17.29 and a median of 32. The time to admission from an earthquake (TAE) was notably greater in the paediatric population than in adults ($p = 0.011$, $p < 0.05$). However, no instances of mortality have been reported in the paediatric cohort. No statistically significant difference was observed between the groups in terms of the time under debris (TUD) and number of fasciotomies. Additionally, the most frequently occurring nerve injury in both groups was peroneal nerve injury (Table 2).

Table 2. The comparison of children and adults regarding general characteristics.

		Children	Adults	P
		(Min–Max)–(Mean ± SD (Median))	(Min–Max)–(Mean ± SD (Median))	
Age		(4–17)–(10.6 ± 4.48)	(19–83)–(39.97 ± 15.98)	[1] 0.000 *
		n (%)	n (%)	
Gender	Male	6 (60%)	15 (50%)	[2] 0.429
	Female	4 (40%)	15 (50%)	
Time-to-admission from the earthquake (TAE) (hours)		(18–144)–(65.1 ± 36.18 (60))	(14–70)–(37.63 ± 17.29 (32))	[3] 0.011 *
Time under the debris (TUD) (hours)		(8–40)–(16.9 ± 12.16 (10))	(2–30)–(9.93 ± 5.82 (8.5))	[3] 0.067
The number of fasciotomy		(0–11)–(3.9 ± 4.33 (2))	(0–10)–(1.93 ± 2.57 (0.5))	[3] 0.261
		n (%)	n (%)	
Fasciotomy	Absent	4 (40%)	15 (50%)	[2] 0.429
	Present	6 (60%)	15 (50%)	
Death	Absent	10 (100%)	25 (83.3%)	-
	Present	0 (0%)	5 (16.7%)	
The reason for death	Cardiac arrest	-	3 (60%)	-
	DIC and Cardiac Arrest	-	1 (20%)	
	Sepsis and DIC	-	1 (20%)	
Nerve Injury	Peroneal nerve injury	6 (60%)	17 (56.7%)	[2] 1.000
	Ulnar nerve injury	1 (10%)	7 (23.3%)	-
	Radial nerve injury	0 (0%)	8 (27.7%)	-
	Medain nerve injury	0 (0%)	7 (23.3%)	-

[1] Student *t* Test, [2] Fisher's Exact Test, [3] Mann–Whitney U Test * $p < 0.05$.

Upon comparing both groups in relation to morbidity, it was observed that the children displayed two instances of DIC and one instance of sepsis. However, adults displayed five instances of DIC, eight distances of ARDS and seven instances of sepsis, although statistical significance could not be determined owing to an inadequate sample size (Table 3).

Analysis of both groups, specifically those who underwent fasciotomy and those who did not, showed no statistically significant difference between the patients who underwent fasciotomy and those who did not, with respect to the manifestation of morbidity criteria such as ARDS and DIC in both groups (Table 4). In the paediatric group, the number of dialysis days ranged from 0 to 10 with a mean of 3.83 ± 4.49, whereas none of the patients who did not undergo fasciotomy required dialysis. Within the adult cohort, the duration of dialysis in patients who had fasciotomy varied from 2 to 30 days, with an average of 9.93 ± 7.47 days. In contrast, non-fasciotomised patients experienced a dialysis duration ranging from 0 to 17 days, with a mean of 2.27 ± 4.61 days. In the adult demographic, there was a notable difference in the duration of dialysis between individuals who underwent fasciotomy and those who did not ($p < 0.05$) (Table 4).

Table 3. The comparison of paediatric and adult morbidity and serum parameters.

		Children	Adults	P
		(Min–Max)–(Mean ± SD (Median))	(Min–Max)–(Mean ± SD (Median))	
Dialysis day		(0–10)–(2.3 ± 3.89 (0))	(0–30)–(6.1 ± 7.24 (4))	[1] 0.085
		n (%)	n (%)	
DIC	Absent	8 (80%)	25 (83.3%)	[2] 0.572
	Present	2 (20%)	5 (16.7%)	
ARDS	Absent	10 (100%)	22 (73.3%)	-
	Present	0 (0%)	8 (26.7%)	
Sepsis	Absent	9 (90%)	23 (76.7%)	-
	Present	1 (10%)	7 (23.3%)	
Amputation	Absent	10 (100%)	28 (93.3%)	-
	Present	0 (0%)	2 (6.7%)	
Serum CPK (median)		(18,790–78,090)–(34,268.1 ± 18,756.8 (28,172))	(2609–56,421)–(23,756.9 ± 12,105.17 (22,943.5))	[1] 0.092
Serum LDH (median)		(438–6986)–(2528.9 ± 2096.58 (1843))	(311–8427)–(1990.3 ± 1950.03 (1203))	[1] 0.399
Serum AST (median)		(74–4415)–(1833.6 ± 1823.47 (943.5))	(27–2618)–(651.63 ± 634.68 (553.5))	[1] 0.070
Serum BUN (median)		(18–122)–(59.9 ± 41.49 (43.5))	(9–221)–(74.23 ± 44.47 (66.5))	[1] 0.295
Serum Creatinine (median)		(0.2–2.3)–(1.04 ± 0.82 (0.6))	(0.27–5.36)–(1.9 ± 1.49 (1.4))	[1] 0.055
Serum Calcium		(5.7–9.9)–(7.6 ± 1.2)	(5.8–9.8)–(7.62 ± 1.01)	[3] 0.966
Serum Phosphor (median)		(3.18–9.09)–(5.49 ± 2.28 (4.4))	(2.18–13.45)–(5.32 ± 2.62 (5))	[1] 0.851
Serum Sodium		(124–140)–(132.2 ± 4.16)	(128–151)–(137.17 ± 5.47)	[3] 0.012 *
Serum Uric Acid		(4.59–14.51)–(8.42 ± 3.73)	(1.51–13.32)–(7.76 ± 3.21)	[3] 0.593

[1] Mann–Whitney U Test, [2] Fisher's Exact Test. [3] Student t Test. CPK: Creatine phosphokinase. LDH: lactate dehydrogenase. AST: Aspartate aminotransferase. BUN: Blood urea nitrogen. * $p < 0.05$.

Table 4. Analysing mortality and morbidity in children and adults based on fasciotomy status.

		Fasciotomy (Children)		P
		Absent	Present	
		(Min–Max)–(Mean ± SD (Median))	(Min–Max)–(Mean ± SD (Median))	
Dialysis day		(0–0)–(0 ± 0 (0))	(0–10)–(3.83 ± 4.49 (2.5))	-
		n (%)	n (%)	
DIC	Absent	4 (100%)	4 (66.7%)	[2] 0.467
	Present	0 (0%)	2 (33.3%)	
ARDS	Absent	4 (100%)	6 (100%)	-
	Present	-	-	
Sepsis	Absent	4 (100%)	5 (83.3%)	[2] 0.600
	Present	0 (0%)	1 (16.7%)	
Amputation	Absent	4 (100%)	6 (100%)	-
	Present	-	-	
Death	Absent	4 (100%)	6 (100%)	-
	Present	-	-	

Table 4. Cont.

			Fasciotomy (Adults)		p
			Absent	Present	
			(Min–Max)–(Mean ± SD (Median))	(Min–Max)–(Mean ± SD (Median))	
Dialysis day			(0–17)–(2.27 ± 4.61 (0))	(2–30)–(9.93 ± 7.47 (8))	[1] 0.000 *
			n (%)	n (%)	
DIC	Absent		13 (86.7%)	12 (80%)	[2] 1.000
	Present		2 (13.3%)	3 (20%)	
ARDS	Absent		13 (86.7%)	9 (60%)	[2] 0.215
	Present		2 (13.3%)	6 (40%)	
Sepsis	Absent		13 (86.7%)	10 (66.7%)	[2] 0.195
	Present		2 (13.3%)	5 (33.3%)	
Amputation	Absent		14 (93.3%)	14 (93.3%)	-
	Present		1 (6.7%)	1 (6.7%)	
Death	Absent		13 (86.7%)	12 (80%)	[2] 0.500
	Present		2 (13.3%)	3 (20%)	

[1] Mann–Whitney U Test. [2] Fisher's Exact Test. * $p < 0.05$.

A significant correlation between an increase in the number of fasciotomy incisions and the development of sepsis was one of the most important findings of the current study. The number of fasciotomy incisions in sepsis patients ranged from 0 to 11, with a mean of 5 ± 4.07. In contrast, non-sepsis patients had a range of 0 to 8 incisions, with a mean of 1.78 ± 2.59. The number of fasciotomy incisions in patients with sepsis was found to be statistically significantly higher than that in those without sepsis ($p = 0.028$; $p < 0.05$) (Table 5). The study found a significant positive correlation between the number of fasciotomy incisions and dialysis days, with a correlation coefficient of 60.1% ($p = 0.000$; $p < 0.05$) (Figure 1).

Table 5. Assessment of morbidity parameters in relation to fasciotomy number.

			The Number of Fasciotomy	
			Min–Max	Mean–SD (Median)
DIC		Absent	0–11	2.03–2.8 (0)
		Present	0–10	4.29–4.27 (3)
		p		0.157
ARDS		Absent	0–11	2.22–3.15 (0)
		Present	0–10	3.25–3.28 (3)
		p		0.244
Sepsis		Absent	0–8	1.78–2.59 (0)
		Present	0–11	5–4.07 (5)
		p		0.028 *
Amputation		Absent	0–11	2.53–3.21 (1)
		Present	0–1	0.5–0.71 (0.5)
		p		0.511

Mann–Whitney U Test. * $p < 0.05$.

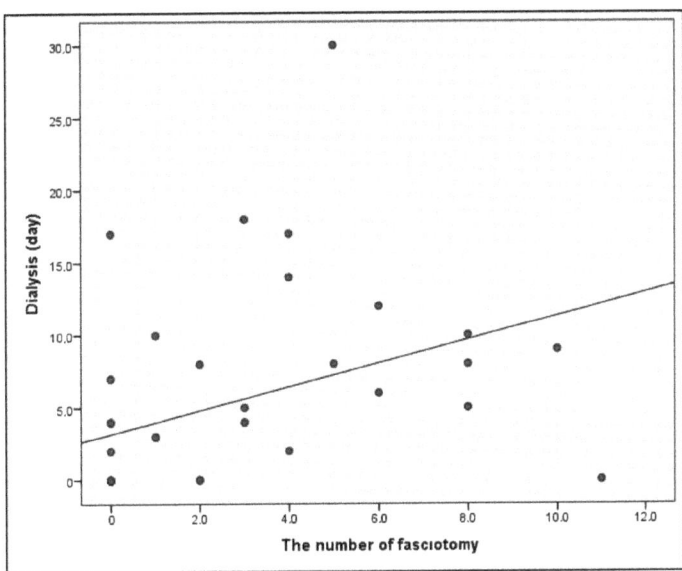

Figure 1. Figure demonstrating the correlation between the number of fasciotomies performed and the duration of dialysis treatment.

4. Discussion

The research findings unveiled a significant revelation indicating that the implementation of fasciotomy in cases of crush-induced AKI did not lead to increased rates of mortality in either the paediatric or adult population. Another significant finding was the strong correlation between the onset of sepsis and the number of fasciotomy incisions. An additional discovery from the investigation indicated that despite delayed hospital admissions among paediatric patients, the rates of mortality and morbidity were statistically comparable to those observed in adults.

In a study conducted by Zhang et al. [18] in 2012, the mortality rate of victims with crush related AKIs in the Wenchuan earthquake was 10.96%, which is in line with our rate of 12.5%. According to the report, 98 fasciotomy procedures were conducted in 68 patients throughout the entire series, accounting for 32.2% of the cases. A total of 91 limbs were subjected to amputation in a cohort of 72 patients, accounting for 34.1% of the sample. In the current study, 21 patients underwent 97 fasciotomy incisions, accounting for 52.5% of the study population. Our amputation rates were far lower than those in the aforementioned study, with only two patients requiring amputation of their fifth toe owing to the advancement of necrosis.

Our findings are consistent with those of a study conducted in 2001 by Sever et al. [13], who found that the highest rates of crush syndrome were observed in patients aged 20–59 years and that both crush syndrome and death rates in children were fairly low. However, there is a lack of consensus in the literature regarding the prognosis of children. After the Kobe earthquake, it was observed that the age group of 30–39 years had the most favourable prognosis, while the rate of death among children was also relatively low [19]. In the wake of the earthquake in Guatemala, the number of fatalities below the age of 20 was relatively low [20]. Based on the aforementioned report, an inverse relationship was observed between age and mortality in children, except for infants, who potentially experienced a different pattern due to co-sleeping with their parents [20]. It is debatable whether children would not have the same chance of survival as adults in a confined location or whether their smaller bodies would provide them with an advantage.

A study conducted by Safari et al. (2011) revealed that the implementation of fasciotomy did not yield a statistically significant effect on the morbidity or mortality rates among individuals with crush-induced AKIs subsequent to the Bam earthquake [21]. This finding was consistent with the results of the present study. Unfortunately, there is a lack of references in the literature regarding which individuals should undergo surgical treatment, when to perform the procedure, and how the procedure should be performed [22]. According to a study conducted by Greaves et al. [23], patients who underwent fasciotomy for crush syndrome face a significant risk of uncontrollable bleeding, sepsis, and wound infection. Hence, the foremost therapeutic approach involves the use of mannitol to reduce compartment pressure, while also highlighting the avoidance of surgical intervention. According to Kang et al. [24], survival rate may increase with prompt intensive care. After fasciotomy, only 13% of individuals with lower-extremity compartment syndrome and foot drop improved, according to Bradley's study [25]. Matsuoka et al. [26] found no evidence that fasciotomy enhanced the results of crushed patients. The International Committee of the Red Cross (ICRC) and the Arbeitsgemeinschaft für Osteosynthesefragen (AO) Foundation's Guidelines for the Management of Limb Injuries in Disasters and Wars recommend performing an urgent fasciotomy between 0 and 8 h after injury if there are clinical signs of compartment syndrome [27]. It has been claimed that the efficacy of fasciotomy eight to twenty-four hours after a disaster is debatable. The decision to perform fasciotomy should be made only after a thorough evaluation of limb viability. In the current study, the duration of time spent beneath the debris for nearly all patients who underwent fasciotomy ranged from 8 to 24 h. There was a male child aged four who was trapped beneath the rubble for a duration of 36 h, alongside a female patient aged 33 years who remained trapped for a period of 30 h. During the course of treatment, the paediatric patient experienced successful recovery through repetitive debridement and skin grafting (Figure 2). Conversely, the female patient developed ARDS and sepsis. However, the patient was ultimately discharged after receiving repetitive vacuum and muscle debridement treatments, as well as skin graft and muscle flap treatments during the follow-up period.

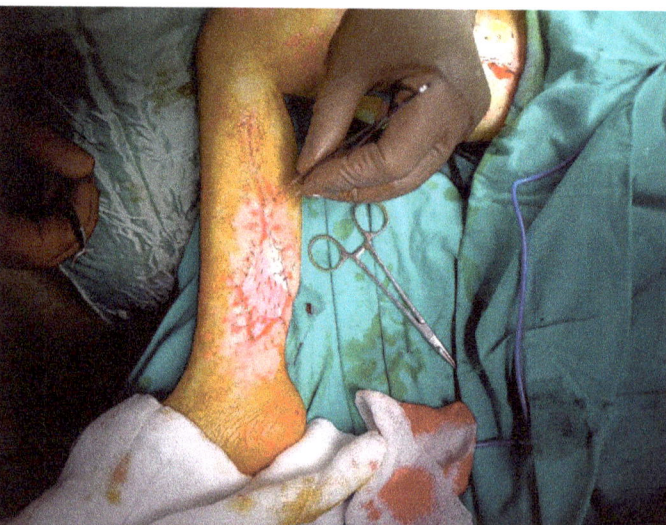

Figure 2. Image presenting the postoperative appearance of male patient, aged four years, after the procedure of skin grafting.

One of the most important findings of the current study is that the risk of developing sepsis increases with the number of fasciotomy incisions, even if the presence of fasciotomy alone is not statistically significant in the development of sepsis. Patients who underwent fasciotomy had a much higher risk of developing sepsis, as reported in 2002 by Erek et al. [28]. Nonetheless, no statistically significant association with mortality was observed. The current study showed that individuals who underwent fasciotomy had a higher frequency of dialysis sessions. However, this factor did not exert any influence on mortality outcomes. In the context of the earthquake that occurred in Turkey in 1999, approximately 70% of patients diagnosed with compartment syndrome underwent routine fasciotomy. Subsequently, 81% of these patients developed sepsis as a result of wound infection [29]. The current study documented the occurrence of sepsis in six of 21 patients who underwent fasciotomy. Acinetobacter Baumannii was detected in wound cultures of four patients, and sepsis resulted in the death of one of these patients. The wound cultures of two patients yielded Staphylococcus aureus, while the wound culture of one patient yielded Pseudomonas aeruginosa. The decline in sepsis rates and the relatively low infection rates observed in patients undergoing fasciotomy, despite a high number of dialysis days, can be attributed to the insights gained from the instructive phrase "Do not perform fasciotomy on every patient!" which was acquired subsequent to the occurrence of the Marmara earthquake in 1999.

Limitations and Strengths

The present study was a retrospective examination of earthquake-affected patients, but the study was subject to a number of restrictions. First, the current study was characterised by its single-centre design, limited sample size, and limited follow-up. The number of participants and their distribution were insufficient to provide a precise depiction of the magnitude of the entire earthquake. Second, because of the retrospective design of the study, standard criteria for AKIs were not used. The diagnosis was confirmed through patient descriptions of crush injuries and the presence of metabolic abnormalities. Third, following the occurrence of the earthquake, the orthopaedic team engaged in rotational shifts within the ED. During this period, it was noted that certain surgeons preferred to perform fasciotomy, while others were more inclined towards providing close follow-up care. The presence of clinician variability in follow-up techniques constitutes an additional factor contributing to the lack of consistency. Fourth, there is a lack of cost-effectiveness analysis. The analysis of healthcare resource utilisation has the potential to provide valuable insights for surgical decision-making and disaster planning. The current study represents a unique contribution to the existing literature, as it examines the impact of fasciotomy on both mortality and morbidity in paediatric and adult patients with AKIs resulting from crush injuries. An additional significant aspect of the study lies in its strong focus on the positive correlation between the number of fasciotomy incisions and increased vulnerability to sepsis development.

5. Conclusions

In conclusion, neither adult nor paediatric patients with crush-induced AKIs showed an increased risk of death after fasciotomy. In addition, the number of fasciotomy incisions was significantly correlated with the development of sepsis. Despite experiencing delays in hospital admission for paediatric patients, the incidence of both crush syndrome and mortality rates among children remained relatively low. It is crucial to conduct prospective studies with a larger number of participants to get more robust and reliable findings.

Author Contributions: Conceptualization, M.Y. and F.G.; methodology, M.Y.; software, M.Y.; validation, M.Y. and F.G.; formal analysis, M.Y.; investigation, M.Y.; resources, F.G.; data curation, M.Y.; writing—original draft preparation, M.Y.; writing—review and editing, F.G.; visualization, M.Y.; supervision, F.G.; project administration, M.Y. All authors have read and agreed to the published version of the manuscript.

Funding: This research received no external funding.

Institutional Review Board Statement: The study was conducted in accordance with the Declaration of Helsinki and approved by the Institutional Review Board (or Ethics Committee) of Fırat University (2023/07-12) on 25 May 2023.

Informed Consent Statement: Informed consent was obtained from all subjects involved in the study. Written informed consent has been obtained from the patient(s) to publish this paper.

Data Availability Statement: Not applicable.

Acknowledgments: We would like to thank Fuat Malkoç for his assistance and guidance in this research.

Conflicts of Interest: The authors declare no conflict of interest.

References

1. Canpolat, N.; Saygılı, S.; Sever, L. Earthquake in Turkey: Disasters and Children. *Turk. Arch. Pediatr.* **2023**, *58*, 119–121. [CrossRef]
2. Bosch, X.; Poch, E.; Grau, J.M. Rhabdomyolysis and acute kidney injury. *N. Engl. J. Med.* **2009**, *361*, 62–72. [CrossRef] [PubMed]
3. Slater, M.S.; Mullins, R.J. Rhabdomyolysis and myoglobinuric renal failure in trauma and surgical patients: A review. *J. Am. Coll. Surg.* **1998**, *186*, 693–716. [CrossRef] [PubMed]
4. Vaillancourt, C.; Shrier, I.; Vandal, A.; Falk, M.; Rossignol, M.; Vernec, A.; Somogyi, D. Acute compartment syndrome: How long before muscle necrosis occurs? *Can. J. Emerg. Med.* **2004**, *6*, 147–154. [CrossRef] [PubMed]
5. Finkelstein, J.A.; Hunter, G.A.; Hu, R.W. Lower limb compartment syndrome: Course after delayed fasciotomy. *J. Trauma* **1996**, *40*, 342–344. [CrossRef]
6. Hope, M.J.; McQueen, M.M. Acute compartment syndrome in the absence of fracture. *J. Orthop. Trauma* **2004**, *18*, 220–224. [CrossRef]
7. Prasarn, M.L.; Ouellette, E.A.; Livingstone, A.; Giuffrida, A.Y. Acute pediatric upper extremity compartment syndrome in the absence of fracture. *J. Pediatr. Orthop.* **2009**, *29*, 263–268. [CrossRef]
8. Ritenour, A.E.; Dorlac, W.C.; Fang, R.; Woods, T.; Jenkins, D.H.; Flaherty, S.F.; Wade, C.E.; Holcomb, J.B. Complications after fasciotomy revision and delayed compartment release in combat patients. *J. Trauma* **2008**, *64*, S153–S161, discussion S161–S152. [CrossRef]
9. Shadgan, B.; Menon, M.; O'Brien, P.J.; Reid, W.D. Diagnostic techniques in acute compartment syndrome of the leg. *J. Orthop. Trauma* **2008**, *22*, 581–587. [CrossRef]
10. Vaillancourt, C.; Shrier, I.; Falk, M.; Rossignol, M.; Vernec, A.; Somogyi, D. Quantifying delays in the recognition and management of acute compartment syndrome. *Can. J. Emerg. Med.* **2001**, *3*, 26–30. [CrossRef]
11. Vanholder, R.; Sever, M.S.; Erek, E.; Lameire, N. Rhabdomyolysis. *J. Am. Soc. Nephrol.* **2000**, *11*, 1553–1561. [CrossRef] [PubMed]
12. Mehta, R.L.; Kellum, J.A.; Shah, S.V.; Molitoris, B.A.; Ronco, C.; Warnock, D.G.; Levin, A. Acute Kidney Injury Network: Report of an initiative to improve outcomes in acute kidney injury. *Crit. Care* **2007**, *11*, R31. [CrossRef] [PubMed]
13. Sever, M.S.; Erek, E.; Vanholder, R.; Akoğlu, E.; Yavuz, M.; Ergin, H.; Tekçe, M.; Korular, D.; Tülbek, M.Y.; Keven, K.; et al. The Marmara earthquake: Epidemiological analysis of the victims with nephrological problems. *Kidney Int.* **2001**, *60*, 1114–1123. [CrossRef] [PubMed]
14. Levi, M. Diagnosis and treatment of disseminated intravascular coagulation. *Int. J. Lab. Hematol.* **2014**, *36*, 228–236. [CrossRef]
15. Schwameis, M.; Schober, A.; Schörgenhofer, C.; Sperr, W.R.; Schöchl, H.; Janata-Schwatczek, K.; Kürkciyan, E.I.; Sterz, F.; Jilma, B. Asphyxia by Drowning Induces Massive Bleeding Due To Hyperfibrinolytic Disseminated Intravascular Coagulation. *Crit. Care Med.* **2015**, *43*, 2394–2402. [CrossRef]
16. Meyer, N.J.; Gattinoni, L.; Calfee, C.S. Acute respiratory distress syndrome. *Lancet* **2021**, *398*, 622–637. [CrossRef]
17. Napolitano, L.M. Sepsis 2018: Definitions and Guideline Changes. *Surg. Infect.* **2018**, *19*, 117–125. [CrossRef]
18. Zhang, L.; Fu, P.; Wang, L.; Cai, G.; Zhang, L.; Chen, D.; Guo, D.; Sun, X.; Chen, F.; Bi, W.; et al. The clinical features and outcome of crush patients with acute kidney injury after the Wenchuan earthquake: Differences between elderly and younger adults. *Injury* **2012**, *43*, 1470–1475. [CrossRef]
19. Tanida, N. What happened to elderly people in the great Hanshin earthquake. *BMJ* **1996**, *313*, 1133–1135. [CrossRef]
20. Glass, R.I.; Urrutia, J.J.; Sibony, S.; Smith, H.; Garcia, B.; Rizzo, L. Earthquake injuries related to housing in a guatemalan village. *Science* **1977**, *197*, 638–643. [CrossRef]
21. Safari, S.; Najafi, I.; Hosseini, M.; Sanadgol, H.; Sharifi, A.; Alavi Moghadam, M.; Abdulvand, A.; Rashid Farrokhi, F.; Borumand, B. Outcomes of fasciotomy in patients with crush-induced acute kidney injury after Bam earthquake. *Iran. J. Kidney Dis.* **2011**, *5*, 25–28. [PubMed]
22. Gerdin, M.; Wladis, A.; von Schreeb, J. Surgical management of closed crush injury-induced compartment syndrome after earthquakes in resource-scarce settings. *J. Trauma Acute Care Surg.* **2012**, *73*, 758–764. [CrossRef] [PubMed]
23. Greaves, I.; Porter, K.M.; Revell, M.P. Fluid resuscitation in pre-hospital trauma care: A consensus view. *J. R. Coll. Surg. Edinb.* **2002**, *47*, 451–457. [PubMed]
24. Kang, P.D.; Pei, F.X.; Tu, C.Q.; Wang, G.L.; Zhang, H.; Song, Y.M.; Fu, P.; Kang, Y.; Kong, Q.Q.; Liu, L.M.; et al. [The crush syndrome patients combined with kidney failure after Wenchuan earthquake]. *Zhonghua Wai Ke Za Zhi* **2008**, *46*, 1862–1864.
25. Bradley, E.L., 3rd. The anterior tibial compartment syndrome. *Surg. Gynecol. Obstet.* **1973**, *136*, 289–297.

26. Matsuoka, T.; Yoshioka, T.; Tanaka, H.; Ninomiya, N.; Oda, J.; Sugimoto, H.; Yokota, J. Long-term physical outcome of patients who suffered crush syndrome after the 1995 Hanshin-Awaji earthquake: Prognostic indicators in retrospect. *J. Trauma* **2002**, *52*, 33–39. [CrossRef]
27. Özkaya, U.; Yalçın, M.B. Deprem yaralanmalı hastada kompartman sendromu ve ezilme (crush) sendromu ayrımı: Fasyotomi kime ve ne zaman. *TOTBİD Dergisi* **2022**, *21*, 312–315. [CrossRef]
28. Erek, E.; Sever, M.S.; Serdengeçti, K.; Vanholder, R.; Akoğlu, E.; Yavuz, M.; Ergin, H.; Tekçe, M.; Duman, N.; Lameire, N. An overview of morbidity and mortality in patients with acute renal failure due to crush syndrome: The Marmara earthquake experience. *Nephrol. Dial. Transplant.* **2002**, *17*, 33–40. [CrossRef]
29. Gunal, A.I.; Celiker, H.; Dogukan, A.; Ozalp, G.; Kirciman, E.; Simsekli, H.; Gunay, I.; Demircin, M.; Belhan, O.; Yildirim, M.A.; et al. Early and vigorous fluid resuscitation prevents acute renal failure in the crush victims of catastrophic earthquakes. *J. Am. Soc. Nephrol.* **2004**, *15*, 1862–1867. [CrossRef]

Disclaimer/Publisher's Note: The statements, opinions and data contained in all publications are solely those of the individual author(s) and contributor(s) and not of MDPI and/or the editor(s). MDPI and/or the editor(s) disclaim responsibility for any injury to people or property resulting from any ideas, methods, instructions or products referred to in the content.

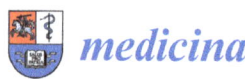

Article

Minimally Invasive Peroneal Tenodesis Assisted by Peroneal Tendoscopy: Technique and Preliminary Results

Rodrigo Simões Castilho [1,*], João Murilo Brandão Magalhães [1], Bruno Peliz Machado Veríssimo [1], Carlo Perisano [2], Tommaso Greco [2] and Roberto Zambelli [1,3]

1. Department of Orthopaedics and Traumatology, Mater Dei Hospital, Belo Horizonte 30170-041, Brazil; brunopmachadov@hotmail.com (B.P.M.V.); zambelliortop@gmail.com (R.Z.)
2. Orthopaedics and Traumatology, Dipartimento di Scienze Dell'invecchiamento, Ortopediche e Reumatologiche Fondazione Policlinico Universitario Agostino Gemelli IRCCS, 00168 Rome, Italy; carlo.perisano@policlinicogemelli.it (C.P.); tommaso.greco01@icatt.it (T.G.)
3. Surgical Department of Faculty of Medical Sciences of Minas Gerais, Belo Horizonte 30170-041, Brazil
* Correspondence: rodrigoscastilho@gmail.com

Abstract: *Introduction:* Peroneal disorders are a common cause of ankle pain and lateral instability and have been described in as much as 77% of patients with lateral ankle instability. Clicking, swelling, pain, and tenderness in the peroneal tendons track are frequent symptoms, but they can be confused with other causes of lateral ankle pain. The management of peroneal disorders can be conservative or surgical. When the conservative treatment fails, surgery is indicated, and open or tendoscopic synovectomy, tubularization, tenodesis or tendon transfers can be performed. The authors present a surgical technique of tendoscopy associated to minimally invasive tenodesis for the treatment of peroneal tendon tears, as well as the preliminary results of patients submitted to this procedure. *Methods:* Four patients with chronic lateral ankle pain who were diagnosed with peroneal brevis pathology were treated between 2020 and 2022 with tendoscopic-assisted minimally invasive synovectomy and tenodesis. Using a 2.7 mm 30° arthroscope and a 3.0 mm shaver blade, the entire length of the peroneus brevis tendon and most parts of the peroneus longus tendon can be assessed within Sammarco's zones 1 and 2. After the inspection and synovectomy, a minimally invasive tenodesis is performed. *Results:* All patients were evaluated at least six months after surgery. All of them reported improvement in daily activities and in the Foot Function Index (FFI) questionnaire (pre-surgery mean FFI = 23.86%; post-surgery mean FFI = 6.15%), with no soft tissue complications or sural nerve complaints. *Conclusion:* The tendoscopy of the peroneal tendons allows the surgeon to assess their integrity, confirm the extent of the lesion, perform synovectomy, prepare the tendon for tenodesis, and perform it in a safe and minimally invasive way, reducing the risks inherent to the open procedure.

Keywords: tendoscopy; tenodesis; peroneal tendon; tendon rupture; tendinopathy; endoscopy; foot and ankle; sports injury; minimally invasive surgery

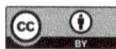

1. Introduction

Chronic disorders of the peroneal tendons are a common cause of posterolateral ankle pain, including ankle lateral instability [1]. In a study among professional football players in America, peroneal tendon pathology was found in 4.0% of all ankle injuries [1]. Moreover, peroneal tendon pathology has been described in 23% to 77% of patients with lateral ankle instability [1,2]. It has been estimated that the range for peroneal tendon tears is between 11% and 37% [3–7], and the peroneal brevis tendon is the most involved (88%) [3,8,9].

The peroneal muscles form the lateral compartment of the lower leg. The peroneus longus (PL) muscle becomes tendinous 3 to 4 cm proximal to the distal fibular tip, and the peroneus brevis (PB) muscle usually extends 0.6 to 2 cm more distally [1]. Both muscles receive their innervation from the superficial peroneal nerve and act as the primary evertors of the foot, and both receive their blood supply from the peroneal artery [3].f At the level of the fibular tip, the PB tendon is located anteromedially to the PL tendon, and both share a common fibro-osseous tunnel formed by the superior peroneal retinaculum (SPR), posterolateral fibrocartilaginous ridge and retro malleolar groove within the fibula. This groove was found to be concave-shaped in 82%, flat in 11%, and convex in 7% in a cadaveric study [1]. With contraction, the peroneal longus tendon compresses the brevis against the fibula [3]. Distal to the fibular tip, the tendons become separated by the lateral calcaneal tubercle to enter their own fibrous tunnel, secured by the inferior peroneal retinaculum. This tubercle is considered prominent in 29% of cadaveric specimens, where it can become a source of pain [1].

The mechanism of peroneal tendon injuries has been classically described as a sudden contraction of the peroneal tendons combined with abrupt involuntary dorsiflexion stress of the ankle. However, a plantarflexion and inversion mechanism of injury has also been described in longitudinal ruptures [2].

Clinical presentation is usually by posterolateral ankle swelling, pain, tenderness in the peroneal track, and functional impairment, symptoms that can be confused with other causes of ankle pain [3,4,10]. Passive plantar flexion and inversion of the foot and active plantar flexion and eversion of the foot may provoke tenderness or pain [1,11]. Clicking, subluxation, and luxation of peroneal tendons may also occur [11,12].

It is important to assess the alignment of the hindfoot since the excess valgus can cause a subperoneal impingement of the peroneal tendons, and the excess varus is associated with peroneal tendon pathologies [3,4].

Different diagnoses can emerge from this clinical picture, the most common being tendonitis, tenosynovitis, subluxation or dislocation, and partial and complete peroneal tears [11,13].

Peroneal tendon abnormalities are traditionally investigated using magnetic resonance imaging (MRI). Some anomalies of the peroneal tendons, such as peroneus quartus or low-lying muscle belly on the peroneus brevis, for example, that were not evident or not diagnosed with MRI can be detected using the peroneal tendoscopy [14]. Ultrasound imaging can also be used, with the advantage of dynamic real-time imaging of the peronei, with a 90% accuracy in diagnosing peroneal tendon tears [4].

The management of peroneal pathologies can be conservative, which includes rest, ice therapy, compression, elevation [13], non-steroidal anti-inflammatory drug (NSAID), immobilization [1,4], shockwave therapy [13] and physical therapy [1,11,13]. If this treatment fails, surgery should be indicated, and the procedure is chosen based on the grading of the lesions. Debridement and synovectomy, tubularization, tenodesis, and tendon transfers with auto or allograft reconstruction using an open approach or endoscopic assisted can be indicated [1,5].

If more than 50% of the cross-sectional area of the tendon is involved, some authors suggest tenodesis of the torn tendon to the healthy one [1]; other authors indicate tenodesis if one of the two tendons is torn, and the other is intact [11].

Endoscopic approaches to tendons around the ankle have been described since 1990 [15,16]. An endoscopic procedure would offer several advantages, such as less morbidity, reduction in postoperative pain, and fewer soft tissue complications [16–19].

The aim of this paper is to present the technique of tendoscopic synovectomy associated to a minimally invasive tenodesis of peroneal tendon tears, and its preliminary results. Our hypothesis is that the minimally invasive peroneal tenodesis provides a good cosmetic result with fewer complications than the traditional open procedure for stenosis.

2. Materials and Methods

After approval of the Institutional Review Board of Ethics in Research, all patients give their informed consent to join the research. Four patients were treated between 2020 and 2022 with this technique, and they were evaluated pre-operatively and at least six months postoperatively. All of them had chronic lateral pain in their ankles, with clinical and imaging (Magnetic Resonance Imaging, MRI) diagnoses of peroneus brevis tendon pathology. All had been submitted to conservative treatment, with medication and physiotherapy, without success. All the procedures were performed by the same two authors using the technique described below. All patients were evaluated at least six months after the operation, and the Foot Function Index (FFI) functional questionnaire was administered by telephone calls [20].

A thorough physical examination was performed on each patient after six months of the surgery. Assessment of edema, scar tissue or scar tenderness, peroneal tendons subluxation or instability, strength, and stabilization capacity were all evaluated at this assessment. Patient standing pattern and gait observation, and all the patients' feelings and opinions regarding the results were registered. This landmark of at least six months was arbitrary, given by the authors to standardize the assessment.

The FFI is a questionnaire developed in English to evaluate foot function in patients who have musculoskeletal injuries. Since evaluation is focused on the foot, the questionnaire has greater accuracy and sensitivity for identifying changes in this area when compared to other available instruments. In assessing the reproducibility of the original FFI, the intraclass correlation coefficient was considered excellent. The questionnaire is divided into blocks of questions: pain and disability, regarding walkability inside the house, need for the use support to walk; difficulty, regarding hardship to walk on different types of floor and ground, climb stairs, walk-in tiptoes, run; pain, in different moments of daily living, such as get up in the morning, walk barefoot, walk with shoes, with orthoses, at the end of the day. All answers are scored, 0 being the least difficulty and 10 being the highest difficulty/limitation [20]. In this research, the highest possible score was 230 points. The more points the patient scores, the greater their disability.

The exclusion criteria were other foot and/or ankle pathologies (instability, arthrosis, fractures), chronic use of corticosteroids, and patient refusal to participate in the research.

Surgical Technique

The patient is placed in lateral decubitus with the affected limb upwards, with a pneumatic tourniquet at the root of the thigh (Figure 1). The type of anesthesia—spinal anesthesia, peripheric nerve block, sedation, or general anesthesia must be individualized and defined prior to the procedure, considering the clinical characteristics of each patient. In this series, all the patients could be submitted to spinal anesthesia and sedation. The main portals for peroneal tendoscopy are performed directly over the peroneal tendons, 2 cm distal and 2 cm proximal to the distal end of the lateral malleolus. However, they can be performed along the entire length of the tendons. The distal portal is performed first, with skin incision with a scalpel and entry into the sheath using a blunt instrument (trocart). A 2.7 mm arthroscope with a 30° inclination is used for this procedure, and the sheath is inflated with 0.9% saline. The proximal portal is performed under direct vision [16]. In this specific case, three portals were used: one proximal, one in the transition between Sammarco's zones A and B [10], and another distal, with the aim to allow full access to the entire length of the peroneus brevis tendon (Figure 2A,B). The Sammarco zones are defined as zone A, which comprises the superior retinaculum of the fibularis; zone B, which comprises the inferior peroneal retinaculum to the peroneal tubercle on the lateral calcaneus; zone C, which comprises the bony groove of the cuboid, and zone D, which is distal to the groove up to the insertion of the peroneus longus at the base of the first metatarsal (Figure 3) [10].

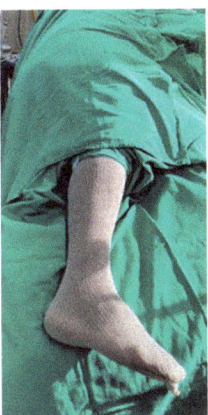

Figure 1. Positioning the patient in lateral decubitus to approach the peroneal tendons.

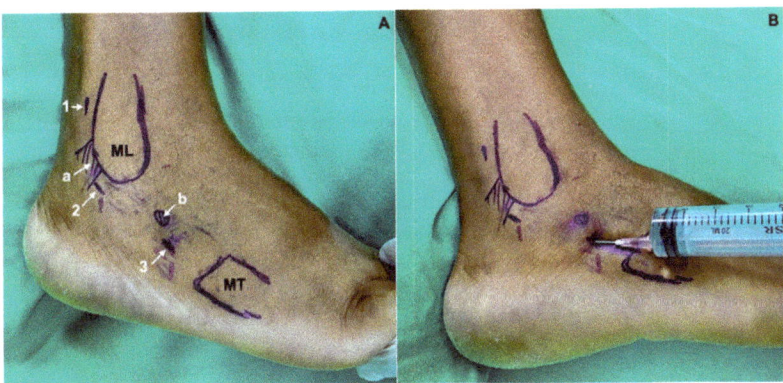

Figure 2. (**A**) Proximal (1), central in the transition of Sammarco's zones a and b (2) and distal (3) arthroscopic portals. Superior Peroneal Retinaculum (a); Peroneal tubercle (b); lateral malleolus (ML); base of fifth metatarsal (MT). (**B**) Sheath being inflated with 0.9% saline. The distension of the sheath in the path of the peroneal tendons should be noted, avoiding infiltration of the serum outside it.

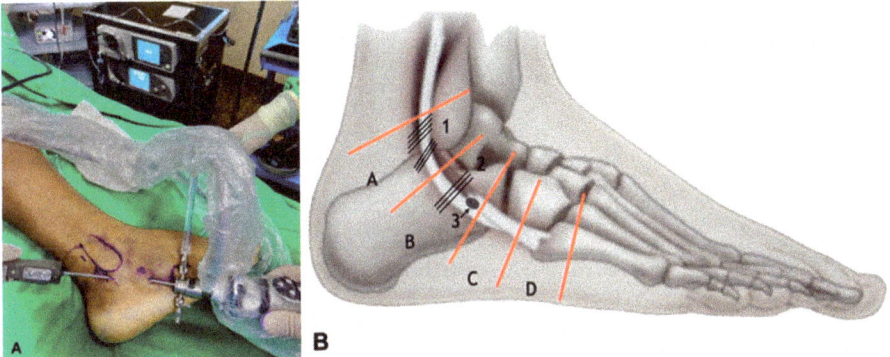

Figure 3. (**A**) Positioning of the arthroscopic instruments for synovectomy in the Sammarco's zone B. (**B**) Schematic drawing of the Sammarco zones: A, B, C, and D. (1) Superior peroneal retinaculum; (2) Inferior Peroneal Retinaculum; (3) Peroneal tubercle.

The shaver blade is then introduced, and the synovectomy of both tendons is performed, as well as their inspection (Figures 3 and 4); if a distal implantation of the peroneus brevis musculature is observed, the removal of this musculature must be performed at this time.

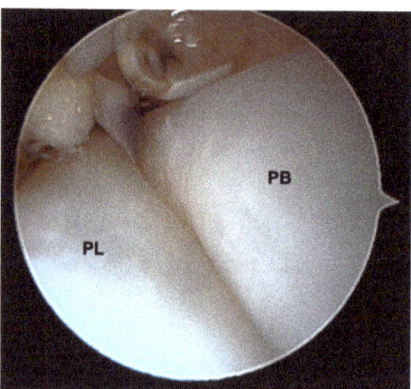

Figure 4. Peroneal Brevis (PB) and Peroneal Longus (PL) position during tendoscopy.

After the synovectomy, the arthroscope is removed, and the portals can be enlarged by approximately 1 cm each, through which the peroneal tendons can then be pulled to perform the tenodesis. Using absorbable threads, the tendons are sutured with two "U" stitches distally and two "U" stitches proximally. Next, the tendon to be removed is sectioned under direct view and extracted (Figure 5).

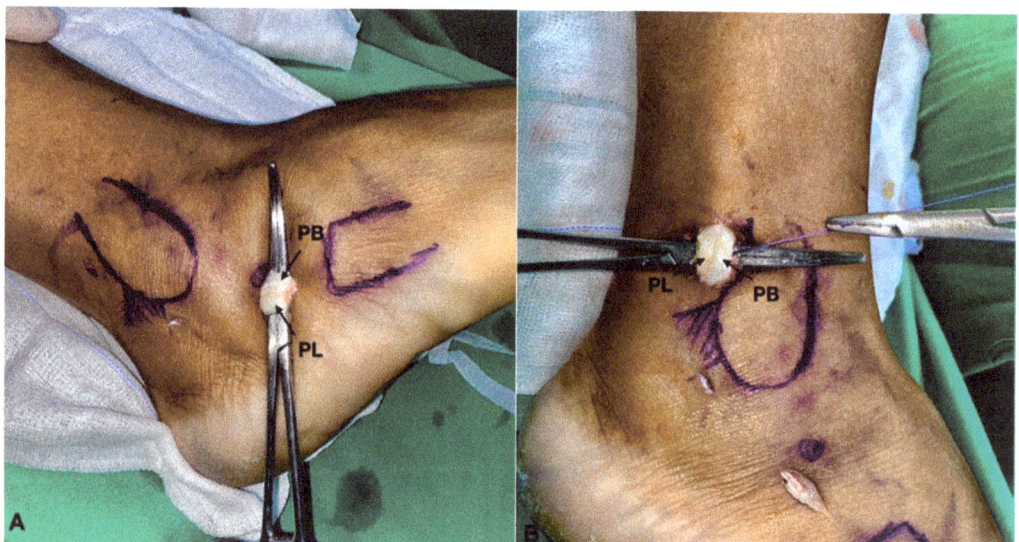

Figure 5. (**A**) Tenodesis is being performed through the distal portal. (**B**) Tenodesis is being performed through the proximal portal. PB: Peroneal Brevis; PL: Peroneal Longus.

At the end of the procedure, the arthroscope can be reintroduced to review the course and, if necessary, optimize the synovectomy. Subsequently, the accesses are sutured (Figure 6), a sterile compressive dressing is applied, and immobilization is performedg with a plaster splint. In the postoperative period, the splint is kept for two weeks until the stitches are removed. Then, the use of a removable immobilization boot is indicated, with progressive protected weight-bearing and active flexion-extension and intrinsic muscle exercises until the sixth week, when the immobilization is removed, and physical therapy rehabilitation is intensified.

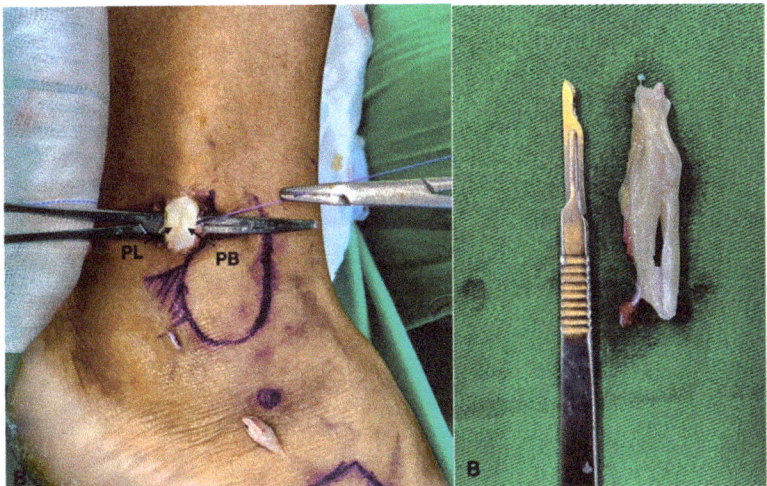

Figure 6. (**A**) Final appearance after the procedure. (**B**) Resected peroneal brevis tendon. PL (peroneal longus); PB (peroneal brevis).

3. Results

In the period between 2020 and 2022, four patients underwent peroneal tendoscopy technique associated with minimally invasive tenodesis. The FFI functional questionnaire was applied with pre- and postoperative information to compare the patients' evolution.

Patients had no complications related to surgical scars or sural nerves (Figure 7). They reported that they had problems in social activities due to pain and that, after the surgical intervention, they had reduced pain and returned to daily living activities. All of them were satisfied after follow-up with physical therapy rehabilitation and strengthening.

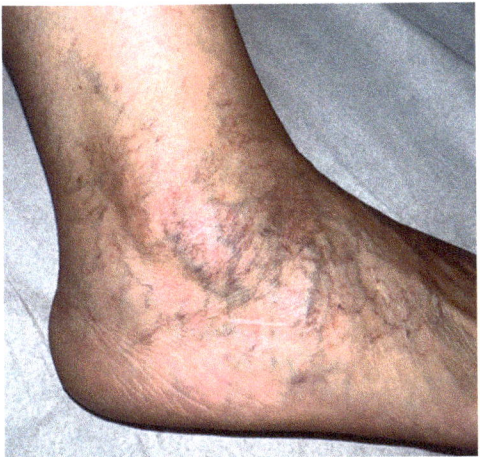

Figure 7. Appearance after 12 months of the procedure.

Analyzing the FFI questionnaire, all patients reported an important functional improvement (pre-mean FFI = 23.86%; post-mean FFI = 6.15%), as shown in Table 1. The results were comparable to those obtained in conventional surgery but with less damage to the soft tissues. No skin complications were observed in the operated cases.

Table 1. Pre and postoperative FFI questionnaire results.

Patient	Age	Side	Time (Months)	FFI Pre	FFI Post
1	64	E	23	74/230 (32%)	16/230 (6.9%)
2	51	E	31	27/230 (11.7%)	20/230 (8.6%)
3	60	E	6	60/230 (26.08%)	6/230 (2.6%)
4	60	D	13	59/230 (25.65%)	15/230 (6.52%)
Mean	58.75	3/1	18.25	23.86%	6.15%

4. Discussion

Peroneal disorders have historically presented challenges in their effective treatment. Traditionally, they have been performed through a long lateral curved incision from the lateral retromalleolar area right down to the fifth metatarsal's base. Such a treatment approach, while conventional, wasn't without its drawbacks. A wide-ranging incidence of complications was reported, with some studies highlighting rates as diverse as 2.4% to 54% [5], such as nerve injuries, infections, postoperative pain, scarring, and stiffness around the ankle joint [18].

Detecting peroneal tendon abnormalities by MRI scan is limited by the quality of the MRI unit and the radiologist's experience. There are some reports showing that the peroneus quartus muscle and/or peroneus brevis low-lying muscle belly may not be identified in the exam [14].

As medicine evolves, so do its methodologies, driven by innovation, research, and patient-centric approaches. The spotlight is now on minimally invasive procedures, heralding a new era in the surgical treatment of peroneal disorders. At the forefront of this revolutionary transition are the techniques of endoscopic synovectomy and minimally invasive tenodesis. These methods are not just transformative in their approach but have also showcased a marked increase in efficacy. Most patients have reported a noticeable reduction in post-operative discomfort, especially evident six months following the surgical intervention.

Peroneal tendons are good candidates for tendoscopic treatment because of their subcutaneous position along the lateral wall of the calcaneus and posterolateral side of the fibula. This technique allows for a unique view of the entire length of the peroneal tendons while also providing a dynamic evaluation of their movement inside the sheath, and it is a useful tool both for the diagnosis and the minimally invasive treatment of different peroneal tendon disorders [18].

To truly appreciate the significance and intricacies of these novel procedures, we must delve deeper into the specifics, particularly the role of tendoscopy. Visualization, accurate and comprehensive, forms the bedrock of successful surgical outcomes. With advancements in tendoscopy, the entire length and circumference of both peroneal tendons can be visualized from the myotendinous junction proximally to 2 cm proximal to their insertions, using a conventional tendoscopy technique [21]. For visualization of the peroneus brevis tendon, Sammarco zones A and B should be considered. Peroneal brevis tendon tears usually occur in the region of the peroneal sulcus at the distal tip of the fibula at Sammarco zone A [8].

Some authors prefer to perform the proximal portal approximately 3.0–3.5 cm proximal to the tip of the lateral malleolus. It provides surgeons with an expansive operative field during tendoscopy, facilitating ease of entry into the superior posterior retinaculum and providing a larger treatment area during tendoscopy [10,19]. This was also our preference, so a wide synovectomy and resection of the distally implanted muscle belly were performed. Furthermore, it ensures the detailed and careful preparation necessary for tenodesis, all while preserving the superior peroneal retinaculum's structural integrity.

The advantages of tendoscopy are common to other arthroscopic procedures in ankle surgery. It can be performed as an outpatient procedure or as a "one-day surgery" hospitalization. Surgical morbidity and postoperative pain are reduced when compared to open procedures [18].

Despite the strategic planning, surgical interventions are not devoid of potential challenges. The main disadvantage of this procedure is that it can be technically demanding in patients with extensive tenosynovitis or a scarred/thickened peroneal sheath [18]. Nerve injuries resulting from peroneal tendoscopy are mainly of the sural nerve or its communicating branch with the superficial peroneal nerve in the distal portal [22] or even of the superficial peroneal nerve in the proximal portal, all of which are iatrogenic. In addition, the risk of injury to the sural nerve due to the extravasation of saline solution outside the peroneal sheath has been reported [11,23,24]. In our series, using the endoscopic approach, we haven't found any nerve complications.

Other complications are reported in the literature. In a study with 30 patients treated for peroneal tendon tears through a long lateral approach, 58% of the patients had scar tenderness, 54% presented lateral ankle swelling, 27% had numbness over the lateral surface of the ankle, and 31% had pain at rest [5].

In a study published in 2020, a case of minimally invasive tenodesis of the peroneus longus tendon was presented [5], but the authors didn't describe synovectomy during their intervention. In our opinion, synovectomy is a crucial step in the treatment of peroneal tendon pathologies. Several authors cite tenosynovitis as a cause of chronic lateral ankle pain [1,10,11,16–19,23–26], thus performing an extensive synovectomy associated with resection of the affected tendon segment and tenodesis from the three steps of the entire treatment of the pathology.

The weaknesses of this study are that it is a case series without a control group to compare the results. Moreover, the number of patients enrolled is still small, and there is a short follow-up period. Prospective comparative studies should be performed to confirm if this combination of procedures is a reliable intervention to treat peroneal tendon disorders.

5. Conclusions

The tendoscopy of the peroneal tendons allows the surgeon to assess their integrity, confirm the extent of the lesion, perform synovectomy, prepare the tendon for tenodesis and perform it in a safe and minimally invasive way, lowering the risks related to the open procedure.

Author Contributions: Idealization, formal analysis, investigation, methodology, visualization, writing-original draft, project administration, R.S.C.; formal analysis, investigation, methodology, writing-review and editing, J.M.B.M.; formal analysis, investigation, methodology, writing-original draft, B.P.M.V.; Data curation, methodology, validation, visualization, writing-review and editing, C.P.; Data curation, methodology, validation, visualization, writing-review & editing, T.G.; idealization, investigation, methodology, supervision, validation, writing-review & editing, R.Z. All authors have read and agreed to the published version of the manuscript.

Funding: This research received no external funding.

Institutional Review Board Statement: The study was conducted in accordance with the Declaration of Helsinki and approved by the Institutional Review Board of Mater Dei Hospital on 18 December 2023. The code is 76480823.4.0000.5128.

Informed Consent Statement: Informed consent was obtained from all subjects involved in the study.

Data Availability Statement: The study data will be available upon request to the corresponding author.

Conflicts of Interest: The authors declare no conflicts of interest.

References

1. Van Dijk, P.A.D.; Kerkhoffs, G.M.M.J.; Chiodo, C.; DiGiovanni, C.W. Chronic Disorders of the Peroneal Tendons: Current Concepts Review of the Literature. *J. Am. Acad. Orthop. Surg.* **2019**, *27*, 590–598. [CrossRef] [PubMed]
2. DiGiovanni, B.F.; Fraga, C.J.; Cohen, B.E.; Shereff, M.J. Associated Injuries Found in Chronic Lateral Ankle Instability. *Foot Ankle Int.* **2000**, *21*, 809–815. [CrossRef] [PubMed]
3. Bahad, S.R.; Kane, J.M. Peroneal Tendon Pathology Treatment and Reconstruction of Peroneal Tears and Instability. *Orthop. Clin. N. Am.* **2020**, *51*, 121–130. [CrossRef] [PubMed]
4. Davda, K.; Malhotra, K.; O'Donnell, P.; Singh, D.; Cullen, N. Peroneal tendon disorders. *EFORT Open Rev.* **2017**, *2*, 281–292. [CrossRef] [PubMed]
5. Nishikawa, D.R.C.; Duarte, F.A.; Saito, G.H.; de Cesar Netto, C.; Fonseca, F.C.P.; de Miranda, B.R.; Monteiro, A.C.; Prado, M.P. Minimally invasive tenodesis for peroneus longus tendon rupture: A case report and review of literature. *World J. Orthop.* **2020**, *11*, 137–144. [CrossRef] [PubMed]
6. Sobel, M.; DiCarlo, E.F.; Bohne, W.H.O.; Collins, L. Longitudinal Splitting of the Peroneus Brevis Tendon: An Anatomic and Histologic Study of Cadaveric Material. *Foot Ankle Int.* **1991**, *12*, 165–170. [CrossRef] [PubMed]
7. Taljanovic, M.S.; Alcala, J.N.; Gimber, L.H.; Rieke, J.D.; Chilvers, M.M.; Latt, L.D. High-Resolution US and MR Imaging of Peroneal Tendon Injuries. *Radiographics* **2015**, *35*, 179–199. [CrossRef]
8. Redfern, D.; Myerson, M. The Management of Concomitant Tears of the Peroneus Longus and Brevis Tendons. *Foot Ankle Int.* **2004**, *25*, 695–707. [CrossRef]
9. Slater, H.K. Acute Peroneal Tendon Tears. *Foot Ankle Clin.* **2007**, *12*, 659–674. [CrossRef]
10. Sammarco, V.J. Peroneal Tendoscopy. *Sports Med. Arthrosc. Rev.* **2009**, *17*, 94–99. [CrossRef]
11. Sharma, A.; Parekh, S.G. Pathologies of the Peroneals: A Review. *Foot Ankle Spec.* **2021**, *14*, 170–177. [CrossRef] [PubMed]
12. Lui, T.H.; Li, H.M. Endoscopic Resection of Peroneus Quartus. *Arthrosc. Tech.* **2019**, *9*, e35–e38. [CrossRef] [PubMed]
13. van Dijk, P.A.; Miller, D.; Calder, J.; DiGiovanni, C.W.; Kennedy, J.G.; Kerkhoffs, G.M.; Kynsburtg, A.; Havercamp, D.; Guillo, S.; Oliva, X.M.; et al. The ESSKA-AFAS international consensus statement on peroneal tendon pathologies. *Knee Surg. Sports Traumatol. Arthrosc.* **2018**, *26*, 3096–3107. [CrossRef] [PubMed]
14. Panchbhavi, V.K.; Trevino, S.G. The Technique of Peroneal Tendoscopy and Its Role in Management of Peroneal Tendon Anomalies. *Tech. Foot Ankle Surg.* **2003**, *2*, 192–198. [CrossRef]
15. Stornebrink, T.; Stufkens, S.A.S.; Appelt, D.; Wijdicks, C.A.; Kerkhoffs, G.M.M.J. 2-Mm Diameter Operative Tendoscopy of the Tibialis Posterior, Peroneal, and Achilles Tendons: A Cadaveric Study. *Foot Ankle Int.* **2020**, *41*, 473–478. [CrossRef] [PubMed]
16. van Dijk, C.; Kort, N. Tendoscopy of the peroneal tendons. *Arthrosc. J. Arthrosc. Relat. Surg.* **1998**, *14*, 471–478. [CrossRef] [PubMed]
17. Monteagudo, M.; Maceira, E.; de Albornoz, P.M. Foot and ankle tendoscopies: Current concepts review. *EFORT Open Rev.* **2016**, *1*, 440–447. [CrossRef] [PubMed]
18. Marmotti, A.; Cravino, M.; Germano, M.; Din, R.D.; Rossi, R.; Tron, A.; Tellini, A.; Castoldi, F. Peroneal tendoscopy. *Curr. Rev. Musculoskelet. Med.* **2012**, *5*, 135–144. [CrossRef]
19. Urguden, M.; Gulten, I.A.; Civan, O.; Bilbasar, H.; Kaptan, C.; Cavit, A. Results of Peroneal Tendoscopy with a Technical Modification. *Foot Ankle Int.* **2019**, *40*, 356–363. [CrossRef]
20. Yi, L.C.; Staboli, I.M.; Kamonseki, D.H.; Budiman-Mak, E.; Arie, E.K. Tradução e adaptação cultural do Foot Function Index para a língua portuguesa: FFI—Brasil. *Rev. Bras. Reumatol.* **2015**, *55*, 398–405. [CrossRef]
21. Hull, M.; Campbell, J.T.; Jeng, C.L.; Henn, R.F.; Cerrato, R.A. Measuring Visualized Tendon Length in Peroneal Tendoscopy. *Foot Ankle Int.* **2018**, *39*, 990–993. [CrossRef] [PubMed]
22. Pereira, B.S.; Pereira, H.; Robles, R.V.; Rivas, A.P.; Nar, Ö.O.; Espregueira-Mendes, J.; Oliva, X.M. The distance from the peroneal tendons sheath to the sural nerve at the posterior tip of the fibula decreases from proximal to distal. *Knee Surg. Sports Traumatol. Arthrosc.* **2019**, *27*, 2852–2857. [CrossRef] [PubMed]
23. Bojanić, I.; Dimnjaković, D.; Bohaček, I.; Smoljanović, T. Peroneal tendoscopy—More than just a solitary procedure: Case-series. *Croat. Med. J.* **2015**, *56*, 57–62. [CrossRef] [PubMed]
24. Lui, T.H. Endoscopic Resection of Peroneal Tubercle. *Arthrosc. Tech.* **2017**, *6*, e1489–e1493. [CrossRef] [PubMed]
25. Rajbhandari, P.; Angthong, C. Peroneal Tendoscopic Debridement and Endoscopic Groove Deepening in the Prone Position. *Arthrosc. Tech.* **2018**, *8*, e11–e16. [CrossRef] [PubMed]
26. Bernasconi, A.; Sadile, F.; Smeraglia, F.; Mehdi, N.; Laborde, J.; Lintz, F. Tendoscopy of Achilles, peroneal and tibialis posterior tendons: An evidence-based update. *Foot Ankle Surg.* **2018**, *24*, 374–382. [CrossRef]

Disclaimer/Publisher's Note: The statements, opinions and data contained in all publications are solely those of the individual author(s) and contributor(s) and not of MDPI and/or the editor(s). MDPI and/or the editor(s) disclaim responsibility for any injury to people or property resulting from any ideas, methods, instructions or products referred to in the content.

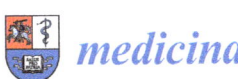

Article

Direct Anterior Approach in Total Hip Arthroplasty for Severe Crowe IV Dysplasia: Retrospective Clinical and Radiological Study

Cesare Faldini [1,2], Leonardo Tassinari [1,2], Davide Pederiva [1,2], Valentino Rossomando [1,2], Matteo Brunello [1,2], Federico Pilla [1,2], Giuseppe Geraci [1,2], Francesco Traina [2,3] and Alberto Di Martino [1,2,*]

[1] I Orthopedic and Traumatology Department, IRCCS Istituto Ortopedico Rizzoli, 40136 Bologna, Italy; cesare.faldini@ior.it (C.F.); leonardo.tassinari@ior.it (L.T.); davide.pederiva@ior.it (D.P.); valentino.rossomando@ior.it (V.R.); matteo.brunello@ior.it (M.B.); federico.pilla@ior.it (F.P.); giuseppe.geraci@ior.it (G.G.)

[2] Department of Biomedical and Neuromotor Science-DIBINEM, University of Bologna, 40126 Bologna, Italy; francesco.traina@ior.it

[3] Orthopedics-Traumatology and Prosthetic Surgery and Hip and Knee Revision, IRCCS Istituto Ortopedico Rizzoli, 40136 Bologna, Italy

* Correspondence: albertocorrado.dimartino@ior.it; Tel.: +39-(05)-16366924

Citation: Faldini, C.; Tassinari, L.; Pederiva, D.; Rossomando, V.; Brunello, M.; Pilla, F.; Geraci, G.; Traina, F.; Di Martino, A. Direct Anterior Approach in Total Hip Arthroplasty for Severe Crowe IV Dysplasia: Retrospective Clinical and Radiological Study. *Medicina* 2024, 60, 114. https://doi.org/10.3390/medicina60010114

Academic Editor: Vassilios S. Nikolaou

Received: 19 October 2023
Revised: 22 December 2023
Accepted: 4 January 2024
Published: 7 January 2024

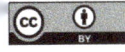

Copyright: © 2024 by the authors. Licensee MDPI, Basel, Switzerland. This article is an open access article distributed under the terms and conditions of the Creative Commons Attribution (CC BY) license (https://creativecommons.org/licenses/by/4.0/).

Abstract: *Background and Objectives*: total hip arthroplasty (THA) for Crowe IV hip dysplasia poses challenges due to severe leg shortening, muscle retraction and bone stock issues, leading to an increased neurological complication, and revision rate. The direct anterior approach (DAA) is used for minimally invasive THA but its role in Crowe IV dysplasia is unclear. This retrospective study examines if DAA effectively restores hip biomechanics in Crowe IV dysplasia patients with <4 cm leg length discrepancy, managing soft tissue and yielding functional improvement, limb length correction, and limited complications. *Materials and Methods*: 19 patients with unilateral Crowe IV hip osteoarthritis and <4 cm leg length discrepancy undergoing DAA THA were reviewed. Surgery involved gradual soft tissue release, precise acetabular cup positioning, and stem placement without femoral osteotomy. *Results*: results were evaluated clinically and radiographically, with complications recorded. Follow-up revealed significant Harris Hip Score and limb length discrepancy improvements. Abductor muscle insufficiency was present in 21%. The acetabular component was accurately placed, centralizing the prosthetic joint's rotation. Complications occurred in 16% of cases, including fractures, nerve issues, and infection. DAA in THA showcased positive outcomes for hip function, limb length, and biomechanics in Crowe IV dysplasia. *Conclusions*: the technique enabled accurate cup positioning and rotation center adjustment. Complications were managed well without implant revisions. DAA is a viable option for Crowe IV dysplasia, restoring hip function, biomechanics, and reducing limb length discrepancy. Larger, longer studies are needed for validation.

Keywords: direct anterior approach; hip dysplasia; Crowe IV; total hip arthroplasty; femoral osteotomy; complications

1. Introduction

Total hip arthroplasty (THA) surgery is a highly effective option for restoring the inflamed state of the hip joint, especially in cases of Crowe IV hip dysplasia. However, achieving hip biomechanics restoration and optimal component positioning in THA for Crowe IV hip dysplasia poses challenges due to severe muscle retraction and poor bone stock resulting from pathologic anatomy [1,2]. Various techniques have been proposed to address these challenges, including proximalization of the center of rotation (COR) for a high hip center THA, which may sacrifice physiological hip biomechanics [3], femoral shortening osteotomy, and extensive soft tissue release to reduce the hip at the true acetabulum [4]. Despite the complexity, many authors argue that positioning the cup at the true acetabulum is associated with better long-term survival rates [5–9], even though it requires a more intricate surgical exposure to facilitate implant reduction at the end of the surgery. Historically, Heuter, Smith-Petersen, and Putti described approaches to the dysplastic hip joint through the sartorius and tensor fasciae latae intermuscular space. Accessing the joint from the anterior allows the surgeon to easily manage redundant capsular tissue and address all pathological alterations of soft tissues by performing a release of the tensor fasciae latae, medius gluteus, rectus anterior muscle, and iliopsoas muscle (Figure 1) [10–12]. At present, a modified version of the original direct anterior approach (DAA) to the hip joint is utilized for minimally invasive THA [12–16]. This approach can be extended proximally and distally to enhance exposure to the pelvis and femur, if necessary. The DAA has gained popularity in THA due to its ability to address hip muscles through an internervous and intermuscular approach. Benefits of this approach include faster healing, reduced pain, and a lower postoperative dislocation rate compared to traditional methods [17,18]. Consequently, the DAA appears to be the most effective approach for THA, at least theoretically.

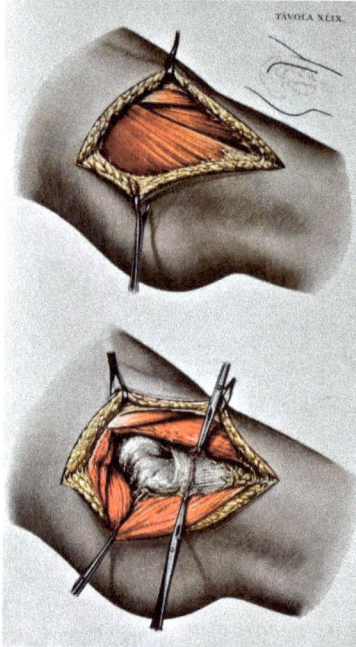
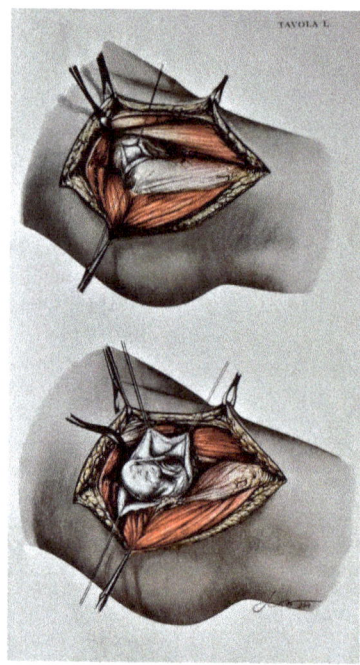

Figure 1. In the original anatomic drawings by Remo Scoto, made on commission by Vittorio Putti himself, the steps of reduction of the hip dislocation through DAA are outlined; the drawings show how DAA is powerful in managing all the pathological elements of DDH in terms of muscular and bony components; moreover, it is possible to fully expose and manage capsule, ligamentum teres at the true acetabulum, and to isolate and section the retracted soft tissues including the psoas muscle (reproduced from the book "Anatomy of congenital dislocation of the hip" by V. Putti, G. Faldini and E. Pasquali, Bologna, Licinio Cappelli Editore, 1935, by permission of Istituto Ortopedico Rizzoli [12]).

Despite the theoretical advantages associated with the use of DAA in Crowe IV dislocated hips, its use has not gained popularity for complex surgery. Only a restricted amount of literature has discussed the role of DAA for THA in DDH patients [19–22], but the heterogeneity in patients' selection and the tendency to perform an adjunctive femoral shortening osteotomy compromise the ability to define the power of DAA alone in such patient populations. The novelty of this study is to report the results of an anterior technique THA in patients suffering from Crowe IV with moderate LLD, acting only on the soft tissues, in a tailored way for the single patient, avoiding the femoral shortening ostetomy. The rationale of the present study is to evaluate the effectiveness of DAA in a homogeneous population of patients with unilateral Crowe IV hip osteoarthritis (OA) requiring a THA. The aims of this study are to investigate (1) whether THA through DAA, with accurate cup placement in the true acetabulum, is a viable and functional approach for maintaining abductor muscles, enhancing hip function, and addressing limb length discrepancy (LLD) without femoral osteotomy. (2) The extent to which this procedure consistently reestablishes the physiological center of rotation of the hip joint at the true acetabulum. (3) The intra and post-operative complications associated with this technique, along with the strategies employed for their management.

2. Materials and Methods

2.1. Patients

This study was approved by the institutional review board and ethical committee, and it was entirely conducted at the authors' Institution (code 347/2021/Oss/IOR). We retrospectively reviewed 19 patients with unilateral hip OA secondary to Crowe IV DDH who underwent a THA through a DDA between January 2016 and December 2020. The dysplastic hips were classified according to the original Crowe classification [23]. Exclusion criteria included patients with neurological diseases compromising ambulation, flaccid (e.g., poliomyelitis) or spastic (e.g., infantile cerebral palsy) paralysis, patients operated on for femoral neck fractures, patients with a radiological LLD greater than 4 cm, or bilateral DDH. The rationale behind the exclusion of patients with LLD above 4 cm is due to our treatment algorithm; indeed, in the major LLD, we perform femoral shortening osteotomy or a progressive distraction and THA at a later stage. All the patients underwent unilateral cementless THA using a DAA with progressive soft tissue release [24], cup positioning at the true acetabulum, and straight or conical stem placement without femoral shortening osteotomy. Surgery was performed by a single experienced surgeon in DAA in a single high-volume center. The implants used for the acetabulum were in all patients a hemispheric cup, coated with 3D-printed porous titanium, and at least two fixation screws were also implanted. Meanwhile, in 8 (42.1%) of the 19 operated patients a conical, short, fixed stem, coated with hydroxyapatite, was used because of the elevated anteversion of the proximal femur, and in the remaining 11 patients (57.9%) a straight, fixed, triple tapered stem, coated in hydroxyapatite, was implanted. In all patients coupling was ceramic-on-ceramic, using a large femoral head diameter. Percutaneous tenotomy at the tendon of the adductor was performed in 4/19 (25%) patients in which a limitation of the hip abduction was observed.

2.2. Surgical Technique

Surgery was performed by DAA in all patients as shown in Video S1. Briefly, the patient lay on a dedicated traction table. The incision started 2 cm distal and 2 cm lateral to the superior inferior iliac spine, and it was extended distally about 7 cm crossing the inguinal fold (Figure 2). The intermuscular plane between the sartorius muscle and the rectus femoris medially, and the tensor fascia latae (TFL) laterally, was identified and developed. After capsulotomy, the femoral neck was exposed: in dysplastic hips, the local anatomical landmarks are not very reliable, therefore, external landmarks were used to correctly perform the neck osteotomy, including femoral shaft positioning and orientation of the patella. After neck osteotomy, a full release of the joint capsule at both the femoral and acetabular sides was required to reduce the hip at the true acetabulum. At the same time, a partial release of the origin of TFL, gluteus minimus (GMi), and gluteus medius (GMe) muscles from the iliac wing, and a release of the iliopsoas tendon at the insertion onto the lesser trochanter, were tailored based on the pathological anatomy of the patients. Release of the muscles was performed starting from the ASIS and extended gradually proximally and deeply to the iliac crest to obtain proper lengthening without compromising the entire origin of the muscles or detaching their insertion at the greater trochanter (Figure 3). The removal of a thick and redundant capsular tissue exposes the false and true acetabulum. The latter is classically hypoplastic and shallow and hosts a hypertrophic pulvinar. Progressive reaming of the true acetabulum was started by using a small reamer to medialize the center of rotation and develop the bone cavity; subsequently, ream size was increased until good stability and sufficient size to host a cup were achieved. Fluoroscopy was then performed to check the correct positioning of the cup in the true acetabulum, before the screw's insertion. In most patients, press fit cup benefited from adjunct screw fixation in the posterior–superior quadrant to increase primary stability, as the bone in the true acetabular area is typically osteopenic due to disuse. To expose the femoral canal through DAA, the limb must be externally rotated, extended, and adducted. The direction of the femoral canal was identified through the sequential use of a chisel and a curved spoon, and then broaching was performed. After the final components were in place, the reduction of the hip was achieved by traction of the lower limb in a close sequence of abduction, internal rotation, and flexion. During the closing, when possible, the TFL, GMi, and GMe were reattached, using stiches, depending on the lengthening obtained. The anterior capsule, usually hypertrophic and redundant, was removed during the true acetabulum exposure or the closure. Percutaneous tenotomy of hip adductors could be performed before surgery or after wound closure if adduction contracture due to limb lengthening limited joint movement as shown in Video S2.

2.3. Post-Operative Management

Postoperative rehabilitation protocol depended on the presence of residual adductor contracture and on the entity of limb lengthening. Physical therapy was aimed at reducing contractures in flexion and adduction, which usually regressed 3 to 6 months after surgery. Ambulation with partial weight bearing (25%) on the operated limb was allowed from the day after surgery. One month postoperatively, 50% weight bearing was granted, while the full load was allowed 8 weeks after surgery. Patients were followed up clinically and radiographically at 1 month, 3 months, 1 year, and then yearly, for a minimum of 2 years postoperative follow-up.

2.4. Clinical Evaluation

Clinical scores and study parameters included the Harris Hip Score (HHS), the evaluation of apparent LLD, and the presence of a Trendelenburg sign and gait. The Harris Hip Score (HHS) [25] in the Italian-validated version was used to quantify parameters such as pain, function, and range of motion of the operated hip on a numerical scale; according to this score, results below 70 are considered poor, between 70 and 79 are discrete, between 80 and 89 are good, and between 90 and 100 are excellent. All patients were tested for LLD before and after surgery, A negative LLD with respect to the contralateral side was expressed with the sign "−", and a positive LLD with the sign "+". Apparent LLD was evaluated by block test using lifts with a 2 mm thickness progression, until the patient felt leg length equality (LLE) [26,27]. All the patients performed a postoperative antero-posterior radiographic control to check implant position.

2.5. Radiographic Evaluation

Radiographic analysis was performed by three independent hip surgeons to keep systematic error rate low. Pelvic tilt and rotation have been verified before further assessments, the tilt was checked measuring the distance between the midportion of the sacrococcygeal joint and the upper border of the symphysis pubis, and the rotation was considered neutral if the coccyx was in line with the symphysis pubis. Parameters included the evaluation of the COR of the native femoral head and THA, true LLD before and after surgery, and implant osteointegration according to Moore for the acetabular component [28] and according to Engh [29] for the femoral component. COR was measured on the horizontal and vertical axis, taking as a reference the apex of the inter-tear drop line on the anteroposterior radiograph of the pelvis [30]; true LLD was measured as the distance between proximal crossing of the femur and lesser trochanter and the bottom part of the pelvic teardrop on an anteroposterior radiograph [31].

2.6. Statistical Analysis

Distribution of variables was reported using means and ranges for normally distributed data. Data were tested for normality using the Shapiro–Wilk test. The paired *t*-test was used to compare pre- and post-operative findings. *p*-values < 0.05 were considered significant. SPSS 17.0 statistical analysis software (SPSS Inc., Chicago, IL, USA) was used to perform statistical analysis.

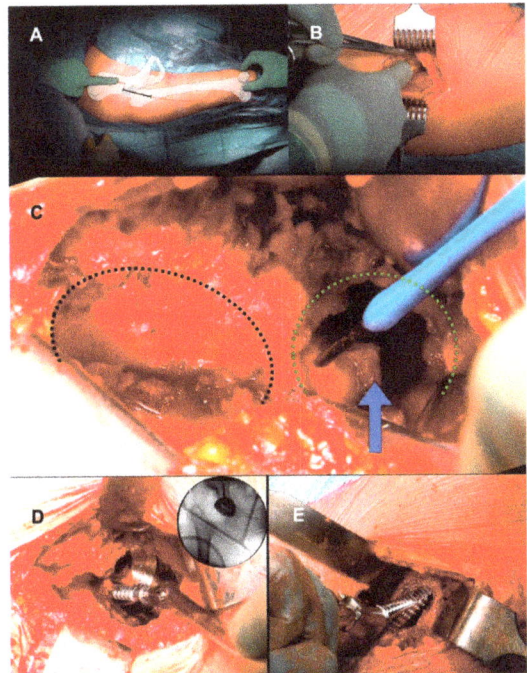

Figure 2. (**A**) Intraoperative photograph of the right hip of a 57-year-old woman with an illustration overlay showing anatomic landmarks for the anterior approach to the hip. The anterior superior iliac spine, the tip of the greater trochanter, the fibular head, and the patella should be included in the surgical field to estimate femoral shaft orientation via palpation of the femoral condyles, which guides neck resection and femoral component positioning. The skin incision begins 2 cm distal and lateral to the anterior superior iliac spine and is directed toward the fibular head for approximately 7–8 cm. (**B**) Elevation of the medial side of the aponeurosis with the use of Kocher forceps and separation of the belly of the tensor fascia latae muscle. A finger is used to develop the intermuscular space between the tensor fascia latae and the sartorius muscles, with the sartorius and the rectus femoris displaced medially and the tensor fascia latae displaced laterally. (**C**) After capsulotomy, the relationship between the false acetabulum (black dashed line) and the true acetabulum (green dashed line) is outlined. The false acetabulum is flat and wide and lies on the surface of the iliac bone. The true acetabulum is small and deficient and is covered by hypertrophic capsular tissue and pulvinar (arrow). Using electrocautery, soft tissue is carefully cleared to achieve complete exposure of the true acetabulum. (**D**) After impaction of the cup in the true acetabulum, two cancellous screws are positioned in the safe zone of the ilium to promote fixation. (**E**) At the femoral level, broach insertion should be performed in line with the femoral canal (15° of anteversion). (Figure drawn by Leonardo Tassinari, MD for this manuscript).

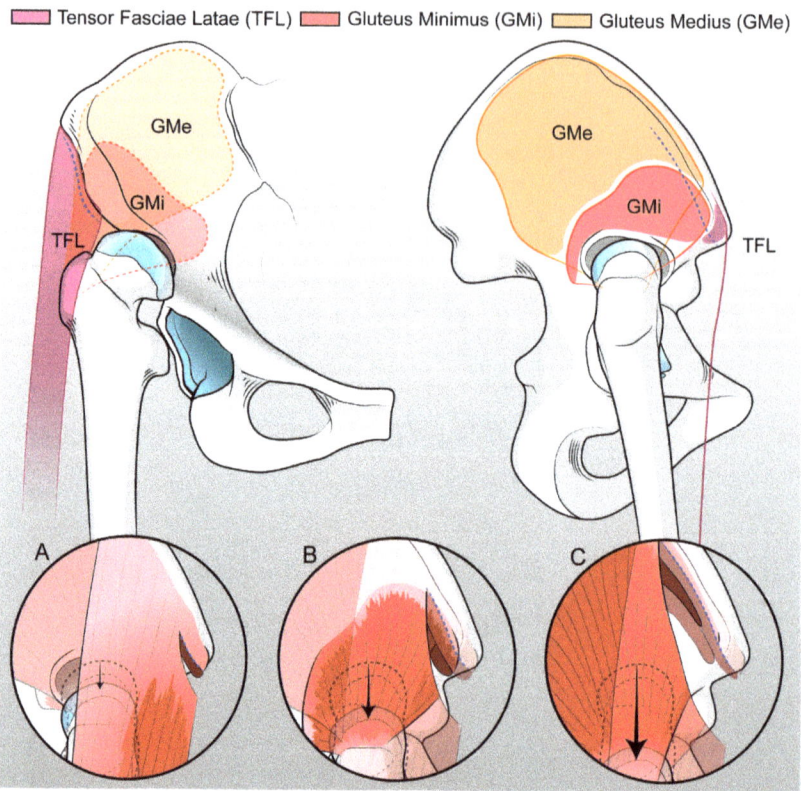

Figure 3. Anterior and lateral view of the hemi-pelvis with the representation of the progressive muscular release in order to obtain the reduction of the femur in the true acetabulum, avoiding femoral shortening osteotomy. The first step includes the detachment of TFL about 1 cm from SIAS (**A**) and the second step consists of the partial release of both TFL and GMi deeply into the iliac crest about 2 cm from SIAS (**B**). Lastly, the third step includes the partial release of the GMe (**C**) (figure drawn by Leonardo Tassinari, MD for this manuscript).

3. Results

3.1. Demographics

The patient population included 15 females and 4 males, with an average age at surgery of 55 years (range 32–71); the average BMI was 26.4 (range 19–34). The average follow-up was 33.4 months (range 24–49).

3.2. Clinical Results

At the last available follow-up, an average HHS improvement of 44.8 points was found, with preoperative values averaging 44.6 points (38–56), and a postoperative average of 89.4 points (82–96) ($p < 0.001$) (Table 1). Abductor muscle insufficiency with positive Trendelenburg gait and sign, which preoperatively was present in all the patients, was observed in 4 out of 19 patients (21%) at the last clinical evaluation. All patients presented an LLD before surgery. The sensation of LLE was obtained at the first follow-up (4 weeks) only in 5 patients (26.3%), in 6 patients (31.5%) at 3 months, in 10 patients (52.6) % at 1 year, and in 12 (63.1%) at the last available evaluation ($p < 0.001$). Apparent LLD at the operated limb decreased from a preoperative average, −3.5 cm (range 2.5–4.3 cm), to −1.2 cm (range 0.5–2.4 cm) at 4 weeks after surgery ($p < 0.001$); at 1 year, it averaged −0.7 cm (0.4–1.4 cm) and decreased up to −0.4 cm (range 0.2–0.8 cm) at the last follow-up.

Table 1. Pre- and post-operative clinical and radiographic findings.

Variable	Pre-Operative Mean (Range)	Post-Operative Mean (Range)	p-Value
Harris Hip Score	44.6 (38–56)	89.4 (82–96)	<0.001
Apparent LLD (cm)	3.5 (2.5–4.3)	1.2 (0.5–2.4)	<0.001
COR (vertical distance, cm)	4.6 (2.8–6.6)	1.9 (1.1–2.4)	<0.002
COR (horizontal distance, cm)	4.4 (4–4.8)	2.4 (1.3–3.4)	<0.0003
True LLD (cm)	3.4 (1.6–4)	0.8 (0.3–1.1)	<0.0001

LLD, limb length discrepancy; COR, center of rotation.

3.3. Radiographic Results

The acetabular component was positioned at the true acetabulum in all the patients, with distalization and medialization of the COR of the prosthetic joint. On the horizontal plane, the distance between the COR and the inter-tear drop line significantly decreased from a preoperative average of 4.4 cm (range 4–4.8) to a postoperative value of 2.4 cm (range 1.3–3.4) ($p < 0.0003$) (Figure 4). The distance between the COR and the apex of the radiographic drop was significantly reduced in the vertical plane ($p < 0.002$), passing from preoperative values of 4.6 cm (range 2.8–6.6) to average postoperative values of 1.9 cm (range 1.1–2.4). True LLD significantly reduced ($p < 0.0001$) from a preoperative average of −3.4 cm (range 1.6–4 cm) at the operated limb to −0.8 cm (range 0.3–1.1 cm) after surgery (Figure 5). At the last available follow-up, no significant loosening of the components or osteolysis was observed. The radiographic evaluation of the acetabular component according to Moore showed at least three signs of osteointegration in all the postoperative radiographs. The radiographic study of the stem according to Engh showed an average total value of 22 out of 27 (range 18.5–27), with an average fixation score equal to 7.5 (range 5–10) and a stability score of 14.5 (range 13.5–17), strongly predictive of osteointegration of the prosthetic components.

3.4. Complications

Our case series was complicated by one intraoperative subtrochanteric fracture, one transient paralysis of the femoral nerve, and one superficial surgical wound infection, accounting for a complication rate of 16%. The single superficial wound infection was from the main incision and was treated with a superficial wound debridement and oral antibiotics for 15 days with complete resolution. The subtrochanteric fracture was managed intraoperatively by metal wiring, which required a distal extension of the surgical incision of about 4 cm. After wiring, use of crutches and a delayed load on the operated limb was required; full load was granted 3 months after the surgery. The patient with transient paralysis of the femoral nerve was a female patient and was treated through a dedicated rehabilitation program with electrostimulation of the quadriceps muscle and targeted strengthening and stretching exercises. The deficit was fully recovered by the sixth postoperative month. Two out of nineteen (10.5%) patients underwent percutaneous adductor tenotomy, respectively, at 6 and 8 months after surgery, because of a severe adductor muscle contracture not improved by postoperative physical therapy; clinically, patients complained of a deficit of hip abduction and symptomatic apparent LLD. None of those patients received intraoperative tenotomy of the adductors. The procedure ensured a rapid improvement of the limitation in hip abduction, and a sensation of LLE. Two patients showed postoperative true LLD values > 1 cm, with limp during ambulation. Both benefited from the use of a shoe lift at the operated limb, achieving a sensation of LLE. No patient required implant revision at the latest available follow-up.

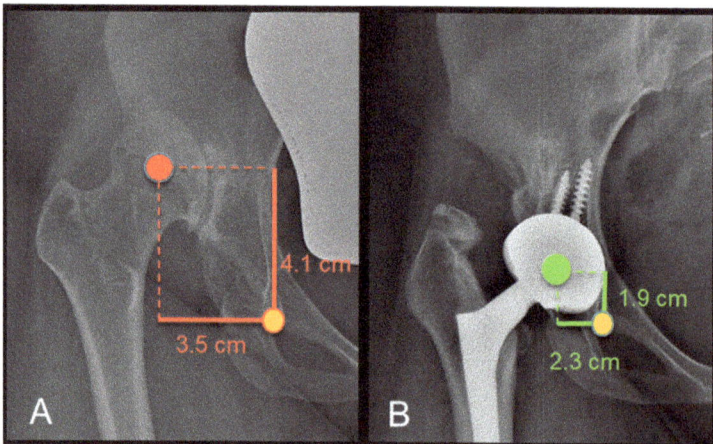

Figure 4. Pre-operative (**A**) and 18 months (**B**) X-rays showing medialization and distalization of the COR with a decrease in both horizontal and vertical distance from the teardrop.

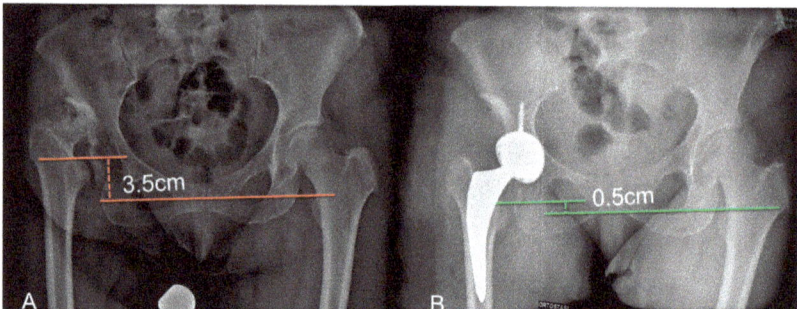

Figure 5. Pre-operative (**A**) and post-operative (**B**) X-rays showing a reduction in anatomical LLD referenced to the lesser trochanter.

4. Discussion

In the current study, patients undergoing THA through the DAA for the treatment of unilateral osteoarthritis secondary to Crowe IV dislocated hip with up to 4 cm limb shortening reported favorable clinical and radiographic outcomes, along with an acceptable complication rate. The management of pathological anatomy through DAA facilitated effective and progressive release of soft tissue contracture, characteristic of the neglected dislocated hip. Tailored soft tissue release for individual patients allowed the restoration of the physiological COR and hip biomechanics, reducing the need for ancillary procedures such as femoral shortening osteotomy. The prosthetic hip's reduction at the true acetabulum was supported by the complete excision of the hypertrophic capsule. Through DAA, the Gluteus Medius (GMi) and Gluteus Maximus (GMe) muscles, instead of being detached from the greater trochanter, could be released from the origin at the iliac wing. Similarly, the Iliopsoas and anterior rectus muscles, dysfunctional and retracted in patients with a chronically dislocated hip, were easily exposed and released when necessary, supporting the proximal femur's reduction toward the true acetabulum [32]. Preserving the insertion of abductor muscles at the greater trochanter promoted positive clinical outcomes with a significant improvement in gluteal function, lateral, and vertical offset restoration [33].

Originally developed by Heuter for managing infections and traumas at the hip [34], the DAA was subsequently used for the open reduction of dislocated dysplastic hips [35].

This approach enables the management of all pathological elements of DDH by performing a tailored soft tissue release based on the severity of the anatomical picture [36]. A notable feature of DAA is its versatility, allowing extension both proximally to expose the false acetabulum and distally to perform a femoral osteotomy or wiring of an intraoperative femoral fracture [15]. In our high-volume department, almost all primary and secondary coxarthrosis cases are treated using DAA. Conditions such as obesity and muscular males are still addressed using this technique. In obese patients, the "bikini" incision is preferred for better postoperative wound management [37]. The implementation of DAA in THA surgery for Crowe IV patients is relatively recent, and reports are limited to case series due to the rarity of the disease and the limited adoption of DAA among hip surgeons. Previous studies, such as that by Oinuma et al. [19], reported satisfactory outcomes in Crowe IV DDH patients undergoing THA replacement for osteoarthritis, with a femoral shortening osteotomy performed in each patient. Another study by Viamont-Guerra et al. [21] reported satisfactory medium- to long-term results in DDH patients undergoing THA through DAA, with four intraoperative femur fractures (21%) and a revision rate of 10% at an average follow-up of 8 years. In our experience, at an average follow-up of 2.7 years, no revisions were necessary, good implant osteointegration was observed, and no patients required femoral shortening osteotomy or femoral head autologous bone grafting to manage the acetabular bone defect. The clinical outcomes were favorable in terms of the Harris Hip Score (HHS), and the intraoperative femoral fracture rate was 5.3%.

Comparing the DAA approach to traditional THA approaches, including lateral, posterolateral, and posterior approaches, has shown excellent outcomes in DDH patients, both in terms of complications and long-term revision rates [38–42]. Traditional techniques are associated with some degree of muscle damage, with postoperative dislocation rates of up to 16.6% [2]. Type IV DDH is linked with hip muscular weakness, potentially predisposing individuals to surgical dislocation [9].

The main limitations of the current study include its retrospective nature, a low sample size, and the absence of a control group with a non-dysplastic patient cohort. Moreover, a larger number of patients and a longer follow-up would be required to confirm the current findings regarding implant failure and long-term complications, as well as for comparison with results in a non-dysplastic population. However, the exclusion of patients with bilateral DDH and LLD above 4 cm makes our conclusions highly specific for a subset of DDH patients. Patients in our study population exhibited positive results in terms of the recovery of apparent LLD, with the resolution of abduction insufficiency and limp due to gluteal insufficiency in most cases. Apparent LLD exhibited a slow but progressive improvement in patients with adduction contracture; rehabilitation therapy, consisting of stretching the adductor muscles, allowed for the achievement of fully active and passive abduction. Two patients with persistent adduction contracture at the operated limb underwent subsequent percutaneous adductor tenotomies at 6 and 8 months after the primary surgery. These results underscore the importance of the correct management of soft tissues to achieve both the restoration of the COR at the true acetabulum and functional results during rehabilitation. The contracture of the adductor muscles is usually managed percutaneously in pediatric patients with a dislocated hip and in the adult population affected by Crowe IV DDH. Given the limitation of joint range of movement due to arthritic degeneration at the false acetabulum, adductor contracture may be underestimated and consequently not managed during THA surgery [9]. In patients with a dysplastic or dislocated hip, adductor contracture significantly alters hip biomechanics, maintaining a condition of forced adduction; after THA, if persistent, adduction contracture increases the shear stress at the implant–bone interface [43], determining limited abduction, increased apparent LLD, the risk of loosening of the acetabular component, and the risk of implant dislocation. Percutaneous adductor tenotomy is sufficient in most patients to manage the residual adduction at the end of THA surgery; alternatively, it is performed preoperatively in patients with an elevated suspicion of adductor contracture [8]. In our experience, we do not perform this procedure routinely on all dysplastic patients. In the case of modest contractures, prosthetic replacement alone is often sufficient to allow acceptable degrees of abduction, especially when there is significant impingement between the femur and ilium. In the case of severe contractions or post-operative intolerance by the patient, this procedure is then performed.

Surgery was aimed at positioning the COR at the true acetabulum in all 19 patients. As reported by Komiyama et al. in a retrospective study of 1079 prosthetic implants in dysplastic patients [30], COR positioning is the main determinant of implants' mechanical complications. Placement of the acetabular cup at the true acetabulum in Crowe IV DDH patients showed better survival rates when compared to COR at the false acetabulum [5]; in fact, positioning the acetabular component at the false acetabulum is associated with an increased risk of aseptic loosening [6,7]. In a study of 49 patients with a 30-year follow-up, Watts et al. [44] showed 68% of failures of the acetabular component in case of proximalization of the COR, compared to 35% of failures in the case of COR at the true acetabulum. Similarly, Linde and Jensen [45] reported 42% of cases of aseptic loosening of the acetabular component when it was implanted at the false acetabulum in a series of 123 THAs in DDH. Stans et al. [46], at an average 16.6-year follow-up (range 5–23), reported a failure rate of the acetabular component in 83.3% of patients when the COR was placed outside the true acetabulum, mostly because of acetabular loosening. However, other authors suggest that a high hip COR in DDH patients showed no significant differences in terms of implant survival when compared to cups placed at the true acetabulum [5,47,48].

Montalti et al. [3] reported the results of a series of 80 modular neck Total Hip Arthroplasties (THAs), 37 of which were performed on Crowe IV hips. At an average 15-year follow-up, they documented excellent clinical and radiographic outcomes, with revision required in only two patients—one due to aseptic cup loosening and the other due to aseptic loosening of the femoral component. Achieving the correct leg length by placing the cup at the false acetabulum without the use of long modular necks is seldom possible. Moreover, if a high hip center THA is performed, a ceramic-on-ceramic coupling is required, limiting the use of polyethylene lips in case of suboptimal cup positioning [48,49].

Patients in the current study demonstrated a good correction of true LLD, with an average postoperative difference of 0.8 cm between the operated and the contralateral healthy limb. Seven patients required the use of a shoe lift to manage LLD, with 63.1% experiencing a sensation of limb length equality. Conversely, LLD due to adductor contracture required intensive rehabilitation therapy with adductor stretching, and in two patients, an additional percutaneous adductor tenotomy was performed to achieve satisfactory clinical results.

During our retrospective study, we observed three complications: one intraoperative subtrochanteric fracture, one transient paralysis of the femoral nerve, and one superficial surgical wound infection. THA surgery in degenerative arthritis secondary to Crowe IV dislocation is associated with a significant number of complications, including neurovascular compromise due to limb lengthening or direct trauma, intraoperative fractures, component loosening, and dislocation [50–53]. Patients in the current study showed an overall acceptable complication rate of approximately 16%, and none of these patients required implant revision surgery at the last follow-up. These data are similar or slightly less compared to the complication rate presented in other studies, including those where other approaches and femoral shortening osteotomy were performed, where the risk of non-union is also to be considered [50,51]. Transient paralysis of the femoral or sciatic nerve, although relatively rare, must be carefully considered in patients with severe flexion contracture who undergo intraoperative limb lengthening. In our cohort of patients, one femoral nerve apraxia and no sciatic nerve paralysis were observed. The risk of paralysis increases in case of limb lengthening above 4 cm [54,55] due to traction of the nerve or compression exerted by the post-surgical hematoma. Somatosensory evoked potential (SSEP) was not routinely used during surgery to check for any nerve injuries; however, a careful control of pre- and post-reduction soft tissue tension was performed to avoid nerve traction. In cases of excessive tension or impossibility of reduction, a rescue procedure was performed, such as femoral shortening osteotomy. Moreover, several strategies are employed to minimize this complication, including proximalization of the COR, nerve isolation, and debridement to avoid traction [19,56]. These procedures were not necessary in our patients because, in all cases, it was possible to place the cup at the true acetabulum through soft tissue management. However, it must be emphasized that true LLD greater than 4 cm represented exclusion criteria for the recruitment of patients in the current study. Beyond this elongation limit, our surgical strategy envisages the gradual distalization of the femur using an external fixation device before THA implant.

5. Conclusions

In conclusion, THA in the Crowe IV dysplastic hip using DAA allows for excellent clinical and radiographic results with an acceptable complication rate. The approach's progressive and patient-specific soft tissue release facilitates the positioning of the cup component at the true acetabulum, eliminating the need for femoral shortening osteotomy.

Supplementary Materials: The following supporting information can be downloaded at: https://www.mdpi.com/article/10.3390/medicina60010114/s1, Video S1: THA by DAA in Crowe IV: surgical technique, Video S2: adductors percutaneous tenotomy.

Author Contributions: Conceptualization, C.F. and F.T.; methodology, V.R. and F.P.; validation, A.D.M.; formal analysis, D.P., L.T. and V.R.; writing—original draft preparation, L.T. and M.B.; writing—review and editing, A.D.M. and G.G.; supervision, A.D.M.; project administration, C.F. and A.D.M. All authors have read and agreed to the published version of the manuscript.

Funding: This research received no external funding.

Institutional Review Board Statement: The study was conducted in accordance with the Declaration of Helsinki and approved by the local Ethics Committee (protocol code 347/2021/Oss/IOR of 23 March 2021).

Informed Consent Statement: Informed consent was obtained from all subjects involved in the study. Written informed consent has been obtained from the patient(s) to publish this paper.

Data Availability Statement: The data presented in this study are available on request from the corresponding author.

Conflicts of Interest: The authors declare no conflicts of interest.

References

1. Husson, J.L.; Mallet, J.F.; Huten, D.; Odri, G.A.; Morin, C.; Parent, H.F. Applications in Hip Pathology. *Orthop. Traumatol. Surg. Res.* **2010**, *96*, S10–S16. [CrossRef] [PubMed]
2. Greber, E.M.; Pelt, C.E.; Gililland, J.M.; Anderson, M.B.; Erickson, J.A.; Peters, C.L. Challenges in Total Hip Arthroplasty in the Setting of Developmental Dysplasia of the Hip. *J. Arthroplast.* **2017**, *32*, S38–S44. [CrossRef] [PubMed]
3. Montalti, M.; Castagnini, F.; Giardina, F.; Tassinari, E.; Biondi, F.; Toni, A. Cementless Total Hip Arthroplasty in Crowe III and IV Dysplasia: High Hip Center and Modular Necks. *J. Arthroplast.* **2018**, *33*, 1813–1819. [CrossRef] [PubMed]
4. Li, Y.; Zhang, X.; Wang, Q.; Peng, X.; Wang, Q.; Jiang, Y.; Chen, Y. Equalisation of Leg Lengths in Total Hip Arthroplasty for Patients with Crowe Type-IV Developmental Dysplasia of the Hip. *Bone Jt. J.* **2017**, *99B*, 872–879. [CrossRef] [PubMed]
5. Sakellariou, V.I.; Christodoulou, M.; Sasalos, G.; Babis, G.C. Reconstruction of the Acetabulum in Developmental Dysplasia of the Hip in Total Hip Replacement. *Arch. Bone Jt. Surg.* **2014**, *2*, 130–136. [PubMed]
6. Bicanic, G.; Barbaric, K.; Bohacek, I.; Aljinovic, A.; Delimar, D. Current Concept in Dysplastic Hip Arthroplasty: Techniques for Acetabular and Femoral Reconstruction. *World J. Orthop.* **2014**, *5*, 412–424. [CrossRef] [PubMed]
7. Pagnano, M.W.; Hanssen, A.D.; Lewallen, D.G.; Shaughnessy, W.J. The Effect of Superior Placement of the Acetabular Component on the Rate of Loosening after Total Hip Arthroplasty: Long-Term Results in Patients Who Have Crowe Type-II Congenital Dysplasia of the Hip. *J. Bone Jt. Surg.* **1996**, *78*, 1004–1014. [CrossRef] [PubMed]
8. Shi, X.-t.; Li, C.-f.; Han, Y.; Song, Y.; Li, S.-x.; Liu, J.-g. Total Hip Arthroplasty for Crowe Type IV Hip Dysplasia: Surgical Techniques and Postoperative Complications. *Orthop. Surg.* **2019**, *11*, 966–973. [CrossRef]
9. Wu, X.; Li, S.H.; Lou, L.M.; Cai, Z.D. The Techniques of Soft Tissue Release and True Socket Reconstruction in Total Hip Arthroplasty for Patients with Severe Developmental Dysplasia of the Hip. *Int. Orthop.* **2012**, *36*, 1795–1801. [CrossRef]
10. Heuter, C. Grundriss Der Chirurgie. In *Grundriss der Chirurgie*; F.C.W. Vogel: Leipzig, Germany, 1883; pp. 129–200.
11. Smith-Petersen, M.N.; Larson, C.B. Complications of Old Fractures of the Neck of the Femur; Results of Treatment of Vitallium-Mold Arthroplasty. *J. Bone Jt. Surg. Am.* **1947**, *29*, 41–48.

12. Putti, V.; Faldini, G.; Pasquali, E. *Anatomy of Congenital Dislocation of the Hip*; Licinio Cappelli Editore: Bologna, Italy, 1935.
13. Cadossi, M.; Sambri, A.; Tedesco, G.; Mazzotti, A.; Terrando, S.; Faldini, C. Anterior Approach in Total Hip Replacement. *Orthopedics* **2017**, *40*, e553–e556. [CrossRef] [PubMed]
14. Lovell, T.P. Single-Incision Direct Anterior Approach for Total Hip Arthroplasty Using a Standard Operating Table. *J. Arthroplast.* **2008**, *23*, 64–68. [CrossRef] [PubMed]
15. Mirza, A.J.; Lombardi, A.V., Jr.; Morris, M.J.; Berend, K.R. A Mini-Anterior Approach to the Hip for Total Joint Replacement: Optimising Results: Improving Hip Joint Replacement Outcomes. *Bone Jt. J.* **2014**, *96B*, 32–35. [CrossRef] [PubMed]
16. Parvizi, J.; Restrepo, C.; Maltenfort, M.G. Total Hip Arthroplasty Performed Through Direct Anterior Approach Provides Superior Early Outcome: Results of a Randomized, Prospective Study. *Orthop. Clin. N. Am.* **2016**, *47*, 497–504. [CrossRef] [PubMed]
17. Nogler, M.M.; Thaler, M.R. The Direct Anterior Approach for Hip Revision: Accessing the Entire Femoral Diaphysis Without Endangering the Nerve Supply. *J. Arthroplast.* **2017**, *32*, 510–514. [CrossRef] [PubMed]
18. Taunton, M.J.; Trousdale, R.T.; Sierra, R.J.; Kaufman, K.; Pagnano, M.W. John Charnley Award: Randomized Clinical Trial of Direct Anterior and Miniposterior Approach THA: Which Provides Better Functional Recovery? *Clin. Orthop. Relat. Res.* **2018**, *476*, 216–229. [CrossRef] [PubMed]
19. Oinuma, K.; Tamaki, T.; Miura, Y.; Kaneyama, R.; Shiratsuchi, H. Total Hip Arthroplasty with Subtrochanteric Shortening Osteotomy for Crowe Grade 4 Dysplasia Using the Direct Anterior Approach. *J. Arthroplast.* **2014**, *29*, 626–629. [CrossRef]
20. Kawasaki, M.; Hasegawa, Y.; Okura, T.; Ochiai, S.; Fujibayashi, T. Muscle Damage After Total Hip Arthroplasty Through the Direct Anterior Approach for Developmental Dysplasia of the Hip. *J. Arthroplast.* **2017**, *32*, 2466–2473. [CrossRef]
21. Viamont-Guerra, M.R.; Chen, A.F.; Stirling, P.; Nover, L.; Guimarães, R.P.; Laude, F. The Direct Anterior Approach for Total Hip Arthroplasty for Severe Dysplasia (Crowe III and IV) Provides Satisfactory Medium to Long-Term Outcomes. *J. Arthroplast.* **2020**, *35*, 1642–1650. [CrossRef]
22. Viamont-Guerra, M.R.; Saffarini, M.; Laude, F. Surgical Technique and Case Series of Total Hip Arthroplasty with the Hueter Anterior Approach for Crowe Type-IV Dysplasia. *J. Bone Jt. Surg. Am.* **2020**, *102*, 99–106. [CrossRef]
23. Jawad, M.U.; Scully, S.P. In Brief: Crowe's Classification: Arthroplasty in Developmental Dysplasia of the Hip. *Clin. Orthop. Relat. Res.* **2011**, *469*, 306–308. [CrossRef] [PubMed]
24. Rodriguez, J.A.; Kamara, E.; Cooper, H.J. Applied Anatomy of the Direct Anterior Approach for Femoral Mobilization. *JBJS Essent. Surg. Tech.* **2017**, *7*, e18. [CrossRef] [PubMed]
25. Banaszkiewicz, P.A. Traumatic Arthritis of the Hip after Dislocation and Acetabular Fractures: Treatment by Mold Arthroplasty: An End-Result Study Using a New Method of Result Evaluation. In *Classic Papers in Orthopaedics*; Springer: London, UK, 2014; pp. 13–17; ISBN 9781447154518.
26. Abraham, W.; Dimon, J., 3rd. Leg Length Discrepancy in Total Hip Arthroplasty. *Orthop. Clin. N. Am.* **1992**, *23*, 201–209. [CrossRef]
27. Sabharwal, S.; Kumar, A. Methods for Assessing Leg Length Discrepancy. *Clin. Orthop. Relat. Res.* **2008**, *466*, 2910–2922. [CrossRef] [PubMed]
28. Moore, M.S.; McAuley, J.P.; Young, A.M.; Engh, C.A. Radiographic Signs of Osseointegration in Porous-Coated Acetabular Components. *Clin. Orthop. Relat. Res.* **2006**, *444*, 176–183. [CrossRef] [PubMed]
29. Engh, C.A.; Bobyn, J.D.; Glassman, A.H. Porous-Coated Hip Replacement. The Factors Governing Bone Ingrowth, Stress Shielding, and Clinical Results. *J. Bone Jt. Surg. Ser. B* **1987**, *69*, 45–55. [CrossRef]
30. Komiyama, K.; Fukushi, J.-i.; Motomura, G.; Hamai, S.; Ikemura, S.; Fujii, M.; Nakashima, Y. Does High Hip Centre Affect Dislocation after Total Hip Arthroplasty for Developmental Dysplasia of the Hip? *Int. Orthop.* **2019**, *43*, 2057–2063. [CrossRef]
31. Della Valle, A.G.; Padgett, D.E.; Salvati, E.A. Preoperative Planning for Primary Total Hip Arthroplasty. *J. Am. Acad. Orthop. Surg.* **2005**, *13*, 455–462. [CrossRef]
32. Glorion, C. Surgical Reduction of Congenital Hip Dislocation. *Orthop. Traumatol. Surg. Res.* **2018**, *104*, S147–S157. [CrossRef]
33. Rüdiger, H.A.; Parvex, V.; Terrier, A. Impact of the Femoral Head Position on Moment Arms in Total Hip Arthroplasty: A Parametric Finite Element Study. *J. Arthroplast.* **2016**, *31*, 715–720. [CrossRef]
34. Hueter, C. Die Methodik Der Resectio Coxae Durch Vorderen Schrägschnitt. (Methode von Schede Und C. Hueter). Verletzungen Und Krankheiten Des Hüftgelenks. Resectio Coxae. In *Grundriss der Chirurgie*; F.C.W. Vogel: Leipzig, Germany, 1880; pp. 935–937.
35. Rachbauer, F.; Kain, M.S.H.; Leunig, M. The History of the Anterior Approach to the Hip. *Orthop. Clin. N. Am.* **2009**, *40*, 311–320. [CrossRef] [PubMed]
36. Faldini, C.; Miscione, M.T.; Chehrassan, M.; Acri, F.; Pungetti, C.; D'Amato, M.; Luciani, D.; Giannini, S. Congenital Hip Dysplasia Treated by Total Hip Arthroplasty Using Cementless Tapered Stem in Patients Younger than 50 Years Old: Results after 12-Years Follow-Up. *J. Orthop. Traumatol.* **2011**, *12*, 213–218. [CrossRef] [PubMed]
37. Corten, K.; Holzapfel, B.M. Direct Anterior Approach for Total Hip Arthroplasty Using the "Bikini Incision". *Oper. Orthop. Traumatol.* **2021**, *33*, 318–330. [CrossRef] [PubMed]
38. Faldini, C.; Brunello, M.; Pilla, F.; Geraci, G.; Stefanini, N.; Tassinari, L.; Di Martino, A. Femoral Head Autograft to Manage Acetabular Bone Loss Defects in THA for Crowe III Hips by DAA: Retrospective Study and Surgical Technique. *J. Clin. Med.* **2023**, *12*, 751. [CrossRef] [PubMed]
39. Sofu, H.; Kockara, N.; Gursu, S.; Issin, A.; Oner, A.; Sahin, V. Transverse Subtrochanteric Shortening Osteotomy During Cementless Total Hip Arthroplasty in Crowe Type-III or IV Developmental Dysplasia. *J. Arthroplast.* **2015**, *30*, 1019–1023. [CrossRef] [PubMed]

40. Mu, W.; Yang, D.; Xu, B.; Mamtimin, A.; Guo, W.; Cao, L. Midterm Outcome of Cementless Total Hip Arthroplasty in Crowe IV-Hartofilakidis Type III Developmental Dysplasia of the Hip. *J. Arthroplast.* **2016**, *31*, 668–675. [CrossRef] [PubMed]
41. Ahmed, E.; Ibrahim, E.G.; Ayman, B. Total Hip Arthroplasty with Subtrochanteric Osteotomy in Neglected Dysplastic Hip. *Int. Orthop.* **2015**, *39*, 27–33. [CrossRef]
42. Li, X.; Lu, Y.; Sun, J.; Lin, X.; Tang, T. Treatment of Crowe Type-IV Hip Dysplasia Using Cementless Total Hip Arthroplasty and Double Chevron Subtrochanteric Shortening Osteotomy: A 5- to 10-Year Follow-Up Study. *J. Arthroplast.* **2017**, *32*, 475–479. [CrossRef]
43. Gofton, J.P. Studies in Osteoarthritis of the Hip. IV. Biomechanics and Clinical Considerations. *Can. Med. Assoc. J.* **1971**, *104*, 1007–1011.
44. Watts, C.D.; Abdel, M.P.; Hanssen, A.D.; Pagnano, M.W. Anatomic Hip Center Decreases Aseptic Loosening Rates after Total Hip Arthroplasty with Cement in Patients with Crowe Type-II Dysplasia: A Concise Follow-up Report at a Mean of Thirty-Six Years. *J. Bone Jt. Surg. Am. Vol.* **2016**, *98*, 910–915. [CrossRef]
45. Linde, F.; Jensen, J. Socket Loosening in Arthroplasty for Congenital Dislocation of the Hip. *Acta Orthop. Scand.* **1988**, *59*, 254–257. [CrossRef] [PubMed]
46. Stans, A.A.; Pagnano, M.W.; Shaughnessy, W.J.; Hanssen, A.D. Results of Total Hip Arthroplasty for Crowe Type III Developmental Hip Dysplasia. *Clin. Orthop. Relat. Res.* **1998**, *348*, 149–157. [CrossRef]
47. Nawabi, D.H.; Meftah, M.; Nam, D.; Ranawat, A.S.; Ranawat, C.S. Durable Fixation Achieved with Medialized, High Hip Center Cementless THAs for Crowe II and III Dysplasia. *Clin. Orthop. Relat. Res.* **2014**, *472*, 630–636. [CrossRef] [PubMed]
48. Traina, F.; De Fine, M.; Biondi, F.; Tassinari, E.; Galvani, A.; Toni, A. The Influence of the Centre of Rotation on Implant Survival Using a Modular Stem Hip Prosthesis. *Int. Orthop.* **2009**, *33*, 1513–1518. [CrossRef] [PubMed]
49. Traina, F.; De Fine, M.; Tassinari, E.; Sudanese, A.; Calderoni, P.P.; Toni, A. Modular Neck Prostheses in DDH Patients: 11-Year Results. *J. Orthop. Sci.* **2011**, *16*, 14–20. [CrossRef] [PubMed]
50. Wang, D.; Li, L.L.; Wang, H.Y.; Pei, F.X.; Zhou, Z.K. Long-Term Results of Cementless Total Hip Arthroplasty With Subtrochanteric Shortening Osteotomy in Crowe Type IV Developmental Dysplasia. *J. Arthroplast.* **2017**, *32*, 1211–1219. [CrossRef]
51. Krych, A.J.; Howard, J.L.; Trousdale, R.T.; Cabanela, M.E.; Berry, D.J. Total Hip Arthroplasty with Shortening Subtrochanteric Osteotomy in Crowe Type-IV Developmental Dysplasia. *J. Bone Jt. Surg.* **2009**, *91*, 2213–2221. [CrossRef]
52. Zhu, B.; Su, C.; He, Y.; Chai, X.; Li, Z.; Hou, Z.; Lou, T.; Yan, X. Combined Anteversion Technique in Total Hip Arthroplasty for Crowe IV Developmental Dysplasia of the Hip. *HIP Int.* **2017**, *27*, 589–594. [CrossRef]
53. Shi, X.-t.; Li, C.-f.; Cheng, C.-m.; Feng, C.-y.; Li, S.-x.; Liu, J.-g. Preoperative Planning for Total Hip Arthroplasty for Neglected Developmental Dysplasia of the Hip. *Orthop. Surg.* **2019**, *11*, 348–355. [CrossRef]
54. Yang, S.; Cui, Q. Total Hip Arthroplasty in Developmental Dysplasia of the Hip: Review of Anatomy, Techniques and Outcomes. *World J. Orthop.* **2012**, *3*, 42–48. [CrossRef]
55. Edwards, B.N.; Tullos, H.S.; Noble, P.C. Contributory Factors and Etiology of Sciatic Nerve Palsy in Total Hip Arthroplasty. *Clin. Orthop. Relat. Res.* **1987**, *218*, 136–141. [CrossRef]
56. Kawai, T.; Tanaka, C.; Kanoe, H. Total Hip Arthroplasty for Crowe IV Hip without Subtrochanteric Shortening Osteotomy—A Long Term Follow up Study. *BMC Musculoskelet. Disord.* **2014**, *15*, 72. [CrossRef] [PubMed]

Disclaimer/Publisher's Note: The statements, opinions and data contained in all publications are solely those of the individual author(s) and contributor(s) and not of MDPI and/or the editor(s). MDPI and/or the editor(s) disclaim responsibility for any injury to people or property resulting from any ideas, methods, instructions or products referred to in the content.

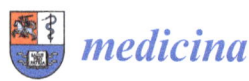

Article

Impact of Syndesmotic Screw Removal on Quality of Life, Mobility, and Daily Living Activities in Patients Post Distal Tibiofibular Diastasis Repair

Isabella-Ionela Sanda [1,2], Samer Hosin [1,3,*], Dinu Vermesan [3], Bogdan Deleanu [3], Daniel Pop [3], Dan Crisan [3], Musab Al-Qatawneh [3], Mihai Mioc [3], Radu Prejbeanu [3] and Ovidiu Rosca [4]

1. Doctoral School, "Victor Babes" University of Medicine and Pharmacy Timisoara, 300041 Timisoara, Romania; isabella.sanda@umft.ro
2. Department of Laboratory Medicine, "Victor Babes" University of Medicine and Pharmacy Timisoara, Eftimie Murgu Square 2, 300041 Timisoara, Romania
3. Department of Orthopedics, "Victor Babes" University of Medicine and Pharmacy Timisoara, 300041 Timisoara, Romania; dinu@vermesan.ro (D.V.); bogdandeleanu@yahoo.com (B.D.); daniellaurentiupop@yahoo.com (D.P.); crisan.dan@gmail.com (D.C.); msb898@gmail.com (M.A.-Q.); mihaillazarmioc@gmail.com (M.M.); raduprejbeanu@gmail.com (R.P.)
4. Department of Infectious Diseases, "Victor Babes" University of Medicine and Pharmacy Timisoara, Eftimie Murgu Square 2, 300041 Timisoara, Romania; ovidiu.rosca@umft.ro
* Correspondence: samerhosin@umft.ro

Abstract: *Background and Objectives:* While numerous studies have been conducted on syndesmotic screw management following distal tibiofibular diastasis repair, a clear consensus remains unclear. This research aims to evaluate whether the postoperative removal of syndesmotic screws leads to improved patient outcomes, specifically in quality of life, mobility, and daily living activities, and whether it offers a cost-effective solution. *Materials and Methods:* Patients with a history of unimalleolar or bimalleolar ankle fractures, classified according to the Danis–Weber and Lauge–Hansen systems, were included. Comprehensive evaluations were made via standardized questionnaires like the SF-36 Health Survey, HADS, and WHOQOL-BREF, distributed approximately 2 months post surgery. A total of 93 patients underwent syndesmotic screw removal while 51 retained the screws (conservative approach). *Results:* Patients who underwent screw removal reported superior satisfaction in mobility, with a score of 7.8, compared to 6.7 in the conservative approach ($p = 0.018$). Similarly, their ability to perform daily activities scored 8.1, higher than the 6.5 from the conservative cohort ($p < 0.001$). Pain levels were also more favorable in the screw removal group, with a score of 5.3 against 6.8 in the conservative group ($p = 0.003$). On the SF-36 physical domain, the screw removal group achieved a mean score of 55.9 versus 53.3 for the conservative group ($p = 0.027$). Notably, the HADS anxiety subscale highlighted reduced anxiety levels in the screw removal cohort with a mean score of 5.8 against 7.3 in the conservative group ($p = 0.006$). However, overall quality of life and recommendations to others showed no significant difference between the groups. *Conclusions:* Syndesmotic screw removal postoperatively leads to marked improvements in patients' mobility, daily activity abilities, and reduced postoperative pain and anxiety levels. However, overall quality of life was similar between the two approaches. The findings offer valuable insights for orthopedic decision making and patient-centered care concerning the management of syndesmotic screws after distal tibiofibular diastasis repair.

Keywords: ankle injuries; tibiofibular ankle syndesmosis; ankle fractures; quality of life

Citation: Sanda, I.-I.; Hosin, S.; Vermesan, D.; Deleanu, B.; Pop, D.; Crisan, D.; Al-Qatawneh, M.; Mioc, M.; Prejbeanu, R.; Rosca, O. Impact of Syndesmotic Screw Removal on Quality of Life, Mobility, and Daily Living Activities in Patients Post Distal Tibiofibular Diastasis Repair. *Medicina* **2023**, *59*, 2048. https://doi.org/10.3390/medicina59122048

Academic Editor: Woo Jong Kim

Received: 16 October 2023
Revised: 10 November 2023
Accepted: 14 November 2023
Published: 21 November 2023

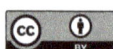

Copyright: © 2023 by the authors. Licensee MDPI, Basel, Switzerland. This article is an open access article distributed under the terms and conditions of the Creative Commons Attribution (CC BY) license (https://creativecommons.org/licenses/by/4.0/).

1. Introduction

Distal tibiofibular syndesmosis, a fibrous joint connecting the tibia and fibula just above the ankle, is integral for weight-bearing and walking [1]. The unique arrangement of ligaments in this region grants stability and permits necessary motion between the two bones [2]. Distal tibiofibular diastasis, which denotes a separation or injury to this joint, can critically compromise ankle function [3,4]. Indeed, according to existing data, such injuries represent approximately 10% of all ankle traumas, with the majority resulting from high-energy mechanisms like falls or motor vehicle accidents [5,6].

Syndesmotic screw fixation has become the gold standard for surgically managing the tibiofibular diastasis, even though other methods such as suture buttons exist and offer good results [7]. By using screws to temporarily hold the tibia and fibula together, this technique aims to ensure proper alignment and healing. Yet, the procedure is not devoid of controversy, primarily surrounding the decision to retain or remove the screws [8–10]. The school of thought supporting retention cites reduced reoperation rates and fewer associated complications [11], whereas proponents for removal argue that it leads to better joint function and decreases potential hardware complications [12].

Notably, the clinical implications of the decision to remove or retain the syndesmotic screw after ankle fixation weigh heavily on patient-reported outcomes [13]. Several patients are likely to express dissatisfaction following syndesmotic screw fixation, the contributing factors often including the medical intervention itself, post-removal pain, decreased range of motion, and limitations in daily activities [14]. Moreover, bone manipulation and generally orthopedic interventions increase the risk for infections that are difficult to treat, such as osteomyelitis [15,16]; thus, some patients may prefer the conservative approach. Some of the literature indicates that patients experience a tangible improvement in these domains after screw removal, although contradictory reports suggest that outcomes might be independent of the screw's presence [17,18]. On the other side, patients that prefer to retain the syndesmotic screw might report lower anxiety levels associated with multiple medical visits and the intervention itself, but they might also have a higher comorbidity index; therefore preferring a more conservative approach [19,20].

The impact of syndesmotic screw fixation on the mechanical properties of bone, particularly its quality and quantity, is an aspect that warrants deeper exploration. Studies on prosthetic designs, such as those highlighted in the referenced works, reveal the significance of balancing material strength and flexibility under varied load conditions. In the context of hand prostheses, the emphasis on lightweight yet sturdy materials to improve functionality and aesthetics [21] mirrors the necessity in ankle surgery to find a balance between stability and the natural movement of bones. Similarly, the review of torsional loads in various engineering applications [22] underscores the importance of considering multidimensional stress factors, which could inform the approach to managing the rotational and axial stresses exerted on the ankle joint post surgery. Furthermore, insights from prosthetic acceptance studies [23], emphasizing the need for adaptability to individual needs, suggest a parallel in surgical decision making, where individual variations in bone structure and healing capacity may influence the choice between screw retention and removal.

Moreover, the economic aspects of this debate are far-reaching. Additional operations for screw removal not only incur direct medical costs but also encompass indirect expenses like patient work absence and rehabilitation. Analysis indicates that the cost of syndesmotic screw removal surgeries averaged EUR 900, compared to only EUR 400 for conservative management [24], a figure which further increases when accounting for the 10%–20% complication rate associated with such procedures [25].

Despite numerous studies on the topic, a consensus remains elusive [26]. Both the orthopedic community and patients stand to benefit from a comprehensive evaluation that not only delves into clinical outcomes but also critically assesses the cost-effectiveness and long-term implications of the decision to remove or retain syndesmotic screws. Building on this background, our study posits that postoperative syndesmotic screw removal yields significant improvements in patients' quality of life, mobility, and ability to perform daily living activities. Furthermore, when the broader economic and societal implications are considered, screw removal may represent a more cost-effective strategy for patient management. The chief aim of this research is to conclusively evaluate these hypotheses and provide an evidence-based recommendation for the management of syndesmotic screws following distal tibiofibular diastasis repair.

2. Materials and Methods

2.1. Study Design and Settings

The present study employed a cross-sectional design; it was conducted at the University Clinic of Orthopedics affiliated with the "Victor Babes" University of Medicine and Pharmacy in Timisoara. Utilizing the clinic's inpatient population database, we identified relevant demographic information and other pertinent clinical data from both digital and paper records. All patient data were safeguarded according to existing privacy laws and accessed by certified physicians and healthcare professionals participating in this research. The orthopedic clinic operates under the Local Commission of Ethics regulations, according to the Article 167 of Law No. 95/2006, Art. 28, Chapter VIII of Order 904/2006; the EU GCP Directives 2005/28/EC; and the International Conference on Harmonisation of Technical Requirements for Registration of Pharmaceuticals for Human Use.

2.2. Participant Selection and Sample Collection

Eligible participants included those with a history of unimalleolar or bimalleolar ankle fractures, identified using International Classification of Diseases (ICD-10) diagnosis codes [27]. The fractures' classifications were, according to the Danis–Weber system, unstable type C [28]. Additionally, the Lauge–Hansen grading system further classified the fractures as SER—supination external rotation fracture; PER—pronation external rotation fracture; SA—supination adduction; and PA—pronation abduction. Other inclusion criteria encompassed patients aged 18 and above with comprehensive medical records and consent for participation. Any missing critical data or absence of a consent form resulted in exclusion from the current study. Patients who developed orthopedic complications were not considered for inclusion. All patients underwent postoperative rehabilitation.

2.3. Data Acquisition and Surveys

For an in-depth understanding of patients' postoperative experiences and quality of life, several standardized questionnaires were provided. All surveys were delivered approximately 2 months after the surgical intervention for distal tibiofibular diastasis repair for the group of patients with conservative management leaving the talofibular screw intact, and 2 months after screw removal for the other group. The SF-36 Health Survey [29] was important in assessing the quality of life, spanning a spectrum of health dimensions, from physical functioning to emotional well-being. The HADS (Hospital Anxiety and Depression Scale) [30] was particularly insightful in shedding light on the mental health aspects, determining the severity of both anxiety and depressive symptoms among participants. The WHOQOL-BREF [31], comprising 26 questions, served as a broader tool to appraise the overall quality of life. In addition to these, an unstandardized survey with 8 specific questions was utilized to determine other areas not covered by the standardized questionnaires, ensuring a holistic patient perspective was captured.

Moreover, the study investigated a range of patient variables, comprising the patients' age with and distinctions based on sex and body mass index, especially identifying those with a BMI over 25.0 kg/m^2 and classifying them as overweight. The environmental and socioeconomic conditions of the participants were recorded by noting their areas of residence, emphasizing those from urban areas. Marital status was considered, and economic conditions were elucidated with an assessment of participants earning an average or above-average income. Educational achievements were recorded by highlighting those with higher education, and employment status focused on those unemployed. Lifestyle habits, which can profoundly impact recovery and rehabilitation, were not overlooked, documenting frequent alcohol consumers and regular smokers. A significant clinical variable was the Charlson Comorbidity Index (CCI), with special attention given to those with a score greater than 2. Regarding the clinical specifics, fracture types were categorized into unimalleolar and bimalleolar. Further classification was conducted based on the Lauge–Hansen system, differentiating fractures into SER (supination external rotation), PER (pronation external rotation), SA (supination adduction), and PA (pronation abduction).

2.4. Statistical Analysis

Data management and analysis were conducted utilizing the statistical software SPSS version 26.0 (SPSS Inc., Chicago, IL, USA). The sample size was calculated based on a convenience sampling method, with a minimum requirement for statistical power of 129 respondents at a 95% confidence level and 5% margin of error. Continuous variables were represented as mean ± standard deviation (SD), while categorical variables were expressed in terms of frequencies and percentages. To analyze the changes between more than two means of continuous variables, Student's t-test was utilized. The Chi-squared test was utilized for the categorical variables. A multivariate regression analysis was performed to determine the risk factors for influenced quality of life. A p-value threshold of less than 0.05 was set for statistical significance. All results were double-checked to ensure accuracy and reliability.

3. Results

From the total sample, 93 patients underwent syndesmotic screw removal while 51 were managed with a conservative approach. Age distribution was similar between the two groups, with the screw removal cohort averaging 32.8 ± years and the conservative approach cohort averaging 33.5 years; this difference was not statistically significant ($p = 0.759$). In terms of gender distribution, 60.2% of the screw removal group were men, compared to 45.1% in the conservative group; this observed difference approached significance but did not reach it ($p = 0.081$). The proportion of overweight individuals, defined by a BMI of greater than 25.0 kg/m^2, was slightly higher in the conservative approach group, at 47.1%, than in the screw removal group, at 38.7%, though the difference was not statistically significant ($p = 0.331$).

Most of the background characteristics such as area of residence (urban vs. rural), relationship status (married vs. other), income levels, education levels, and employment status revealed no significant differences between the two groups. The same was observed for habits such as frequent alcohol consumption and smoking. Moreover, there was no significant difference in the Charlson Comorbidity Index (CCI) > 2 between the two groups. Fracture type, categorized as unimalleolar or bimalleolar, showed similar distributions between the groups and did not present statistically significant differences ($p = 0.762$). The Lauge–Hansen classification, which differentiates fractures based on patterns such as supination external rotation (SER), pronation external rotation (PER), supination adduction (SA), and pronation abduction (PA), also did not show significant differences between the groups ($p = 0.185$), as presented in Table 1.

Participants were asked about their satisfaction with overall mobility since the surgical procedure. Those who underwent syndesmotic screw removal reported an average satisfaction score of 7.8, which was significantly higher than the 6.7 reported by the conservative approach cohort ($p = 0.018$). When questioned on the perceived impact of the screw removal (or retention) on their ability to perform daily living activities, the screw removal group rated this aspect at 8.1, significantly higher than the 6.5 from the conservative approach group ($p < 0.001$). In terms of pain or discomfort experienced post surgery, the screw removal group averaged a score of 5.3, which was significantly lower, indicating less pain or discomfort, than the 6.8 reported by the conservative approach group ($p = 0.003$).

However, not all results favored the screw removal procedure. When asked if they would recommend their respective treatment approach to someone else with a similar condition, both groups displayed almost equal confidence, with the screw removal group scoring 7.6 and the conservative approach scoring 7.4 ($p = 0.591$). Similarly, there was no significant difference between the two groups when asked about the impact of the surgical procedure on their quality of life: the screw removal group scored 6.9, and the conservative approach scored 7.1 ($p = 0.714$).

Table 1. Comparison of the study cohort background characteristics.

Variables	Screw Removal (n = 93)	Conservative Approach (n = 51)	p-Value *
Age, years	32.8 ± 12.5	33.5 ± 14.1	0.759
Sex (men, %)	56 (60.2%)	23 (45.1%)	0.081
Overweight (>25.0 kg/m^2)	36 (38.7%)	24 (47.1%)	0.331
Area of residence (urban)	58 (62.4%)	28 (54.9%)	0.382
Relationship status (married)	62 (66.7%)	37 (72.5%)	0.466
Level of income (average or higher)	53 (57.0%)	29 (56.9%)	0.988
Level of education (higher education)	66 (71.0%)	31 (60.8%)	0.212
Occupation (employed)	51 (54.8%)	32 (62.7%)	0.358
Frequent alcohol consumption	10 (10.8%)	8 (15.7%)	0.392
Frequent smoker	25 (26.9%)	17 (33.3%)	0.415
CCI > 2	8 (8.6%)	3 (5.9%)	0.556
Fracture type			0.762
Unimalleolar	24 (25.8%)	12 (23.5%)	
Bimalleolar	49 (52.7%)	24 (47.1%)	
Lauge–Hansen classification			0.185
SER	42 (45.2%)	17 (33.3%)	
PER	30 (32.3%)	14 (27.5%)	
SA	10 (10.8%)	11 (21.6%)	
PA	11 (11.8%)	8 (15.7%)	

* Chi-squared or Fisher's exact test; CCI—Charlson Comorbidity Index; SER—supination external rotation fracture; PER—pronation external rotation fracture; SA—supination adduction; PA—pronation abduction.

Nevertheless, participants' confidence in their decision varied significantly. Those who opted for screw removal expressed higher confidence in their choice, scoring 8.9, compared to 7.8 by those who chose conservative treatment ($p = 0.013$). The patients' perception of limitations in daily activities due to the surgical procedure also showed significant differences, with the screw removal group averaging a score of 5.6 and the conservative approach group scoring higher at 6.9 ($p = 0.016$), indicating more perceived limitations. Lastly, in terms of patient information regarding the advantages and disadvantages of screw removal versus retention, the scores were close between groups, with 8.4 for the screw removal cohort and 8.0 for the conservative approach, and this difference was not statistically significant ($p = 0.222$), as presented in Table 2.

For the physical domain of the SF-36 survey, patients in the screw removal group reported a mean score of 55.9, which was significantly higher than the 53.3 reported by the conservative approach group ($p = 0.027$), as seen in Table 3 and Figure 1. This suggests that those who underwent screw removal experienced a better physical health status compared to those who opted for the conservative approach. Regarding the mental domain of the survey, the difference between the groups was not statistically significant. The screw removal group scored an average of 54.9, slightly higher than the 53.0 of the conservative approach group, but the p-value of 0.140 indicated that this difference was not significant. Therefore, both groups had comparable mental health statuses postoperatively. The total score on the SF-36, which encompasses both physical and mental health domains, showed a mean of 56.4 for the screw removal group and 55.1 for the conservative approach group. This difference was not statistically significant ($p = 0.349$), implying that, when considering overall health status and quality of life, the two groups were largely comparable.

Table 2. Unstandardized survey results.

Questions	Screw Removal (n = 93)	Conservative Approach (n = 51)	p-Value *
Q1: How satisfied are you with your overall mobility since the surgical procedure?	7.8 ± 2.5	6.7 ± 2.9	0.018
Q2: To what extent do you believe the removal (or retention) of the syndesmotic screw impacted better your ability to perform daily living activities?	8.1 ± 2.1	6.5 ± 3.0	<0.001
Q3: How often do you experience pain or discomfort in the area of the surgical procedure?	5.3 ± 2.7	6.8 ± 3.2	0.003
Q4: Would you recommend the same treatment approach to someone else with a similar condition? (1 being not likely, 10 being highly likely)	7.6 ± 1.9	7.4 ± 2.6	0.591
Q5: How has this surgical procedure impacted your quality of life? (higher is better)	6.9 ± 3.3	7.1 ± 2.8	0.714
Q6: How confident are you in your decision (either removal or retention of the screw)?	8.9 ± 1.6	7.8 ± 2.4	0.013
Q7: Have you noticed any limitations in daily activities due to the surgical procedure?	5.6 ± 2.9	6.9 ± 3.3	0.016
Q8: On a scale of 1 to 10, how would you rate the information provided to you regarding the pros and cons of screw removal versus retention?	8.4 ± 1.8	8.0 ± 2.0	0.222

* Student's t-test.

Table 3. SF-36 survey results.

Scores (Mean ± SD)	Screw Removal (n = 93)	Conservative Approach (n = 51)	p-Value *
SF-36—Physical	55.9 ± 6.6	53.3 ± 6.8	0.027
SF-36—Mental	54.9 ± 7.2	53.0 ± 7.6	0.140
SF-36—Total	56.4 ± 7.8	55.1 ± 8.2	0.349

* Student's t-test; SD—standard deviation; SF-36—short-form survey (higher scores indicate better health status and quality of life).

The physical domain of the WHOQOL-BREF survey showed that the screw removal group had a mean score of 64.8, which was higher than the 60.9 ± 11.6 reported by the conservative approach group. Although this difference suggests a better physical quality of life for the screw removal group, the p-value of 0.064 indicated that this difference was marginally outside the conventional threshold of statistical significance. For the mental domain, the conservative approach group reported a mean score of 66.4, which was higher than the 62.3 from the screw removal group. This difference, with a p-value of 0.082, was also marginally nonsignificant, suggesting that there might be a trend towards a better mental quality of life in the conservative approach group, but this was not conclusively demonstrated.

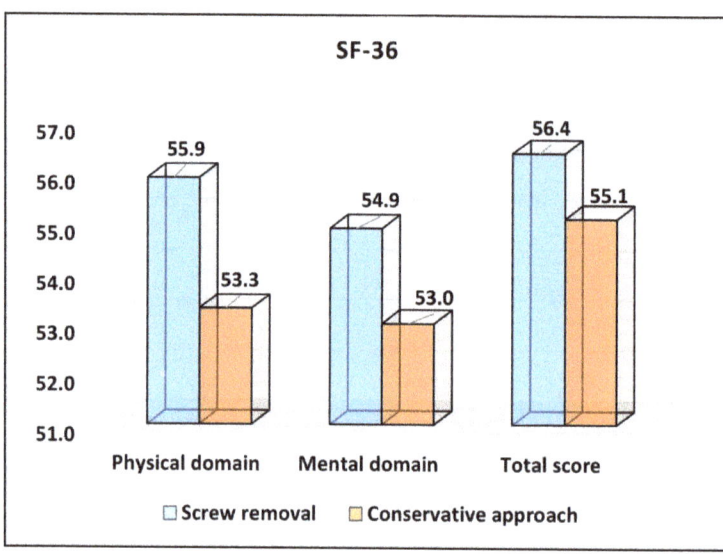

Figure 1. Analysis of the SF-36 questionnaire results.

In the social domain, there was a statistically significant difference between the two groups. The conservative approach group had a higher average score of 65.5 than the 60.8 from the screw removal group, with a p-value of 0.039, as presented in Table 4 and Figure 2. This indicates that patients in the conservative approach group reported a better social quality of life postoperatively. The environmental domain showed no significant difference between the two groups. The screw removal group reported a score of 63.8, while the conservative approach group reported 62.0, with a p-value of 0.399, indicating that the environmental quality of life was comparable between the two treatments.

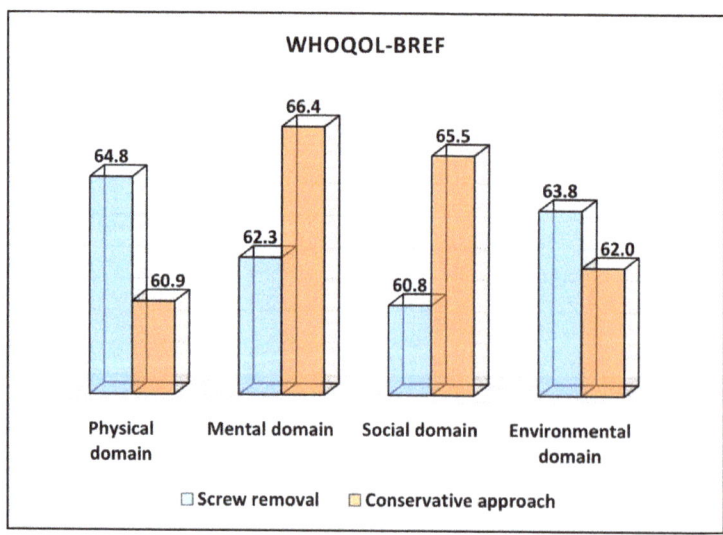

Figure 2. Average values of domain scores on the WHOQOL-BREF questionnaire.

Table 4. WHOQOL-BREF survey results.

WHOQOL-BREF (Mean ± SD)	Screw Removal (n = 93)	Conservative Approach (n = 51)	p-Value *
Physical domain	64.8 ± 12.2	60.9 ± 11.6	0.064
Mental domain	62.3 ± 13.8	66.4 ± 12.8	0.082
Social domain	60.8 ± 12.9	65.5 ± 13.1	0.039
Environmental domain	63.8 ± 11.6	62.0 ± 13.3	0.399

* Student's t-test; SD—standard deviation; WHOQOL-BREF—brief version of the World Health Organization Quality of Life survey (higher scores indicate better quality of life).

Starting with the anxiety subscale of the HADS, the group that underwent screw removal reported a mean score of 5.8. In contrast, the conservative approach group had a higher mean score of 7.3. This difference was statistically significant, with a p-value of 0.006, suggesting that patients who underwent screw removal experienced, on average, lower levels of anxiety compared to those who followed the conservative approach. Regarding the depression subscale, the screw removal group had a mean score of 6.3, which was marginally lower than the 6.9 reported by the conservative approach group. However, with a p-value of 0.109, this difference was not statistically significant, indicating that both groups had similar levels of depression postoperatively. When considering the total HADS score, which combines both anxiety and depression components, the screw removal group showed a mean score of 12.1. This was slightly lower than the 13.0 from the conservative approach group. Nevertheless, the difference was not statistically significant, as evidenced by a p-value of 0.252, as described in Table 5 and Figure 3.

Table 5. HADS survey results.

HADS (Mean ± SD)	Screw Removal (n = 93)	Conservative Approach (n = 51)	p-Value *
Anxiety	5.8 ± 3.4	7.3 ± 2.5	0.006
Depression	6.3 ± 2.3	6.9 ± 1.8	0.109
Total score	12.1 ± 4.6	13.0 ± 4.3	0.252

* Student's t-test; SD—standard deviation; SF-36—short-form survey (higher scores indicate higher levels of anxiety or depression).

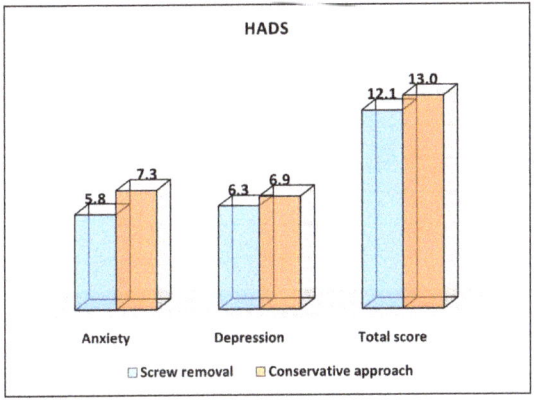

Figure 3. Analysis of the HADS questionnaire results.

Female patients, in contrast to males, demonstrated a 0.8 hazard ratio (HR), which means they had a 20% reduced risk of presenting with a low score on the SF-36 physical domain. This relationship bore statistical significance, given that the 95% confidence interval (CI) spanned from 0.6 to 1.1 and was solidified with a p-value of 0.014. Consequently, being female could conceivably be associated with a better perception of physical health in this specific patient group. Furthermore, anxiety levels, as per the HADS scale, revealed an intriguing pattern. For every unit increase in anxiety score, the likelihood of a lower score in the SF-36 physical domain surged by 60% (HR = 1.6), a finding corroborated by a 95% CI ranging from 1.2 to 3.1 and a significant p-value of 0.006. This suggests that elevated anxiety levels might substantially compromise the perceived physical quality of life.

The WHOQOL-BREF, employed to gauge quality of life across various domains, also unveiled noteworthy observations. Specifically, each unit elevation in the physical domain score corresponded to an 80% amplified risk (HR = 1.8) of a depressed SF-36 physical score. This relationship was robust, denoted by its CI from 1.3 to 2.5 and a highly significant p-value of less than 0.001. The mental domain of the same scale indicated that every unit increase was linked to a 50% heightened risk (HR = 1.5) of a lower SF-36 physical score, with its 95% CI spanning 1.1 to 2.8 and a p-value of 0.013, as seen in Table 6 and Figure 4. Moreover, patients with a Charlson Comorbidity Index (CCI) exceeding 2 were found to be twice as likely (HR = 2.0) to report lower scores on the SF-36 physical domain. This association's strength is highlighted by the CI, which ranged from 1.1 to 3.6, and a p-value of 0.024, indicating the potential influence of multiple comorbidities on the perceived physical health quality of life.

Table 6. Regression analysis for low SF-36 scores on the physical domain.

Independent Variables	HR—Exp (B)	95% CI	p-Value
Gender (Female vs. Male)	0.8	0.6–1.1	0.014
Age (Per year increase)	1.02	0.97–1.19	0.132
Overweight (>25.0 kg/m^2)	1.4	1.0–1.9	0.072
Area of residence (Urban vs. Rural)	1.1	0.8–1.4	0.621
Relationship status (Relationship vs. Single)	0.9	0.6–1.3	0.466
Level of income (Average or higher vs. Below average)	1.2	0.9–2.6	0.201
Level of education (Higher vs. Below higher)	1.1	0.8–1.5	0.499
Occupation (Employed vs. Unemployed)	0.9	0.7–1.1	0.173
Frequent alcohol consumption (Yes vs. No)	0.8	0.6–1.2	0.091
Frequent smoker (Yes vs. No)	1.2	0.9–1.6	0.212
Fracture type (Unimalleolar vs. Bimalleolar)	1.2	0.9–2.2	0.193
HADS—Anxiety (Per unit increase)	1.6	1.2–3.1	0.006
HADS—Depression (Per unit increase)	1.1	0.9–2.0	0.218
WHOQOL-BREF Physical domain	1.8	1.3–2.5	<0.001
WHOQOL-BREF Mental domain	1.5	1.1–2.8	0.013
WHOQOL-BREF Social domain	1.6	0.9–2.2	0.095
WHOQOL-BREF Environmental domain	1.4	1.0–1.9	0.068
Charlson Comorbidity Index (CCI > 2)	2.0	1.1–3.6	0.024

HR—hazard ratio; CI—confidence interval; SF—short form; data in this table analyze both study groups.

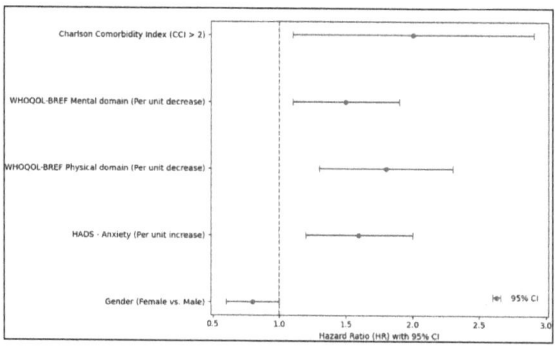

Figure 4. Regression analysis results.

4. Discussion

4.1. Literature Findings

The debate surrounding the optimal management of syndesmotic screws post distal tibiofibular diastasis repair continues to perplex the orthopedic community [32,33]. Grounded in this context, our study sought to elucidate the impact of screw removal on quality of life, mobility, and activities of daily living in postoperative patients. The findings suggest that there are indeed significant differences in specific patient-reported outcomes depending on whether the syndesmotic screws are removed or retained.

When investigating mobility and daily living activities post surgery, participants who underwent screw removal indicated a perceptibly improved satisfaction score in contrast to those who favored the conservative approach. This result aligns with the theory that screw removal may alleviate some of the mechanical restrictions that syndesmotic screws could impose [13,34]. Such outcomes underscore the potential advantages of screw removal in fostering enhanced mobility, a cornerstone for improved rehabilitation and overall quality of life. However, even though the reduced pain or discomfort reported by the screw removal group further solidifies this stance, screw removal can also determine various complications such as infection of early loss of reduction, therefore worsening the quality of life and mobility [13].

However, our study also highlighted areas where there was little discernment between the two groups. For instance, both groups were equivocal in their willingness to recommend their respective treatments to peers, suggesting that despite the measurable differences in certain outcomes, overall satisfaction may be influenced by various factors not exclusively related to the presence or absence of the screw. Intriguingly, the assessment of overall quality of life did not demonstrate a statistically significant difference between the groups. This parity, when juxtaposed against the marked differences in mobility and pain scores, might reflect the multi-faceted nature of the quality of life construct. It emphasizes that while physical factors play a pivotal role, psychological, social, and environmental variables also hold considerable weight.

Diving deeper into the psychological aspects, the anxiety subscale of the HADS presented an illuminating pattern. The group that underwent screw removal reported significantly reduced anxiety levels compared to their counterparts. Such findings could be indicative of the mental relief afforded by the removal of the syndesmotic screw, perhaps due to a perceived return to a more 'natural' state or the elimination of potential future surgery for screw-related complications. In contrast, levels of depression did not differ significantly between the groups, highlighting that while interventions might ameliorate certain psychological aspects, they may not offer relief for all mental health concerns postoperatively.

Our findings also resonate with a broader context when scrutinizing the gender-based disparities. Female participants seemed to have a better perception of physical health, as indicated by the SF-36 physical domain, suggesting possible gender-specific differences in postoperative adaptation or pain perception. Nevertheless, this is in contrast with the existing literature showing that women have lower thresholds to pain than their male counterparts [35,36]. This result reiterates the need for personalized care tailored to specific demographic subsets. Moreover, the profound influence of anxiety on perceived physical quality of life underscores the intrinsic link between mental and physical health in postoperative rehabilitation.

Drawing parallels with other studies, it is noteworthy that the tangible benefits of screw removal affect mobility and pain, thus aligning with the previous literature and increasing the reliability of our findings. Nevertheless, it should not be omitted that other studies report no significant mobility changes after syndesmotic screw removal [37]. While the debate persists, this research, by critically evaluating both clinical outcomes and broader economic implications, casts a more holistic light on the decision making process surrounding syndesmotic screw management.

It is imperative to consider the potential effects of syndesmotic screw removal on bone architecture, which bears significant relevance for orthopedic decision making and patient-centered care. The mechanical integrity of the distal tibiofibular joint, influenced by factors such as bone density, shape, and overall architecture, is crucial for determining the success of syndesmotic screw procedures. The current literature, although not entirely conclusive, suggests that screw removal can influence the microstructure and mechanical properties of the bone, potentially impacting its ability to withstand normal physiological loads and stresses [38]. This aspect is particularly important in the context of long-term bone health and the prevention of osteoarthritis or other degenerative conditions. The decision to remove or retain the syndesmotic screw, therefore, must be made with a comprehensive understanding of these biomechanical implications, alongside patient-specific factors such as age, bone quality, activity level, and personal preferences. Our study's findings, emphasizing the importance of physical and psychological outcomes, should thus be contextualized within this broader framework of bone architecture considerations to guide more nuanced and individualized patient care strategies.

4.2. Study Limitations

The current study possesses several inherent limitations. Firstly, the cross-sectional design used restricts the capability to infer causal relationships between variables, limiting our conclusions to associations observed at one specific point in time. While the study relied on the clinic's inpatient population database for demographic and clinical data, the possibility of inconsistencies between digital and paper records cannot be completely ruled out. The sample size, determined through a convenience sampling method, might not wholly represent the broader population of individuals with unimalleolar or bimalleolar ankle fractures, potentially introducing selection bias. The exclusion of patients with missing data or those who developed orthopedic complications could lead to the omission of certain clinical scenarios from our analysis. Another notable limitation of our study is the relatively short follow-up period of approximately two months post surgery, which may not sufficiently capture long-term outcomes and potential complications associated with distal tibiofibular diastasis repair, thereby limiting our ability to comprehensively assess the enduring effects of the treatment strategies employed. Moreover, even though a variety of standardized questionnaires were utilized, the reliance on self-reported data poses a risk of recall bias. Lastly, the study's findings are based on data from a single center, which could limit the generalizability of results to other settings or populations.

5. Conclusions

This study provided a comprehensive analysis of the outcomes related to the management of syndesmotic screws post distal tibiofibular diastasis repair. The postoperative removal of syndesmotic screws was found to have a favorable impact on several patient-centered outcomes. Specifically, patients who underwent screw removal exhibited enhanced mobility, superior ability to execute daily activities, and experienced reduced levels of postoperative pain and anxiety than those who adopted a conservative approach by retaining the screws. Notably, these benefits did not translate into a significant difference in the overall quality of life between the two groups. Despite these advancements in our understanding, the decision to remove or retain the screw should be personalized and tailored to individual patient needs, considering the multifaceted nature of postoperative recovery. The insights gleaned from this study augment the current orthopedic knowledge and serve as a significant reference for delivering patient-centric care in the context of distal tibiofibular diastasis repair.

Author Contributions: Conceptualization, S.H.; methodology, S.H.; software, O.R.; validation, D.V.; formal analysis, D.V. and I.-I.S.; investigation, D.C. and M.A.-Q.; resources, D.C. and M.A.-Q.; data curation, O.R.; writing—original draft preparation, S.H., B.D. and R.P.; writing—review and editing, D.P., I.-I.S. and M.M.; visualization, D.P., I.-I.S. and M.M.; supervision, B.D. and R.P.; project administration, B.D. and R.P. All authors have read and agreed to the published version of the manuscript.

Funding: This research received no external funding.

Institutional Review Board Statement: The study was conducted according to the guidelines of the Declaration of Helsinki and approved by the Ethics Committee of the Clinic of Orthopedics affiliated with the "Victor Babes" University of Medicine and Pharmacy in Timisoara, on 16 February 2022 (approval number 38).

Informed Consent Statement: Written informed consent was obtained from the patients to publish this paper.

Data Availability Statement: Data available on request.

Conflicts of Interest: The authors declare no conflict of interest.

References

1. Yuen, C.P.; Lui, T.H. Distal Tibiofibular Syndesmosis: Anatomy, Biomechanics, Injury and Management. *Open Orthop. J.* **2017**, *11*, 670–677. [CrossRef] [PubMed]
2. Carto, C.; Lezak, B.; Varacallo, M. Anatomy, Bony Pelvis and Lower Limb: Distal Tibiofibular Joint (Tibiofibular Syndesmosis). In *StatPearls [Internet]*; StatPearls Publishing: Treasure Island, FL, USA, 2023. Available online: https://www.ncbi.nlm.nih.gov/books/NBK547655/ (accessed on 8 August 2023).
3. Pogliacomi, F.; De Filippo, M.; Casalini, D.; Longhi, A.; Tacci, F.; Perotta, R.; Pagnini, F.; Tocco, S.; Ceccarelli, F. Acute syndesmotic injuries in ankle fractures: From diagnosis to treatment and current concepts. *World J. Orthop.* **2021**, *12*, 270–291. [CrossRef] [PubMed]
4. Hunt, K.J. Syndesmosis injuries. *Curr. Rev. Musculoskelet. Med.* **2013**, *6*, 304–312. [CrossRef] [PubMed]
5. Magan, A.; Golano, P.; Maffulli, N.; Khanduja, V. Evaluation and management of injuries of the tibiofibular syndesmosis. *Br. Med. Bull.* **2014**, *111*, 101–115. [CrossRef] [PubMed]
6. Cao, M.-M.; Zhang, Y.-W.; Hu, S.-Y.; Rui, Y.-F. A systematic review of ankle fracture-dislocations: Recent update and future prospects. *Front. Surg.* **2022**, *9*, 965814. [CrossRef]
7. Yawar, B.; Hanratty, B.; Asim, A.; Niazi, A.K.; Khan, A.M. Suture-Button Versus Syndesmotic Screw Fixation of Ankle Fractures: A Comparative Retrospective Review Over One Year. *Cureus* **2021**, *13*, e17826. [CrossRef]
8. Corte-Real, N.; Caetano, J. Ankle and syndesmosis instability: Consensus and controversies. *EFORT Open Rev.* **2021**, *6*, 420–431. [CrossRef]
9. Baxter, S.; Farris, E.; Johnson, A.H.; Brennan, J.C.; Friedmann, E.M.; Turcotte, J.J.; Keblish, D.J. Transosseous Fixation of the Distal Tibiofibular Syndesmosis: Comparison of Interosseous Suture and Endobutton Across Age Groups. *Cureus* **2023**, *15*, e40355. [CrossRef]
10. Sipahioglu, S.; Zehir, S.; Isikan, U.E. Syndesmotic screw fixation in tibiofibular diastasis. *Niger. J. Clin. Pr.* **2018**, *21*, 692–697. [CrossRef]
11. Kapadia, B.H.; Sabarese, M.J.; Chatterjee, D.; Aylyarov, A.; Zuchelli, D.M.; Hariri, O.K.; Uribe, J.A.; Tsai, J. Evaluating success rate and comparing complications of operative techniques used to treat chronic syndesmosis injuries. *J. Orthop.* **2020**, *22*, 225–230. [CrossRef]
12. Walley, K.C.; Hofmann, K.J.; Velasco, B.T.; Kwon, J.Y. Removal of Hardware After Syndesmotic Screw Fixation: A Systematic Literature Review. *Foot Ankle Spéc.* **2017**, *10*, 252–257. [CrossRef] [PubMed]
13. Schepers, T. To retain or remove the syndesmotic screw: A review of literature. *Arch. Orthop. Trauma Surg.* **2011**, *131*, 879–883. [CrossRef] [PubMed]
14. Ijezie, N.; Fraig, H.; Abolaji, S. Outcomes of the Routine Removal of the Syndesmotic Screw. *Cureus* **2022**, *14*, e26675. [CrossRef] [PubMed]
15. Zeng, M.; Xu, Z.; Song, Z.Q.; Li, J.X.; Tang, Z.W.; Xiao, S.; Wen, J. Diagnosis and treatment of chronic osteomyelitis based on nanomaterials. *World J. Orthop.* **2023**, *14*, 42–54. [CrossRef] [PubMed]
16. Ribeiro, M.; Monteiro, F.J.; Ferraz, M.P. Infection of orthopedic implants with emphasis on bacterial adhesion process and techniques used in studying bacterial-material interactions. *Biomatter* **2012**, *2*, 176–194. [CrossRef]
17. Moon, Y.J.; Kim, D.H.; Lee, K.B. Is it necessary to remove syndesmotic screw before weight-bearing ambulation? *Medicine* **2020**, *99*, e19436. [CrossRef]
18. Schnetzke, M.; Vetter, S.Y.; Beisemann, N.; Swartman, B.; Grützner, P.A.; Franke, J. Management of syndesmotic injuries: What is the evidence? *World J. Orthop.* **2016**, *7*, 718–725. [CrossRef]
19. Kujanpää, T.; Jokelainen, J.; Auvinen, J.; Timonen, M. Generalised anxiety disorder symptoms and utilisation of health care services. A cross-sectional study from the "Northern Finland 1966 Birth Cohort". *Scand. J. Prim. Health Care* **2016**, *34*, 151–158. [CrossRef]
20. Mao, W.; Shalaby, R.; Agyapong, V.I.O. Interventions to Reduce Repeat Presentations to Hospital Emergency Departments for Mental Health Concerns: A Scoping Review of the Literature. *Healthcare* **2023**, *11*, 1161. [CrossRef]
21. Buccino, F.; Bunt, A.; Lazell, A.; Vergani, L.M. Mechanical Design Optimization of Prosthetic Hand's Fingers: Novel Solutions towards Weight Reduction. *Materials* **2022**, *15*, 2456. [CrossRef]

22. Buccino, F.; Martinoia, G.; Vergani, L.M. Torsion—Resistant Structures: A Nature Addressed Solution. *Materials* **2021**, *14*, 5368. [CrossRef]
23. Millstein, S.G.; Heger, H.; Hunter, G. Prosthetic Use in Adult Upper Limb Amputees: A Comparison of the Body Powered and Electrically Powered Prostheses. *Prosthet. Orthot. Int.* **1986**, *10*, 27–34. [CrossRef] [PubMed]
24. Hosin, S.; Vermesan, D.; Prejbeanu, R.; Crisan, D.; Al-Qatawneh, M.; Pop, D.; Mioc, M.; Bratosin, F.; Feciche, B.; Hemaswini, K.; et al. Avoiding the Removal of Syndesmotic Screws after Distal Tibiofibular Diastasis Repair: A Benefit or a Drawback? *J. Clin. Med.* **2022**, *11*, 6412. [CrossRef] [PubMed]
25. Bragg, J.T.; Masood, R.M.; Spence, S.S.; Citron, J.E.; Moon, A.S.; Salzler, M.J.; Ryan, S.P. Predictors of Hardware Removal in Orthopaedic Trauma Patients Undergoing Syndesmotic Ankle Fixation with Screws. *Foot Ankle Orthop.* **2023**, *8*, 24730114231198841. [CrossRef] [PubMed]
26. Desouky, O.; Elseby, A.; Ghalab, A.H. Removal of Syndesmotic Screw After Fixation in Ankle Fractures: A Systematic Review. *Cureus* **2021**, *13*, e15435. [CrossRef] [PubMed]
27. Steindel, S.J. International classification of diseases, 10th edition, clinical modification and procedure coding system: Descriptive overview of the next generation HIPAA code sets. *J. Am. Med. Inform. Assoc.* **2010**, *17*, 274–282. [CrossRef] [PubMed]
28. Fonseca, L.L.D.; Nunes, I.G.; Nogueira, R.R.; Martins, G.E.V.; Mesencio, A.C.; Kobata, S.I. Reproducibility of the Lauge-Hansen, Danis-Weber, and AO classifications for ankle fractures. *Rev. Bras. De Ortop.* **2017**, *53*, 101–106. [CrossRef]
29. Lins, L.; Carvalho, F.M. SF-36 total score as a single measure of health-related quality of life: Scoping review. *SAGE Open Med.* **2016**, *4*, 2050312116671725. [CrossRef]
30. Snaith, R.P. The Hospital Anxiety And Depression Scale. *Health Qual. Life Outcomes* **2003**, *1*, 29. [CrossRef]
31. Vahedi, S. World Health Organization Quality-of-Life Scale (WHOQOL-BREF): Analyses of Their Item Response Theory Properties Based on the Graded Responses Model. *Iran. J. Psychiatry* **2010**, *5*, 140–153.
32. Huang, C.T.; Huang, P.J.; Lu, C.C.; Shih, C.L.; Cheng, Y.M.; Chen, S.J. Syndesmosis Changes before and after Syndesmotic Screw Removal: A Retrospective Radiographic Study. *Medicina* **2022**, *58*, 445. [CrossRef]
33. Pogliacomi, F.; Artoni, C.; Ricciboni, S.; Calderazzi, F.; Vaienti, E.; Ceccarelli, F. The management of syndesmotic screw in ankle fractures. *Acta Biomed.* **2018**, *90*, 146–149. [CrossRef]
34. Kim, J.; Kwon, M.; Day, J.; Seilern und Aspang, J.; Shim, J.; Cho, J. The Impact of Suture Button Removal in Syndesmosis Fixation. *J. Clin. Med.* **2021**, *10*, 3726. [CrossRef]
35. Dao, T.T.; LeResche, L. Gender differences in pain. *J. Orofac. Pain* **2000**, *14*, 169–195. [PubMed]
36. Dingemans, S.A.; Birnie, M.F.N.; Sanders, F.R.K.; Bekerom, M.P.J.v.D.; Backes, M.; van Beeck, E.; Bloemers, F.W.; van Dijkman, B.; Flikweert, E.; Haverkamp, D.; et al. Routine versus on demand removal of the syndesmotic screw; a protocol for an international randomised controlled trial (RODEO-trial). *BMC Musculoskelet. Disord.* **2018**, *19*, 35. [CrossRef] [PubMed]
37. Briceno, J.; Wusu, T.; Kaiser, P.; Cronin, P.; Leblanc, A.; Miller, C.; Kwon, J.Y. Effect of Syndesmotic Implant Removal on Dorsiflexion. *Foot Ankle Int.* **2019**, *40*, 499–505. [CrossRef] [PubMed]
38. Boyle, M.J.; Gao, R.; Frampton, C.M.A.; Coleman, B. Removal of the syndesmotic screw after the surgical treatment of a fracture of the ankle in adult patients does not affect one-year outcomes. *Bone Jt. J.* **2014**, *96-B*, 1699–1705. [CrossRef] [PubMed]

Disclaimer/Publisher's Note: The statements, opinions and data contained in all publications are solely those of the individual author(s) and contributor(s) and not of MDPI and/or the editor(s). MDPI and/or the editor(s) disclaim responsibility for any injury to people or property resulting from any ideas, methods, instructions or products referred to in the content.

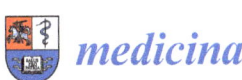 medicina

Article

The Association of Acetabulum Fracture and Mechanism of Injury with BMI, Days Spent in Hospital, Blood Loss, and Surgery Time: A Retrospective Analysis of 67 Patients

Rafał Wójcicki [1], Tomasz Pielak [1], Piotr Marcin Walus [1,*], Łukasz Jaworski [2], Bartłomiej Małkowski [3], Przemysław Jasiewicz [4], Maciej Gagat [5,6], Łukasz Łapaj [7] and Jan Zabrzyński [1,2]

1. Department of Orthopaedics and Traumatology, Faculty of Medicine, J. Kochanowski University in Kielce, 25-001 Kielce, Poland
2. Department of Orthopaedics and Traumatology, Faculty of Medicine, Collegium Medicum in Bydgoszcz, Nicolaus Copernicus University in Toruń, 85-092 Bydgoszcz, Poland
3. Department of Urology, Oncology Centre Prof. Franciszek Łukaszczyk Memorial Hospital, Bydgoszcz, 2 dr I. Romanowskiej St., 85-796 Bydgoszcz, Poland
4. Department of Anesthesiology, Faculty of Medicine, Collegium Medicum in Bydgoszcz, Nicolaus Copernicus University in Toruń, 85-092 Bydgoszcz, Poland
5. Department of Histology and Embryology, Faculty of Medicine, Nicolaus Copernicus University in Torun, Collegium Medicum in Bydgoszcz, 85-067 Bydgoszcz, Poland
6. Faculty of Medicine, Collegium Medicum, Mazovian Academy in Płock, 09-402 Płock, Poland
7. Department of General Orthopaedics, Musculoskeletal Oncology and Trauma Surgery, University of Medical Sciences, 61-701 Poznan, Poland
* Correspondence: walus.md@gmail.com; Tel.: +48-507563441

Abstract: *Background and Objectives*: The objective of this retrospective study was to investigate the association between acetabulum fractures; the mechanism of injury; and variables such as BMI, duration of hospital stay, blood loss, and surgery time. By exploring these factors, we aim to enhance our understanding of them and their impact on the healing process and the subsequent management of pelvic fractures. *Materials and Methods*: This study included 67 of 136 consecutive patients who were admitted for pelvic ring fracture surgery between 2017 and 2022. The data were collected prospectively at a single trauma center. The inclusion criteria were acetabulum fractures and indications for operative treatment. The exclusion criteria were non-operative treatment for acetabular and pelvic ring fractures, fractures requiring primary total hip arthroplasty (THA), and periprosthetic acetabular fractures. Upon admission, all patients underwent evaluation using X-ray and computed tomography (CT) scans of the pelvis. *Results*: The present study found no statistically significant differences between the examined groups of patients with pelvic fractures in terms of BMI, surgery duration, length of hospital stay, and blood transfusion. However, two notable findings approached statistical significance. Firstly, patients who experienced a fall from height while sustaining a pelvic fracture required a higher number of blood transfusions (2.3 units) than those with other mechanisms of injury which was close to achieving statistical significance ($p = 0.07$). Secondly, patients undergoing posterior wall stabilization required a significantly lower number of blood transfusions than those with other specific pelvic injuries (0.33 units per patient), approaching statistical significance ($p = 0.056$). *Conclusions*: The findings indicated that factors such as BMI, time of surgery, blood loss, and the duration of hospital stay were not directly correlated with the morphology of acetabular fractures, the presence of additional trauma, or the mechanism of injury. However, in the studied group, the patients whose mechanism of trauma involved falling from height had an increased number of blood transfusions compared to other groups. Moreover, the patients who had surgery due to posterior wall acetabulum fracture had decreased blood transfusions compared to those with other Judet and Letournel types of fractures. Additionally, they had the shortest duration of surgery.

Keywords: acetabulum; fracture; pelvis; BMI; transfusion

Citation: Wójcicki, R.; Pielak, T.; Walus, P.M.; Jaworski, Ł.; Małkowski, B.; Jasiewicz, P.; Gagat, M.; Łapaj, Ł.; Zabrzyński, J. The Association of Acetabulum Fracture and Mechanism of Injury with BMI, Days Spent in Hospital, Blood Loss, and Surgery Time: A Retrospective Analysis of 67 Patients. *Medicina* **2024**, *60*, 455. https://doi.org/10.3390/medicina60030455

Academic Editor: Woo Jong Kim

Received: 6 February 2024
Revised: 7 March 2024
Accepted: 8 March 2024
Published: 9 March 2024

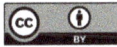

Copyright: © 2024 by the authors. Licensee MDPI, Basel, Switzerland. This article is an open access article distributed under the terms and conditions of the Creative Commons Attribution (CC BY) license (https:// creativecommons.org/licenses/by/ 4.0/).

1. Introduction

Pelvic fractures pose significant challenges for orthopedic surgeons, requiring extensive knowledge and experience to navigate safely among the organs, vital vessels, and nerves located in the pelvic bone area [1–4]. The surgical treatment of these fractures is complicated by the frequent occurrence of additional injuries, many of which can be fatal [5–9]. This is primarily due to the high-energy nature of these traumas [10–14]. Given these challenges, it is crucial to identify and manage concomitant injuries, consider the mechanism of trauma, and take into account personal details such as body mass index (BMI) to ensure appropriate treatment.

Previous studies have demonstrated that obese patients have higher rates of complications and longer hospital stays following pelvic fractures [15]. However, conflicting results exist regarding the association between decreased BMI and increased failure of internal fixation. Additionally, the duration of hospitalization after sustaining a pelvic fracture can vary significantly, with a time period of a few days to several weeks [16–18].

The aim of this retrospective study was to investigate the association between acetabulum fractures; the mechanism of injury; and variables such as BMI, duration of hospital stay, blood loss, and surgery time. By exploring these factors, we aim to enhance our understanding of these accompanying factors of pelvic fractures and their impact on the healing process and the subsequent management.

2. Materials and Methods

2.1. General Characteristics

This study included 67 of 136 consecutive patients who were admitted for pelvic ring fracture surgery between 2017 and 2022. Patients included in the study who suffered from acetabular fractures qualified for operative treatment. The data were collected prospectively at a single trauma center. All patients underwent operative treatment using De Puy Synthes implants for pelvic fixation. Upon admission, all patients underwent evaluation using X-ray and computed tomography (CT) scans of the pelvis.

Demographic data were collected, including sex, age (in years), body mass index (BMI), date of injury, type of fracture, mechanism of trauma, concomitant trauma in other regions and the pelvic ring, date of surgery, surgical approach with stabilization methods, surgery duration, blood transfusions, and number of days spent in the hospital. Acetabulum fractures were classified according to the Letournel and Judet system (A+T—anterior column with posterior hemi-transverse fracture, AC—anterior column, BC—both column, PC—posterior column, PC+W—posterior column+posterior wall, PW—posterior wall, T—transverse, and T+P—transverse with posterior wall fracture), while pelvic ring fractures were classified according to the Young and Burgess system (LC—lateral compression, APC—anterior–posterior compression, and VS—vertical shear). The surgical approaches used for acetabulum fractures were the ilio-inguinal and Kocher–Langenback approaches. The ilio-inguinal approach was mainly used in the anterior wall and anterior column fixation. In the posterior wall and posterior column fixation, the Kocher–Langenback approach was mainly used. In the case of one patient with anterior and posterior wall/column fractures, both approaches were used during a single operation.

2.2. Inclusion Criteria

The inclusion criteria were acetabulum fractures and indications for operative treatment, namely instability (hip dislocation associated with posterior wall or column displacement and anterior wall or column displacement) and incongruity (fractures through the roof or dome; displaced dome fragment; transverse or T-type fractures; both column types with incongruity; retained bone fragments; soft-tissue interposition). Patients who suffered from acetabular fractures with intra-articular displacement <3 mm were initially qualified for conservative treatment. The exclusion criteria were non-operative treatment for acetabular and pelvic ring fractures, fractures requiring primary total hip arthroplasty (THA), and periprosthetic acetabular fractures.

2.3. Ethics

The study was conducted in accordance with the Declaration of Helsinki guidelines for human experiments. Prior to the study, permission was obtained from the local Bioethics Committee (approval number KB 645/2022). Written informed consent was obtained from all patients or their relatives upon admission to the hospital to include them in scientific studies.

2.4. Statistical Analysis

All group comparisons and statistical analyses were conducted by two independent investigators using Prism 9 software (GraphPad). A p-value of less than 0.05 was considered statistically significant. Nominal variables were described by the number of observations and their distribution. The normality of variables was assessed using the Shapiro–Wilk test. Relationships between the studied parameters were evaluated using Spearman's rank correlation coefficient. Non-parametric tests, such as the Mann–Whitney U test and analysis of variance, were used to compare the data.

3. Results

Out of the initial 136 patients who underwent operative treatment for pelvic ring fractures between 2017 and 2022, a total of 67 patients fulfilled the inclusion criteria and were included in this study. The inclusion criteria required patients to have an acetabulum fracture, either with or without concomitant pelvic ring injury.

The studied cohort had a mean body mass index (BMI) of 26.25 (ranging from 18 to 39). The mean duration of surgery was 153 min, ranging from 60 to 270 min. The average number of blood transfusions received was 1.58 units, with a range of 0 to 5 units. The mean length of hospital stay was 5.25 days, ranging from 2 to 34 days.

In the study cohort, 15 patients (22.3%) were female, and 52 patients (77.6%) were male. Statistical analysis showed no significant differences between male and female populations in terms of BMI ($p = 0.11$), duration of surgery ($p = 0.92$), blood transfusion ($p = 0.31$), and length of hospital stay ($p = 0.47$) (Figure 1A–D).

In the female subgroup, the mean BMI was 27.87 (ranging from 21 to 39), while in the male subgroup, it was 25.79 (ranging from 18 to 32). The average surgery duration for females was 152 min (varying between 60 and 245 min), and for males, it was 153.5 min (range of 65 to 270 min). The mean length of hospital stay for females was 7.26 days (ranging from 2 to 34 days), whereas for males, it was 4.67 days (ranging from 2 to 31 days). Additionally, the mean amount of blood transfused for females was 1.86 units (ranging from 0 to 4 units), while for males, it was 1.5 units (ranging from 0 to 5 units).

The participants were categorized into various groups based on the mechanism of injury and the type of fracture according to the Judet and Letournel classification (Tables 1 and 2). Within the studied population, there were 3 patients with anterior column with posterior hemi-transverse fractures, 14 patients with anterior column fractures, 11 patients with both column fractures, 10 patients with posterior column fractures, 4 patients with posterior column and posterior wall fractures, 6 patients with posterior wall fractures, 10 patients with transverse acetabulum fractures, and 9 patients with transverse fractures with posterior wall involvement.

Table 1. Characteristics of pelvic fractures classified according to the Judet and Letournel systems, including BMI, length of hospital stay, blood transfusion, and surgery duration.

	A + T	AC	BC	PC	PC + W	PW	T	T+P	p-Value
Mean BMI (kg/cm^2)	26.0	26.5	26.5	24.8	24.8	29.5	26.4	27.4	$p = 0.4003$
Mean days in hospital (days)	4.0	5.6	3.9	11.6	3.3	2.8	3.7	3.9	$p = 0.8152$
Mean blood transfusion (units)	2.3	1.3	2.4	1.1	1.7	0.3	1.7	2.0	$p = 0.0563$
Mean time of surgery (minutes)	145.0	159.6	183.6	119.5	126.3	105.0	186.5	152.8	$p = 0.0193$

Table 2. Categorization of pelvic fractures classified according to the mechanism of injury with BMI, length of hospital stay, blood transfusion, and surgery duration.

	Fall from Height	Industrial	Fall from Standing Height	Pedestrian	Traffic Accident	Unknown	p-Value
Mean BMI (kg/cm^2)	26.6	23.6	26.6	28.5	25.8	26.7	$p = 0.4752$
Mean days in hospital (days)	5.2	3.0	6.9	18.0	4.7	3.1	$p = 0.2533$
Mean blood transfusion (units)	2.3	2.0	1.1	2.0	1.37	1.2	$p = 0.0721$
Mean time of surgery (minutes)	172.8	158.3	148.0	147.5	157.6	110.0	$p = 0.1799$

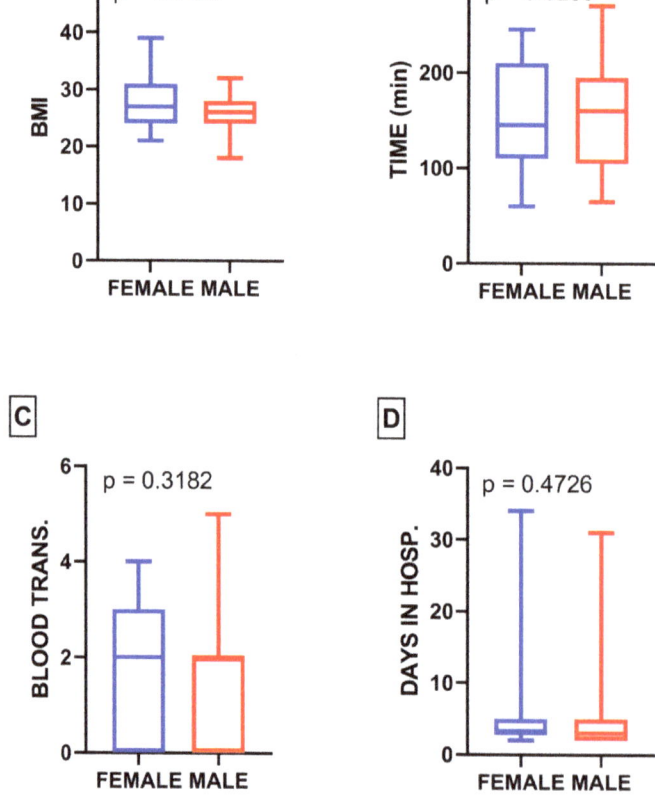

Figure 1. (A) Comparison of BMI between male and female subgroups; (B) comparison of surgery duration between male and female subgroups; (C) comparison of blood transfusion between male and female subgroups; (D) comparison of length of hospital stay between male and female subgroups.

The mechanism of injury presented a diverse range, with 16 patients experiencing falls from height, 3 patients involved in industrial accidents, 10 patients experiencing falls from standing height, 2 patients with pedestrian injuries, 27 patients involved in traffic accidents, and 9 patients with an unknown mechanism of injury.

The classification based on the mechanism of injury did not reveal any statistically significant differences when analyzing BMI ($p = 0.47$), length of hospital stay ($p = 0.25$), surgery duration ($p = 0.17$), and blood transfusion ($p = 0.07$) (Figure 2A–D).

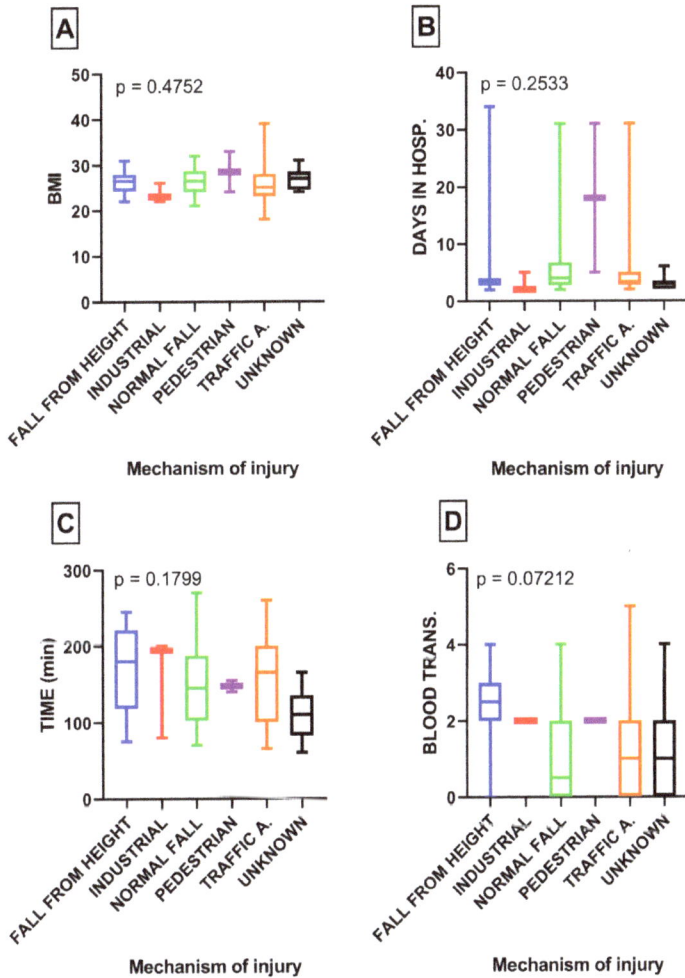

Figure 2. (**A**) Comparison of BMI in subgroups with various mechanisms of injury; (**B**) comparison of length of hospital stay in subgroups with various mechanisms of injury; (**C**) comparison of surgery duration in subgroups with various mechanisms of injury; (**D**) comparison of blood transfusion in subgroups with various mechanisms of injury.

However, the variable of blood transfusion approached significance, with falls from height showing a tendency toward increased blood transfusion requirements ($p = 0.07$) (Figure 2D).

When analyzing the population according to the Judet and Letournel classification, no significant differences were observed in BMI ($p = 0.40$), length of hospital stay ($p = 0.81$), blood transfusion ($p = 0.056$), and concomitant injury ($p = 0.38$) within certain subgroups. However, posterior wall stabilization demonstrated the lowest rate of blood transfusion and approached statistical significance ($p = 0.056$) (Figure 3A–E). Notably, the posterior wall stabilization group exhibited the shortest surgery duration ($p = 0.01$) (Figure 3D).

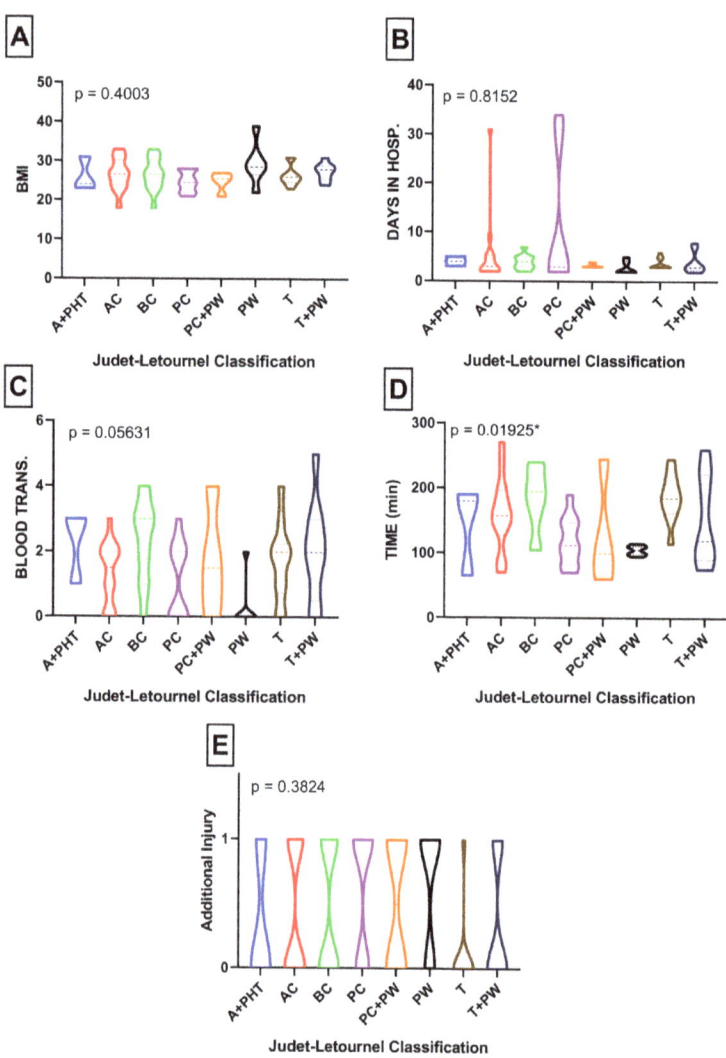

Figure 3. (**A**) Comparison of BMI according to Judet and Letournel subdivisions; (**B**) comparison of length of hospital stay according to Judet and Letournel subdivisions; (**C**) comparison of blood transfusion according to Judet and Letournel subdivisions; (**D**) comparison of surgery duration according to Judet and Letournel subdivisions; (**E**) comparison of additional injury in specific Judet and Letournel subdivisions. * Statistically significant result.

Within the studied cohort, 28 patients had an additional injury. When analyzing the relationship between acetabular fractures and the additional injuries involving the spine, head, chest, abdomen, and upper/lower limbs, no significant differences were found in terms of blood transfusion ($p = 0.28$), BMI ($p = 0.88$), length of hospital stay ($p = 0.65$), and surgery duration ($p = 0.43$) (Figure 4A–D).

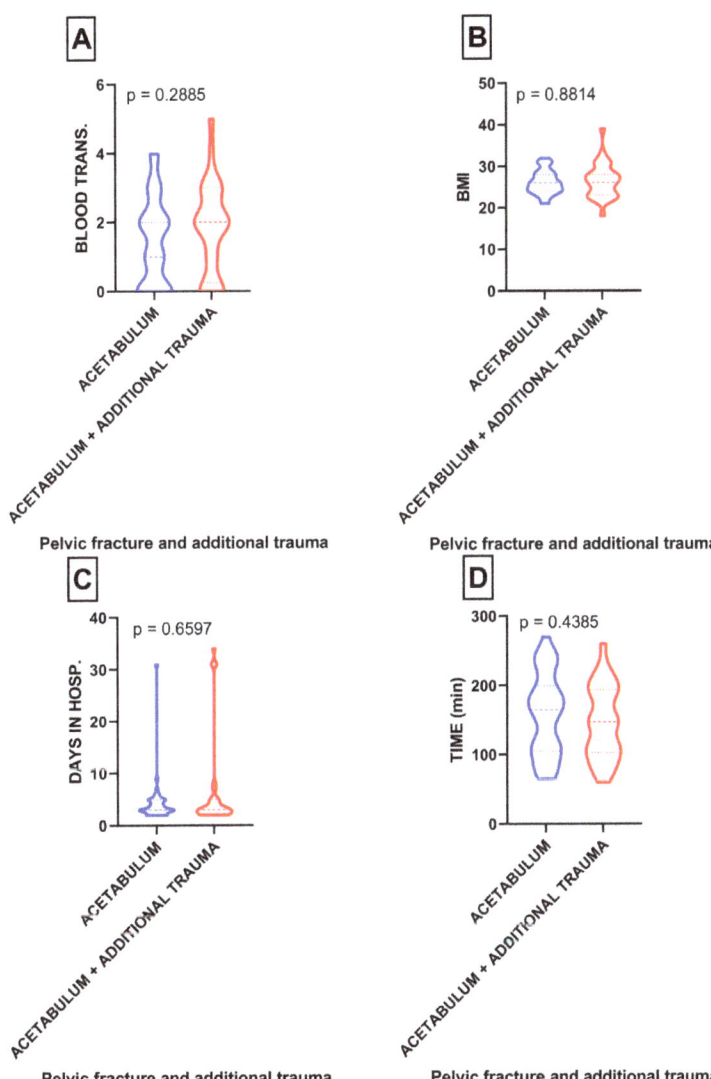

Figure 4. (**A**) Comparison of blood transfusion in patients with acetabulum fractures with or without concomitant trauma; (**B**) comparison of BMI in patients with acetabulum fractures with or without concomitant trauma; (**C**) comparison of length of hospital stay in patients with acetabulum fractures with or without concomitant trauma; (**D**) comparison of surgery duration in patients with acetabulum fractures with or without concomitant trauma.

Among the participants, only seven patients had an additional pelvic ring injury, specifically LC II, LC III, and APC II injuries. When comparing exclusively acetabulum fractures with acetabulum fractures accompanied by a concomitant pelvic ring injury, no statistically significant differences were observed in terms of blood transfusion ($p = 0.28$), surgery duration ($p = 0.43$), BMI ($p = 0.75$), and length of hospital stay ($p = 0.24$) between these two groups (Figure 5A–D).

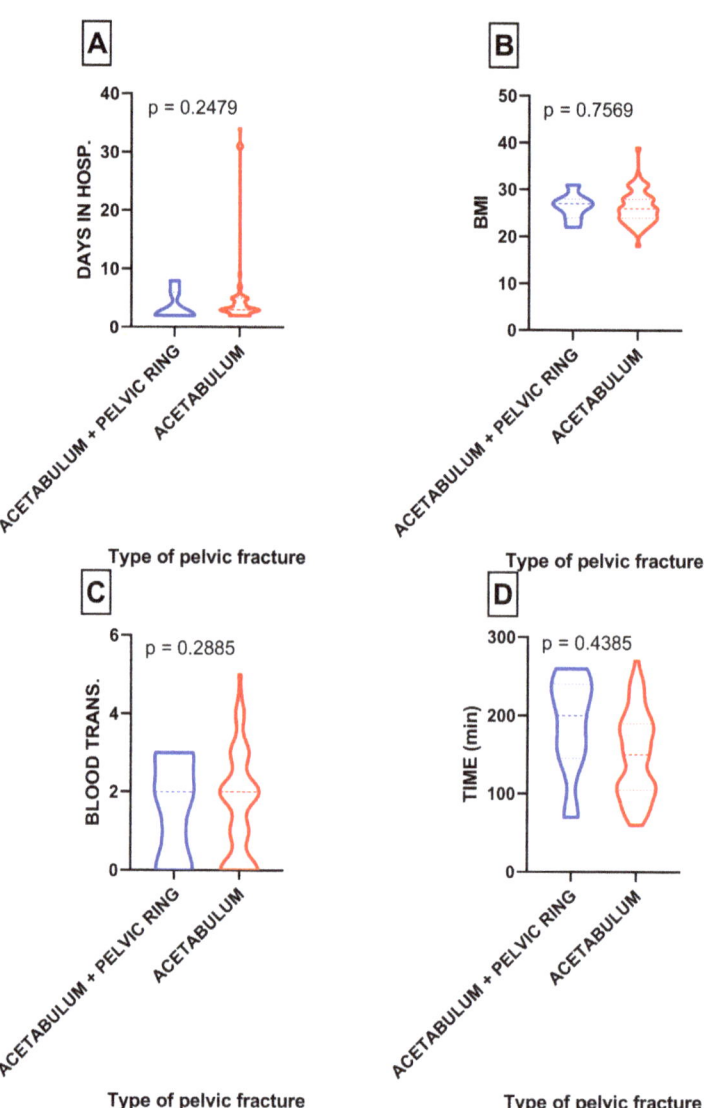

Figure 5. (**A**) Comparison of length of hospital stay in patients with acetabulum fractures with or without pelvic ring fracture; (**B**) comparison of BMI in patients with acetabulum fractures with or without concomitant pelvic ring fracture; (**C**) comparison of blood transfusion in patients with acetabulum fractures with or without concomitant pelvic ring fracture; (**D**) comparison of surgery duration in patients with acetabulum fractures with or without pelvic ring fracture.

The Spearman rho correlation analysis between BMI and surgery duration ($p = 0.31$), blood transfusion ($p = 0.42$), and length of hospital stay ($p = 0.20$) did not reveal a statistically significant relationship (Figure 6A–C).

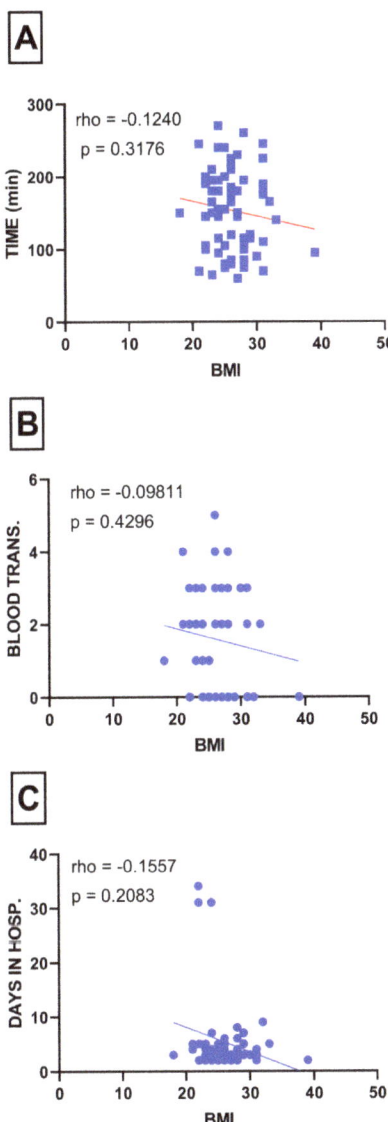

Figure 6. (**A**) Correlation between surgery duration and BMI; (**B**) correlation between blood transfusion and BMI; (**C**) correlation between length of hospital stay and BMI.

4. Discussion

The present study found no statistically significant differences among the examined groups of patients with pelvic fractures in terms of BMI, surgery duration, length of hospital stay, and blood transfusion. However, two notable findings approached statistical significance. Firstly, patients who had experienced a fall from height while sustaining a pelvic fracture required a higher number of blood transfusions (2.3 units) than those with other mechanisms of injury (Figure 2D), which was close to achieving statistical significance ($p = 0.07$). This finding is likely attributed to the high prevalence of concomitant injuries associated with falls from height, which are known to be high-energy traumas [18].

Secondly, patients undergoing posterior wall stabilization required a significantly lower number of blood transfusions than those with other specific pelvic injuries (0.33 units per patient), approaching statistical significance ($p = 0.056$). This result is consistent with the findings of Magnussen et al., who demonstrated that patients with posterior wall fractures required fewer blood transfusions than patients with other types of pelvic fractures classified according to Judet and Letournel [19]. This finding may be linked to the fact that patients in the posterior wall fracture group had the shortest mean surgery duration of 105 min among the studied population (Table 2). Additionally, the higher BMI observed in patients with posterior wall fractures could also be a contributing factor. Frisch et al. demonstrated that a higher BMI significantly reduces the likelihood of perioperative blood transfusion in total hip arthroplasty and total knee arthroplasty [20]. There are several current publications concerning BMI, blood loss, and perioperative transfusions in orthopedic surgeries, and these studies advocate for lower transfusion rates in obese and overweight patients [21–24]. Thus, our results indicating lower blood transfusion requirements in the group with the highest BMI align with these previous findings.

Furthermore, an interesting correlation was found between BMI and fracture type in the Judet and Letournel classification, similar to the findings of Waseem et al. They also reported that patients with posterior wall fractures had the highest BMI [25]. In our study, patients with posterior wall fractures had a mean BMI of 29.5, further supporting this association (Table 1).

It is not surprising that patients with both column fractures required the highest number of blood transfusions and had longer mean surgery durations (Table 1). Magnussen et al. also reported that patients with both column fractures required the highest amount of blood transfusions in their study population [19], which aligns with our findings.

In all patient groups, except for those with industrial injuries, the BMI of our study population was classified as "overweight." Therefore, it is important to note that a high BMI has been associated with various complications in patients with pelvic fractures. Waseem et al. reported that obese patients with pelvic fractures were at a higher risk of almost every complication studied, including deep vein thrombosis, iatrogenic nerve injuries, pneumonia, and wound infection [26]. Similarly, Morris et al. observed that obese patients treated operatively for pelvic fractures experienced more complications than non-obese patients, and even among those managed conservatively, obese patients had a higher percentage of complications [27].

Some of our findings are consistent with the study conducted by Abdelrahman et al., which involved 2112 individuals with traumatic pelvic fractures [16]. In both studies, a higher proportion of males were found to have sustained pelvic fractures compared to females, with percentages of 22% vs. 78% and 23% vs. 77%, respectively [16]. Similar results were also reported by Gosh et al. and Cuthbert et al., according to which males accounted for 75% and 72% of the studied population with pelvic fractures, respectively [10,18].

Furthermore, our study identified similar leading causes of pelvic fractures as those reported by Abdelrahman et al., with falls from height, traffic accidents, and pedestrian incidents being the major causes [16]. Cuthbert et al. also presented comparable results, highlighting falls from height and pedestrian incidents as the two leading causes of pelvic fractures [10]. Interestingly, Abdelrahman et al. did not include falls from standing height as a specific cause of traumatic pelvic injuries requiring surgery in their study, whereas in our study, this category ranked as the second leading cause (Table 1).

Another interesting finding that contradicts other studies is the duration of hospital stay. In our studied population, the mean hospital stay for males was 4.8 days, while for females, it was 7.3 days. In contrast, Abdelrahman et al. reported a mean duration of 15 days in their population [16]. Comparable results were obtained by Gosh et al., with a mean duration of 14.4 days, although their study included both conservatively treated pelvic fractures [18].

Regarding the frequency of specific types of fractures in the Judet and Letournel classification, our analysis revealed a different pattern from that in the current literature.

Trikha et al. and Fakru et al. reported the posterior wall fracture as the most common type of acetabular fracture, whereas in our studied population, the dominant injury was anterior column fractures. This finding is particularly intriguing considering that all three studies (i.e., our study, Fakru et al.'s study, and Trikha et al.'s study) identified traffic accidents as the main cause of acetabular fractures [28,29]. Providing a satisfactory explanation for these discrepancies seems challenging at this point.

On the other hand, Vipulendran et al. found that the leading types of acetabular fractures were anterior column, anterior column + transverse, and both column fractures [30]. This finding is somewhat consistent with our study, where both column and anterior column fractures were the two leading types. Additionally, posterior column fracture was the least common type in Vipulendran et al.'s study, which correlates with our results, where it was identified as the second-to-last type [30]. However, in their studied population, falls from standing height were identified as the leading cause of pelvic injury (50%), in contrast to the studies by Trikha et al. and Fakhru et al., where traffic accidents were the main causes (77.4% and 85.3%, respectively, compared to 30% in our study). These substantial differences in fracture types among the studied populations may indicate potential problems with the accurate identification of fracture types. Further studies are needed to investigate whether this discrepancy is a significant concern.

Nevertheless, it is important to acknowledge the limitations of this study. One limitation is the restricted sample size, primarily consisting of the local population. As a retrospective study, there may be biases that could influence our results. Additionally, all data were collected by a single operative team at a single trauma center, and all procedures were performed by a surgical team consisting of two operators who regularly conducted pelvic surgeries interchangeably. Since only two operators were performing acetabular fixations in our studied population, the operators' bias needs to be strongly addressed. The lack of a larger number of operators may have limited the breadth of our data to some extent.

Acetabular surgeries still remain one of the most complex procedures in the orthopedic field. Therefore, only a few surgeons decide to be trained in this area. The reason why our trauma center has been performing such a substantial number of pelvic fixation surgeries is that we agree to admit and treat patients from other major trauma centers. Therefore, a potential solution to most of the limitations of our study could be to train a greater number of orthopedic surgeons in pelvic surgeries.

Undoubtedly, further studies, particularly multicenter prospective studies, are necessary to improve our understanding and management of factors that influence appropriate treatment across a diverse population. Therefore, as a final remark, we emphasize the importance of a comprehensive evaluation of patients with pelvic fractures to achieve optimal outcomes.

5. Conclusions

This study provides valuable insights into pelvic fractures and their association with the investigated factors. The findings indicate that factors such as BMI, time of surgery, blood loss, and duration of hospital stay are completely correlated with the morphology of acetabular fractures, the presence of additional trauma, and the mechanism of injury. However, in the studied group, patients whose mechanism of trauma involved falling from height had an increased number of blood transfusions compared to other groups. Moreover, patients who had surgery due to posterior wall acetabulum fractures had decreased blood transfusions compared to other Judet and Letournel types of fractures. Additionally, they had the shortest duration of surgery.

Author Contributions: Conceptualization, J.Z. and R.W.; methodology, J.Z.; software, Ł.J.; validation, B.M. and P.J.; formal analysis, J.Z.; investigation, P.M.W.; resources, R.W. and T.P.; data curation, M.G.; writing—original draft preparation, R.W.; writing—review and editing, P.M.W.; visualization, Ł.Ł.; supervision, J.Z.; project administration, R.W. All authors have read and agreed to the published version of the manuscript.

Funding: This research received no external funding.

Institutional Review Board Statement: This study was conducted in accordance with the Declaration of Helsinki guidelines for human experiments. Prior to the study, permission was obtained from the local Bioethics Committee at Nicolaus Copernicus University in Torun (approval number KB 645/2022).

Informed Consent Statement: Informed consent was obtained from all subjects involved in the study.

Data Availability Statement: No new data were created or analyzed in this study. Data sharing is not applicable to this article.

Conflicts of Interest: The authors declare no conflict of interest.

References

1. Morgan, O.; Davenport, D.; Enright, K. Pelvic injury is not just pelvic fracture. *BMJ Case Rep.* **2019**, *12*, e232622. [CrossRef] [PubMed]
2. Dunn, E.L.; Berry, P.H.; Connally, J.D. Computed Tomography of the Pelvis in Patients with Multiple Injuries. *J. Trauma Acute Care Surg.* **1983**, *23*, 378. [CrossRef]
3. Chaumoître, K.; Portier, F.; Petit, P.; Merrot, T.; Guillon, P.O.; Panuel, M. CT imaging of pelvic injuries in polytrauma patients. *J. Radiol.* **2000**, *81*, 111–120. [PubMed]
4. Davis, D.D.; Foris, L.A.; Kane, S.M.; Waseem, M. Pelvic Fracture. In *StatPearls*; StatPearls Publishing: Treasure Island, FL, USA, 2023.
5. Holstein, J.H.; Culemann, U.; Pohlemann, T. What are Predictors of Mortality in Patients with Pelvic Fractures? *Clin. Orthop. Relat. Res.* **2012**, *470*, 2090–2097. [CrossRef] [PubMed]
6. Kobziff, L. Traumatic pelvic fractures. *Orthop. Nurs.* **2006**, *25*, 235–241; quiz 242–243. [CrossRef]
7. Skitch, S.; Engels, P.T. Acute Management of the Traumatically Injured Pelvis. *Emerg. Med. Clin. N. Am.* **2018**, *36*, 161–179. [CrossRef]
8. Guerado, E.; Medina, A.; Mata, M.I.; Galvan, J.M.; Bertrand, M.L. Protocols for massive blood transfusion: When and why, and potential complications. *Eur. J. Trauma Emerg. Surg.* **2016**, *42*, 283–295. [CrossRef]
9. Coppola, P.T.; Coppola, M. Emergency department evaluation and treatment of pelvic fractures. *Emerg. Med. Clin. N. Am.* **2000**, *18*, 1–27. [CrossRef]
10. Cuthbert, R.; Walters, S.; Ferguson, D.; Karam, E.; Ward, J.; Arshad, H.; Culpan, P.; Bates, P. Epidemiology of pelvic and acetabular fractures across 12-mo at a level-1 trauma centre. *World J. Orthop.* **2022**, *13*, 744–752. [CrossRef]
11. Rondanelli, A.M.; Gómez-Sierra, M.A.; Ossa, A.A.; Hernández, R.D.; Torres, M. Damage control in orthopaedical and traumatology. *Colomb. Med.* **2021**, *52*, e4184802. [CrossRef]
12. Trainham, L.; Rizzolo, D.; Diwan, A.; Lucas, T. Emergency management of high-energy pelvic trauma. *JAAPA* **2015**, *28*, 28–33. [CrossRef] [PubMed]
13. Rommens, P.M. Focus on high energy pelvic trauma. *Eur. J. Trauma Emerg. Surg.* **2018**, *44*, 153–154. [CrossRef]
14. Atif, M.; Hasan, O.; Baloch, N.; Umer, M. A comprehensive basic understanding of pelvis and acetabular fractures after high-energy trauma with associated injuries: Narrative review of targeted literature. *J. Pak. Med. Assoc.* **2020**, *70* (Suppl. S1), S70–S75.
15. Karunakar, M.A.; Shah, S.N.; Jerabek, S. Body mass index as a predictor of complications after operative treatment of acetabular fractures. *J. Bone Jt. Surg. Am.* **2005**, *87*, 1498–1502. [CrossRef]
16. Abdelrahman, H.; El-Menyar, A.; Keil, H.; Alhammoud, A.; Ghouri, S.I.; Babikir, E.; Asim, M.; Muenzberg, M.; Al-Thani, H. Patterns, management, and outcomes of traumatic pelvic fracture: Insights from a multicenter study. *J. Orthop. Surg. Res.* **2020**, *15*, 249. [CrossRef] [PubMed]
17. Buller, L.T.; Best, M.J.; Quinnan, S.M. A Nationwide Analysis of Pelvic Ring Fractures: Incidence and Trends in Treatment, Length of Stay, and Mortality. *Geriatr. Orthop. Surg. Rehabil.* **2016**, *7*, 9–17. [CrossRef] [PubMed]
18. Ghosh, S.; Aggarwal, S.; Kumar, V.; Patel, S.; Kumar, P. Epidemiology of pelvic fractures in adults: Our experience at a tertiary hospital. *Chin. J. Traumatol.* **2019**, *22*, 138–141. [CrossRef]
19. Magnussen, R.A.; Tressler, M.A.; Obremskey, W.T.; Kregor, P.J. Predicting Blood Loss in Isolated Pelvic and Acetabular High-Energy Trauma. *J. Orthop. Trauma* **2007**, *21*, 603–607. [CrossRef]
20. Frisch, N.; Wessell, N.M.; Charters, M.; Peterson, E.; Cann, B.; Greenstein, A.; Silverton, C.D. Effect of Body Mass Index on Blood Transfusion in Total Hip and Knee Arthroplasty. *Orthopedics* **2016**, *39*, e844–e849. [CrossRef]
21. Cao, G.; Yang, X.; Yue, C.; Tan, H.; Xu, H.; Huang, Z.; Quan, S.; Yang, M.; Pei, F. The effect of body mass index on blood loss and complications in simultaneous bilateral total hip arthroplasty: A multicenter retrospective study. *J. Orthop. Surg.* **2021**, *29*, 23094990211061210. [CrossRef]
22. Cao, G.; Chen, G.; Yang, X.; Huang, Q.; Huang, Z.; Xu, H.; Alexander, P.G.; Zhou, Z.; Pei, F. Obesity does not increase blood loss or incidence of immediate postoperative complications during simultaneous total knee arthroplasty: A multicenter study. *Knee* **2020**, *27*, 963–969. [CrossRef] [PubMed]
23. Aggarwal, V.A.; Sambandam, S.; Wukich, D. The Impact of Obesity on Total Hip Arthroplasty Outcomes: A Retrospective Matched Cohort Study. *Cureus* **2022**, *14*, e27450. [CrossRef] [PubMed]

24. Aggarwal, V.A.; Sambandam, S.N.; Wukich, D.K. The impact of obesity on total knee arthroplasty outcomes: A retrospective matched cohort study. *J. Clin. Orthop. Trauma* **2022**, *33*, 101987. [CrossRef]
25. Waseem, S.; Lenihan, J.; Davies, B.M.; Rawal, J.; Hull, P.; Carrothers, A.; Chou, D. Low body mass index is associated with increased mortality in patients with pelvic and acetabular fractures. *Injury* **2021**, *52*, 2322–2326. [CrossRef]
26. Sems, S.A.; Johnson, M.; Cole, P.A.; Byrd, C.T.; Templeman, D.C.; Minnesota Orthopaedic Trauma Group. Elevated body mass index increases early complications of surgical treatment of pelvic ring injuries. *J. Orthop. Trauma* **2010**, *24*, 309–314. [CrossRef] [PubMed]
27. Morris, B.J.; Richards, J.E.; Guillamondegui, O.D.; Sweeney, K.R.; Mir, H.R.; Obremskey, W.T.; Kregor, P.J. Obesity Increases Early Complications After High-Energy Pelvic and Acetabular Fractures. *Orthopedics* **2015**, *38*, e881–e887. [CrossRef]
28. Fakru, N.; Faisham, W.; Hadizie, D.; Yahaya, S. Functional Outcome of Surgical Stabilisation of Acetabular Fractures. *Malays. Orthop. J.* **2021**, *15*, 129–135. [CrossRef]
29. Trikha, V.; Ganesh, V.; Cabrera, D.; Bansal, H.; Mittal, S.; Sharma, V. Epidemiological assessment of acetabular fractures in a level one trauma centre: A 7-Year observational study. *J. Clin. Orthop. Trauma* **2020**, *11*, 1104–1109. [CrossRef]
30. Vipulendran, K.; Kelly, J.; Rickman, M.; Chesser, T. Current concepts: Managing acetabular fractures in the elderly population. *Eur. J. Orthop. Surg. Traumatol.* **2021**, *31*, 807–816. [CrossRef]

Disclaimer/Publisher's Note: The statements, opinions and data contained in all publications are solely those of the individual author(s) and contributor(s) and not of MDPI and/or the editor(s). MDPI and/or the editor(s) disclaim responsibility for any injury to people or property resulting from any ideas, methods, instructions or products referred to in the content.

MDPI
St. Alban-Anlage 66
4052 Basel
Switzerland
www.mdpi.com

Medicina Editorial Office
E-mail: medicina@mdpi.com
www.mdpi.com/journal/medicina

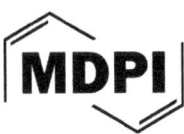

Disclaimer/Publisher's Note: The statements, opinions and data contained in all publications are solely those of the individual author(s) and contributor(s) and not of MDPI and/or the editor(s). MDPI and/or the editor(s) disclaim responsibility for any injury to people or property resulting from any ideas, methods, instructions or products referred to in the content.

www.ingramcontent.com/pod-product-compliance
Lightning Source LLC
LaVergne TN
LVHW070232100526
838202LV00015B/2122